OCULAR EMERGENCIES

Editor:

ROBERT A. CATALANO, MD
Vice President for Medical Affairs
Olean General Hospital
Olean, New York

Formerly Acting Chairman, Department of Ophthalmology
Associate Professor of Ophthalmology and
Associate Professor of Pediatrics
Albany Medical College
Ophthalmologist-in-Chief
Albany Medical Center Hospital
Albany, New York

Associate Editor:

MICHAEL BELIN, MD
Associate Professor, Department of Ophthalmology
Albany Medical College
Albany, New York

W. B. SAUNDERS COMPANY
Harcourt Brace Jovanovich, Inc.

Philadelphia, London, Toronto, Montreal, Sydney, Tokyo

W. B. SAUNDERS COMPANY
Harcourt Brace Jovanovich, Inc.

The Curtis Center
Independence Square West
Philadelphia, Pennsylvania 19106

Library of Congress Cataloging-in-Publication Data

Ocular emergencies / edited by Robert Catalano ; assisting editor, Michael Belin.
   p. cm.
   ISBN 0-7216-3647-0
   1. Ophthalmic emergencies.   2. Eye—Wounds and injuries.
I. Catalano, Robert A.   II. Belin, Michael.
   [DNLM: 1. Emergencies.   2. Eye Diseases—diagnosis.   3. Eye Diseases—
therapy.   4. Eye Injuries.   5. Orbit—Injuries.   WW 166 0207]
RE48.038   1992
617.7′025—dc20
DNLM/DLC
for Library of Congress   91-35980
                                                                                            CIP

Editor: Joan T. Meyer

OCULAR EMERGENCIES   ISBN   0-7216-3647-0

Copyright © 1992 by W. B. Saunders Company.

All rights reserved. No part of this publication may be reproduced or transmitted in any form or by any means, electronic or mechanical, including photocopy, recording, or any information storage and retrieval system, without permission in writing from the publisher.

Printed in Mexico.

Last digit is the print number: 9   8   7   6   5   4   3   2   1

This book is dedicated to my family,
for their unending understanding, patience, and support.

Madeline
Christopher
Ruth
Thomas
Matthew

It is also dedicated to the following teachers
for their dedication and guidance.

George Butterstein
Joseph Calhoun
Ida Catalano
Richard Gorman
Robert Mollenhauer

NOTICE

Ophthalmology is an ever-changing field. Standard safety precautions must be followed, but as new research and clinical experience broaden our knowledge, changes in treatment and drug therapy become necessary or appropriate. The editors of this work have carefully checked the generic and trade drug names and verified drug dosages to assure that the dosage information in this work is accurate and in accord with the standards accepted at the time of publication. Readers are advised, however, to check the product information currently provided by the manufacturer of each drug to be administered to be certain that changes have not been made in the recommended dose or in the contraindications for administration. This is of particular importance in regard to new or infrequently used drugs. It is the responsibility of the treating [physician], relying on experience and knowledge of [the patient], to determine dosages and the best treatment for their [patient]. The editors cannot be responsible for misuse or misapplication of the information in this work.

CONTRIBUTORS

ROBERT A. CATALANO, M.D., Editor
Vice President for Medical Affairs, Olean General Hospital, Olean, New York; Former Acting Chairman and Associate Professor, Department of Ophthalmology, Albany Medical College, Albany, New York
Examination of the Eye; Diagnostic Testing; Special Considerations in the Pediatric Patient; Eyelid Injuries; Blunt Injuries and Fractures of the Orbit; Blunt Ocular Injuries; Burns of the Eye; Nonpenetrating, Noninfectious Emergencies of the Cornea and Ocular Lens; Glaucoma Emergencies; Nontraumatic Orbital Disorders; Neuro-Ophthalmologic and Nontraumatic Retinal Emergencies; Sudden and Unexpected Loss of Vision; Functional and Psychotic Ophthalmologic Disorders; Appendix: Common Abbreviations in Ophthalmology

MICHAEL W. BELIN, M.D., Associate Editor
Associate Professor, Department of Ophthalmology, Albany Medical College, Albany, New York; Director, Corneal and External Disease Service, Albany Medical College, Albany, New York
Burns of the Eye; Foreign Bodies and Penetrating Injuries to the Eye; Nonpenetrating, Noninfectious Emergencies of the Cornea and Ocular Lens; Ocular Infections and Inflammation; Antibiotics, Steroids, and Tetanus Immunization

FREDERICK A. EAMES, M.D.
Assistant Professor, Department of Radiology, Albany Medical College, Albany, New York; Assistant Attending Radiologist, Albany Medical Center Hospital, Albany, New York
Diagnostic Testing

DAVID LITOFF, M.D.
Fellow, Corneal and External Disease Service, Department of Ophthalmology, University of Iowa Hospitals and Clinics, Iowa City, Iowa
Ocular Infections and Inflammation

DALE R. MEYER, M.D.

Assistant Professor, Department of Ophthalmology, Albany Medical College, Albany, New York; Director, Oculoplastic and Orbital Surgery Service, Albany Medical College, Albany, New York

Evaluation and Management of Nontraumatic Disorders of the Lacrimal Drainage System

JAMES L. SCOTT, M.D.

Associate Professor, Department of Emergency Medicine, and Assistant Dean of Student Affairs, George Washington University, Washington, D.C.

Burns of the Eye

PETER ZLOTY, M.D.

Assistant Professor, Department of Ophthalmology, Albany Medical College, Albany, New York; Director, General Eye Service, Albany Medical College, Albany, New York

Antibiotics, Steroids, and Tetanus Immunization

ILLUSTRATED BY LAURIE MAIMONE

ACKNOWLEDGMENTS

It is with pleasure and gratitude that I recognize the many individuals who made this publication possible. Particular thanks go to Laurie Maimone, whose artistic talents are superseded only by her gracious ability to work tirelessly on short notice, and Joe Fisher, my photographer, who exceeded every expectation placed on him by a demanding individual. I am also indebted to Judy Whalen, who critically reviewed the entire manuscript and offered numerous helpful comments and suggestions, and Tiffany Redmond, whose ability to remain cheerful after retyping the same chapter ten times is legendary. Finally, I am pleased to acknowledge the insight and assistance of the three individuals at W. B. Saunders who shared in bringing this project to fruition: Joan Meyer, Richard Zorab, and Marjorie Price. From inception through production, I could not have had a better team.

PREFACE

Each year as new physicians begin their training, I am reminded that the joy of medicine lies in establishing a diagnosis, formulating a treatment plan, and observing the beneficial effects of one's actions. This book was conceived to provide new ophthalmology and emergency room residents the tools to achieve this goal.

The first section of the book reviews examination techniques and diagnostic modalities that are useful in emergency situations. Particular attention is directed toward the appropriate use of different tests, and findings that might be expected in common disorders. A separate chapter is devoted to special considerations and techniques that are useful when dealing with pediatric patients.

The remainder of the book discusses the treatment of ocular and orbital emergencies. These emergency treatments are separated into two sections: traumatic and nontraumatic. Within each section, further categorization is used to guide the reader to the appropriate diagnosis and treatment. A general overview of infectious disorders, antibiotic and corticosteroid treatments, and tetanus immunization is presented in the final section of the book.

Traumatic conditions are classified according to the particular structure involved. Penetrating injuries, blunt injuries, and burns are all treated separately. Nontraumatic disorders are differentiated into those whose cause is readily apparent, and those that present with nonspecific and non-localizing symptoms. Readily apparent conditions are reviewed in chapters that list disorders by a specific structure or etiology. Twelve common symptoms and one sign are discussed in the chapter on neuro-ophthalmologic and retinal disorders. An additional chapter is devoted to the patient who presents with sudden loss of vision, and another chapter to functional visual disorders.

Cross-referencing and overlapping information are used extensively in the book. Antibiotic suggestions are given when a disorder is specifically discussed and are also generally reviewed in the last chapter. When a certain disorder is listed under more than one differential diagnosis, the reader is directed to the section where it is most fully discussed. Finally, up-to-date references are listed at the end of each chapter. This will allow the book to serve as a resource for publications pertaining to the disorders discussed.

The principal intent of this book is to provide a ready reference for the practical hands-on management of patients with ocular and orbital emergencies. The ophthalmologist and emergency room physician should use it to direct their evaluation of patients with ophthalmologic disorders and to develop optimal therapeutic plans.

ROBERT A. CATALANO, M.D.

CONTENTS

I EXAMINATION, DIAGNOSTIC TESTS, AND PEDIATRIC PATIENTS

1
Examination of the Eye 3
Robert A. Catalano

2
Diagnostic Testing 45
Robert A. Catalano and Frederick A. Eames

3
Special Considerations in the Pediatric Patient 91
Robert A. Catalano

II OCULAR AND ORBITAL TRAUMA

4
Eyelid Injuries 109
Robert A. Catalano

5
Blunt Injuries and Fractures of the Orbit 131
Robert A. Catalano

6
Blunt Ocular Injuries 153
Robert A. Catalano

7
Burns of the Eye 179
Michael W. Belin, Robert A. Catalano, and James L. Scott

8
Foreign Bodies and Penetrating Injuries to the Eye 197
Michael W. Belin

III NONTRAUMATIC OCULAR AND ORBITAL EMERGENCIES

9
Evaluation and Management of Nontraumatic Disorders of the Lacrimal Drainage System 217
Dale R. Meyer

10
Nonpenetrating, Noninfectious Emergencies of the Cornea and Ocular Lens 237
Michael W. Belin and Robert A. Catalano

11
Glaucoma Emergencies 261
Robert A. Catalano

12
Nontraumatic Orbital Disorders 289
Robert A. Catalano

13
Neuro-Ophthalmologic and Nontraumatic Retinal Emergencies 335
Robert A. Catalano

14
Sudden and Unexpected Loss of Vision 395
Robert A. Catalano

15
Functional and Psychotic Ophthalmologic Disorders 441
Robert A. Catalano

IV INFECTIONS/ANTIBIOTICS/CORTICOSTEROIDS/TETANUS

16
Ocular Infections and Inflammation 461
David Litoff and Michael W. Belin

17
Antibiotics, Steroids, and Tetanus Immunization 497
Peter Zloty and Michael W. Belin

Appendix: Common Abbreviations in Ophthalmology 513
Robert A. Catalano

Index 523

Examination, Diagnostic Tests, and Pediatric Patients

1

Examination of the Eye

Robert A. Catalano

Ocular emergencies demand a disciplined, methodical approach. The routine described in this chapter begins with an ophthalmic and medical history and ends with an eight-part examination of the eye. None of the steps should be bypassed. An abbreviated history may lead to erroneous hypotheses and the use of inappropriate or unnecessary tests; failure to obtain a baseline visual acuity may lead to questions regarding the quality of care rendered; and omission of intraocular pressure measurement or retinal examination, unless contraindicated, may not uncover an unrelated glaucoma or intraocular tumor. The practiced physician can cite numerous examples in which a thorough history and examination resulted in optimal patient care; the malpractice attorney can cite numerous cases in which its curtailment did not.

The ocular examination must also be conducted in the proper sequence. For example, measuring the intraocular pressure prior to the slit lamp examination in a patient with a red eye risks infectious contamination of the instrument used to measure the pressure. If the pupils have been dilated with a cycloplegic agent (a drug that widens the pupils and prevents the lenses from focusing), pupillary responses and near vision cannot be tested. Corneal sensitivity cannot be assessed after the instillation of topical anesthetics. The proper sequence to conduct the eye examination is summarized in Table 1–1. The ten steps are discussed in this chapter. Diagnostic tests are reviewed in Chapter 2, and special considerations in the pediatric patient are presented in Chapter 3.

TABLE 1-1. THE TEN-PART EYE EXAM

Ophthalmic history
Chief complaint
History of present illness
Past ocular history
Family history of ophthalmic disorders

Systemic history
General medical history
Current medications
Allergies

Assessment of vision (each eye tested separately except for stereopsis testing)
Corrected/uncorrected visual acuity
Distance/near visual acuity
Contrast sensitivity vision*
Color vision*
Photostress recovery test*
Stereopsis (depth perception) testing*

External examination
Orbit
Eyelids
Lacrimal system

Pupils
Pupillary responses
Relative afferent pupillary defect
Paradoxical pupillary reaction

Ocular alignment and motility
Versions, vergences, and ductions
Ocular rotations into the cardinal positions of gaze
Ocular alignment
Dissimilar image and target tests*
Sensory assessment*
Oculocephalic and caloric testing*
Forced duction and active force generation testing*

Visual field examination
Examination techniques
Amsler grid
Visual field defects

Slit lamp examination
Eyelids
Conjunctiva and sclera
Cornea and tear film
Anterior chamber
Iris
Ocular lens
Gonioscopy*

Measurement of intraocular pressure
Indentation tonometry**
Applanation tonometry**
Digital measurement

Fundus examination
Direct ophthalmoscopy
Indirect ophthalmoscopy
Contact lens exam*
Ophthalmodynamometry*

*Optional techniques for selected disorders.
**Deferred in the presence of active infection.

THE OPHTHALMIC HISTORY

The *chief complaint* is the patient's reason for seeking medical care. If it is very specific (e.g., "I splashed bleach in my eye"), the examination and treatment can be readily directed. If the complaint is a symptom (e.g., "I woke up with double vision"), a differential diagnosis must be developed. This book is designed to assist physicians in both cases. The treatment of readily apparent conditions is detailed in the chapters that list disorders by a specific structure or etiology (Chapters 4 through 11 and 16). The workup for patients who present with common symptoms (usually a disturbance of vision or pain in or about the eyes) is reviewed by symptom in Chapters 13 and 14.

Regardless of whether the patient presents with a specific complaint or a symptom, the *history of present illness* should provide sufficient information for the examiner to reconstruct a sequence of events. The physician should ascertain the following information, which can be remembered as what, where, when, and how and the four "P's."

What occurred?
Where did it occur?
When did it occur?
How did it occur?

	Is it:	Progressive or static?
		Persistent or transient?
	Were there any:	Precipitating influences?
		Associated signs or symptoms Present?

Additionally, any instituted treatment, including self-treatment, should be carefully documented. This is particularly important when antibiotics have been applied prior to obtaining microbiologic cultures.

The *past ocular history* should elicit any preexisting cause for decreased vision in an eye with an acute problem—for example, amblyopia, previous trauma, surgery, or infection. The ocular history also elicits whether the patient is using or has ever used any medications for the eyes, topically or systemically, and the name of the disorder being treated. For most ocular drugs, the color of the bottle top correlates with the type of medication (Table 1–2). Any previous episodes similar to the current disorder should be thoroughly reviewed, with emphasis on the effectiveness of the treatments. An ocular surgical history should also be recorded.

The *family history* specifically elicits whether other family members ever had a condition similar to that of the patient. Detailing the cataract history of every grandparent is not as productive as concentrating on persons with poor vision of undetermined cause and heritable ophthalmic disorders. If the family history is unavailable, it should be recorded as such rather than misleadingly as a negative history.

TABLE 1-2. BOTTLE TOP COLORS OF EYE MEDICATIONS

COLOR	PHARMACOLOGIC PROPERTY	ACTION(S)
Green	Cholinergic	Treats glaucoma
		Constricts pupil
Red	Anticholinergic	Dilates pupil
	Sympathomimetic	Treats glaucoma (some)
White	Corticosteroid (milky solution)	Reduces inflammation
	Antibiotic (clear solution)	Treats infection
	Artificial tears (clear solution)	Treats dry eye conditions
Yellow	Beta blocker	Treats glaucoma
Blue	Beta blocker	Treats glaucoma

THE SYSTEMIC HISTORY

The *general medical/surgical history* reviews the relevant organ systems of the body. Information regarding the frequency of bowel movements and painful urination is irrelevant to the ophthalmic evaluation. Rather, attention should be directed to abnormalities in the cardiac, cerebrovascular, respiratory, and immune systems, as well as any history of collagen vascular disease and benign or malignant tumors, which can present with neuro-ophthalmologic symptoms (see Chapters 13 and 14). Knowledge of a preexisting condition may modify the treatment of an ophthalmic disorder.

A review of *current medications* may reveal a disorder about which the patient was unaware (e.g., some elderly patients are unaware that their "fluid pill" is treating hypertension). Information about current medications helps prevent the use of incompatible pharmaceuticals and identifies any medications that may have an adverse effect on the eyes. Concerns regarding the latter can often be answered by the federal Food and Drug Administration, which maintains a National Registry of Drug-induced Ocular Side Effects. Suspected adverse drug responses should also be reported to this agency.

A review of medicinal *allergies* is always appropriate prior to administering any pharmaceutical, including intravenous fluorescein. Many patients do not distinguish allergic from toxic effects. Signs of true allergy—itching, hives, rashes, respiratory distress, and cardiovascular collapse—should always be elicited. In patients with pruritic "red eyes," a history of environmental allergies is relevant.

ASSESSMENT OF VISION

Acuity is the most widely recognized and understood measure of visual function. Of the various charts available to test acuity, the most frequently employed is the Snellen acuity chart, composed of rows of letters that decrease in size as one descends the chart (Figure 1-1). Acuity is recorded as an unre-

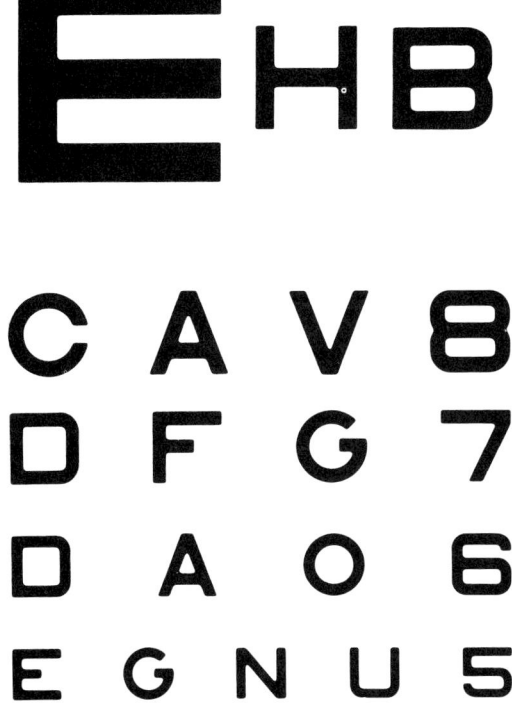
FIGURE 1-1. Snellen distant visual acuity chart.

duced fraction based on a normal viewing distance of 20 feet. The numerator of the fraction is the viewing distance; the denominator represents the distance at which a person without a need for corrective lenses can resolve the same-sized letter. For example, an individual with 20/200 vision can resolve at 20 feet the same-sized letter that an individual without ocular abnormality can recognize 200 feet away. In most parts of the world, acuities are given in metric equivalents. Table 1–3 lists these and also gives an estimate of the percentage loss of central vision corresponding to a given level of acuity.

Near-vision charts (Figure 1–2) are held at 14 in (35 cm) and illuminated at approximately three times the usual room illumination. A similar Snellen notation, or comparable Jaeger or American type-point notations of acuity, are used (Table 1–4). In patients over age 40 years, reading glasses or a hand-held +3.00 lens should be used when checking near vision.

The standard Snellen chart is not without criticism; the letters vary in resolvable difficulty (letters with oblique lines and curves are more difficult to resolve), the progression of letter size is irregular, and the spacing and number of letters on each line is inconsistent. More recently developed charts use an equal number of letters on each line, of approximately equal difficulty, with a

TABLE 1-3. DISTANCE VISUAL ACUITY CONVERSIONS AND PERCENTAGE OF LOSS OF CENTRAL VISION: SNELLEN OPTOTYPES

BRITISH (ft)	METRIC (m)	% LOSS	BRITISH (ft)	METRIC (m)	% LOSS
20/15	6/5	0	20/80	6/24	45
20/20	6/6	0	20/100	6/30	50
20/25	6/7.5	5	20/150	6/50	70
20/30	6/10	10	20/200	6/60	80
20/40	6/12	15	20/300	6/90	85
20/50	6/15	25	20/400	6/120	90
20/60	6/20	35	20/800	6/240	95
20/70	6/22	40			

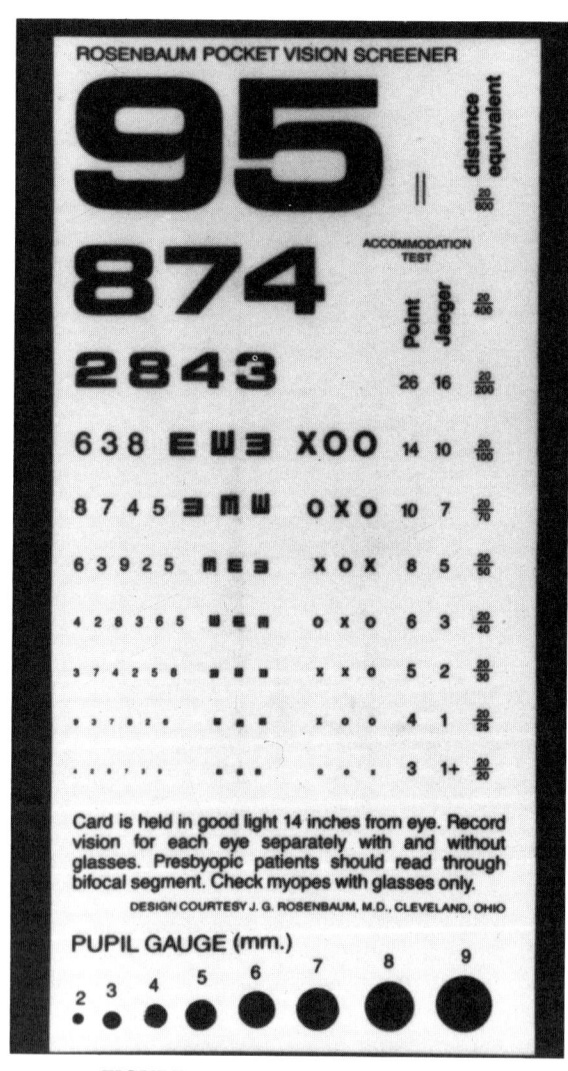

FIGURE 1-2. Near visual acuity chart.

TABLE 1-4. NEAR-VISUAL ACUITY CONVERSIONS AND PERCENTAGE OF LOSS OF CENTRAL VISION

SNELLEN (in)	JAEGER	AMERICAN POINT-TYPE	% LOSS
14/14	1	3	0
14/18	2	4	0
14/21	3	5	5
14/24	4	6	7
14/28	5	7	10
14/35	6	8	50
14/40	7	9	55
14/45	8	10	60
14/60	9	11	80
14/70	10	12	85
14/80	11	13	87
14/88	12	14	90
14/112	13	21	95
14/140	14	23	98

geometric progression of letter height from line to line (Figure 1–3). These charts are called *Log MAR,* because they are based on a logarithmic scale of the minimal angle of resolution.

Charts have also been developed to assess a different parameter of vision, *contrast sensitivity* (Figure 1–4). Reduced contrast sensitivity occurs in patients with optic neuritis, glaucoma, diabetic retinopathy, and compressive lesions of

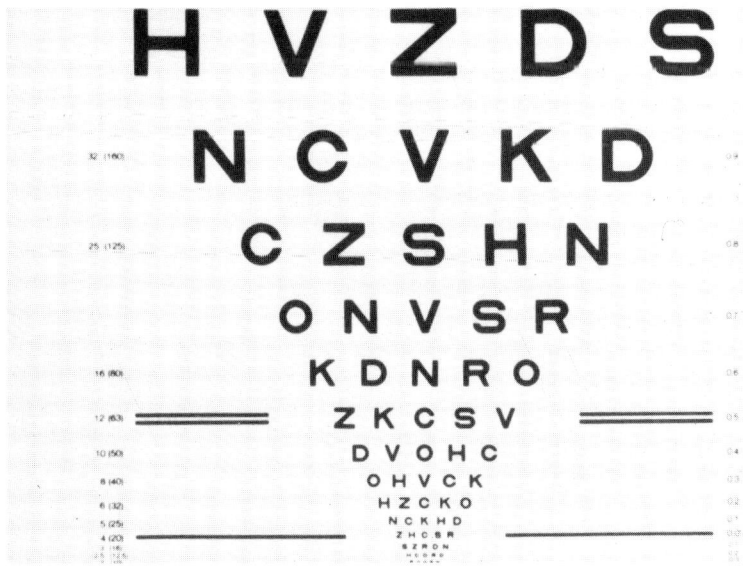

FIGURE 1–3. Log MAR visual acuity chart.

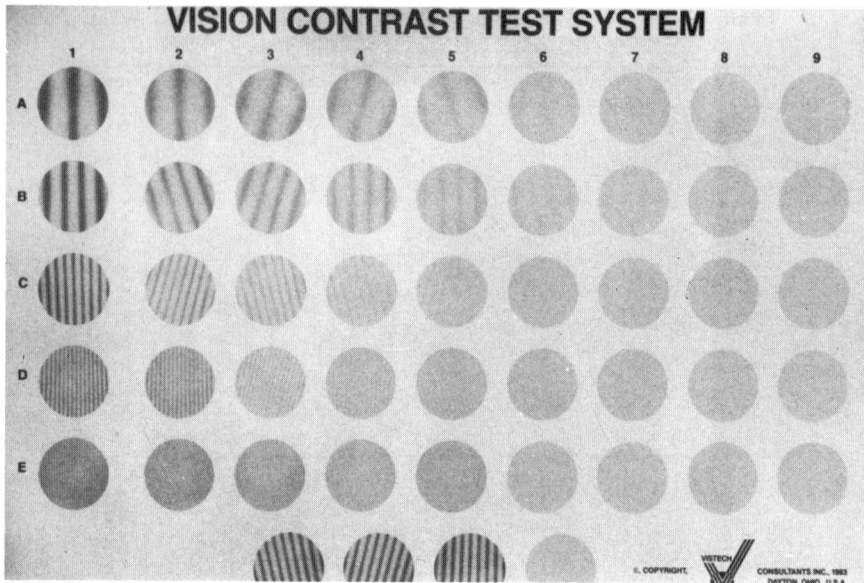

FIGURE 1-4. Contrast sensitivity vision chart.

the optic nerve and chiasm. Differences in contrast sensitivity have also been noted in amblyopia.

Common excuses for not recording a visual acuity are that the patient is too young or his or her vision is too poor to read the vision chart. These are never credible reasons; the only patients for whom a measure of acuity cannot be obtained are those in a comatose or delirious state. The acuity in preverbal children can be recorded in terms of their ability to fixate and follow a specific-sized object at a specific distance. The generation of nystagmus when an infant or malingerer views a rotating optokinetic drum is another (albeit crude) measure of vision. Special charts have been designed for use with children and illiterate individuals (see Chapter 2). Adults with poor vision can be moved closer to the chart until they just see the top (20/400) line. Their vision is then recorded in terms of the distance in feet/the Snellen letter size viewed (e.g., the acuity of a patient who can just resolve the top line at a distance of 5 feet from the chart is recorded as 5/400). Several different measures are available for adults with markedly reduced vision, including the ability to count fingers presented by the examiner (at a stated distance) or recognize hand movements or light. The visual quadrants where these are perceived should also be recorded. The abbreviations used to describe these levels of acuity are: CF (count fingers), HM (hand motion), LP (light perception), and NLP (no light perception). Because the term *blind* has legal and social connotations, the acuity should never be recorded as "blind." The federal government defines *legal blindness* as a best corrected visual acuity in the better eye of 20/200 or less, or a field of vision of 20° or less.

Each eye is tested individually to measure acuity. Vision can be tested with and without correction, at distance and at near. For most situations, the best corrected vision at distance is of primary importance. A near visual acuity is less reproducible but should be used when circumstances prevent the determination of distance acuity. If a patient's corrective lenses are not available, a pinhole (PH) can be used to try to ascertain the best possible acuity. If the patient's vision improves when he or she looks through a pinhole, a reduction in acuity is likely secondary to a refractive error (need for glasses). Acuity is recorded in terms of the lowest line an individual can read. A plus notation denotes that the patient recognized a certain number of letters on the next line and a minus that he or she missed a certain number of letters on it. The notations and abbreviations used to record visual acuity are listed in Table 1–5.

Color vision is tested when the history, signs, or symptoms suggest an optic nerve or retinal abnormality. Special pseudoisochromatic plates are available (Figure 1–5), including illiterate charts for children, to test the ability to discriminate different hues. Different hues are juxtaposed on each plate in such a way that the normal eye recognizes a pattern or number. The absence of this recognition signifies a hereditary deficit, optic nerve or retinal abnormality. More detailed color vision tests are available but are not usually used in the acute setting.

When the visual acuity is reduced but better than 20/80, the *photostress recovery test* is used to differentiate between macular and optic nerve disease. The test is performed monocularly after obtaining the best corrected acuity for each eye. The patient fixates a bright light held 1 in (2.5 cm) in front of the eye for 10 seconds. Normally the retinal cones require less than 60 seconds to recover from this bleaching. With optic nerve disease, the recovery is normal, but with a maculopathy, the recovery time can be prolonged up to 180 seconds. When the starting visual acuity is less than 20/80, the test loses its accuracy.

Depth perception (stereopsis) can be tested using the Titmus (Figure 1–6) or the TNO random dot test. Each test presents slightly disparate polarized objects to the two eyes, grouped with objects without disparity. When the disparate objects are viewed through Polaroid glasses, they are seen to project out of the plane of the test, toward the observer. Groups of figures are arranged such that the amount of disparity in the odd object decreases as one descends through the chart. In this way, the degree of stereopsis can be quantitated. The smallest stereoscopic target subtends approximately 20 seconds of arc. These tests have only limited use in most emergency evaluations but can be useful in diagnosing functional visual loss. Depth perception requires the normal functioning of both eyes and the central visual pathway. An excellent result on stereopsis testing is incompatible with monocular or binocular visual loss.

TABLE 1-5. NOTATIONS AND ABBREVIATIONS USED TO RECORD VISUAL ACUITY

VA = visual acuity
cc = with correction
sc = without correction
PH = acuity looking through a pinhole
NI = no improvement
W = wears (spectacle correction)
PC = present correction (spectacle)
J = Jaeger notation (near vision)
+ = convex lens used to treat hyperopia
− = concave lens used to treat myopia

RE = right eye
LE = left eye
OD = oculus dexter: right eye
OS = oculus sinister: left eye
OU = oculi uterque: both eyes
D = distance acuity
N = near acuity
E = E game
Pics = Allen pictures
SPH = spherical lens

Acuity notations in infants
F+F = fixate and follow
CSM = central, steady, maintained fixation
C(S)M = central, unsteady, maintained fixation (nystagmus)
CS(M) = central, steady, but not maintained fixation (amblyopia)
GCM = good, central, maintained fixation
G(C)M = eccentric but maintained fixation
GC(M) = good, central, but not maintained fixation (amblyopia)

Acuity notations in older children and adults
20/50−1 = missed one letter on 20/50 line
20/50+2 = resolved 20/50 line and two letters on 20/40 line
20/30 Pics = 20/30 on Allen chart
20/25 E = 20/25 on E game
CF at 1′ = count fingers at 1 foot
HM at 3′ = hand motion at 3 feet

LP = light perception
NLP = no light perception
LP c proj = light perception with projection
Quadrants:
ST = superotemporal
IT = inferotemporal
SN = superonasal
IN = inferonasal

Example:

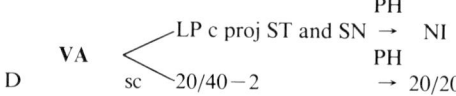

This indicates that without correction, the distance vision in the right eye is light perception with projection in the superotemporal and superonasal quadrants. In the left eye, the patient could read all but two letters on the distant 20/40 line. No improvement in vision of the right eye was obtained looking through a pinhole, but the vision in the left eye improved to 20/20.

THE EXTERNAL EXAMINATION

The orbit should be examined for proptosis (protrusion of an eye), enophthalmos (recession of an eye within the orbit), pulsations, or periorbital changes. An exophthalmometer (Figure 1–7) is used to measure protrusion of the eyes. Measurements are made of the distance between the lateral orbital rim and the anterior surface of the eye. A difference of 2 mm or more between the eyes is considered abnormal. To ensure accurate serial measurements, the same base setting of the exophthalmometer must always be used for a given

1—Examination of the Eye 13

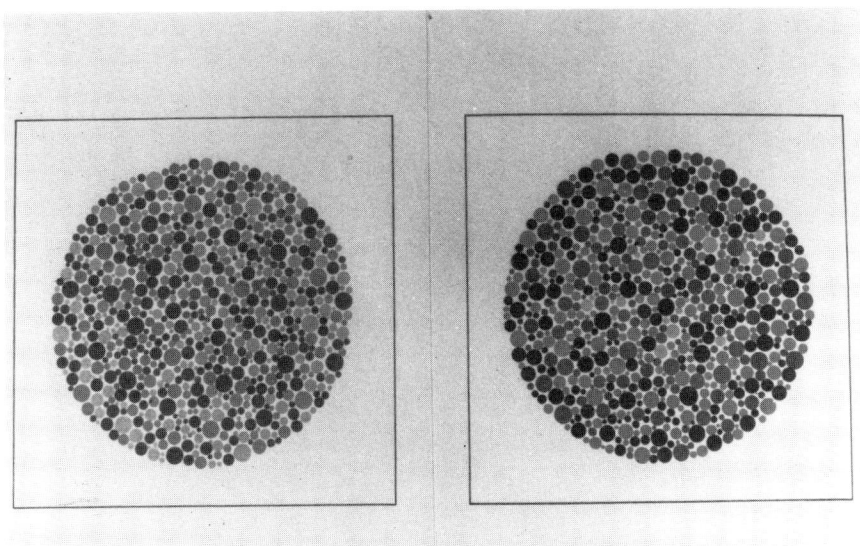

FIGURE 1-5. Color vision plate.

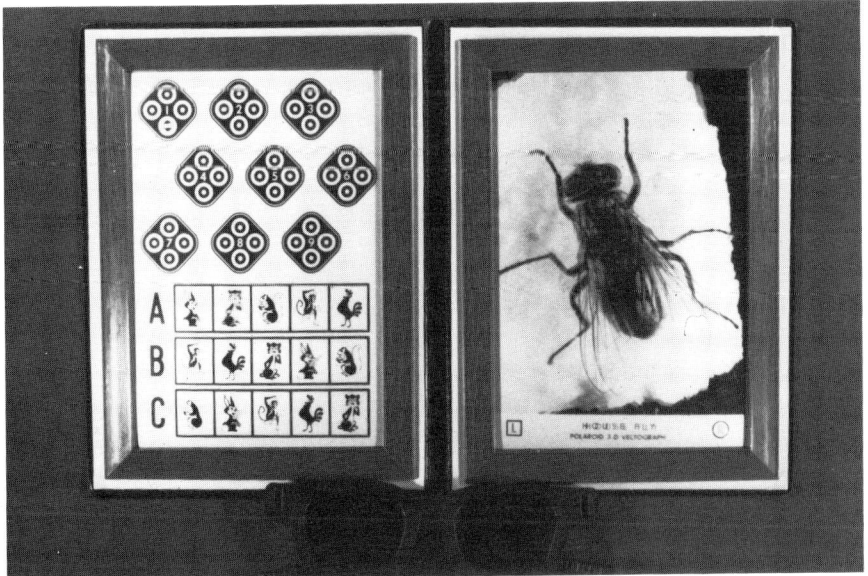

FIGURE 1-6. Titmus depth perception chart.

14   I—Examination, Diagnostic Tests, and Pediatric Patients

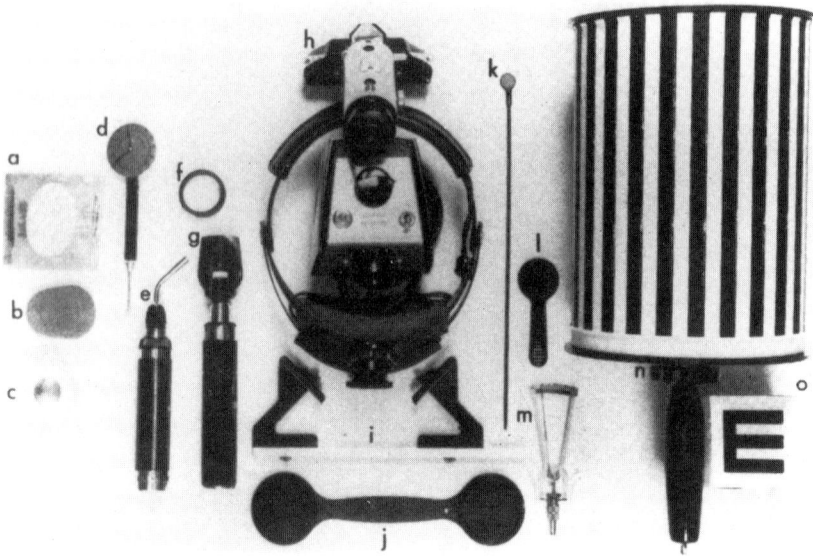

FIGURE 1-7. Basic equipment for examination and emergency treatment of the eye: (a) sterile patch, (b) elastoplast patch, (c) role of Micropore paper tape, (d) ophthalmodynamometer, (e) transilluminator, (f) lens for indirect ophthalmoscope, (g) direct ophthalmoscope, (h) indirect ophthalmoscope, (i) exophthalmometer, (j) occluder and Maddox rod, (k) test object for confrontation fields, (l) multipinhole, (m) Schiotz tonometer, (n) optokinetic drum, (o) E-game test box. (From: Paton D, Goldberg MF: *Management of ocular injuries.* Philadelphia, WB Saunders Co, 1976, p 6, with permission.)

patient. The ends of the instrument are symmetrically apposed to the lateral orbital margins (Figure 1-8). The examiner stands directly in front of the patient and aligns the two fine lines in the mirror (to avoid a parallax error). When the patient looks directly ahead, the cornea can be seen in the mirror and its anterior extent measured using the ruler imprinted over the mirror.

Palpation of the orbit can detect masses, orbital rim fractures, and subcutaneous emphysema. Orbital rim fractures are suspected when "step-offs," or asymmetries of the bony orbits, are found; orbital floor or medial wall fractures are suspected when subcutaneous emphysema (crepitus) is present (see Chapter 5). Palpation should be performed with the eyes open and gaze directed straight ahead. The anterior orbit is palpated with the examiner's fingers placed between the patient's eye and the orbital rim. Auscultation for orbital bruits can be performed by placing the bell of a stethoscope over closed eyelids. Pulsation of the globe is most apparent when observing the patient from a lateral position.

The *eyelids* are inspected for symmetry of position, function, apposition to the globe, and inflammation. Unilateral ptosis (drooping of the upper eyelid) is measured by the difference in size between the two palpebral fissures. Alter-

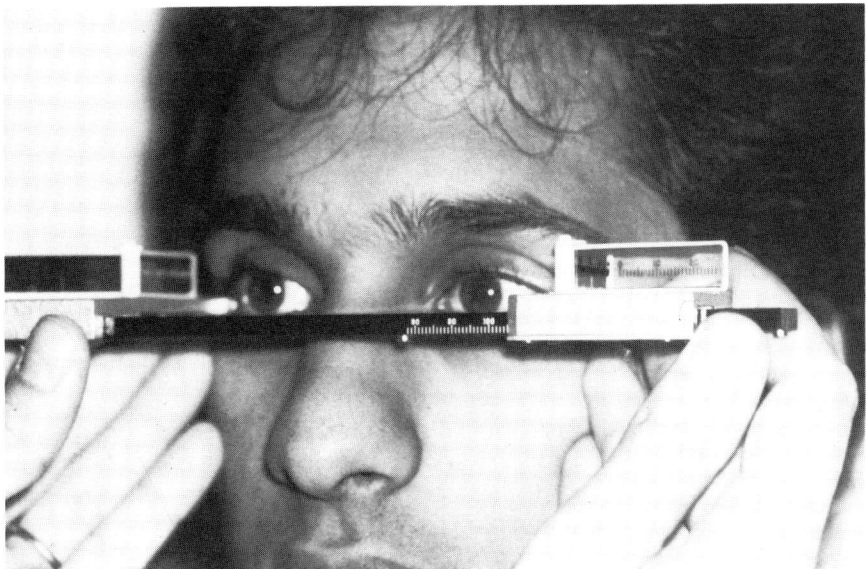

FIGURE 1-8. Use of the Hertel exophthalmometer.

natively, it is recorded as the number of millimeters of corneal coverage by the eyelid. Levator function is measured by applying firm pressure to the brow (to prevent elevation of the eyelid by frontalis contraction) and measuring the difference in interpalpebral width between downward and upward gaze. A difference of 4 mm or less is considered poor function; an increase of 8 mm or more indicates good function. The normal span is approximately 15 mm.

Additional eyelid malpositions include eyelid eversion *(ectropion)* and inturning *(entropion)* (see Figures 9-5 and 9-6). *Dermatochalasis* is redundancy of the skin of the eyelid. It usually accompanies aging and is associated with herniation of orbital fat through the orbital septum. *Blepharochalasis,* most frequently seen in young women, is a relaxation and wrinkling of the skin due to loss of elastic tissue from repeated episodes of inflammation. *Trichiasis,* a condition in which the eyelashes are misdirected and rub against the cornea (see Figure 9-7), can cause symptoms of ocular irritation, foreign body sensation, tearing, and red eye. *Distichiasis* is an extra row of eyelashes, usually originating near the openings of the meibomian glands; it is usually asymptomatic. *Epicanthus* is a skin fold that runs from the upper to the lower eyelid, covering the medial canthal angle. It is frequently present in infants and young children. Because less sclera (white) is seen on the inside than the outside of the eye, epicanthal folds give a child the appearance of having crossed eyes (pseudoesotropia). *Epiblepharon* is a redundant fold of skin near the lid margin of the lower eyelid. Like epicanthus, it can be prominent in infancy and regress during the first years of life. Occasionally, epiblepharon causes the medial eyelashes of the lower eyelid to turn in against the cornea, a condition that requires surgical correction.

Common masses in the eyelid include *hordeola* (styes), infections of the Zeiss glands or lash follicles, and *chalazia,* chronic lipogranulomas of the meibomian glands that follow acute infections in these glands (see Chapter 16). Multiple tumors can occur on the eyelids, including basal, squamous, and sebaceous cell carcinomas, melanomas, keratoacanthomas, papillomas, and hemangiomas. *Xanthelasma* refers to flat, sharply demarcated lipid deposits in the eyelids, occasionally related to hypercholesterolemia.

The *lacrimal system* is evaluated in patients with inadequate tear secretion, as well as those with obstruction, inflammation, or infection of the tear drainage system. The *Schirmer's test* uses a 0.5 mm by 3.5 mm strip of Whatman no. 41 filter paper to test baseline tear secretion. An end of the strip is placed in the lower fornix for 5 minutes while the patient sits with eyes open in subdued light (Figure 1–9). Normally 15 mm or more of the strip will be wetted in 5 minutes. When there is wetting of less than 5 mm, considered hyposecretion, a *Jones dye test* can be performed. The first part of this two-part test is performed by instilling 2% fluorescein solution into the conjunctival sac. The patient is instructed to bend the head forward, and after 5 minutes a cotton pledget is placed under the inferior turbinate of the nose to detect the presence of any fluorescein. The second part of the test is performed when no dye is

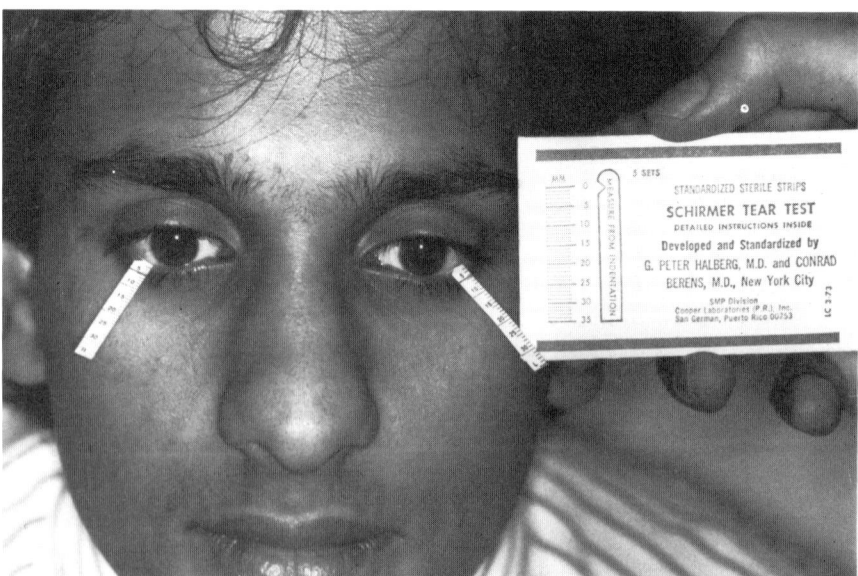

FIGURE 1–9. Schirmer test.

recovered. The lacrimal system is irrigated and rechecked for fluorescein under the inferior turbinate. If the system cannot be irrigated, a total obstruction is present. If dye is recovered with irrigation, a partial obstruction, likely at the level of the lacrimal sac or duct, is present. If clear saline is recovered, an abnormality in the functioning of the "lacrimal pump" is suggested. Other tests that can be performed are reviewed in Chapter 9.

Physical examination of the orbit is reviewed in Chapter 12.

THE PUPILS

The *pupillary light reflex* describes constriction of the pupils to light and the *pupillary near reflex* constriction due to fixation of the eyes on a near object. The latter reflex is associated with convergence and accommodation of the eyes. Pupillary responses should be evaluated in both bright and dim illumination, with the patient's gaze directed toward a distant object. Common abbreviations and notations to describe pupillary responses are listed in Table 1–6. Abnormalities of the pupil, particularly asymmetry in pupil size (anisocoria) and shape, are reviewed in Chapter 13.

A *relative afferent pupillary defect* (RAPD) is characterized by bilateral pupillary dilation with continuous light stimulation to an affected eye. The swinging flashlight test, used to detect a RAPD, is performed in a dim room by alternately illuminating the eyes (Figure 1–10). A penlight is directed obliquely

TABLE 1–6. NOTATIONS AND ABBREVIATIONS USED TO RECORD PUPILLARY RESPONSES

RRL   = round, reactive to light
RAPD   = relative afferent pupillary defect; graded from 0 (no RAPD) to 4+ (brisk RAPD)
4 → 2   = 4 mm wide pupils in dim illumination, constricting to 2 mm in bright illumination
0 to 4+ = briskness of light and near responses, graded from 0 (no response) to 4+ (brisk)

Examples
Pupils: 4 → 2 RRL s RAPD
        5 → 3 RRL c RAPD

This indicates that the right pupil is 4 mm wide in dim illumination and constricts to 2 mm in bright illumination. It is also without an afferent pupillary defect. The left pupil is 5 mm wide in dim illumination, constricts to 3 mm, and has a relative afferent pupillary defect.

Pupils:	Size	Light response	Near response	RAPD
	4 → 2	4+	4+	0
	5 → 3	3+	3+	2+
or:	4/5 → 2/3	4+/3+	4+/3+	0/2+

This indicates that the right pupil responds more briskly by both the light and near reflex than the left pupil. This also grades the relative afferent pupillary defect in the left eye as 2+.

RELATIVE AFFERENT PUPILLARY DEFECT

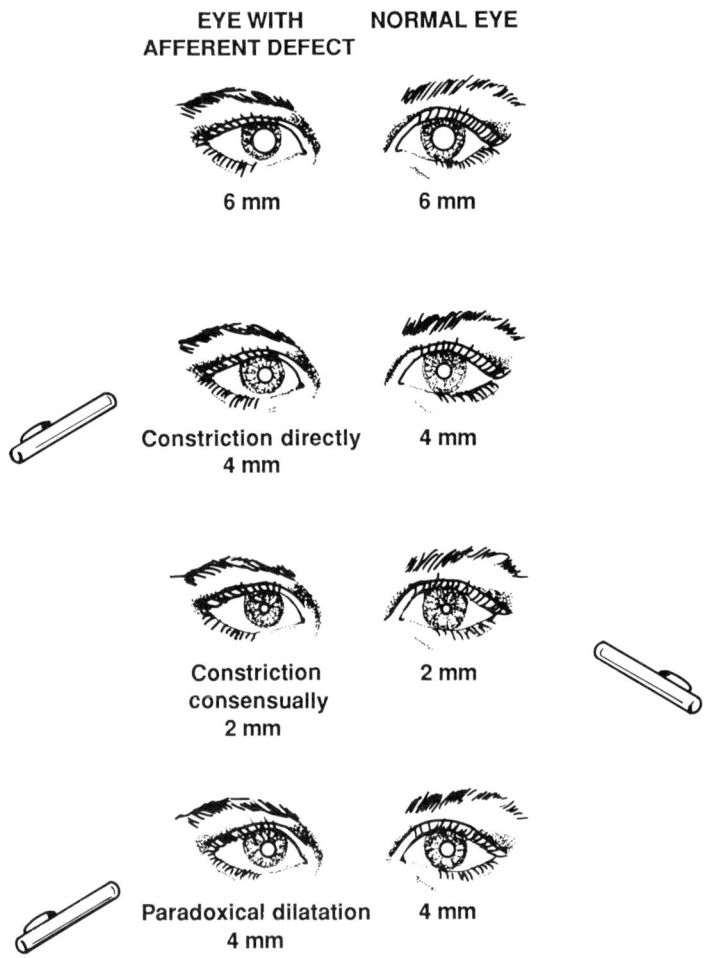

FIGURE 1-10. Swinging flashlight test demonstrating a relative afferent pupillary defect in the left eye.

in one eye and then the other from below. Constriction of the iris in the illuminated eye is a direct response; constriction of the opposite iris is a consensual response. In the absence of a RAPD, pupillary constriction does not vary in either eye when they are alternately illuminated. With a RAPD, however, both pupils constrict when light is directed into the unaffected eye and dilate when it is directed into the affected eye.

The presence of a RAPD is useful in localizing a defect in the visual pathway anterior to the optic chiasm and in determining whether a reduction in visual acuity is due to an optic nerve or a macular disorder. A subtle RAPD can occur with central serous retinopathy and rarely with other maculopathies, but no macular abnormality can account for a profound RAPD. Similarly, the presence of a cataract or a nontotal hyphema never explains a brisk RAPD. A RAPD can be seen in an amblyopic eye even when the visual acuity is not markedly diminished, but similar to a maculopathy, a RAPD in amblyopia is generally very subtle.

A *paradoxical pupillary reaction* is defined as pupillary dilation on exposure to light and constriction when the light is removed or dilation with near vision and constriction with distance vision. It is best detected by shining a penlight obliquely on the pupils and then turning off the room lights. If pupils constrict rather than dilate, the reaction is confirmed. A paradoxical pupillary reaction is most frequently noted in patients with congenital stationary night blindness, characterized by night blindness, decreased vision, and normal or only mildly abnormal color vision, or congenital achromotopsia, characterized by a complete absence of color vision, visual acuity worse than 20/200, and photophobia. Nystagmus (usually pendular), a normal fundus appearance, electroretinogram abnormalities, and lack of progression are characteristics of both. A paradoxical pupillary reaction can also occur with Leber's congenital amaurosis, dominant optic atrophy, and old bilateral optic neuritis. Rare associations include syphilis, tumors of the quadrigeminal region, and barbiturate intoxication.

OCULAR ALIGNMENT AND MOTILITY

There are six extraocular muscles, named according to their location and the direction they traverse to insert on the globe (see Figure 5–2). For each muscle, there is a singular position of the eye for which it acts as the primary mover (see Figure 5–3). (The anatomy of the extraocular muscles is reviewed in Chapter 5.) The six positions corresponding to the six muscles are called the *cardinal positions of gaze*. In testing *ocular rotations*, the strength of each muscle is checked individually by sequentially rotating the eye through the cardinal positions. The reduced ability of an eye to rotate into a specific gaze suggests a congenital strabismus syndrome, a cranial nerve palsy, or an extraocular muscle restriction.

Ductions describe monocular movements. Adduction is movement of the eye nasally; abduction is a temporal movement. *Versions* and *vergences* describe binocular movements. Versions, also called conjugate movements, are movements of the two eyes in the same direction, at the same time, and of approximately the same magnitude. Dextroversion describes movement of both eyes to the right and levoversion movement to the left. Vergences are binocular movements in which the eyes move in opposite directions, or disju-

the two eyes. Both tests are also useful in detecting any incomitance in a deviation. As the eyes are rotated into the different cardinal positions of gaze, the patient is asked to identify where the image separation becomes greater. Paresis or restriction of a specific extraocular muscle can be identified by the patient's response that the separation of images is greater when the eyes are moved in the direction of action of the affected muscle. This is particularly useful in the workup of diplopia (see Chapter 13). *Dissimilar target tests* present different targets to the two eyes that the patient is asked to superimpose. These tests generally require specific equipment that is not available in the emergency setting; they are useful in determining the position of gaze in which the maximum deviation occurs.

An evaluation of the sensory status of the eyes also uses special tests, which are only used for specific indications; these include Worth's four dot test, the afterimage test, Bagolini's striated glass test, and the four diopter base-out test. The principal use for these tests in the emergency setting is to prove functional visual loss (see Chapter 15).

Oculocephalic (doll's head) testing and *caloric testing* are used in patients with gaze palsies to determine if the palsy is of supranuclear origin. Both tests rely on the vestibular system's ability to drive the eyes in a particular direction. The doll's head test is performed in conscious patients. While the patient fixates an object, the examiner rotates his head horizontally or vertically. Caloric testing is performed on unconscious patients and those with potential neck injuries. Cold or warm water is irrigated in an ear canal with the patient's head elevated 30° above the horizontal. Cold water irrigation produces a nystagmus with the fast phase in the opposite direction of the irrigated ear; hot water produces the inverse (the fast phase is ipsilateral). The mnemonic COWS can be used to remember the direction of the fast phase (cold, opposite; warm, same). Bilateral cold water irrigation produces a nystagmus with the fast phase up; bilateral warm irrigation produces the opposite. If the eyes can be made to deviate in the direction of the gaze palsy, the disorder is of supranuclear origin (above the cranial nerve nucleus to extraocular muscle pathways).

Forced duction and *active force generation testing* are used when an infranuclear gaze palsy exists to differentiate a neurogenic from a restrictive ocular motor disorder. In a forced duction test, the anesthetized eye is mechanically moved into various positions of gaze to detect any resistance to passive movement. Any resistance is considered a positive result. The test is performed by grasping the conjunctiva and episclera near the limbus with two forceps held 180° apart (Figure 1-11). The eye is moved into positions suspected of being restricted as a result of mechanical factors. The test can be performed under general or local anesthesia. Awake patients are asked to look in the direction the eye is being moved to eliminate resistance caused by extraocular muscle contraction in the opposite direction. Care is taken not to press the globe into the orbit, as this can give a false-negative result in the face of true restriction. The active forced generation test is useful in determining the residual function

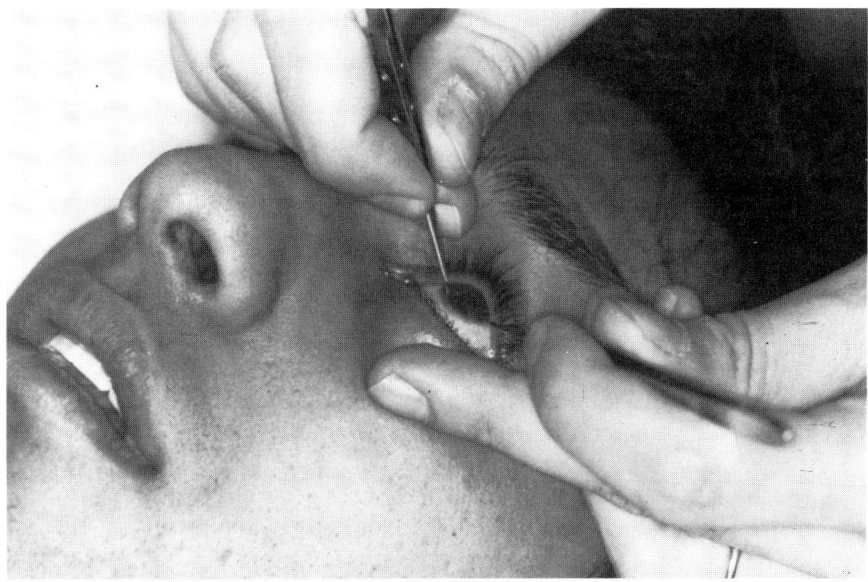

FIGURE 1-11. Forced duction testing.

of a paretic muscle. The eye is stabilized with a single forceps and the patient asked to look in the direction of the gaze palsy. If the examiner detects a tug on the forceps, some residual function of the paretic muscle exists. The forceps is always placed 180° opposite to the direction of movement. A corneal abrasion can occur if a forceps, placed in the line of movement, slips. Neither of these tests should be performed if there is any suspicion of a ruptured globe.

VISUAL FIELD EXAMINATION

Multiple tests are available to assess the field of vision. The majority of these are used to detect or monitor glaucoma and are beyond the scope of this chapter. Two screening tests, however, can be useful in the emergency setting.

Confrontational visual field testing requires only that the examiner have a normal visual field. Several different steps are useful in obtaining the maximum information. The examiner faces the patient from about 20 in (50 cm) away and closes one eye; the facing eye of the patient is similarly occluded by paper tape or the patient's hand. Each individual fixates the other's nose. The patient is asked to count the number of fingers presented to him or her in the superior and inferior zones temporally and nasally. If the patient is successful, the examiner presents fingers in more than one field. The ability to discern hand motion is used for patients unable to count fingers. Specific visual field deficits are reviewed in Chapter 13.

24   I—Examination, Diagnostic Tests, and Pediatric Patients

A relative visual field defect can be detected by asking a patient to compare the clarity of the examiner's two hands, presented simultaneously to their temporal and nasal, or superior and inferior, fields. Color comparison can be performed similarly, using red objects. Patients with chiasmal disorders note that the color of the object held in their temporal field appears washed out. The patient can also be asked to fixate one red object while a second similar article is held peripherally. Normally he or she will report that the peripheral object appears less red. Patients with central visual deficits report the opposite.

An *Amsler grid* is used to detect irregularities in the central 20° of the visual field (Figure 1–12). The grid is composed of intersecting horizontal and vertical lines and contains a central fixation dot. Each square on the grid is 5 mm in size and subtends a visual angle of 1° at a viewing distance of 12 in (30 cm). The test is performed monocularly in moderate illumination. It should always be completed prior to ophthalmoscopy or the instillation of dilating or cycloplegic drops.

The patient is asked to fixate the central dot of the grid. A reply that the central spot is not visible suggests the presence of a central scotoma (area of blindness). If the center spot can be fixated, the patient is asked if all four sides are visible. The inability to perceive a side suggests a scotoma encroaching on the central area (due to glaucoma, a macular, or an optic nerve disorder). Next, the patient is asked if there are any defects or areas where the grid is not visible. An affirmative response locates paracentral scotomas. The final question asks if the

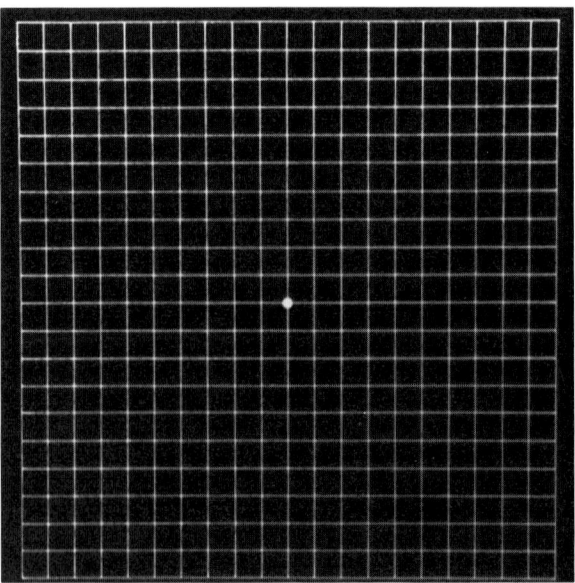

FIGURE 1–12.   Amsler grid.

horizontal and vertical lines are straight and parallel. Any distortion or bending of the lines is called metamorphopsia and suggests a foveal disturbance. With micropsia (the perception of objects as smaller than their true size), the parallel lines are usually noted to bend inward. With macropsia (objects appear larger than their true size), the lines usually bend outward. The luminance of the test can be lowered by having the patient wear Polaroid filters. Although filters can increase the sensitivity of the test, they are not routinely used.

SLIT LAMP EXAMINATION

A slit lamp is a binocular microscope positioned vertically on an adjustable table for examination of the eye (Figure 1–13). The combination of superb illumination, magnification, and a stereoscopic view has made it the instrument

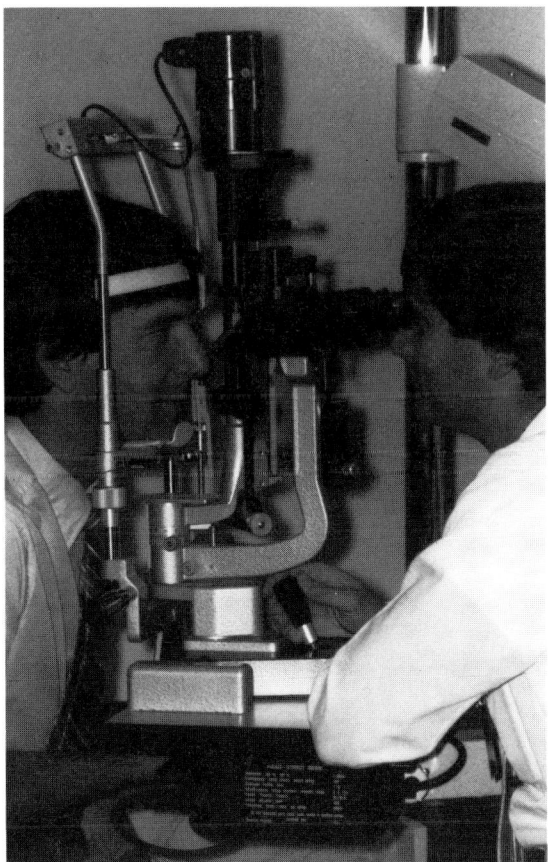

FIGURE 1–13. Slit lamp examination using the Haag-Streit model 900 slit lamp.

of choice for examining the anterior eye. Its name is derived from a special feature of the illumination system that projects the light beam as a slit, which can be varied in width, height, and angle of projection. Magnification is that of a simple microscope, with the optics designed such that the image is direct and virtual. Stereopsis is the appreciation of seeing an object in depth; it is achieved by viewing the object slightly disparately with each eye.

Proper use of the slit lamp requires knowledge of four possible illumination/observation techniques (Figure 1–14):

1. ***Direct focal illumination***
   Technique: Light is directed from an oblique angle and focused as a narrow slit on the various parts of the anterior eye. Particles that lie within the light path scatter light rays and are visible as bright objects against a dark background. Scatter is best appreciated with the observation and illumination arms angled from each other. The flare of protein in the aqueous is best seen when these two are separated by a right angle; other angles are better for larger particles.
   Advantages and uses: Direct illumination is useful for visualizing opacities in otherwise transparent media (see Figure 7–6). It can also be used to view solid objects on the eyelids and sclera if the beam is broadened and reduced in intensity. Its major advantage is that it provides accurate determination of depth.

SLIT LAMP ILLUMINATION TECHNIQUES

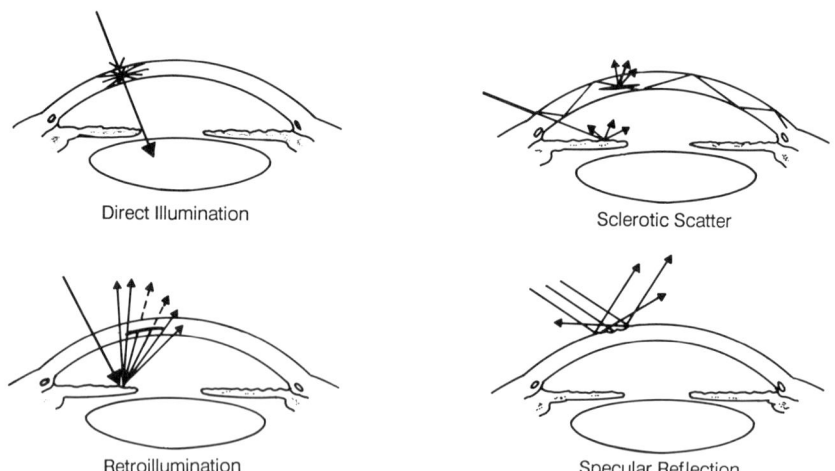

FIGURE 1–14. Slit lamp illumination techniques. (Modified from Tate GW Jr, Safir A: The slit lamp: history, principles and practice. In Tasman W, Jaeger EA: *Duane's clinical ophthalmology.* Philadelphia, JB Lippincott, 1979, Figure 59–38.)

2. *Retroillumination*
   Technique: The microscope is focused on the part of the eye to be examined, but the beam of light is focused on a posterior structure. Light is reflected from the posterior structure and transmitted back to the microscope through the first tissue. The slit is laterally displaced so that light will not fall directly on the object of regard.
   Advantages and uses: This technique is useful for detecting irregularities of the corneal epithelium, corneal edema and neovascularization, inflammatory deposits (keratic precipitates) on the posterior surface of the cornea, and iris transillumination, such as occurs with albinism and pigmentary glaucoma (see Figure 7–7).
3. *Sclerotic scatter*
   Technique: The microscope is focused on the cornea, while the light beam is focused directly on the limbus (the junction of the cornea and sclera). Light will be reflected between the anterior and posterior surfaces of the cornea, illuminating the entire circumcorneal area. Some retroillumination also occurs from light reflected onto posterior surfaces.
   Advantages and uses: This technique is used to visualize corneal opacities and corneal edema. It is also useful in the fitting of contact lenses.
4. *Specular reflection*
   Technique: Specular reflection requires that the angle of illumination of the light beam equal its angle of reflection (and observation). The slit is directed from the temporal side of the eye, and the microscope is positioned nasally. The angle formed by the two arms is approximately 50° to 60°, and the visual axis of the patient's eye is directed between the two.
   Advantages and uses: This technique is used to examine the anterior and posterior surfaces of the cornea and anterior surface of the lens. Individual surface cells, particularly the corneal endothelium, can be visualized.

During the slit lamp examination, the *eyelids* can be examined for any misdirection of the eyelashes, or the puncta (openings to the tear drainage system; see Figure 9–1), or inflammation within the eyelid glands or lash follicles.

The *conjunctiva and sclera* are examined for evidence of inflammation, abnormal vascularization or pigmentation, or degeneration. Evaluation of the palpebral conjunctiva requires eversion of the eyelids (see Figures 8–2 and 8–3). Lymphoid hyperplasia of the palpebral conjunctiva appears as translucent, dome-shaped protuberances *(follicles)* with a lacy vascularization between the elevations (Figure 1–15). Follicles represent active germinal centers and occur in adenoviral, herpetic, and toxic keratoconjunctivitis (from antivirals, miotics, adrenergics, atropine, or shedding of *Molluscum contagiosum*), chlamydial infections, Newcastle's disease, and benign lymphoid hyperplasia of childhood. They are always more prominent in the lower cul-de-sac. *Papillae* are thickened, polygonal elevations with central fibrovascular cores that erupt onto the surface to form a spokelike pattern of vessels. They are better appreciated on

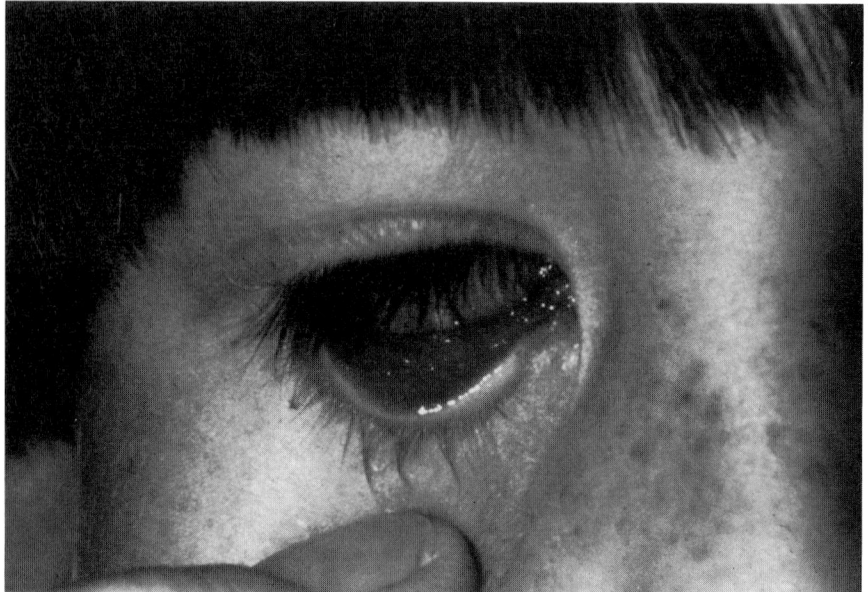

FIGURE 1-15. Follicular conjunctival reaction.

the palpebral conjunctiva of the upper eyelid. Small papillae are a nonspecific sign of inflammation. Giant papillae occur more specifically with vernal conjunctivitis, the use of contact lenses or ocular prostheses, or the protruding ends of nylon sutures (Figure 1-16). Transudation of inflammatory cells and fibrin through the conjunctival blood vessels produces *pseudomembranes* and *membranes* (see Figure 16-9). The difference between these is one of degree. True membranes are more adherent and cause bleeding when stripped from the conjunctiva. These inflammatory collections occur most frequently in conjunctivitis due to adenovirus, herpes simplex virus, beta-hemolytic streptococcus, gonococcus, neonatal chlamydial infection, diphtheria, Candida, vernal conjunctivitis, ocular pemphigoid, and Stevens-Johnson syndrome.

Several benign conjunctival degenerations should also be noted. *Pinguecula* are yellowish-white subconjunctival elevations comprised of degenerated elastic tissue. They are located nasally and temporally in the bulbar conjunctiva between the palpebral fissures; they encroach upon but do not cross the limbus. *Pterygia* are more exuberant hypertrophic proliferations of fibrovascular tissue, located in the same area, that extend onto the cornea (Figure 1-17). Their name is derived from their winged shape. The main factor in the development of pinguecula and pterygia appears to be ultraviolet (actinic) exposure. Excision of pterygia is indicated only if they threaten the visual axis, interfere with contact lens wear, or become inflamed (rare). As many as 40% of excised pterygia recur, often worse than the primary growth. Dermoid tumors,

1—Examination of the Eye 29

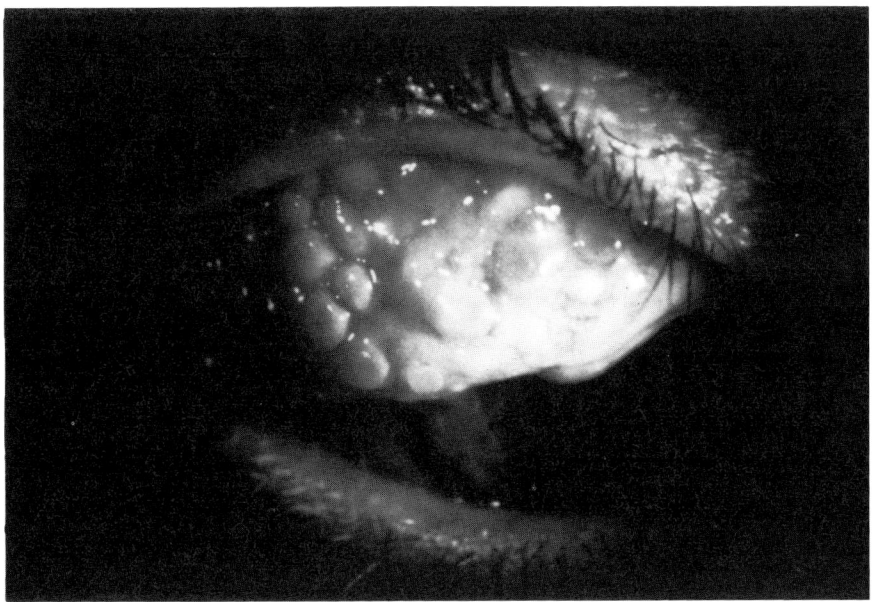

FIGURE 1-16. Giant papillary conjunctival reaction.

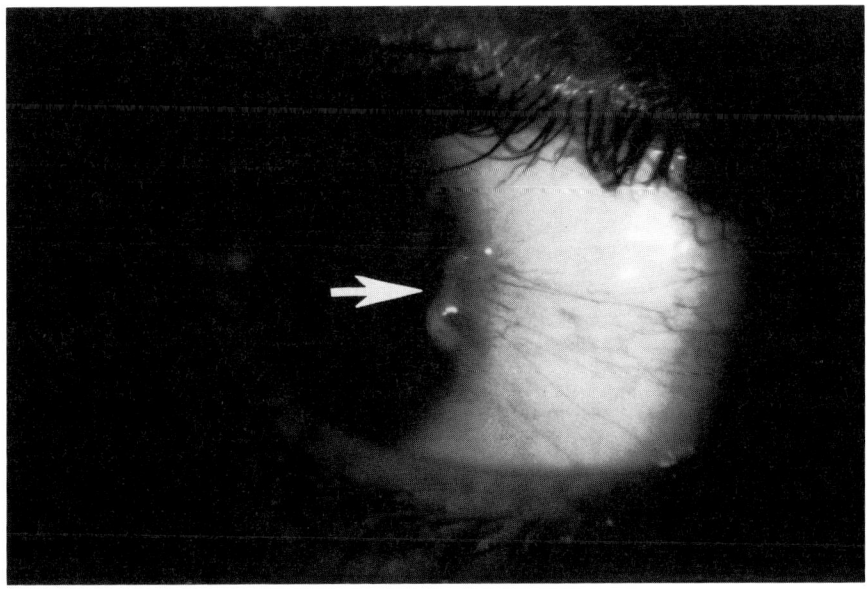

FIGURE 1-17. Pterygium.

papillomas, pigmentations, and angiomatous lesions can also be fully evaluated at the slit lamp. Inflammation of the sclera or episclera is differentiated by the blanching of blood vessels by topical vasoconstrictors and movement of the vessels with a cotton swab in episcleritis (see Chapter 16).

The *cornea* is examined for abnormalities of the epithelium, stroma, or endothelium (see Chapters 10 and 16). Two dyes, fluorescein and rose bengal, are especially useful in the diagnosis of external corneal disorders. Fluorescein sodium 2% is applied topically or from an impregnated paper strip to examine the integrity of the corneal epithelium. Defects appear as bright yellow-green when illuminated with the cobalt blue light of the slit lamp (see Figure 16-15). Fluorescein is also used in performing the Jones test and applanation tonometry. Whereas fluorescein stains denuded epithelial basement membrane and stroma, rose bengal 1% stains devitalized cells. This dye demonstrates devitalized cells in the dry eye syndrome especially well. Either dye stains soft contact lenses; these should be removed prior to instillation of any dye. The thickness of the cornea can be measured with a pachymeter, an accessory instrument that can be used with most slit lamps.

Examination of the *tear film* includes timing its dissolution and assessing the completeness of corneal wetting, the adequacy of the tear lake, and the presence of oily or soapy concretions or debris within the tears. The tear film breakup time, measured as the time before disruption in the tear film appears after a blink, is observed after the instillation of fluorescein dye. Disruption within 10 seconds suggests a tear dysfunction. The tear film should also be examined for its ability to wet the cornea completely after each blink, and the height of the tear lake should be noted. Debris or concretions in the tear film suggest an abnormality of tear composition, chronic inflammation, or infection.

The *anterior chamber* of the eye is the area between the posterior surface of the cornea and the anterior surface of the iris and lens. Its depth is appreciated by making the slit lamp beam a long, narrow slit and observing the distance between cornea and iris from an oblique angle. Inflammatory or red blood cells, pigmentary granules, and proteinaceous material (flare) are more easily visualized by using a small, narrow slit of light or a small cylindrical dot of light in a darkened room. Two techniques are helpful in visualizing cells and pigment granules. The first is to keep the illumination and observation arms steady and waiting for cells to pass through the light beam due to natural convection currents in the aqueous (cells will be illuminated as they pass through the light beam). The second technique is to oscillate the illumination beam gently from side to side while holding the observation arm steady.

The *iris* can be examined for transillumination defects by directing the light beam indirectly into the pupil and reflecting the light off the retina (retroillumination). Iris lesions and nodules are best evaluated by directing the light to the side of the lesion. The complete extent of the *ocular lens* is within the focal length of the slit lamp. The lens is examined for the presence of opacities (cataracts), which can occur in or under the anterior or posterior lens capsule, or in the lens cortex, or nucleus. The color of the lens should be noted and a sketch made of the location and shape of significant opacities.

Gonioscopy is a technique for examining the anterior chamber angle. Because the opaque sclera and corneal limbus prevent direct inspection of this area, one of several different lenses can be used to visualize the angle. Each lens has advantages. The Zeiss goniolens (Figure 1-18 and 11-3) can be placed comfortably on the eye without the need for a gel-coupling medium. Zeiss lens gonioscopy places only minimum pressure on the eye and does not distort the cornea. The Zeiss lens can also be used to apply pressure to the center of the cornea, which is occasionally successful in terminating an early acute angle closure glaucoma attack. Goldmann three-mirror gonioscopy requires a coupling agent but has the advantage of also providing visualization of the peripheral and posterior retina (Figure 1-19). Koeppe lens gonioscopy is performed with the patient in the recumbent position, without the use of a slit lamp. A dome-shaped Koeppe lens is placed on the eye, and the anterior chamber is visualized using a hand-held Barkan light and a binocular scope. Its advantage is that a lens can be placed on each eye, with rapid comparisons made between the two eyes.

The notations and abbreviations used to record findings on the slit lamp examination are given in Table 1-9.

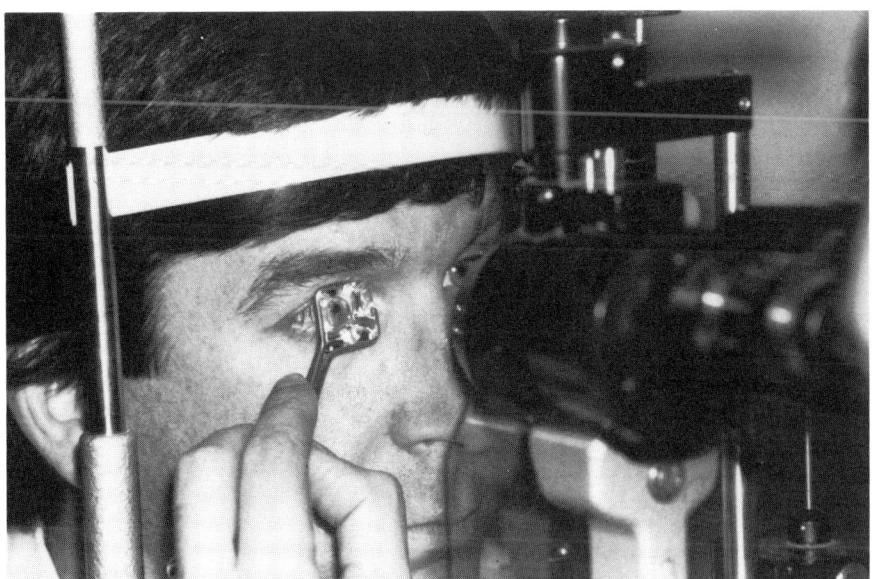

FIGURE 1-18. Zeiss goniolens examination of the anterior chamber angle.

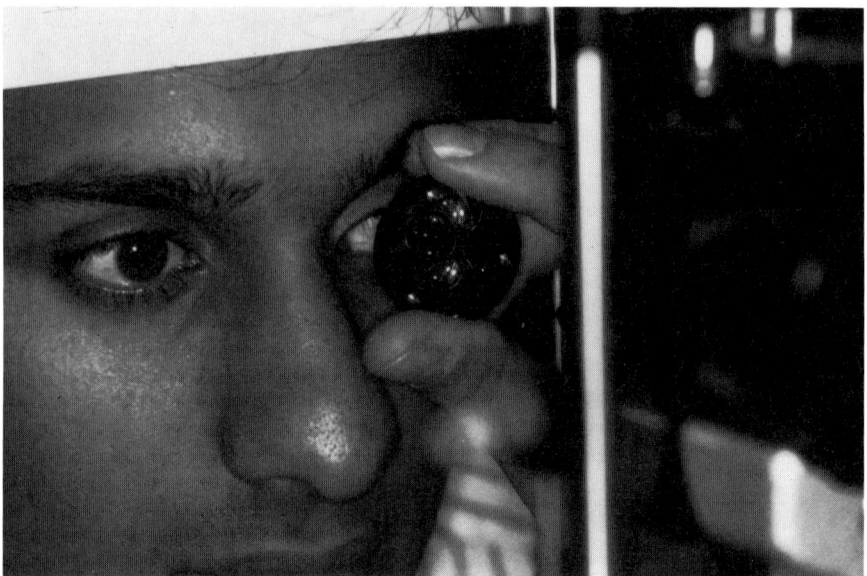

FIGURE 1-19. Goldmann three-mirror lens examination of the anterior chamber angle.

MEASUREMENT OF INTRAOCULAR PRESSURE (TONOMETRY)

A tonometer is an instrument used to measure intraocular pressure (IOP). Schiotz tonometry is based on indentation of the globe. A scale on the tonometer measures the amount of indentation for a given weight of the plunger (Figure 1-20). Charts are available for converting these scale readings to intraocular pressures based on the weight of the plunger (Table 1-10). The advantage

TABLE 1-9. NOTATIONS AND ABBREVIATIONS USED TO RECORD FINDINGS ON SLIT LAMP EXAMINATION

C,C,S	= cornea, conjunctiva, and sclera
AC	= anterior chamber
D + C	= deep and clear
cells	= presence of red or white blood cells in the anterior chamber of the eye; graded on a scale of 0 to 4+
flare	= presence of proteinaceous material in the anterior chamber
K	= keratometer reading (refractive power of the cornea)
KP	= keratic precipitates (accumulations of inflammatory cells on the posterior (endothelial) surface of the cornea)
hyphema	= layering of red blood cells in the anterior chamber (eight ball = complete filling of anterior chamber)
hypopyon	= layering of inflammatory cells in the anterior chamber

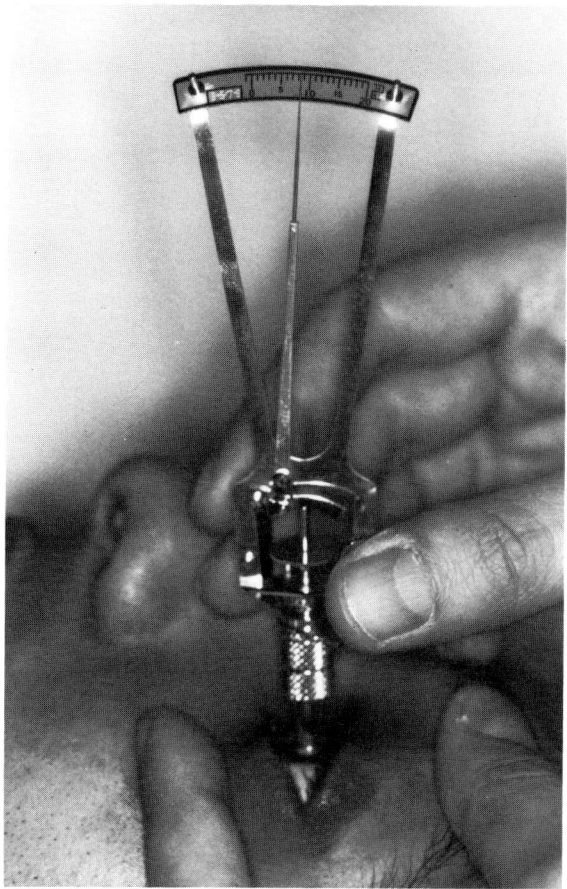

FIGURE 1-20. Schiotz tonometry.

of Schiotz tonometry is that it can be performed with minimal training and instrumentation. The patient should be recumbent, and a topical anesthetic must be used. Care must be exercised not to apply pressure on the globe when spreading the eyelids and to maintain a vertical alignment of the instrument.

Applanation tonometers do not indent the globe; rather, they measure the force necessary to flatten a given area (3.06 mm) of the cornea. The Goldmann applanation tonometer is standard equipment on both the Haag-Streit and Zeiss slit lamp (Figure 1-21). It has the advantage of being less affected by gravity or scleral rigidity than the Schiotz tonometer. A prism incorporated within the tonometer head divides the produced image of a ring into an upper and lower half. Applanation tonometry is performed by instilling topical anesthetic and fluorescein dye into the eye, directing maximum illumination to the tonometer tip, and aligning the inner parts of the ring while observing through

TABLE 1-10. INTRAOCULAR PRESSURE (mm Hg) BY SCHIOTZ TONOMETRY

TONOMETER SCALE READING	PLUNGER WEIGHT (g)			
	5.5	7.5	10.0	15.0
0.0	41.4	59.1	81.7	127.5
0.5	37.8	54.2	75.1	117.9
1.0	34.5	49.8	69.3	109.3
1.5	31.6	45.8	64.0	101.4
2.0	29.0	42.1	59.1	94.3
2.5	26.6	38.8	54.7	88.0
3.0	24.4	35.8	50.6	81.8
3.5	22.4	33.0	46.9	76.2
4.0	20.6	30.4	43.4	71.0
4.5	18.9	28.0	40.2	66.2
5.0	17.3	25.8	37.2	61.8
5.5	15.9	23.8	34.4	57.6
6.0	14.6	21.9	31.8	53.6
6.5	13.4	20.1	29.4	49.9
7.0	12.2	18.5	27.2	46.5
7.5	11.2	17.0	25.1	43.2
8.0	10.2	15.6	23.1	40.2
8.5	9.4	14.3	21.3	38.1
9.0	8.5	13.1	19.6	34.6
9.5	7.8	12.0	18.0	32.0
10.0	7.1	10.9	16.5	29.6
10.5	6.5	10.0	15.1	27.4
11.0	5.9	9.1	13.8	25.3
11.5	5.3	8.3	12.6	23.3
12.0	4.9	7.5	11.5	21.4
12.5	4.4	6.8	10.5	19.7
13.0	4.0	6.2	9.5	18.1
13.5		5.6	8.6	16.5
14.0		5.0	7.8	15.1
14.5		4.5	7.1	13.7
15.0		4.1	6.4	12.6
15.5			5.8	11.4
16.0			5.2	10.4
16.5			4.7	9.4
17.0			4.2	8.5
17.5				7.7
18.0				6.9
18.5				6.2
19.0				5.6
19.5				4.9
20.0				4.5

the slit lamp (Figure 1-22). Hand-held applanation tonometers (see Figure 3-6), noncontact pneumotonometers, and electronic tonometers are also available.

Digital measurement is crude but can give an approximation of intraocular pressure when the above instrumentation is unavailable. The technique involves palpating (balloting) the globe with the eyelids closed. With the

1—Examination of the Eye   35

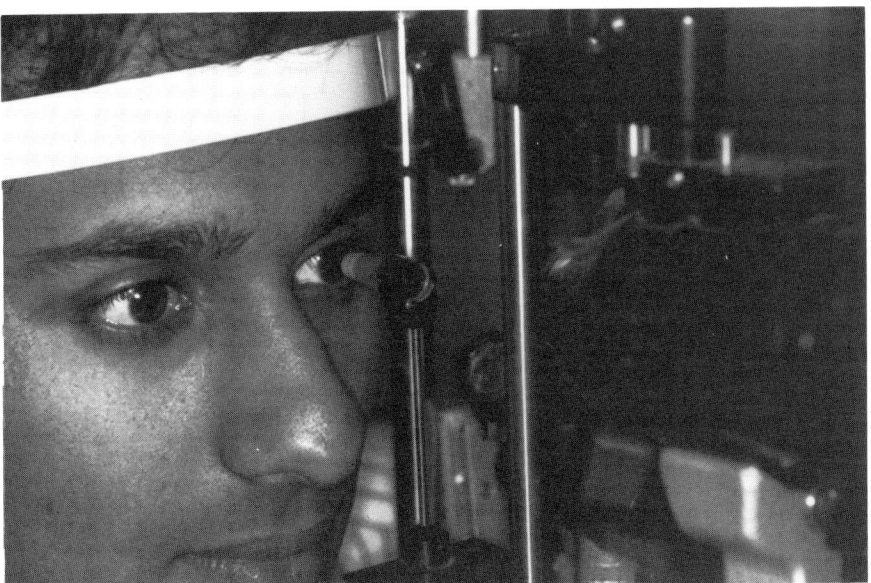

FIGURE 1-21. Goldmann applanation tonometry at the slit lamp.

patient looking down, the examiner uses two fingers placed between the globe and superior orbit (Figure 1-23). A small amount of sponginess to the globe is normal. Firmness to the degree that indentation cannot be easily performed is consistent with elevated intraocular pressure. Molding of the globe to the indenting finger and movement of the internal structures of the eye are consistent with a soft (hypotonic) eye.

The notations and abbreviations used to record findings on tonometry are given in Table 1-11.

APPLANATION TONOMETRY

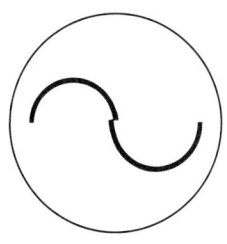
Correct Amount of Fluorescein
Correct Apposition

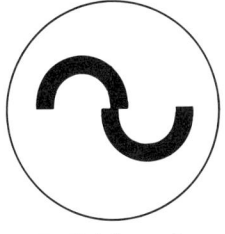
Too Much Fluorescein
Too Much Overlap

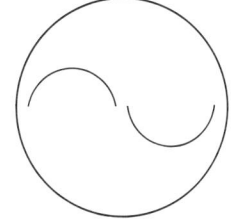
Too Little Fluorescein
Semicircles Not Apposed

FIGURE 1-22. Proper position of the semicircles for the measurement of intraocular pressure by tonometry.

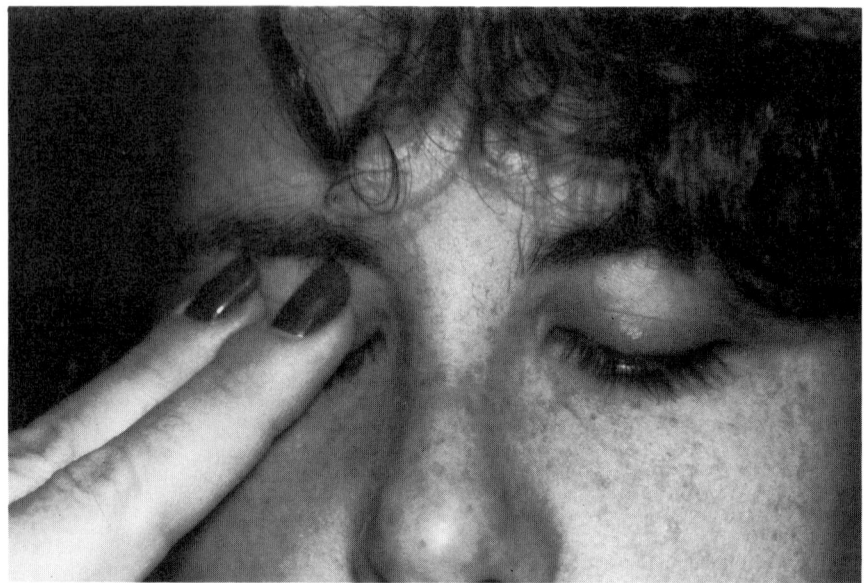

FIGURE 1-23. Digital tonometry.

TABLE 1-11. NOTATIONS AND ABBREVIATIONS USED TO RECORD FINDINGS ON VISUAL FIELD EXAMINATION AND TONOMETRY

Visual field
VF = visual field
Conf = confrontational visual field

Tonometry
T = tonometry
T_{AP} = applanation tonometry
$T_{SCH\ 5.5}$ = Schiotz tonometry with a 5.5 gm weight
FT = finger tension
TT = tactile tension (same as above)
IOP = intraocular pressure

Examples

$$VF \begin{matrix} \text{full to conf} \\ \text{full to conf} \end{matrix}$$

The visual field was full to confrontation in both eyes.

$$T_{AP} \begin{matrix} 12 \\ 13 \end{matrix}$$

The intraocular pressure in the right eye measured by applanation tonometry was 12 mm Hg; in the left eye, it was 13 mm Hg.

FUNDUS EXAMINATION

Examination of the fundus of the eye, the inner posterior aspect of the globe, begins with inspecting the vitreous. Depending on the presenting signs and symptoms, one should search for pigment granules, inflammatory or red blood cells, or a posterior vitreous detachment. The anterior vitreous can be visualized through the slit lamp, but the posterior vitreous is best seen with the direct ophthalmoscope focused in front of the retina.

After examination of the vitreous, attention is turned to the optic disk, retina, and retinal vasculature. The optic disk, or optic nerve head, is approximately 1.5 mm in diameter. Other structures in the fundus are often measured in terms of disk diameters (DD). The normal disk is pink in color, with the exception of the physiologic cup, which appears as a white depression in the center of the disk. The cup-to-disk ratio refers to the relative size of the horizontal diameter of the cup to the disk diameter and is given in terms of the nearest 0.1. Less than 3% of the normal population have a ratio greater than 0.6. Large cups and asymmetries of greater than 0.2 between the eyes are suggestive of glaucoma. The edges of the disk are normally flat and sharp. Elevation and blurring of the disk margin and obscuration of blood vessels are consistent with disk edema from inflammation or elevated intracranial pressure (see Figure 14–14).

The anatomic macula is an ill-defined zone approximately 3.5 DD (5.5 mm) in size, located approximately 2 DD (3 mm) temporal and 0.5 DD (0.75 mm) inferior to the center of the optic disk. The fovea is a central depression within the macula, approximately 1 DD in diameter. The foveola is the capillary-free zone in the center of this, approximately 0.3 DD in diameter. This capillary-free zone is best appreciated on fluorescein angiography (see Figure 2–17). Yellowish xanthophyll pigment is present in an area of the retina extending about 2 DD nasal and temporal to the foveola and to the arching temporal vessels above and below this area. The area where this pigment is present is often loosely referred to as the macula (although the designation is anatomically incorrect). The macula is inspected for the presence of edema, exudates, and hemorrhages in patients with a sudden loss of vision (see Chapter 14). The remaining retina is examined for the presence of lesions, tears, detachments, hard (yellow, lipid) and soft (nerve fiber layer) infarcts, exudates, hemorrhages, and drusen (hyaline excrescences of the retinal pigment epithelium).

The central retinal artery bifurcates into superior and inferior branches and then, respectively, into nasal and temporal branches. Branches of the central retinal vein parallel those of the artery. The central retinal vein is occasionally seen pulsating. Whereas this is a physiologic finding in over half the population, pulsation of the central retinal artery is pathologic. Arterial pulsation indicates reduced perfusion to the eye caused by either elevated intraocular or arterial pulse pressure. The vasculature is also evaluated for signs of arteriolar sclerosis, including attenuation of arterioles, arteriovenous crossing changes, changes in the vascular light reflex (irregularities in caliber, copper and silver-wire broadening of the light reflex), arteriolar sheathing, and tortuosity (Figure 1-24). Dilation of the veins, with boxcar formation of the blood column, suggests venous stasis; neovascularization and intraretinal microvascular changes suggest diabetic retinopathy (see Chapter 14).

Four types of instruments are used to examine the fundus: the direct and indirect ophthalmoscope and contact and noncontact retinal lenses. *Direct ophthalmoscopy* is accomplished in a stepwise fashion. The physician approaches the patient temporally using his or her left eye to examine the left eye of the patient (correspondingly for the right eye). The physician peers through the observer aperture of the scope while directing the light beam toward the patient's pupil. The examiner's index finger should be on the focusing wheel of lenses as he or she comes closer to the patient (Figure 1-25). With proper focusing of the red reflex, the retina will become visible. When a large retinal vessel is located, it is followed either nasally or temporally to the optic disk, which is usually examined first. Examination of the retinal vessels follows in the same manner. The macular area is examined by asking the patient to look toward the light, followed by an examination of the peripheral retina.

Indirect ophthalmoscopy requires specialized equipment and training and is usually the domain of the ophthalmologist. Its use requires the alignment of the observer's eyes, light source, an indirect lens, and the patient's eye (Figure 1-26). Its advantages are many. Stronger illumination allows visualization through opacities that the direct ophthalmoscope cannot penetrate. A wider

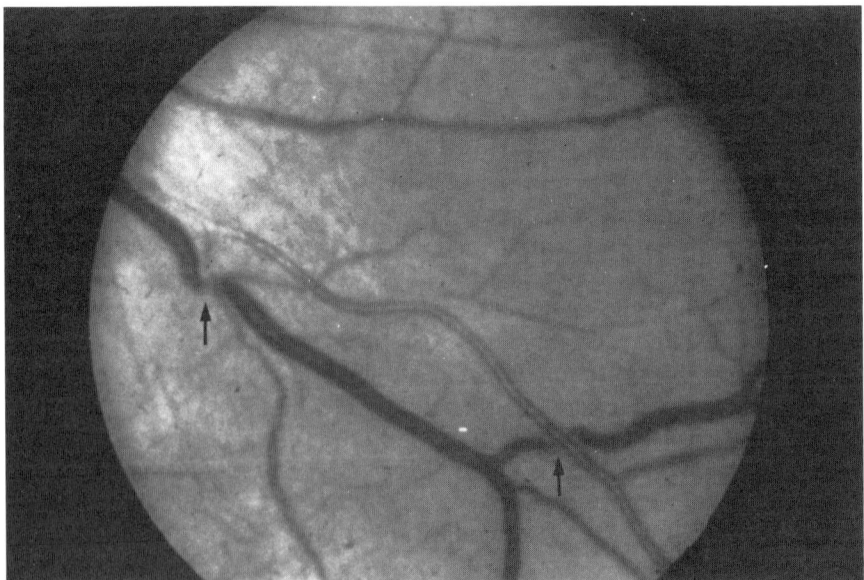

FIGURE 1-24. Hypertensive retinopathy. Note the arteriovenous crossing changes (arrows) and the copper wire arterial reflex.

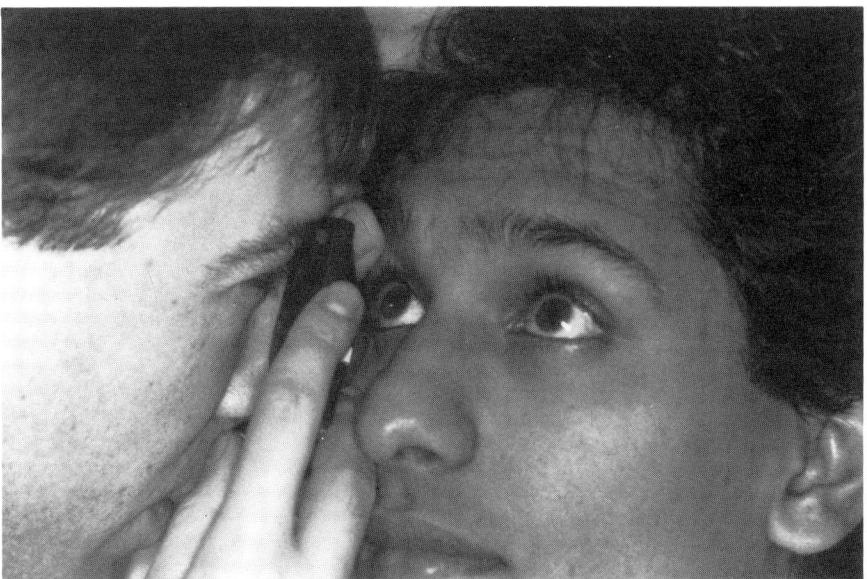

FIGURE 1-25. Method of direct ophthalmoscopy.

field of the retina can be visualized, and with the use of scleral depression, the entire retina can usually be examined. Perhaps its greatest advantage is that lesions can be visualized in depth. A disadvantage is that magnification is minimal. Fourteen, 20, and 30 diopter lenses give $4\times$, $3\times$, and $2\times$ magnification, respectively—compared to the direct ophthalmoscope, which gives $15\times$ magnification. The 20 diopter lens is most commonly used. It should be held with the convex side facing the observer; in the proper position, the two light reflexes formed on it are of the same size. Scleral depression is performed by indenting the posterior globe with a hand-held or thimblelike depressor. The patient is asked to look opposite the area to be examined while the depressor is situated on the eyelid over the area to be depressed. Placing the depressor above the tarsal plate of the eyelid reduces discomfort. As the patient looks toward the depressor, the globe is gently indented. Due to the anatomy of the orbital bones and requisite positioning, the novice will find it easiest to see the peripheral retina (ora serata) in the superior nasal quadrant.

Several *contact and noncontact retinal lenses* are also available for examining the retina at the slit lamp: the Goldmann lens, the Hruby lens (an attachment to many slit lamps), and several hand-held lenses, such as the Volk 90 diopter lens. These provide highly magnified, well-illuminated, three-dimensional views of the fundus. The notations and abbreviations used to record findings on the fundus examination are given in Table 1–12.

Ophthalmodynamometry is a special technique performed in conjunction with auscultation and palpation of the neck vessels in patients with signs or symptoms of carotid vascular disease. It compares the ophthalmic artery pres-

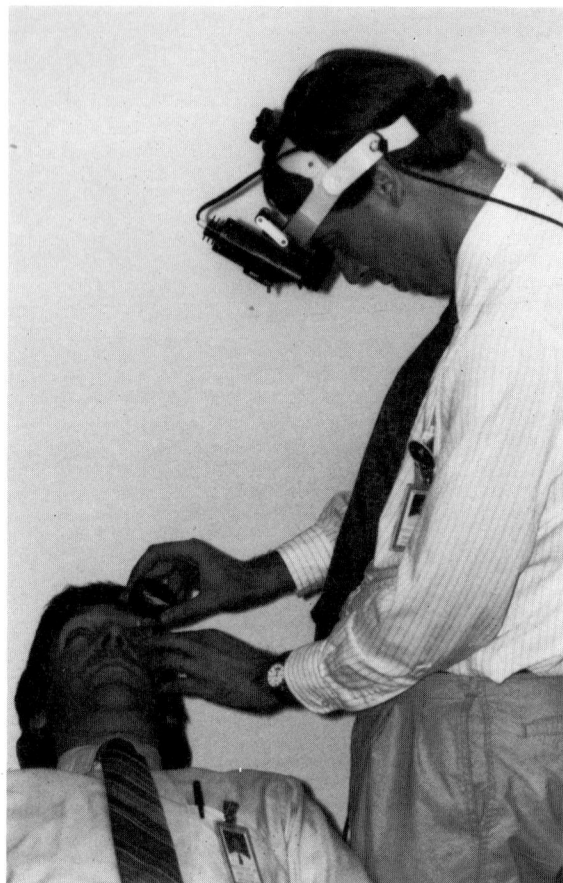

FIGURE 1–26. Method of indirect ophthalmoscopy.

sure of the two eyes. Asymmetry suggests that a 70% to 90% stenosis is present in the carotid system with the lower pressure. A normal finding does not rule out carotid artery disease; symptomatic atheromatous disease (e.g., amaurosis fugax) can occur with minimal stenosis. The test is performed after the intraocular pressure (IOP) has been measured. This measurement is necessary for the conversion of the scale reading on the instrument to millimeters of mercury (mm Hg) of pressure. The two-person technique is recommended

TABLE 1–12. NOTATIONS AND ABBREVIATIONS USED TO RECORD FINDINGS ON FUNDUS EXAMINATION

D = optic disk	C/D = cup to disk ratio	HE = hard exudate
M = macula	DD = disk diameters	SE = soft exudate
V = vessels	F = fundus	

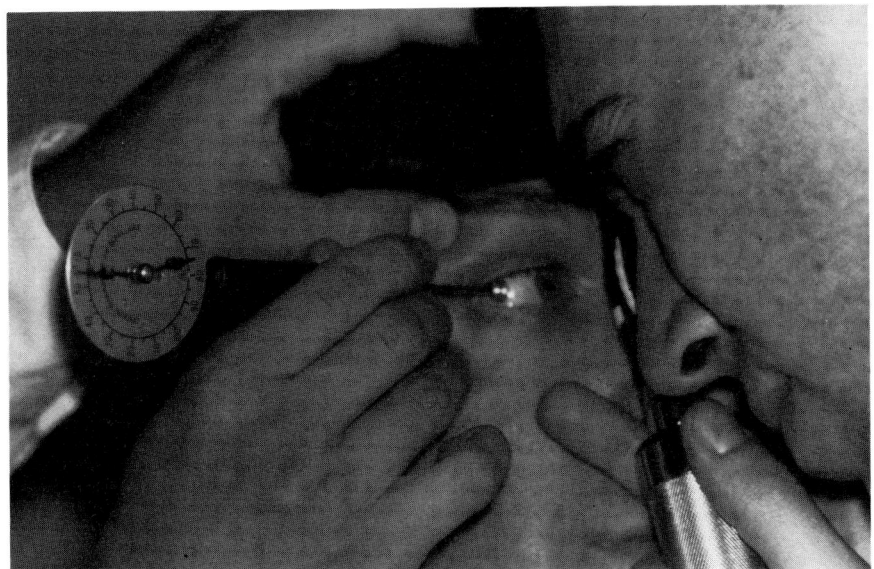

FIGURE 1-27. Two-person technique of ophthalmodynamometry.

(Figure 1-27). The first person views the patient's central retinal artery through a direct ophthalmoscope while the second applies the instrument to the lateral sclera. With the patient seated, pressure is slowly increased until the retinal arteries are observed to pulsate. When this occurs, the reading on the instrument dial represents the ophthalmic artery diastolic pressure. Pressure is increased until the retinal arterioles collapse; this reading is the systolic pressure. The readings are given in grams of applied pressure. A formula to convert scale readings to mm Hg is given in Table 1-13. The average ophthalmic artery systolic pressure varies between 60 mm Hg and 85 mm Hg and diastolic pres-

TABLE 1-13. BEDAVANIJA'S FORMULA FOR CONVERTING READINGS ON OPHTHALMODYNAMOMETRY TO MILLIMETERS OF MERCURY*

$$\text{mm Hg} = 0.87 \times g + T_{corr}$$

where: g = scale reading on the ophthalmodynamometer
T_{corr} = corrected value for intraocular pressure (IOP) based on initial IOP and applied force:

Initial IOP	T_{corr}
12.0	18.0
14.0	19.0
16.0	19.5
18.0	20.5
20.0	21.5

*From: Sanborn GE, Miller NR, Maguire M, Kumar AJ: Clinical angiographic correlation of ophthalmodynamometry in suspected carotid artery disease. *Arch Ophthalmol* 99:1811, 1981.

sure between 30 mm Hg and 40 mm Hg. If an asymmetry of greater than 20% is present between the two eyes in either the systolic or diastolic pressure, carotid stenosis proximal to the ophthalmic artery is suggested. Ophthalmodynamometry can also be used to evaluate increased intracranial pressure, which is suggested if the diastolic pressure on ophthalmodynamometry is 10 mm Hg to 15 mm Hg higher than the brachial diastolic pressure.

INDICATIONS FOR OPHTHALMOLOGIC REFERRAL

Many ocular disorders can be adequately managed by emergency and primary care physicians. Certain conditions, however, should be evaluated by an ophthalmologist. At times it is necessary to call upon the ophthalmologist only for follow-up; occasionally immediate referral is required. The following list notes conditions where ophthalmologic referral is suggested:

Findings on the history that merit referral
Loss of vision, whether transient or sustained.
Distortion of vision (metamorphopsia).
Constriction or loss of the visual field.
Diplopia in any field of gaze.
The perception of flashes of light or new floaters.
Abnormal sensitivity to light.

Findings on the ocular examination that merit referral
Any ocular disorder that results in a sustained reduction of vision or loss of the visual field.
Perforating injury to the eye or orbit.
Laceration involving the eyelid margin.
Imbedded corneal foreign body.
Blood in the anterior chamber.
Inflammation within the eye.
Irregular, asymmetric, or poorly reacting pupil.
Relative afferent pupillary defect.
Restricted ocular movements with diplopia.
Metamorphopsia on Amsler grid testing.
Elevated intraocular pressure.
Blood in the vitreous.
Evidence of diabetic or hypertensive retinopathy.
Absence of findings but persistent eye pain or visual complaints.

REFERENCES

Crawford JS, Pashby RC: Lacrimal system disorders. *Int Ophthalmol Clin* 24:39, 1984.
Deutsch TA, Feller DB: *Paton and Goldberg's Management of Ocular Injuries.* Philadelphia, WB Saunders, 1985, pp 1–8.

Freeman HM: Examination of the traumatized eye. In Miller D, Stegman R (eds): *Treatment of anterior segment ocular trauma.* Montreal, Medicopea, 1986, pp 95–119.
Hecht SD: Evaluation of the lacrimal drainage system. *Ophthalmology* 85:1250, 1978.
Klein OG: The initial evaluation in ophthalmic injury. *Otolaryngol Clin North Am* 12:303, 1979.
Nelson LB, Catalano RA: *Atlas of ocular motility.* Philadelphia, WB Saunders, 1989, pp 2–43.
Richard JM (ed): *A manual for the beginning ophthalmology resident.* 3d ed. San Francisco, American Academy of Ophthalmology, 1980.
Sanborn GE, Miller NR, Maguire M, Kumar AJ: Clinical angiographic correlation of ophthalmodynamometry in suspected carotid artery disease. *Arch Ophthalmol* 99:1811, 1981.
Thompson HS, Corbett JJ, Cox TA: How to measure the relative afferent pupillary defect. *Surv Ophthalmol* 26:39, 1981.

2

Diagnostic Testing

Robert A. Catalano
Frederick A. Eames

Numerous modalities are available to assist the physician in evaluating ocular emergencies. Rapid developments have occurred in many areas but especially in computed tomography (CT) and magnetic resonance imaging (MRI). The vast superiority of these newer methods has rendered many older diagnostic studies, such as optic canal tomograms, radioisotope orbital scanning, pneumoencephalography, and orbitography (the injection of radiopaque dye into the orbital tissues) largely obsolete. This chapter emphasizes newer modalities and techniques; older methods are mentioned for completeness only.

ULTRASOUND

Human tissues transmit, absorb, refract, and reflect sound waves. Ultrasonography (echography) records these effects of tissues on sound. The ultrasound transducer contains a piezoelectric crystal, which is capable of both emitting sound and capturing reflected vibrations (echos). Captured sound is converted to electrical potentials, which are displayed on a cathode ray oscilloscope. The images on the oscilloscope can be photographed, to provide a permanent record of any findings. Three different imaging techniques—the A-scan, B-scan, and Doppler sonography—have been developed for ophthalmologic use.

A-scans detect changes in tissue elasticity or density (acoustic impedance) and record the distance of interfaces from a stationary transducer. The A-scan probe emits an unfocused beam that penetrates as deep as 15 cm and receives reflected sound waves from a cylindrical section of tissue 3 mm to 5 mm wide.

Changes in impedance are displayed as spikes on the oscilloscope (Figure 2–1). The number, location, height, and motion of the spikes give information regarding different tissue characteristics. A paucity of spikes within a structure, for example, suggests a homogeneous composition. The height of the spike is a reflection of the acoustic density of the tissue, which varies with its cellular composition. Fast-flickering spike movements indicate vascularity. A-scans are particularly useful in differentiating tissue reflectivity, a characteristic of great importance in evaluating orbital lesions. High internal reflectivity is seen in tissues containing numerous thick interfaces (septae). Most normal tissues in the orbit, with the exception of the extraocular muscles and optic nerve, have high internal reflectivity, in contradistinction to most lesions, which are more homogeneous and exhibit lower internal reflectivity. The A-scan transducer can also be used to compress orbital lesions, distinguishing firm masses from elastic ones. Most cysts and vascular lesions (e.g., varices and lymphangiomas) are soft and easily compressible.

B-scan units emit focused sound waves and produce cross-section images of tissue (Figure 2–2). B-scan ultrasonography is performed by sweeping a motorized transducer in a linear fashion across the eye. Increases in acoustic impedance are characterized by a brighter signal. The integration of many beam positions allows a much greater area to be depicted than is possible with the A-scan and creates a two-dimensional picture of the eye and orbit (A-scans are one-dimensional). The B-scan is useful in determining a lesion's shape and its proximity to normal ocular structures. Even under the most optimal gray scale conditions, however, the brightness of the B-scan signal cannot be quantitated. The differential reflectivity of orbital lesions, a prime use of A-scan ultrasonography, cannot be evaluated with the B-scan.

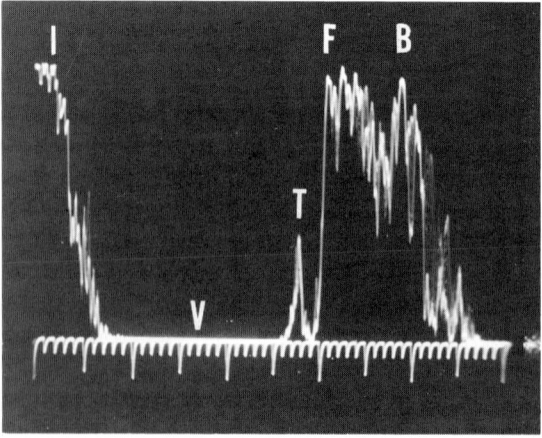

FIGURE 2–1. A-scan ultrasonogram of malignant melanoma (I = initial spike, V = vitreous, T = tumor, F = fundus, B = bone spike).

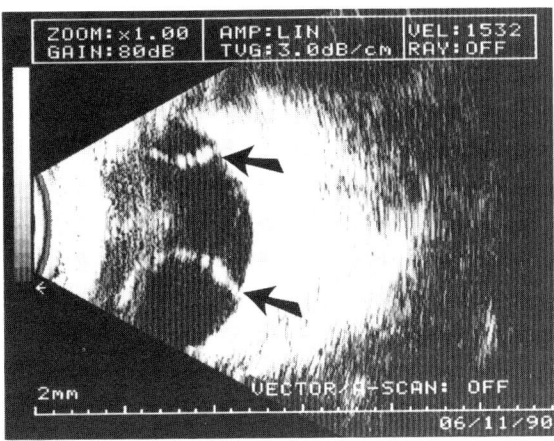

FIGURE 2-2. B-scan ultrasonogram demonstrating choroidal detachments (arrows) that extend from the iris root anteriorly to the vortex veins posteriorly.

Doppler techniques detect whether blood is moving toward or away from the transducer. The velocity of blood flow is proportional to the induced shift in frequency in the recaptured sound waves. Electronic circuitry converts these induced shifts into audible signals. Doppler techniques are useful in evaluating occlusive vascular disease and vascular abnormalities. Color Doppler imaging (CDI), a relatively new technique, displays color-encoded Doppler flow information throughout a two-dimensional gray scale image. CDI provides selective analysis of Doppler spectra in small vessels and may be useful in the diagnosis and management of vascular intraocular tumors.

The typical ultrasound evaluation uses each scanning method. The B-scan localizes and defines the configuration of the lesion. The A-scan then quantitates tissue characteristics. Standard echography is performed in eight meridians, using both paraocular and transocular approaches. To scan paraocularly, the transducer is placed over closed eyelids and angled so that sound projects between the globe and bony orbital wall. Methylcellulose is used as a coupling agent. Paraocular approaches are used to evaluate the anterior portion of the orbit. To scan transocularly, the probe is placed on the eye. Because the ocular lens refracts, reflects, and attenuates the sound beam, the patient is asked to look away from where the transducer is applied (toward the meridian to be examined). The sound beam is also aimed perpendicular to the structure to be investigated. Transocular approaches are used to evaluate the posterior orbit.

To visualize the anterior chamber and lens on B-scan ultrasonography, an immersion technique is necessary. This can be accomplished by use of a water bath or a balloon stand-off of soft prophylactic latex partially filled with saline. The latter method places much less pressure on the eye. Some machines incorporate a water bath in the transducer; this allows scanning of the anterior segment through closed eyelids, a distinct advantage in evaluating recently traumatized eyes. Most ocular ultrasounds are performed at 8000 to 20,000 hertz. The use of lower frequencies (5000 Hz) may be beneficial in the presence of hemorrhage or inflammation.

Ultrasonography offers no advantages to CT scanning for orbital disorders. It can, however, uniquely image ocular disorders. Proceeding from the front of the eye, ultrasonography can demonstrate hyphema, iridodialysis, vitreous in the anterior chamber, lens rupture or dislocation, the integrity of the zonules, vitreous hemorrhage, retinal or choroidal detachment, and retained foreign bodies. In traumatized eyes, a preoperative ultrasound can assist in planning the extent of the primary repair and localizing any foreign bodies. It may be the only way to evaluate the integrity of the posterior eye. Ultrasound should not be performed preoperatively in severely lacerated eyes; in these cases, it can be used intraoperatively or postoperatively.

PLAIN FILM RADIOGRAPHY

Plain film radiography is an inexpensive, readily available modality that can be used to diagnose or screen for many commonly encountered orbital disorders. It is the study of choice to determine the configuration and number of any metallic foreign bodies. Plain films also demonstrate the majority of orbital and facial fractures, many ocular and orbital tumors, congenital bony malformations, and disorders of the paranasal sinuses. Specific pathologic findings include the following:

Calcification: retinoblastoma, meningioma, varix, hemangioma, choroidal osteoma, degeneration (phthisis) of the globe.

Hyperostosis: meningioma, fibrous dysplasia.

Orbital enlargement: benign or malignant neoplasm in childhood and benign tumor in adulthood.

Orbital erosion: malignant tumor.

Sphenoid wing elevation, hypoplasia, or absence: unilateral coronal synostosis, neurofibromatosis, other cranial dysplasia.

Loss of the oblique (innominate line): sphenoid ridge meningioma, metastatic carcinoma.

Orbital emphysema. fracture through a paranasal sinus.

The usual orbital series of X rays provides five views, most of them described according to the relationship of the central X-ray beam (central ray) to the line that connects the outer canthus of the eye to the external auditory meatus (the canthomeatal or orbitomeatal line):

1. *Caldwell view,* produced by placing the patient's face against the film plate and directing the central ray 15° upward from the canthomeatal line,

from a posterior to anterior position. The orbital margins, medial wall, ethmoid and frontal sinuses, sphenoid wings and ridge, superior orbital fissure, lacrimal fossa, and posterior orbital floor are well visualized (Figure 2–3).

2. *Waters view,* taken with the patient's chin and nose against the film plate and head extended until the central ray is directed 37° above the canthomeatal line. This provides an excellent view of the orbital roof and floor and the maxillary antrum. It is the ideal view to screen for an orbital floor or zygomatic (tripod) fracture (Figure 2–4).

3. *Lateral view,* obtained by placing the side of the face against the radiograph and directing the central ray parallel to the orbital floors. It is useful in evaluating abnormalities of the nasopharynx and sella turcica, as well as the orbital roof, and frontal and maxillary sinuses (Figure 2–5).

4. *Submentovertex (base, subaxial, Hirtz's) view,* obtained by hyperextending the neck such that the top of the head lies against the film plate. This position places the canthomeatal line parallel to the film plate. The central ray is then directed perpendicular to both. This view demonstrates the posterior lateral wall of the orbit, the sphenoid wings, the sphenoid and ethmoid sinuses, basal foramina, pterygoid fossa, zygomatic arches, and nasopharynx (Figure 2–6).

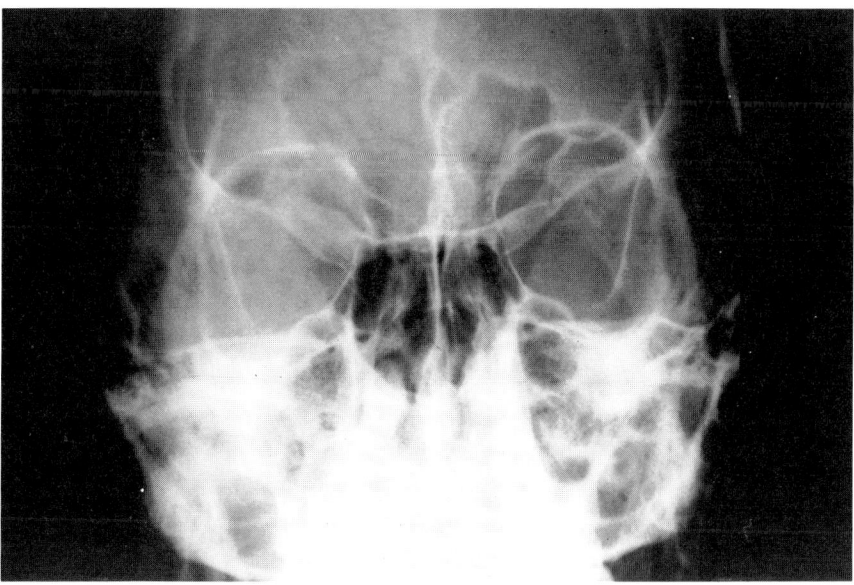

FIGURE 2–3. Caldwell projection plain film radiograph.

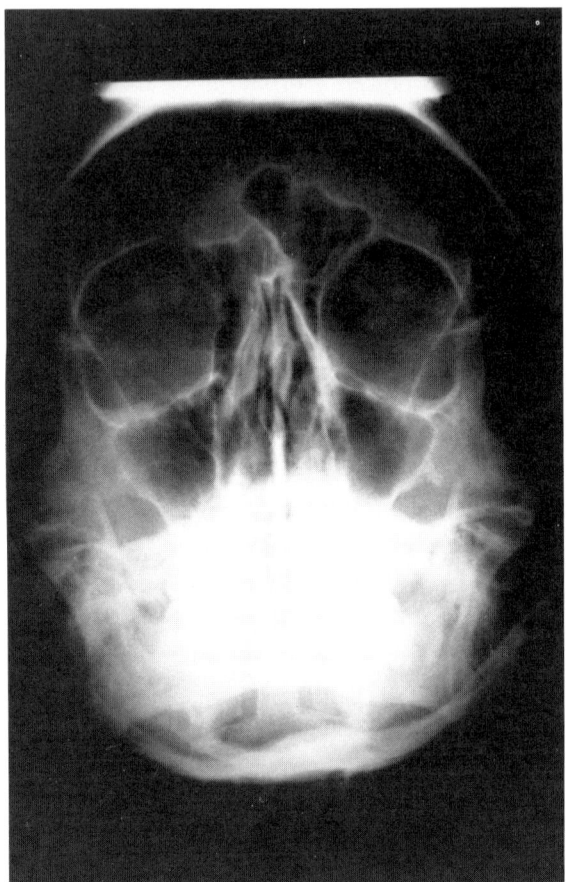

FIGURE 2-4. Waters view plain film radiograph.

5. *Oblique (Rhese) views,* produced by placing the face obliquely against the film plate such that one orbit and cheek lies against the plate. The central ray is directed 40° lateral to the anteroposterior axis of the head and 15° upward from the canthomeatal line. Prior to the development of CT, this view was used to demonstrate the optic foramen, which is visible in this projection in the inferolateral quadrant of the orbit (Figure 2-7).

Tomography is a radiographic technique that blurs unwanted portions of the image to provide a sharper image at a given plane. It has been replaced by CT. Previously it was used to demonstrate enlargement of an optic canal, suggesting an optic nerve glioma (see Figure 12-11), or bone destruction, suggesting a lacrimal gland or other orbital tumor, or to evaluate maxillo-facial fractures.

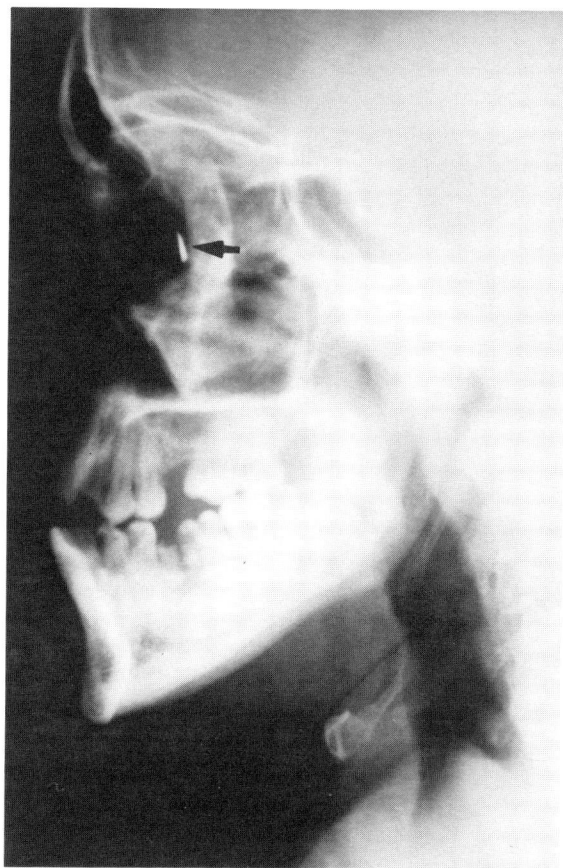

FIGURE 2-5. Lateral projection plain film radiograph, demonstrating an intraorbital foreign body (arrow).

COMPUTED TOMOGRAPHY AND MAGNETIC RESONANCE IMAGING

Computed tomography (CT) is based on the principle that atoms with higher atomic numbers absorb proportionately more ionizing radiation. The development of machines that can deliver a focused band of radiation and computer software that can analyze the difference in radiation transmitted through contiguous tissues with different atomic compositions has resulted in the production of detailed CT images. The CT scanner reconstructs data points, or pixels (picture elements), based on the attenuation coefficient of a volume of tissue (a voxel, or volume element). The computer relates these attenuation coefficients to a suitably graduated gray scale, which is displayed on a cathode ray tube

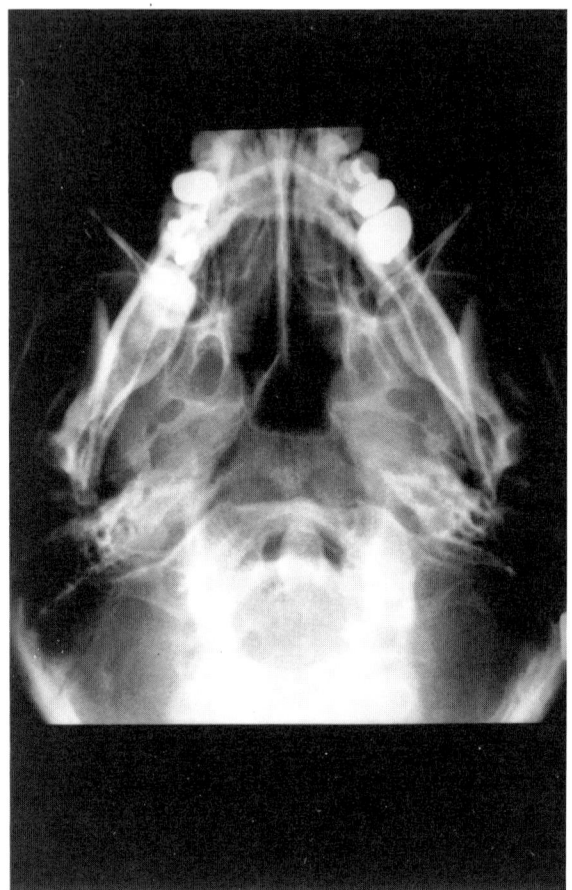

FIGURE 2-6. Submentovertex projection plain film radiograph.

(CRT). An important characteristic of CT scanning is that the CRT display can be modified so that the extremes of the gray scale represent pixels having very small differences in attenuation coefficients. The term *window width* refers to the range of the gray scale. *Window level* refers to the attenuation coefficient that the operator sets as the midpoint of this range.

Attenuation coefficients are given in terms of Hounsfield units. Table 2-1 lists attenuation coefficients for different orbital tissues. A window width of 200 Hounsfield units to 500 Hounsfield units and a window level of -10 units to 30 units encompasses most of the densities of structures in and around the orbit. For evaluating orbital bones, however, higher levels (200 units) with wider widths (2000 units to 4000 units) are required. Algorithms (kernels) are preset programs, available on newer machines, that can be used to highlight specific tissues (e.g., "bone window," "soft tissue window").

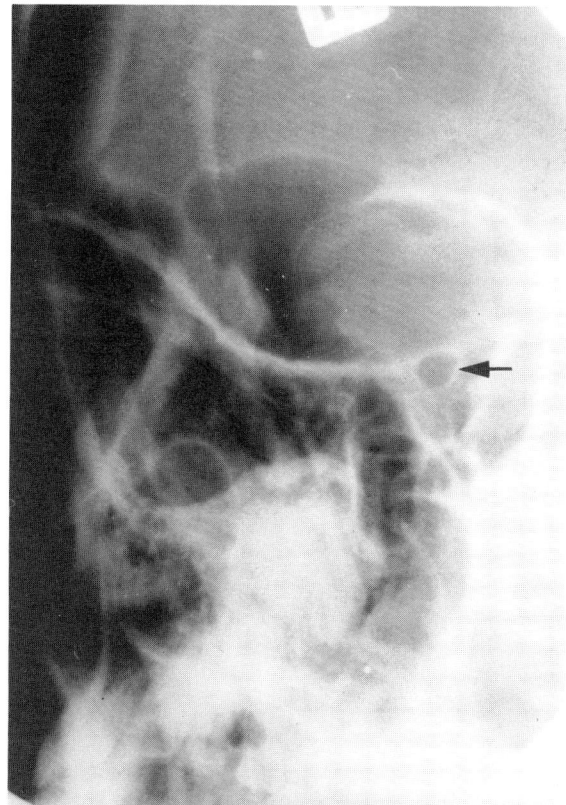

FIGURE 2-7. Oblique (Rhese) projection plain film radiograph, demonstrating the optic canal (arrow).

Axial, coronal, and reconstructed coronal and sagittal images can be obtained by CT (Figures 2–8 through 2–10). The plane of axial CT imaging is usually described relative to Reid's line (also called the anthropologic baseline or infraorbital-meatal line), which extends from the inferior orbital rim to the upper margin of the external auditory meatus. Routine cranial axial CT is per-

TABLE 2-1. ATTENUATION COEFFICIENTS

TISSUE	COEFFICIENT (H)
Air	−1000
Orbital fat	−100
Water	0
Extraocular muscle	35
Dense bone	1000

H = Hounsfield unit.

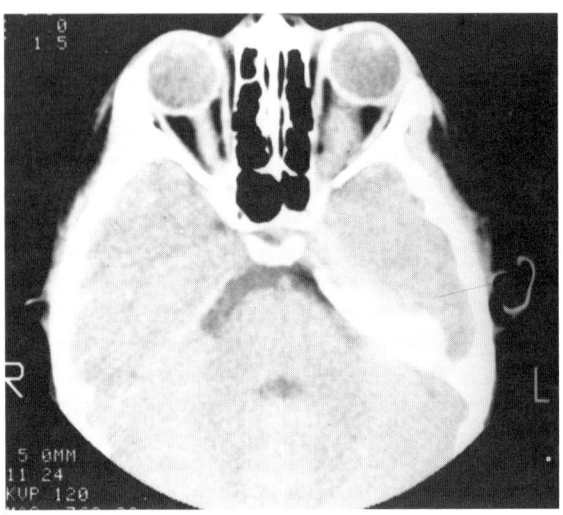

FIGURE 2–8. Axial CT, demonstrating an optic nerve glioma in the left eye.

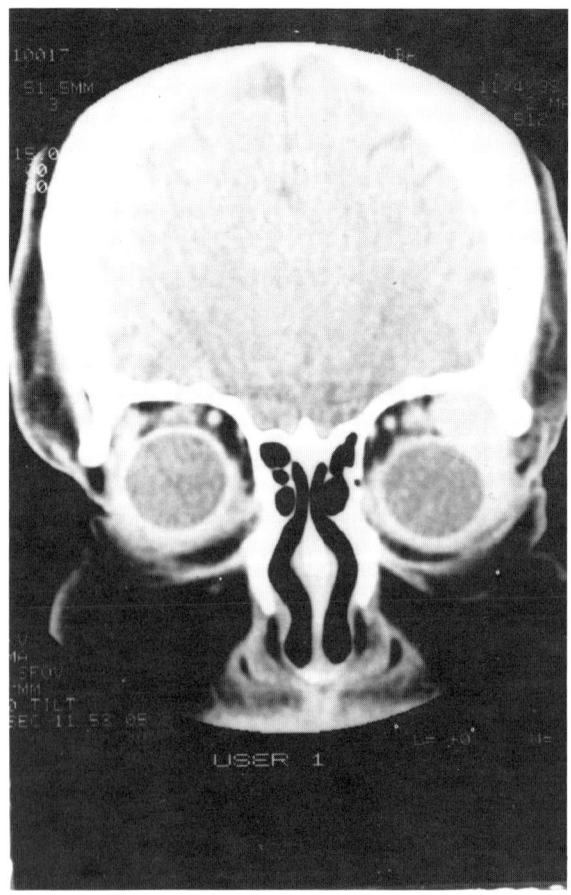

FIGURE 2–9. Coronal CT, demonstrating an orbital lymphoma molding about the left eye.

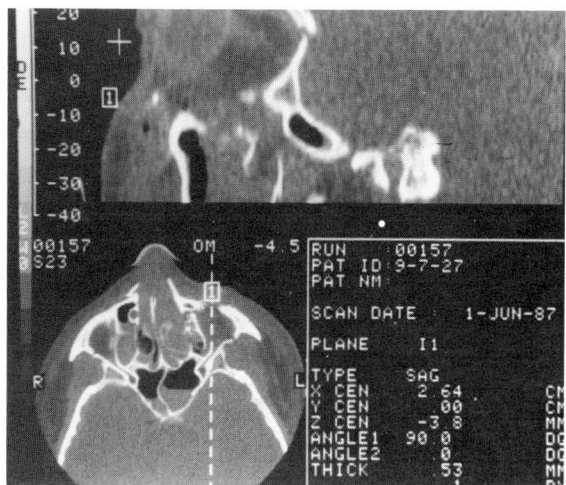

FIGURE 2-10. Reconstructed sagittal CT.

formed at an angle of 25° to 30° positive to Reid's line (Figure 2-11). Routine orbital CT, however, should be parallel to Reid's line, with the globes in neutral position (Figure 2-12). For optimal visualization of the optic nerve, an angle of −20° to −30°, with the globe in upward gaze, is sometimes used. The field of view of newer machines can be narrowed (targeted) to increase resolution. Orbital scans are usually targeted by a factor of 1.5 to 3, producing larger

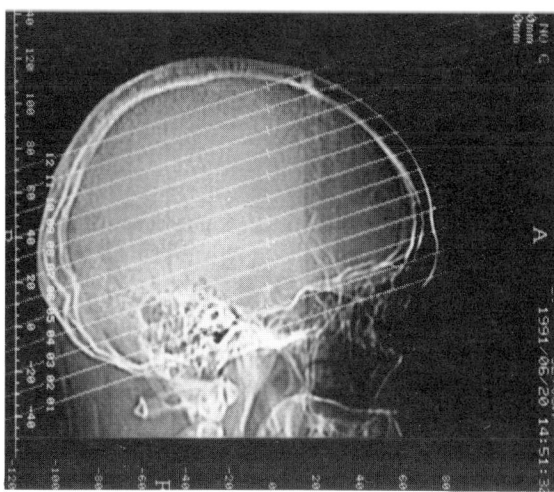

FIGURE 2-11. Sectioning performed at 25° to 30° positive to Reid's (infraorbital-meatal line) used for routine axial CT scanning.

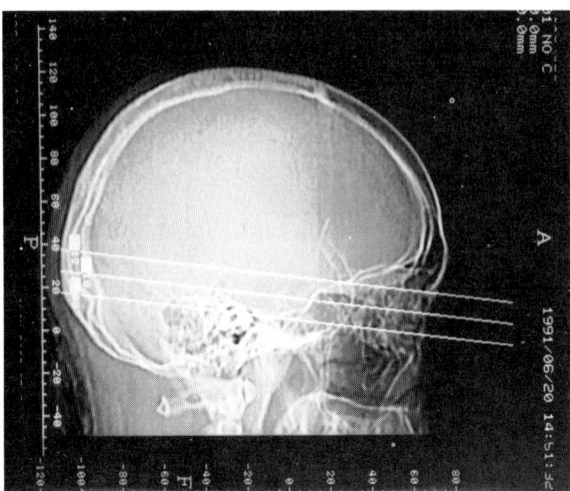

FIGURE 2-12. Sectioning parallel to Reid's line used for orbital CT scanning.

images whose quality is superior to those simply magnified. Slice thickness varies by machine from 1.5 mm to 5.0 mm. Thin 1.5 mm slices should be used when localizing foreign bodies or investigating the optic canal, optic nerve, or extraocular muscles. Coronal scans should be of the same thickness as axial scans. Direct coronal images provide much greater detail than reconstructed images. Direct sagittal scans are technically difficult to obtain but may be of use preoperatively in evaluating orbital floor fractures. Iodinated intravenous contrast is often useful but usually not mandatory (because of the inherent high-contrast structures of the orbit) in evaluating orbital masses or inflammatory processes. Its use is required, however, to visualize any intracranial extension of such processes. Nonenhanced scans are almost always sufficient in cases of orbital trauma, foreign body localization, thyroid ophthalmopathy, congenital lesions, or bony processes.

Magnetic resonance imaging (MRI) is based on the principle that atomic nuclei with odd numbers of protons or neutrons act as small magnets when placed in a strong magnetic field. Nuclear magnetic resonance is produced by polarizing these nuclei under a large static magnetic field and then subjecting them to a radiofrequency (RF) pulse emitted from a coil lying within the magnetic field. The RF pulse causes the polarized atoms to absorb energy, resonate, and realign themselves against the static magnetic field. When the RF pulse terminates, the excited nuclei flip back to their original alignment and relax to a state of equilibrium. This relaxation is accompanied by a release of electromagnetic energy, which is detected as the MR signal by a receiving coil oriented perpendicular to the strong magnetic field axis. The use of a surface coil allows for a gain in the signal-to-noise ratio (SNR). This greatly improves image quality, resulting in the ability to visualize lesions as small as 0.4 mm × 0.4 mm × 3 mm. Surface coil images are usually obtained by using the body coil as the excitation coil and the surface coil as the receiver. The superficial location of the eye and orbit is ideally suited for this technology.

Several MRI parameters are used to produce an image. Relaxation times are based on the time required for excited atoms to become realigned with the static magnetic field, after termination of the RF pulse. Two relaxation times are described. The T_1 (longitudinal or spin lattice) time measures the time required for the bulk of excited atoms to realign along the original axis. T_1 is a function of the interactions of excited nuclei with other nuclei in the environment. Tissues with a high water content have longer T_1 values than fatty tissues. The T_2 (transverse spin-spin) time is the mean relaxation time based on interactions between excited proton spins and is a measure of the effect excited nuclei have on each other. The *proton density* is a measure of the number of protons per unit volume of tissue. Relaxation times and proton density are the principal determinants of relative image contrast. By varying the echo (TE) and repetition (TR) times of the radiofrequency pulses, scans can be tailored to image primarily the T_1 or T_2 relaxation time or the proton density. Such scans are usually referred to as T_1 weighted (TR $\leq$ 600 msec; TE 20–60 msec), T_2 weighted (longer TR and TE sequences), or proton density (long TR and short TE sequences) scans. The terms *saturation recovery, inversion recovery, spin echo,* and *gradient echo* describe various algorithms that can be applied to the RF pulse to produce a T_1- or T_2-weighted image. Numerous algorithms are being developed to alter the RF pulse sequence in ways that will reduce imaging time and increase accuracy.

The signal intensity produced by different tissues depends on whether T_1 or T_2 weighting is used. Fat, white matter and melanotic melanomas are relatively bright on T_1 scans (Figure 2–13) but dark on T_2 scans (Figure 2–14). The opposite occurs for cerebrospinal fluid, the vitreous, edema, abscesses, demyelination, and most other tumors. Air, cortical bone, and calcium give no MR signal. T_1 scans can be easily distinguished from T_2 scans by looking at the vitreous. If the vitreous is hypointense, the scan is T_1 weighted. For most ocular and orbital imaging, T_1-weighted images provide the most contrast and detail.

Several contrast agents are under investigation for use in MRI. Each preferentially reduces the relaxation time of one tissue relative to another, thereby accentuating tissue differentiation. The only agent approved for use in the United States is gadolinium-diethylene triamine pentacetic acid (Gd-DTPA). Gd-DTPA contrast produces a hyperintense signal on a T_1-weighted scan in areas where the blood-brain barrier has broken down. It is also useful in the diagnosis of intraorbital gliomas, hemangiomas, metastases, and meningiomas. The last, in particular, enhance brightly with Gd-DTPA. Such enhancement is even better visualized with fat-suppression scan techniques, which diminish the very hyperintense fat signal (Figure 12–15).

58 I—Examination, Diagnostic Tests, and Pediatric Patients

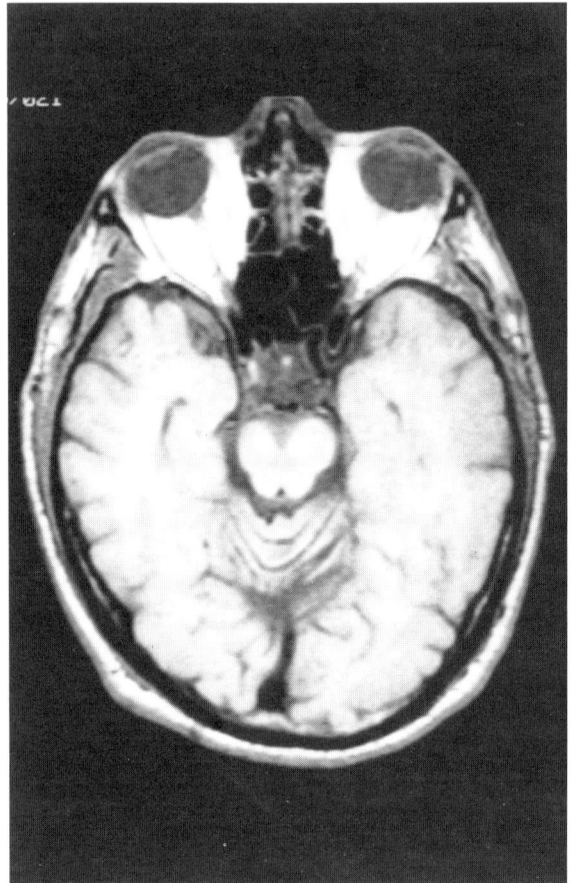

FIGURE 2-13. T_1-weighted MRI scan.

OTHER IMAGING TECHNIQUES

Cerebral angiography involves injecting contrast material intra-arterially and recording vascular images with either plain film radiography or digital techniques. Digital subtraction angiography (DSA) subtracts bone structures, enhancing the image produced by intravascular contrast (Figure 2-16). DSA is generally faster than plain film angiography and utilizes a lower concentration of contrast. Plain film angiography, however, produces the highest resolution images and remains the gold standard in cerebrovascular imaging. Digital techniques can also be used with intravenously administered contrast (intravenous DSA), but large amounts of contrast are needed, and the image quality is often

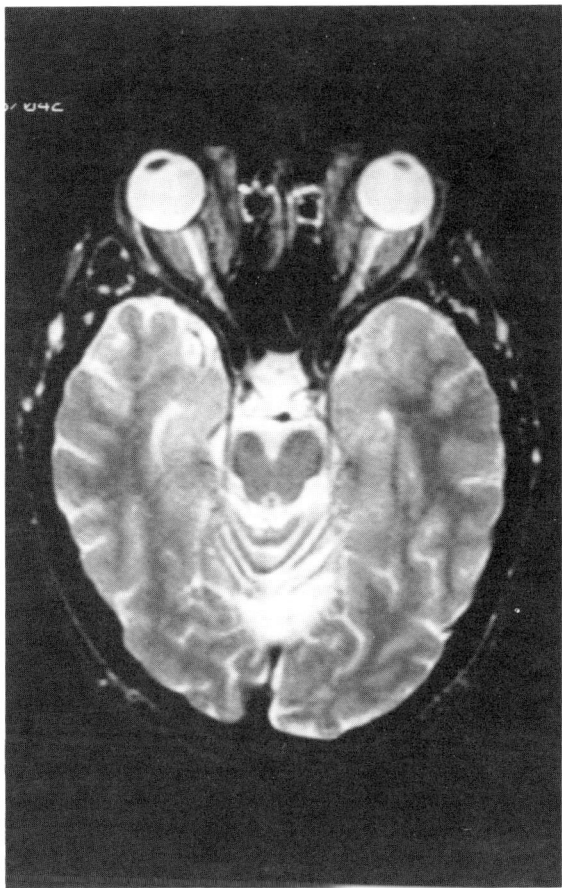

FIGURE 2–14. T_2-weighted MRI scan.

poor. Selective intra-arterial angiography is always preferred for diagnostic accuracy but carries the risk of vascular accident or embolic event (approximately 1/500).

Cerebral angiography is used to visualize aneurysms, arteriovenous malformations, and the vasculature of intracranial tumors. In conjunction with arteriography, balloon or embolization techniques can be used to occlude aneurysms and carotid-cavenous sinus fistulas or decrease the blood supply of intracranial tumors prior to their surgical removal. Embolization materials include steel springs, silastic microspheres, gelatin sponges, polyvinyl alcohol, and n-butyl-cyanoacrylate (NBCA).

Magnetic resonance angiography (MRA) is a rapidly developing technique that shows great potential for completely noninvasive vascular imaging. Cur-

60   I—Examination, Diagnostic Tests, and Pediatric Patients

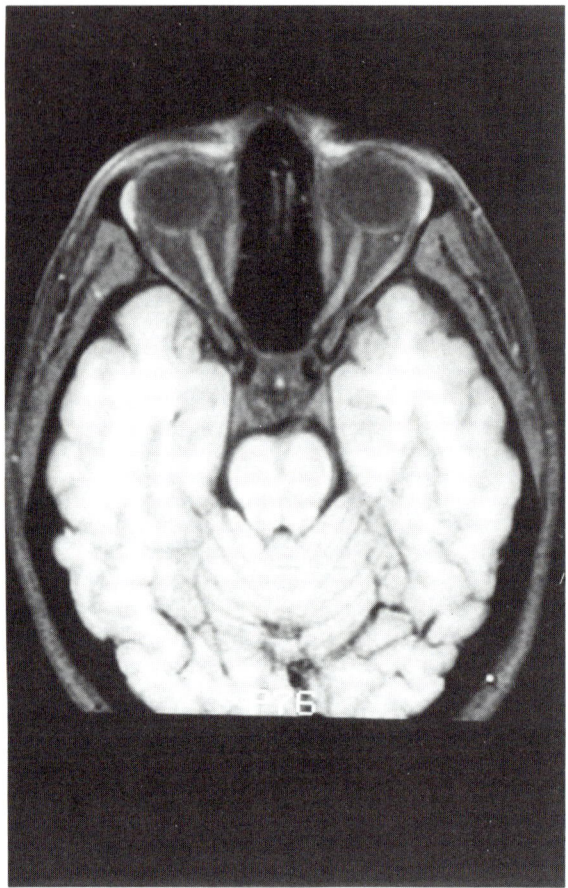

FIGURE 2-15. Fat-suppression MRI demonstrating the intracanalicular portion of the optic nerve.

rently its relatively poor resolution severely limits its role in evaluating orbital pathology.

In *orbital venography,* contrast material is injected into a superficial orbital vein (usually a forehead vein), and blood flow is evaluated through the superior ophthalmic vein using plain film radiography. Although useful in evaluating cavernous sinus or orbital venous thrombosis, this technique has been largely replaced by CT and MRI.

Dacryocystography is performed by injecting an oil-based, iodinated, viscous substance into the lacrimal drainage system. The anatomy and patency of the lacrimal drainage system are recorded using plain film radiography (with or without digital subtraction techniques; see Figure 9–10). Dacryoliths (lacri-

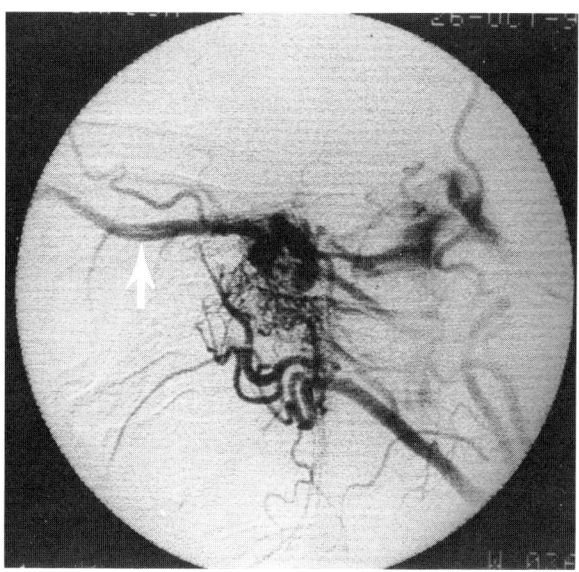

FIGURE 2-16. Intra-arterial digital subtraction angiography, demonstrating a dural and orbital arteriovenous malformation. Note the dilated superior ophthalmic vein (arrow).

mal "stones") and lacrimal masses are well demonstrated. Similar to venography, CT and MRI have eliminated most of the indications for this procedure.

Fluorescein angiography (FA) is based on the principle that sodium fluorescein, excited to a higher energy state by light energy of between 465 nm and 490 nm, will spontaneously decay to a lower state by emitting light energy of between 520 nm and 530 nm. This reaction can be visualized and photographed as fluorescein travels through the vasculature of the eye. Blue filtered light is used to excite the molecule, and a green filter, placed in front of a film carrier, transmits emitted light to photographic film. Typically, 5 mL of 10% sodium fluorescein is injected into the antecubital vein, and photography is begun when the fluorescein reaches the retinal arteries (about 10 seconds after injection). Using black and white film, fluorescent activity is recorded as a bright white image (Figure 2-17).

Fluorescein angiography is useful in detecting abnormal vascular permeability in the eye, particularly when evaluating diabetic retinopathy and syndromes associated with the development of neovascular membranes between the choroid and retina. In the acute setting, fluorescein angiography is used when the history and physical findings suggest a treatable cause of sudden loss of vision, such as an exudative maculopathy emanating from a subretinal membrane that spares the foveal avascular zone (see Chapter 14).

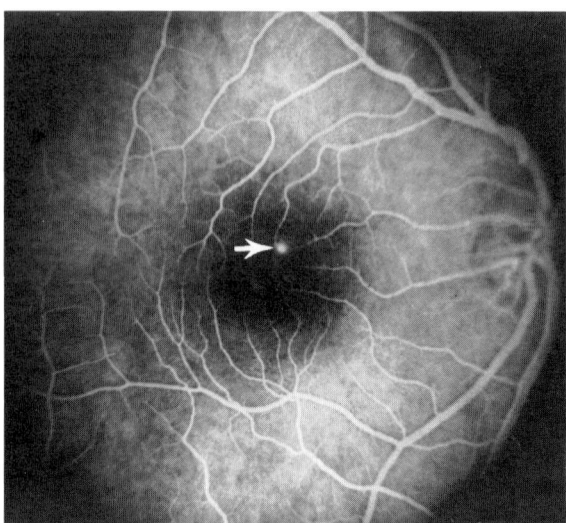

FIGURE 2-17. Fluorescein angiogram demonstrating pinpoint leakage of fluid from a break in Bruch's membrane (arrow).

ADVANTAGES AND DISADVANTAGES OF DIFFERENT IMAGING TECHNIQUES

The proper selection of imaging studies is always important, and it is especially so in the acute setting. Table 2-2 lists the advantages of the common imaging techniques, and Table 2-3 notes their limitations.

It is particularly useful to know when CT is preferable to MRI, and vice versa. Although any recommendation is likely to change in this rapidly evolving field, a few suggestions appear unchanging. When bony detail is necessary, CT is decidedly more appropriate. Orbital and facial fractures, bony erosions, and hyperostosis from tumors are more clearly demonstrated by CT. MRI allows better visualization of most intracranial abnormalities, especially those involving the brain stem or posterior fossa, and demonstrates demyelination in multiple sclerosis. In general, CT is the method of choice for most orbital studies because of its speed, convenience, availability, and high spatial resolution. Orbital MRI is limited by slightly lower spatial resolution and much more motion-related artifact. Fat-suppression techniques, surface coils, and fast scan methods may change this recommendation. MRI may localize nonmetallic foreign bodies better than CT, and the use of contrast agents such as Gd-DTPA may render MRI preferable to CT in evaluating meningiomas, hypervascular lesions, and metastatic disease. Table 2-4 summarizes the preferred imaging modality by location and disorder.

SUGGESTED STUDIES BY OCULAR, ORBITAL, OR VISUAL DISORDER

Ocular and Orbital Trauma

Depending on the integrity of the globe, *ocular trauma* is best evaluated with ultrasound or CT. Ultrasound demonstrates the status of intraocular structures and the presence of intraocular hemorrhage or foreign bodies, although it cannot be used preoperatively for severely lacerated eyes. CT may demonstrate abnormalities in the integrity of the eye (Figure 2–18), orbital emphysema (Figure 2–19), and the location of foreign bodies (see Figure 8–8).

Plain film radiography is useful in screening patients with ocular trauma for *orbital or facial fractures*. The Waters view is particularly useful in demonstrating orbital floor and zygomatic fractures (see Figure 5–10). The "teardrop sign" refers to the radiographic appearance of orbital tissue that has prolapsed into the maxillary sinus. Additional signs include an air fluid level from accompanying hemorrhage, complete opacification of the maxillary sinus, and orbital emphysema. The Caldwell view is useful in evaluating fractures of the medial orbital wall, superior and lateral orbital rim, and frontal sinuses. Ethmoid fractures can sometimes be visualized on this projection, but usually the contiguity of multiple overlying structures impedes their assessment. The lateral projection is useful in assessing orbital roof fractures, fractures involving the sphenoid and frontal sinuses, and the status of the pterygoid plates in LeFort fractures. The submentovertex view is useful in evaluating zygomatic arch (e.g., tripod) fractures. All of the plain film projections require particular positioning of the patient, which may not be possible if cervical or cranial trauma is associated. Of even greater importance is the soft tissue detail afforded by CT. For these reasons, CT is generally suggested in orbital and facial trauma, particularly prior to any surgical repair (see also Chapter 5).

The failure to diagnose a *retained foreign body* accounts for a substantial number of trauma-related malpractice suits. Foreign bodies are not uncommon with even minor facial lacerations or soft tissue injuries; additionally, foreign bodies can perforate the globe without significant pain, and entrance wounds that are small and through the sclera may not be readily apparent. For these reasons and because the majority of foreign bodies are radiopaque, plain film radiography is commonly used to screen for foreign bodies if the history is suggestive. The majority of lawsuits arise when foreign bodies cannot be ruled out with certainty by plain film radiography and a second diagnostic modality is not used (ARGUS, April 1991, p. 16). For this reason, ultrasound or CT should be performed if there is uncertainty. It should also be remembered that streak artifacts on CT may obscure the presence of multiple foreign bodies. A confirmatory CT or ultrasound should be performed after the removal of a magnetic foreign body to rule out additional foreign bodies that were obscured by artifacts on the original scan. Wooden and certain plastic foreign bodies may

Text continues on page 67

TABLE 2-2. ADVANTAGES OF DIFFERENT IMAGING TECHNIQUES

TECHNIQUE	ADVANTAGES
Ultrasound	Ideal for imaging ocular disorders, including: traumatic ocular injuries, ocular tumors, retinal or choroidal detachments, and intraocular foreign bodies
Plain film radiography	Best technique to demonstrate the shape and number of foreign bodies Less expensive than CT or MRI Detects most orbital wall and facial fractures
Computed tomography	Better definition of bone, orbital fractures, and metastatic disease to the bony orbit than MRI The spatial relationship of a foreign body to the globe can be demonstrated well Metallic foreign bodies less than 1 mm in size (except aluminum) can be detected The exact extent of orbital wall fractures and incarceration of tissue can be visualized Thinner sections than MRI possible Scanning times are shorter, resulting in less motion artifact (an individual scan requires less than 5 seconds)
Magnetic resonance imaging	Direct scanning in multiple anatomic planes (axial, coronal, sagittal, and oblique) is possible without repositioning the patient Has greater sensitivity to tissue contrast than CT Changes in normal anatomic patterns, nonmagnetic foreign bodies, and demyelination are better visualized No ionizing radiation is used Excellent for postoperative evaluation of globes in which silicone or perfluorocarbon was injected Ideal for imaging the optic canal, optic chiasm, and relative location of perichiasmal tumors Better characterization of hemorrhages and ocular melanomas than CT Vascular lesions with flowing blood are void of any MR signal allowing for their easy detection Newer techniques can separate venous from arterial lesions Superficial location of the eye allows the use of surface coils, improving image quality
Cerebral angiography	Useful in visualizing aneurysms, arteriovenous malformations, and the vasculature of intracranial tumors

TABLE 2-3. LIMITATIONS OF DIFFERENT IMAGING TECHNIQUES

TECHNIQUE	LIMITATIONS
Ultrasound	An immersion technique is necessary to visualize the anterior chamber and lens Injected silicone or perfluorocarbon greatly distorts B-scan image
Plain film radiography	The relationship of foreign bodies to the globe is poorly delineated; without special techniques, it cannot be determined if a foreign body is within the eye or how near it is to the globe The juxtaposition of multiple overlying structures prevents the easy determination of muscle entrapment in medial wall fractures
Computed tomography	Direct coronal CT scanning is possible but requires complex positioning, which may not be advisable in traumatized patients Direct sagittal CT scanning is difficult to perform An object with a very high attenuation coefficient and volume can cause streaks and Hounsfield artifacts, resulting in localization artifacts Confirmatory scanning is necessary after the removal of a foreign body because artifacts on the original scan from large foreign bodies can obscure smaller foreign bodies Radiation of 2 rads to 3 rads in typical orbital scan
Magnetic resonance imaging	Cannot be used if there is suspicion of a metallic foreign body Cannot be used in patients with cardiac pacemakers or magnetizable aneurysmal clips Makeup containing iron oxide pigment obscures images Soft tissue changes in the orbit, including injuries to the extraocular muscles and optic nerve, can be obscured by the high-intensity signal from fat Chemical shift artifacts obscure details at fat-water interfaces Does not readily demonstrate orbital fractures, calcifications, or metastatic disease to the bony orbit Minimum required time to complete scanning is usually 10 minutes to 30 minutes, and image quality is degraded by motion artifacts. This is particularly a problem in the orbit due to ocular movement. More rapid scanning techniques are being devised. Claustrophobia can interfere with completion of a study
Cerebral angiography	Risk of vascular accident or embolic event, as well as local complications (hematoma, arterial thrombosis)

TABLE 2-4. PREFERRED IMAGING MODALITIES

LOCATION/DISORDER	PREFERRED MODALITY
Eye	
Leukocoria	Ultrasound > CT > MRI
Congenital anomaly	Ultrasound > CT > MRI
Retinal detachment	Ultrasound > CT > MRI
Foreign body	Ultrasound > CT > Plain film
Melanoma	Ultrasound > MRI
Optic nerve	
Glioma	MRI > CT > Ultrasound > Tomography
Meningioma	Gd-DTPA MRI ≥ CT
Orbit	
Orbital walls	CT > plain film
Soft tissue	Surface coil MRI > CT
Inflammation	CT > MRI
Cavernous sinus/optic chiasm/parasellar	MRI > CT cisternography
Brain stem/posterior fossa	MRI > CT
Intracerebral	
Tumors	MRI > CT
Infarction	MRI > CT
Hemorrhage	CT > MRI
Demyelination	MRI > CT

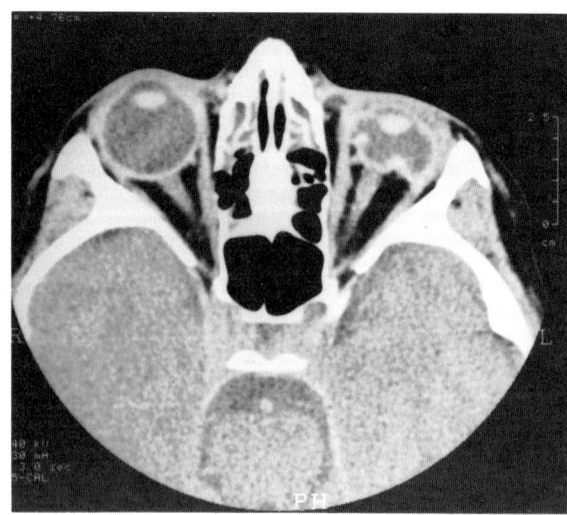

FIGURE 2-18. CT demonstrating ruptured left globe with loss of intraocular contents.

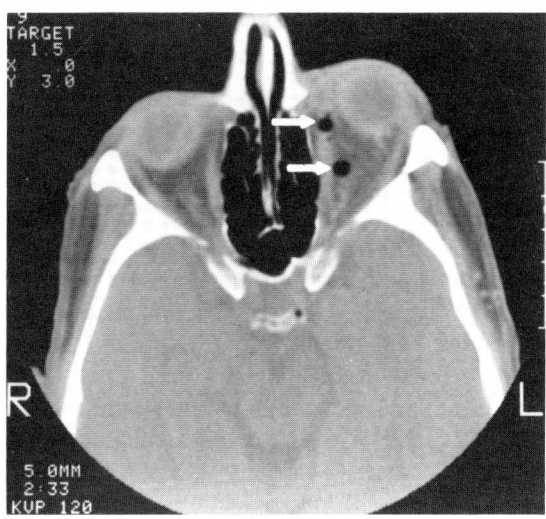

FIGURE 2-19. CT demonstrating intraorbital air (orbital emphysema) following trauma to the left orbit (arrows).

be entirely radiolucent. If the history suggests these possibilities, MRI should be performed.

Plain film radiography is the best technique to visualize the shape and number of metallic foreign bodies (Figures 2-5 and 8-10), but it does not clearly demonstrate the relationship of the foreign body to the globe. CT and MRI are vastly superior in this capability (see Chapter 8).

Ocular Tumors

Malignant melanoma is the most common intraocular tumor in adults, and retinoblastoma is the most common in children. Multiple modalities are used to distinguish these from less common ocular tumors.

Ophthalmoscopy, fluorescein angiography, ultrasound, and neuroimaging techniques are used to diagnose uveal melanomas. FA demonstrates fluorescence of deep intralesional vessels during the arteriovenous stage and staining of the tumor mass in the late stages. FA is particularly useful in differentiating melanomas from subretinal hemorrhages. Tumor findings on A-scan ultrasonography include a high-amplitude initial echo, low internal reflectivity, and spontaneous vascular pulsations (Figure 2-1). The highly reflective anterior border is also prominent on B-scan ultrasound. Additional B-scan findings include acoustic hollowness, choroidal excavation, and orbital shadowing. Metastatic carcinomas usually appear solid, without choroidal excavation by ultrasound. On CT, melanomas appear as hyperdense, sharply marginated masses that enhance slightly. Despite these characteristics, misdiagnoses still occur. The misdiagnosis of a choroidal nevus (but not a hemorrhagic lesion) for a melanoma may be lessened by the property of melanomas to shorten both T_1 and T_2 MRI relaxation times. Because of this relative shortening of relaxation times, malignant melanomas appear hyperintense on T_1 and proton-weighted images and hypointense on T_2-weighted images. Hemorrhagic lesion can act similarly. A recent study demonstrated that choroidal nevi are not visualized with MRI; hemangiomas appear hypointense on T_1 and hyperintense on T_2-weighted images, and metastases appear hyperintense on both T_1 and T_2 scans (Peyman and Mafee, 1987). Neither FA nor ultrasound depicts tumors involving the ciliary body well, but ultrasound may be superior to MRI for posterior lesions less than 3 mm in thickness.

Retinoblastoma is difficult to evaluate by ultrasound because its density is similar to clotted blood in the vitreous. A round, solid, retinal mass in an infant is suggestive of retinoblastoma, especially when it contains scattered high-amplitude spikes, consistent with calcification. Plain film radiography and CT (Figure 2–20) can also reveal calcification; over 90% of tumors show calcification on CT scans (Char, 1984). Because of the poorly developed vasculature of most retinoblastomas, these tumors enhance only slightly to moderately, in contrast to persistent hyperplastic primary vitreous (PHPV), which enhances markedly (especially centrally, in the region of Cloquet's canal). The mass in toxocariasis does not generally enhance, but the adjacent uveal-scleral coat does enhance slightly and is diffusely or locally thickened. On MRI, most retinoblastomas have a similar behavior as melanomas, and paramagnetic contrast agents may allow even better differentiation. MRI is also helpful in differ-

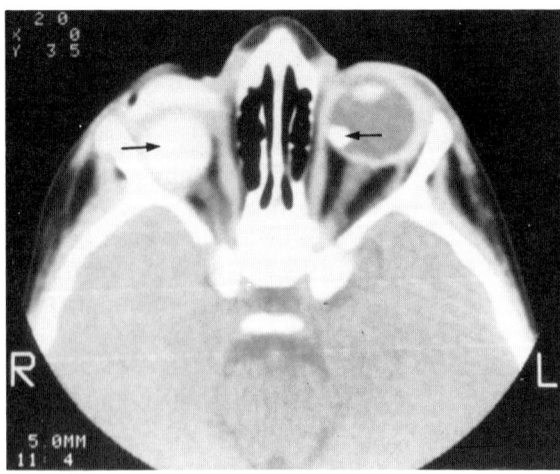

FIGURE 2–20. CT demonstrating calcification in retinoblastoma (arrows).

entiating retinoblastoma from Coats' disease. In Coats' the subretinal exudate is hyperintense on both T_1 and T_2 images.

Proton MRI is becoming more widely used in the diagnosis of intraocular tumors, especially when it is performed with surface coils. Investigational MRI techniques that show promise for differentiating intraocular tumors from benign conditions include sodium-23 and phosphorus-31 MR spectroscopy.

Other Choroidal and Retinal Disorders

Choroidal and retinal detachments can be differentiated by ultrasound or neuroimaging techniques. With B-scan ultrasound, CT, and MRI, retinal detachments are depicted as V shaped, with the leaves of the detachment anchored to the optic disc. In contrast, choroidal detachments usually do not reach the optic disc because the short posterior ciliary arteries anchor the choroid anterior to the optic nerve (Figures 2–2 and 2–21). A-scan ultrasound reveals one or two high echo spikes from the surface of a detachment followed by a sonolucent area. The difference in intensity between subretinal fluid and the vitreous is an additional CT and MRI finding.

Hemorrhagic collections vary in intensity on MRI, depending on the state of hemoglobin. Acute choroidal hematomas and vitreous hemorrhage appear hypointense on both T_1- and T_2-weighted images (Figure 2–22), whereas chronic (beyond 9 days to 14 days) hematomas appear hyperintense on both images. Choroidal hemangiomas are best recognized by their bright enhance-

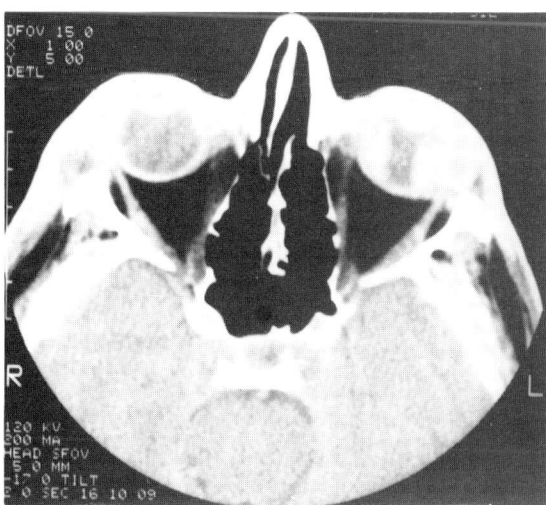

FIGURE 2–21. CT demonstrating choroidal detachments in the left eye.

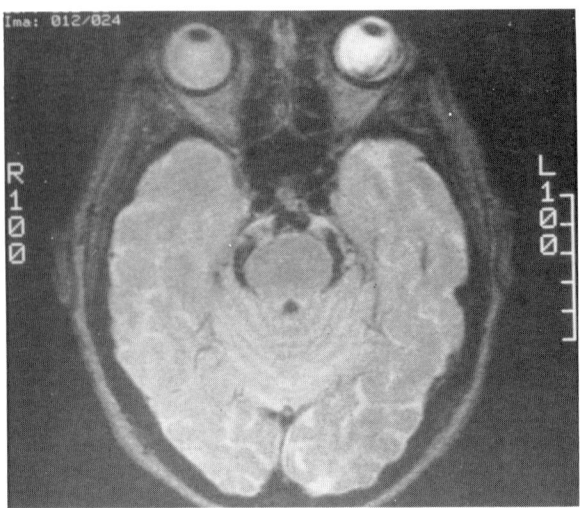

FIGURE 2-22. T$_2$-weighted image demonstrating a vitreous hemorrhage in the left eye.

ment on contrast-enhanced CT. Inflammatory diseases of the choroid or sclera (uveitis, scleritis) demonstrate diffuse thickening and enhancement on CT. This diffuse involvement is suggestive against a neoplastic lesion. The presence and size of ocular colobomas, staphylomas, microophthalmos with cyst, and morning glory optic nerve anomaly can also be assessed by CT or MRI (Figure 2–23).

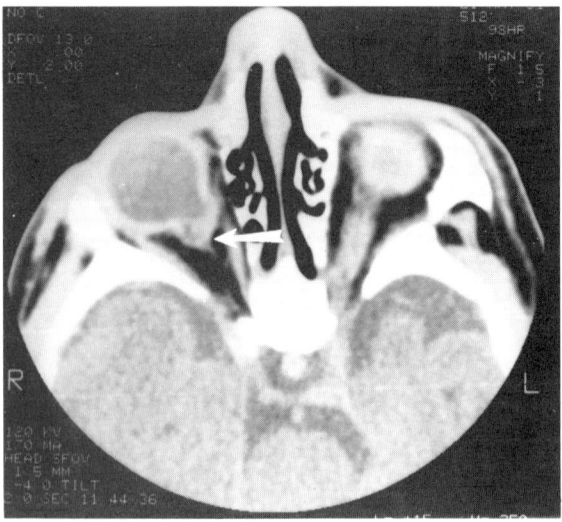

FIGURE 2-23. Congenital coloboma with cyst in the right eye of an infant (arrow). The plane is not true axial; the inferior globe and inferior rectus muscle is seen in the left orbit.

Optic Nerve and Sheath Disorders

Prior to the advent of CT and MRI, diagnostic evaluation of the optic nerve was limited to information attainable by ultrasonography or plain film tomography. By ultrasound, the optic nerve appears as an acoustically hollow space, bounded on both sides by a single walled outline. Inflammatory edema separates the meningeal sheaths and creates a doubling of this outline. This can be seen with optic neuritis, papilledema, and other causes of orbital inflammation or congestion (pseudotumor, thyroid orbitopathy). With optic nerve gliomas, the homogeneity of the optic nerve increases, further lowering its acoustic reflectivity. Plain film tomography, or Rhese (oblique) views, can demonstrate the size of the optic foramina. A diameter greater than 6.5 mm and asymmetry of more than 1 mm is consistent with optic nerve glioma (see Figure 12–11). The lateral projection may also demonstrate erosion of the chiasmatic sulus (J-shaped sella).

CT evaluation of the optic nerve involves multiplanar views and contrast enhancement. MRI has the advantage of being able to scan sagittally directly along the long axis of the orbit to illustrate the intracanalicular portion of the nerve (Figure 2–15). Flat, calcified meningiomas are better appreciated by CT than with noncontrast MRI, but the detection of calcification is often not crucial, and MRI better demonstrates any intracranial extension of tumor. A characteristic, but not pathognomonic, sign of meningioma is the presence of a central lucent line in a widened optic nerve (tram track sign; Figure 2–24). This finding has also been reported with optic neuritis and pseudotumor. Sclerotic changes at the orbital apex are an indication of intracranial extension of the meningioma.

MRI is clearly the study of choice for optic nerve gliomas. A characteristic

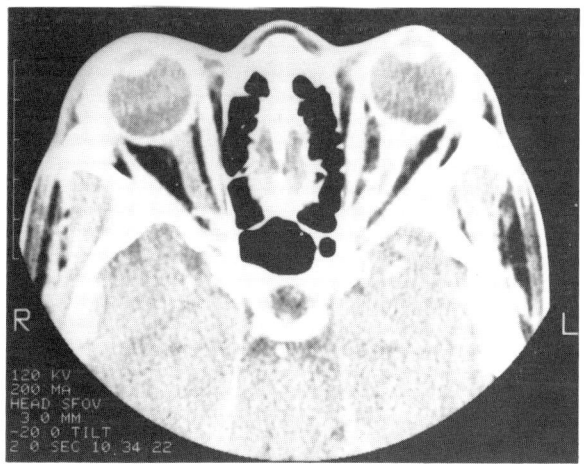

FIGURE 2–24. CT demonstrating meningioma of the left optic nerve.

feature is downward kinking of the elongated nerve. These tumors are hypointense relative to the white matter on T_1-weighted images; those associated with arachnoidal hyperplasia can be delineated further by the hyperintensity of the arachnoid on long TR/TE images. Both gliomas and meningiomas mildly to moderately enhance on contrast CT and MRI. Slight enlargement and enhancement of the optic nerve is also seen in optic neuritis.

Optic nerve hypoplasia can be confirmed by sagittal and coronal T_1-weighted MRI imaging. Hypoplastic nerves appear thin and demonstrate signal attenuation compared to normal nerves. Acute optic neuritis and radiation-induced optic neuropathies can be diagnosed in some affected patients by Gd-DTPA contrast enhancement of the optic nerve.

Nontraumatic Orbital Disorders

Coleman, Lizzi, and Jack (1977) demonstrated that orbital masses could be differentiated based on their ultrasonographic transmission and boundary properties. The criteria they suggested are presented in Table 2–5.

Orbital rhabdomyosarcoma, neuroblastoma, leukemia, and histiocytosis X can cause bone destruction, which is visible on plain film radiography and CT. Neuroblastoma can often be differentiated from rhabdomyosarcoma by its relatively high CT attenuation values; it also rarely extends posterior to the orbital septum. Cavernous hemangiomas appear as well-demarcated, round or oval, homogeneous masses with smooth margins on CT and MRI. Because their intratumoral circulation may be slow, they enhance variably, as compared to capillary hemangiomas, which have a rapid blood flow and enhance brightly. Occasionally calcifications in cavernous hemangiomas can be seen on CT. Lymphangiomas appear as poorly demarcated, heterogeneous masses of increased density on CT; they are hyperintense on both T_1- and T_2-weighted MRI images. Lymphoid tumors tend to be localized to one area. They also mold to the globe and other structures without significantly displacing them (see Figure 12–24). There are no specific neuroradiologic signs differentiating

TABLE 2–5. ULTRASONIC DIFFERENTIATION OF ORBITAL MASSES

BOUNDARY	DENSITY	TRANSMISSION	POSSIBLE TUMORS
Round	Solid	Poor	Meningioma, glioma, neurofibroma
Round	Cystic	Good	Mucocele, dermoid, cavernous hemangioma
Irregular	Solid	Good	Angiomatous tumor (diffuse hemangioma, lymphangioma)
Irregular	Solid	Poor	Infiltrative tumor (lymphoma, metastatic carcinoma, pseudotumor)

(Adapted from: Coleman DJ, Dallow RL: *Orbital Ultrasonography.* In Tasman W, Jaeger EA: *Duane's Clinical Ophthalmology.* Philadelphia, J.B. Lippincott Company, 1976, figure 27–3.)

malignant from benign lymphoid tumors. Orbital metastases appear as poorly marginated masses with greater density than orbital fat or the optic nerve by CT but isodense to the extraocular muscles and vascular structures. They usually enhance mildly to moderately. Metastatic disease to the bony orbit will often show bone destruction on plain film radiography and CT.

Orbital inflammation includes thyroid ophthalmopathy, pseudotumor, and myositis. A characteristic finding of thyroid disease is widening of an extraocular muscle with sparing of its tendon. This can be visualized by ultrasound, CT, or MRI (see Figure 12-17). Potential compression of the optic nerve at the orbital apex is better demonstrated by MRI. Ultrasound can also demonstrate an increased volume of orbital fat, with mottled heterogeneity, in thyroid disease and cellulitis. Myositis and pseudotumors may have a similar ultrasonic appearance. Contrast enhancement of the sclera (ring sign) is characteristic of pseudotumor (see Figure 12-4).

Orbital cellulitis and abscesses cause diffuse inflammation and edema. Ultrasound in cellulitis demonstrates an increased volume in the orbital fat, which also has a diffusely mottled appearance. Acutely, an abscess appears as a focal area of mottling on ultrasound; with chronicity, it appears cystic and filled with moderate amplitude echos from inflammatory debris. CT can demonstrate the location and extent of disease in the orbit and paranasal sinuses. Preseptal cellulitis is characterized on CT by diffuse soft tissue swelling in the eyelid and conjunctiva, anterior to the orbital septum (Figure 2-25). Orbital cellulitis is recognized when the tissue posterior to the septum becomes involved (Figure 2-26). Intraorbital abscesses can also be well delineated; if

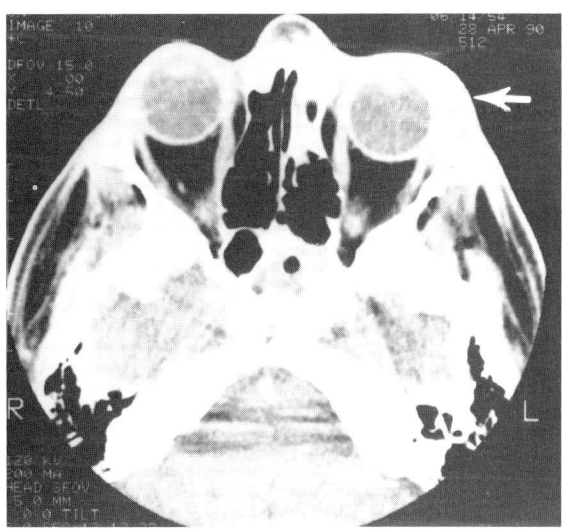

FIGURE 2-25. CT demonstrating preseptal cellulitis (arrow).

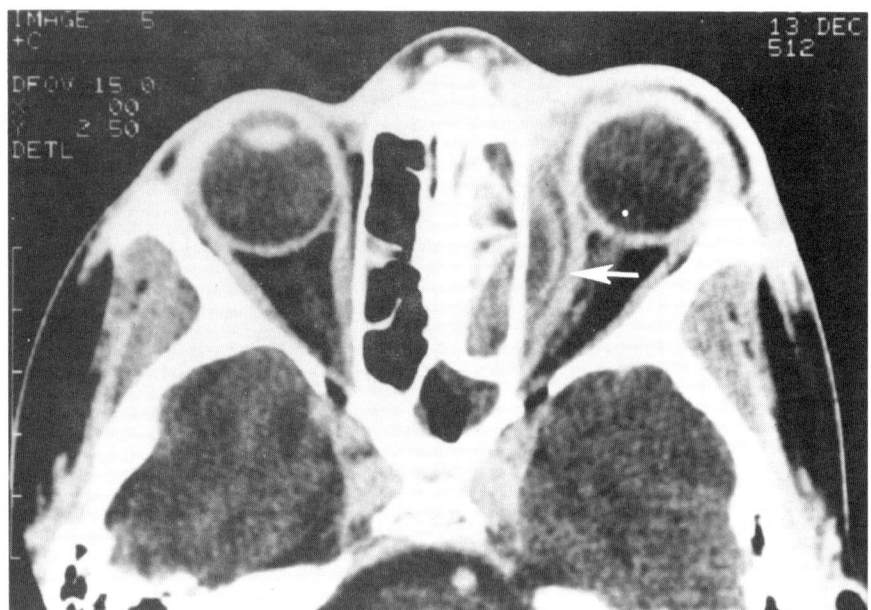

FIGURE 2–26. CT demonstrating orbital cellulitis involving the left orbit. Note the ethmoid sinusitis and inward bowing of the medial rectus muscle (arrow).

they occur adjacent to the globe, thickening of the scleral-uveal coat will be seen. The CT and MRI criteria for distinguishing a subperiosteal orbital abscess from reactive inflammatory edema, however, have not been well established (see Chapter 12).

Vascular malformations of the orbit are imaged by arteriography, CT, or MRI. Orbital arteriovenous malformations (AVMs), dural AVMs, and traumatic fistulas require selective external and internal carotid angiography for accurate evaluation. Orbital tumors can be suggested on carotid angiography by displacement and stretching of the ophthalmic and other arteries and the presence of a "tumor blush." Ultrasound is of limited value in evaluating vascular malformations, but the Doppler phenomenon may be of use in capillary hemangiomas and arteriovenous shunts.

Disorders of Ocular Motility

Restrictions of ocular motility can occur acutely with traumatic entrapment of the extraocular muscles in orbital wall fractures and semiacutely in thyroid eye disease, orbital pseudotumor and myositis, and orbital cellulitis (see above).

Disorders of the Sella Turcica, Cavernous Sinus, and Optic Chiasm

Suspected suprasellar and parasellar masses on enhanced CT scans can be further evaluated by contrast cisternography or MRI. To perform the former, 5 mL to 7 mL of nonionic, water-soluble contrast is injected into the lumbar subarachnoid space. The contrast is brought to the head under fluoroscopic control by tilting the table and flexing the patient's head. Axial and/or coronal CT is then performed within 30 minutes, through the area of interest. MRI is rapidly replacing positive contrast cisternography for these evaluations, except when it is contraindicated (e.g., previous metallic clipping of an aneurysm).

Pituitary microadenomas are usually hypodense and nonenhancing on CT. With MRI, they demonstrate prolonged T_1 and T_2 relaxation times. In contrast, macroadenomas usually enhance and may contain calcification. The CT findings of pituitary apoplexy (sudden expansion of the gland) depend on whether it is the result of hemorrhage or necrosis. With hemorrhage, increased density is seen within the mass; with necrosis, the attenuation decreases. Meningiomas in the parasellar region, like their counterparts in the orbit, are readily evaluated by CT, on which the tumor often has higher attenuation values than the surrounding brain (due to psammomatous calcification), or by MRI. Using either modality, homogeneous enhancement is the rule. Craniopharyngiomas demonstrate a combination of cystic, solid, and calcific components on CT. The solid portions and rim of the cystic portions enhance. Parasellar aneurysms should be considered when the CT demonstrates an enhancing lesion in this area with destruction of the lateral wall of the sella. Differentiation is possible with angiography and MRI. Gliomas of the optic chiasm are suspected when CT demonstrates enlargement of the chiasm and obliteration of the suprasellar cistern. These are better evaluated by MRI, on which they demonstrate high intensity.

Cavernous sinus thrombosis is evaluated with axial and coronal CT scanning following high-dose contrast infusion. The contrast-enhanced arteries stand out against the low attenuation of the thrombosed sinus. Dilation of the superior ophthalmic vein is another, albeit nonspecific, sign. On MRI, the thrombosed sinus appears enlarged and hyperintense compared to the normal cavernous sinus. Orbital venography is the gold standard for confirming this diagnosis but is rarely utilized.

Disorders of the Brain Stem and Posterior Fossa

CT of the brain stem is of limited use due to the induction of artifacts by surrounding bone. CT cisternography is superior to routine CT and pneumoencephalography, but MRI is clearly the modality of choice. MRI can detect foci of demyelination, tumors, lacunar infarctions, and traumatic changes. The Arnold-Chiari malformation, an important and often treatable cause of oculomotor disturbances, is much better appreciated on sagittal MRI than any other modality. Acoustic neuromas are now also routinely evaluated by MRI.

Intracerebral Disorders

Intracerebral tumors are most often identified on CT as mass lesions, with or without contrast enhancement or peritumoral edema. Hydrocephalus and distortion of the neuroaxis may be present, depending on the tumor's location. Astrocytomas are usually isodense to hypodense to normal brain tissue; more aggressive tumors (glioblastoma multiforme) demonstrate greater enhancement and peritumor edema. Meningiomas are usually hyperdense and may show calcification. Metastatic tumors may be multiple and occasionally contain intratumoral hemorrhage. They are generally hypodense unless they contain hemorrhage, and they nearly always enhance. MRI characterizes tumors better than CT, except when calcification or bone abnormalities are present. On long TR/TE images, both primary and metastatic neoplasms have a high signal intensity, except for hemorrhagic masses and melanoma. More aggressive tumors also demonstrate more irregular borders and greater disruption of the blood-brain barrier. The latter accounts for the increased signal intensity when Gd-DTPA contrast is used.

Nonhemorrhagic cerebral infarctions may demonstrate no change in density on CT during the most immediate 48-hour period. They start to become hypodense during the following 2 weeks and after this time are permanently hypodense (Figure 2–27). MRI can image edema within hours of a nonhemmor-

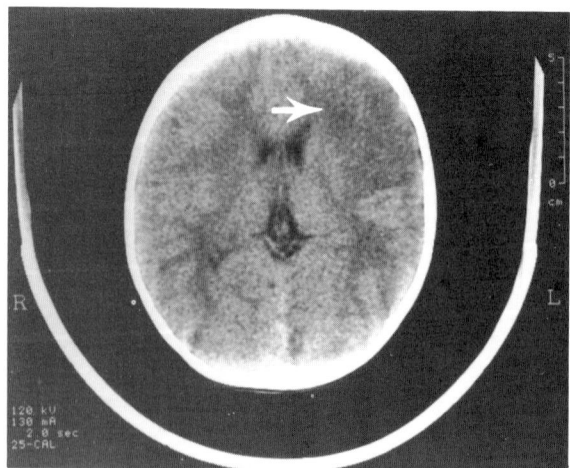

FIGURE 2–27. CT demonstrating cerebral infarction, 2 weeks after the event (arrow).

rhagic event. Hemorrhagic infarctions are immediately visible on CT as higher density areas (Figure 2-28). These decrease in density with time due to degradation and absorption of hemoglobin.

The initial CT scan in *whiplash (shaken) injuries in infants* may be normal or demonstrate only subtle abnormalities. Sequential scanning days to weeks later, however, may demonstrate intrahemispheric subdural hematomas (see Figure 3-10). Subsequent imaging studies may also demonstrate evidence of diffuse atrophy or hydrocephalus.

Multiple sclerosis plaques in the brain stem and cerebral cortex are best appreciated by MRI. On T_2-weighted and proton density scans, they appear bright; on T_1-weighted scans, they are darker than the surrounding tissue. They are present acutely and may resolve over time. Plaques are not usually seen in the optic nerve, even when acute optic neuritis is present.

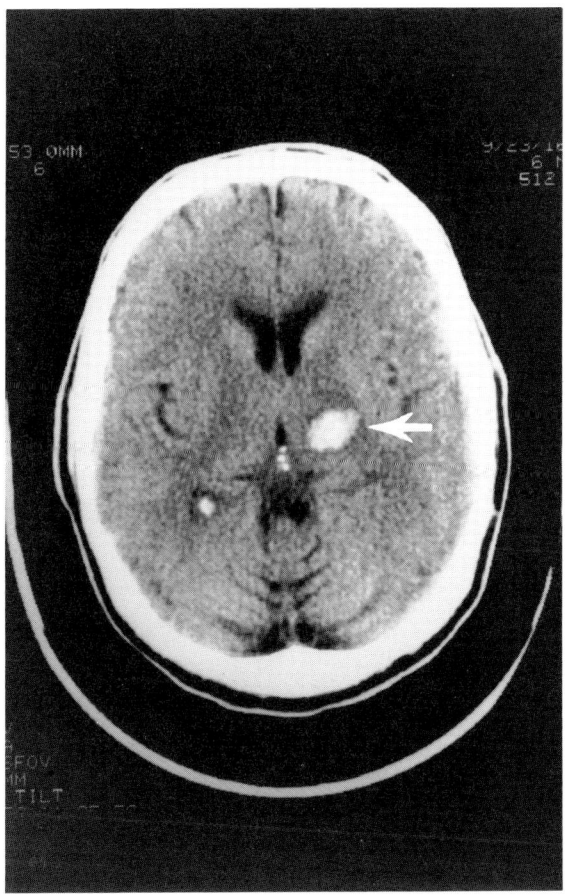

FIGURE 2-28. CT demonstrating acute left thalamic hemorrhage in a hypertensive individual (arrow).

Intracranial aneurysms, when large, may have a rim of mural calcification, which is detectable by CT. The lumen and wall also enhance on contrast infusion. CT and MRI can detect the presence of large thrombi, which may give a better indication of the true size of the aneurysm than angiography. Dynamic contrast CT and MRI also demonstrate rapidly flowing blood (an area of signal void on MRI). Cerebral angiography still demonstrates the neck of the aneurysm, its location, and the presence of smaller aneurysms better than CT or MRI. It remains the modality of choice prior to planning intervention.

Carotid-cavernous fistulas can be localized on angiography in most cases by vertebral artery injection with compression of the carotid ipsilateral to the fistula. Detachable balloon-occlusion techniques have been developed to treat these during angiography.

ASSOCIATED RISKS AND COSTS OF DIFFERENT NEUROIMAGING TECHNIQUES

The radiation hazards of an orbital CT, orbital series of skull X rays (four projections), and head CT are similar. Each gives approximately 2 rads to 3 rads. The dose to the eye per orbital CT is 1.2 rem (Grossman, 1991). This compares to the cataract threshold of 500 rem. The approximate costs of these and other current diagnostic modalities are given in Table 2–6.

Iodinated intravascular contrast agents are necessary or helpful for many imaging techniques. Patients with a known allergy can be premedicated with oral steroids if a contrast study is strongly indicated. Alternatively or addition-

TABLE 2–6. COST OF DIAGNOSTIC TESTS*

TEST	COST
Ultrasound A-scan	$ 225
Ultrasound B-scan	225
Orbital series (4 X rays)	230
Orbital CT	869
Orbital MRI	1334
Cerebral angiography	2188
Fluorescein angiography	175
Gram's stain	19
Giemsa stain	46
Blood agar culture	36
Sabouraud's culture	33
Chlamydia culture	35

*Effective July 1991 at a major academic health center in upstate New York.

ally, allergic reactions can be treated with oral or intravenous diphenhydramine (Benadryl) if mild, or subcutaneous or intravenous epinephrine if severe. Such patients should receive nonionic/low osmolality contrast agents, as these have been shown to have approximately a sixfold lower incidence of severe reactions.

Local and systemic complications of fluorescein angiography—gastrointestinal disturbances, anaphylaxis, respiratory or cardiac arrest, and death—have been well documented. Fluorescein angiography is contraindicated in the ipsilateral arm to a previous axillary lymph node dissection (e.g., radical mastectomy). In the presence of compromised lymphatic drainage, FA can result in a severe lymphangitis. A retrospective review has suggested that FA during pregnancy does not result in a high incidence of birth anomalies (Halperin, Olk, Soubrane, and Coscas, 1990), but the safety of it in pregnancy has not been incontrovertibly documented. FA should be considered only when the vision is threatened and treatment depends on the angiographic findings. Even then, the patient should be fully informed of the risks and benefits of the procedure.

LABORATORY STUDIES

Laboratory studies for external diseases of the eye include stains of smears and scrapings, and cultures. Obtaining these requires only minimal instrumentation, but proper technique should be followed (see Chapter 16).

Smears and scrapings are obtained to identify bacteria, fungi, and characteristics of the exudate. *Conjunctival* specimens are taken from the palpebral conjunctiva by scraping with a Kimura or Lindner platinum spatula (see Figure 16-13) or loop. The spatula should be sterilized over an alcohol lamp and allowed to cool prior to use. The lower conjunctival fornix is scraped several times in the same direction, taking care to avoid the lid margin and canthal areas, where saprophytic corynebacteria and staphylococci live. The exudate is evenly smeared on a glass slide and fixed by gently passing the slide over the flame several times or immersing it in absolute alcohol for 5 minutes. Material can also be expressed from the meibomian glands, lacrimal canaliculi, and lacrimal sac for staining and culture, and directly obtained from draining orbital abscesses.

Corneal scrapings are obtained under topical anesthesia (proparacaine hydrochloride 0.5%) from the base and edges of a corneal ulcer, using a Kimura spatula or the beveled tip of a 23-gauge needle. The workup of exogenous *endophthalmitis* requires anterior chamber and vitreous aspirates; endogenous (metastatic) endophthalmitis, however, can often be adequately evaluated using smears and cultures from blood and nonocular seeding sites.

The Gram's stain is the most frequently used microbiologic stain; Giemsa is the preferred cellular stain. Acid-fast and special fungal stains are also used based on clinical suspicions (Table 2-7). Gram's stain demonstrates bacteria

TABLE 2-7. MICROBIOLOGIC STAINS AND CULTURE MEDIA FOR INFECTIOUS AGENTS

AGENT	STAIN	CULTURE MEDIA
General bacteria	Gram's	Blood, general nutrient
Neisseria species	Gram's	Chocolate, Thayer-Matin
Anaerobes	Gram's	Thioglycolate
Hemophilus	Gram's	Blood, chocolate
Mycobacteria/nocardia	Ziehl-Neelson	Lowenstein-Jensen
Fungi	Giemsa (hyphae)	Sabouraud's
	Gram's (yeasts)	Brain-heart
	Periodic acid-Schiff (PAS) with Gridley modification	
	Gomori-methenamine-silver	
Viruses	Papanicolaou	Viral cultures
Chlamydia	Giemsa	McCoy cell
Acanthamoeba	Calcofluor white	Nonnutrient agar with *E. coli* overlay

and yeast well. Using this stain, bacteria can be differentiated based on their size, shape, and Gram's stain characteristic (gram-positive or negative) (Figure 2-29). The procedure for Gram's stain is reviewed in Table 2-8. The Giemsa stain demonstrates fungal hyphae, yeasts, and the intracytoplasmic inclusion bodies of chlamydial inclusion conjunctivitis (Figure 2-30). Giemsa is also the

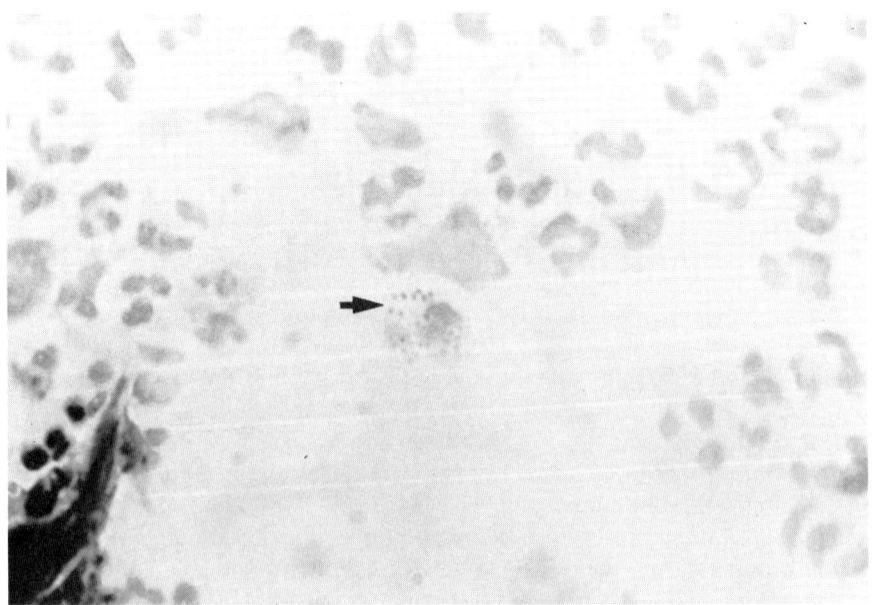

FIGURE 2-29. Gram-negative intracellular diplococci (gonococci) at arrow ($\times$ 1000).

TABLE 2-8. PROCEDURE FOR GRAM'S STAIN

1. Allow slide to air dry.
2. Fix slide by gently passing over alcohol lamp two or three times or (preferably) flooding with absolute methyl alcohol for 5 minutes.
3. Flood slide with gentian violet 2% for 30 seconds.
4. Rinse with water.
5. Flood slide with Gram's iodine solution; after 30 seconds, tip slide to drain (*do not* rinse residual iodine solution).
6. Tilt slide again, and pour 95% alcohol over the surface for 1 second to 2 seconds only, to decolorize the slide.
7. Rinse immediately with water.
8. Flood slide with safranin 1% for 30 seconds to counterstain the slide.
9. Rinse slide, blot dry, and examine under oil emersion.

stain of choice for cytologic studies of both normal and inflammatory cells (Figure 2-31). The procedure for the Giemsa stain is outlined in Table 2-9. Multiple special fungal stains have also been developed (Figure 2-32); of these the calcofluor white stain also demonstrates Acanthamoeba but requires a fluorescent microscope.

Microbiological culture media include chocolate, blood, brain-heart or beef-heart, and Sabouraud's agars and thioglycolate and general nutrient (PABA,

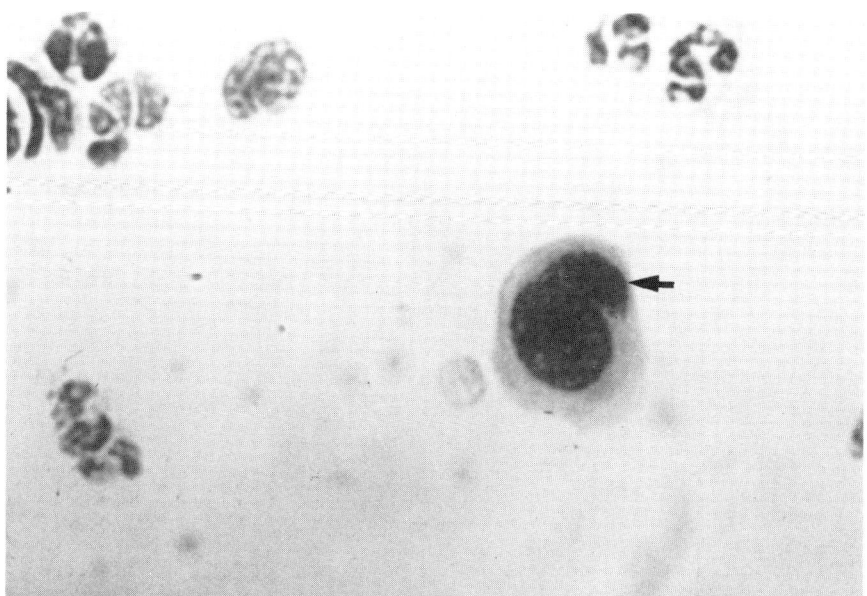

FIGURE 2-30. Giemsa stain of basophilic inclusion within the cytoplasm of an epithelial cell (arrow) in chlamydial inclusion conjunctivitis ($\times$ 1000).

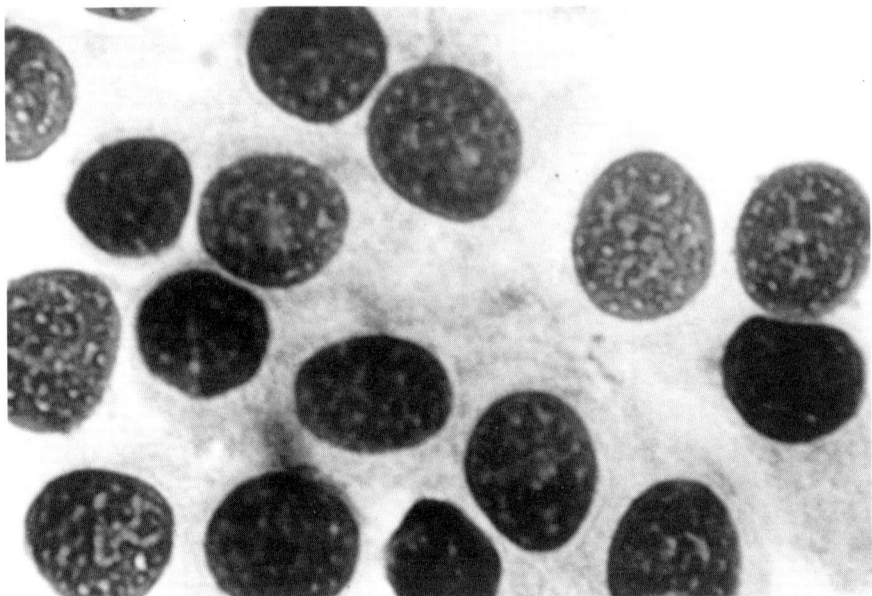

FIGURE 2–31. Giemsa stain of normal conjunctival epithelial cells ($\times$ 400).

trypticase soy) broths. Their use is reviewed in Table 2–7. Special chlamydial and viral cultures are also available. To obtain specimens for viral cultures, calcium alginate– or dacron-tipped swabs must be used. The specimen should be placed immediately in refrigerated transport media and taken to the laboratory within 24 hours for inoculation. The specimen should not be frozen, and the physician should note the specimen site and suspected pathogen.

A wide spectrum of antibodies, labeled with enzymes, fluorochromes, radioisotopes, and inert metals, is also available with activity against numerous microbial antigens. Enzyme and fluorescent labels are most commonly used because they are rapid and sensitive and provide a visual result. Enzyme-linked immunosorbent assay (ELISA) "sandwich" techniques have been developed for the rapid and relatively inexpensive detection of herpes virus (Herpchek, Dupont Diagnostics, Wilmington, Delaware), adenovirus (Adenoclone, Cam-

TABLE 2–9. PROCEDURE FOR GIEMSA STAIN

1. Immediately fix the slide by dipping in absolute methyl alcohol for 5 minutes (*not* by *flaming*). Do *not* air dry.
2. Prepare fresh Giemsa stain (mix 1 drop of stock Giemsa stain to 20 drops of a sterile buffer).
3. Place the slide in a Coplin jar filled with Giemsa stain and incubate at 37° for 1 hour.
4. Rinse slide twice with 95% ethyl alcohol.
5. Blot dry and examine under oil emersion.

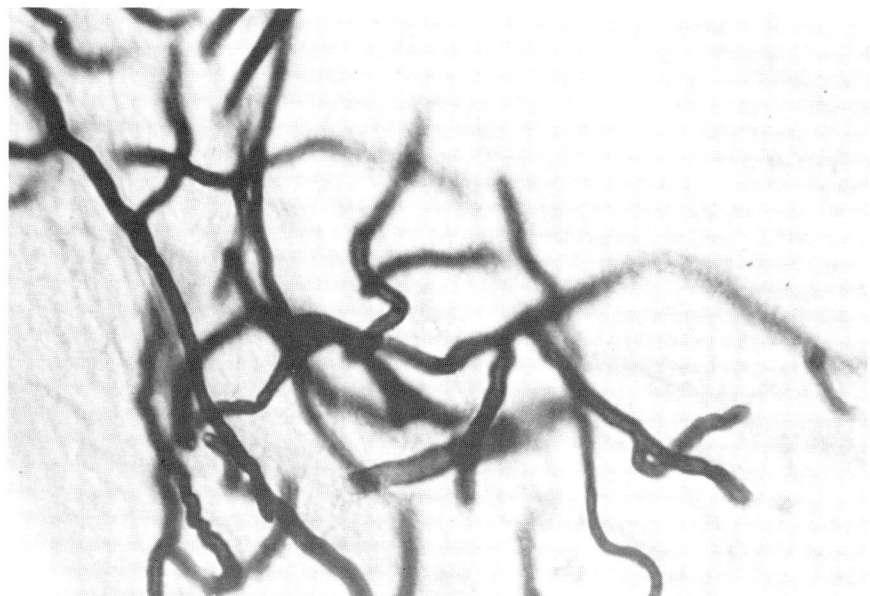

FIGURE 2-32. Gomori-methenamine-silver stain of *Fusarium solani*, a filamentous fungus with fine septa (× 1000).

bridge BioScience, Hopkinton, Massachusetts), and chlamydia (Chlamydiazyme, Abbott Laboratories, North Chicago, Illinois). Each of these tests appears highly sensitive and specific.

LABORATORY STUDIES IN UVEITIS

Several laboratory studies are useful in differentiating the etiology of uveitis, but their use is often misunderstood. A directed approach, dependent on historical and clinical findings, is suggested. Extensive laboratory testing is usually performed only for bilateral or severe recurrent uveitis.

The first step in the evaluation of uveitis is to obtain a uveitis history. It is important to understand whether the uveitis is acute, chronic, or recurrent and if it is unilateral or bilateral. The history should determine whether there are any associated systemic conditions, particularly arthritis, gastrointestinal disorders, dermatologic disorders, and venereal diseases. Finally, the personal history should detail the patient's sex, age, race, geographic background, illicit drug use, and association with pets. Table 2-10 lists the uveitic entities to consider based on historical information.

The second step is to establish the anatomic location of the primary inflammation. *Uveitis* is a general term referring to inflammation of the uvea (one of

TABLE 2-10. HISTORICAL ASSOCIATIONS OF UVEITIS

HISTORICAL INFORMATION	POTENTIAL UVEITIC ENTITIES
Age	
Childhood/youth (0–21 years)	Juvenile rheumatoid arthritis, toxocariasis, Pars planitis
Middle age (21–60 years)	Histoplasmosis, toxoplasmosis, pars planitis, Vogt-Koyanagi-Harada and Behcet's syndromes, acute multifocal posterior pigment epitheliopathy (AMMPE)
Elderly (over 60 years)	Masquerade syndrome, reticulum cell sarcoma, malignant melanoma, herpes zoster
Race	
Black	Sarcoidosis, sickle cell disease
Caucasian	Reiter's syndrome, ankylosing spondylitis
Oriental	Vogt-Koyanagi-Harada syndrome, Behcet's syndrome
Mediterranean	Behcet's syndrome
Sex	
Male	Ankylosing spondylitis, Reiter's syndrome, Behcet's syndrome, Eales's disease
Female	Juvenile rheumatoid arthritis, sarcoidosis
Geographic background	
Ohio, Mississippi valleys	Ocular histoplasmosis
Southeastern United States	Sarcoidosis
Mediterranean	Behcet's syndrome
Japan	Vogt-Koyanagi-Harada syndrome
San Joaquin Valley	Coccidioidomycosis
Pets	
Cat	Toxoplasmosis
Dog	Toxocariasis
Birds	Psittacosis
Personal history	
Drug abuse	Candida retinitis
Venereal disease	Syphilitic iritis or chorioretinitis
AIDS	Cytomegalovirus retinitis, toxoplasmosis, herpes zoster ophthalmicus, tuberculosis, candida retinitis, acute retinal necrosis, cryptococcus
Onset/course	
Insidious/chronic	Juvenile rheumatoid arthritis, candida and toxoplasmosis retinitis, pars planitis
Sudden (pain and injection)	Ankylosing spondylitis, Vogt-Koyanagi-Harada, Behcet's and Reiter's syndromes

(Modified from: Nozik RA: Laboratory testing in uveitis. *Focal points: Clinical Modules for Ophthalmologists.* San Francisco, American Academy of Ophthalmology, 1983, p 2, with permission.)

the three coats of the eye). More specific terms describe inflammation of the iris (iritis), ciliary body (cyclitis), iris and ciliary body (iridocyclitis), pars plana (pars planitis), and choroid (choroiditis). Additional terms describe inflammation in nonuveal ocular structures, including the retina (retinitis), vitreous (vitritis), the vasculature of the retina (vasculitis, periphlebitis), and the retinal pigment epithelium (epitheliitis).

Uveitis is associated with over 100 disease syndromes. Although a complete description of these is beyond the scope of this chapter, the workup for certain common entities, based on the patient's age and sex and the location of the primary inflammation, is presented in Table 2–11. Two disorders that should always be considered in the patient with uveitis (because they are common and can be specifically treated) are syphilis and tuberculosis. An FTA-ABS sero-

TABLE 2–11. SUGGESTED UVEITIS WORKUP

Age	PATIENT Sex	Race	PRIMARY SITE	POTENTIAL DISORDER	SUGGESTED TESTS
Child	M/F	B/W	Iridocyclitis	Syphilis	FTA-ABS, VDRL
	M/F	B/W		Tuberculosis	PPD, chest X ray, ESR
	F	B/W		Juvenile rheumatoid arthritis	ANA, knee X ray, ESR
Adult	M/F	B/W	Iridocyclitis	Syphilis	As above
	M/F	B/W		Tuberculosis	As above
	F	B		Sarcoidosis	Chest X ray, skin test anergy, gallium scan, serum ACE level, serum calcium level, Kveim test
	M	W		Ankylosing spondylitis/ Reiter's syndrome	Sacroiliac joint X ray, HLA-B27, ESR
Child	M/F	B/W	Chorioretinitis	Toxocariasis	ELISA for toxocara, ESR, CBC (for eosinophilia)
	M/F	B/W		Toxoplasmosis	Serologic tests, indirect FA test, hemagglutination test
	M/F	B/W		Tuberculosis	As above
Adult	M/F	B/W	Chorioretinitis	Toxoplasmosis	Serologic tests, indirect FA test, hemagglutination test
	M/F	B/W		Histoplasmosis	Histoplasma skin test chest X ray, HLA-B7
	M/F	B/W		Syphilis	As above
	M/F	B/W		Tuberculosis	As above
	F	B		Sarcoidosis	As above
	M/F	B/W		Cytomegalovirus/ herpes zoster ophthalmicus/ acute retinal necrosis	Serologic tests for AIDS

Abbreviations: M/F = male or female; M = male; F = female; B/W = black or white; B = black; W = white; FTA-ABS = fluorescent treponemal antibody absorption test; VDRL = venereal disease research lab test; PPD = purified protein derivative (tuberculin skin test); ANA = antinuclear antibody test; ESR = erythrocyte sedimentation rate; HLA = human leukocyte antigen; FA = fluorescent antibody test; ELISA = enzyme-linked immunosorbent assay; CBC = complete blood count; ACE = angiotensin converting enzyme.

logic test can confirm whether the patient ever had syphilis, and a VDRL can determine its state of activity. Both should be ordered if this possibility is considered. Any previous systemic infection with tuberculosis is diagnosed with a tuberculin PPD-2 skin test, and chest X ray.

Human leukocyte antigen (HLA) testing is used to detect the presence of specific cell surface markers called histocompatibility antigens. Several uveitic entities are associated with specific HLA antigens: B27 (ankylosing spondylitis, Reiter's syndrome, juvenile rheumatoid arthritis); B5 (Behcet's syndrome); B7 (histoplasmosis); DRW2 (macular histoplasmosis); BW22J (Vogt-Koyanagi-Harada syndrome); and B29 (birdshot choroiditis). HLA typing is expensive and often nonspecific; it should be reserved for specific conditions when other tests have been inconclusive. Invasive procedures should also be used judiciously. An anterior chamber tap can be considered when the differential includes reticulum cell sarcoma, bacterial or fungal endophthalmitis, iris or ciliary body melanoma, phacolytic glaucoma (see Chapter 10), sarcoidosis (angiotensin converting enzyme level), and toxocariasis (ELISA test). A vitreous tap should be performed in all cases of suspected bacterial or fungal endophthalmitis and considered for reticulum cell sarcoma.

REFERENCES

Ultrasound

Atta HR, Byrne SF: The findings of standard echography for choroidal folds. *Arch Ophthalmol* 106:1234, 1988.

Byrne SF: Standardized echography: I. A-scan examination procedures. *Int Ophthalmol Clin* 19(4):267, 1979.

Byrne SF, Glaser JS: Orbital tissue differentiation with standardized echography. *Ophthalmology* 90:1071, 1983.

Coleman DJ: Reliability of ocular and orbital diagnosis with B-scan ultrasound. II. Orbital diagnosis. *Am J Ophthalmol* 74:708, 1972.

Coleman DJ, Dallow RL, Smith ME: Immersion ultrasonography: Simultaneous A-scan and B-scan. *Int Ophthalmol Clin* 19(4):67, 1979.

Coleman DJ, Franzen LA: Vitreous surgery: Preoperative evaluation and prognostic value of ultrasonic display of the vitreous. *Arch Ophthalmol* 92:375, 1974.

Coleman DJ, Jack RL, Franzen LA: High resolution B-scan ultrasonography of the orbit. I. The normal orbit. *Arch Ophthalmol* 88:358, 1972.

Coleman DJ, Jack RL, Franzen LA: Ultrasonography in ocular trauma. *Am J Ophthalmol* 75:279, 1973.

Coleman DJ, Lizzi FL, Jack RL: *Ultrasonography of the Eye and Orbit.* Philadelphia, Lea & Febiger, 1977.

Lieb WE, Shields JA, Cohen SM, et al: Color Doppler imaging in the management of intraocular tumors. *Ophthalmology* 97:1660, 1990.

Ossoinig KC: Quantitative echography—the basis of tissue differentiation. *J Clin Ultrasound* 2:33, 1974.

Ossoinig KC: Standardized echography: Basic principles, clinical applications, and results. *Int Ophthalmol Clin* 19(4):127, 1979.

Ossoinig KC: Echographic differentiation of vascular tumors in the orbit. *Doc Ophthalmol Proc Ser* 29:283, 1981.

Ossoinig KC, Cennamo G, Byrne SF: Echographic differential diagnosis of optic nerve lesions. *Doc Ophthalmol Proc Ser* 29:327, 1981.

Shammas HJF, Minckler DS, Ogden C: Ultrasound in early thyroid orbitopathy. *Arch Ophthalmol* 98:277, 1980.

Plain Film Radiography

Burrows EH, Leeds NE: *Neuroradiology.* New York, Churchill Livingstone, 1981.
Lloyd GA: *Radiology of the Orbit.* Philadelphia, WB Saunders, 1975, pp 197–210.
Rao VM, Gonzalez CF: Plain film radiography and tomography of the orbit. In Gonzalez CF, Becker MH, Flanagan JC (eds): *Diagnostic Imaging in Ophthalmology.* New York, Springer-Verlag, pp 1–17.
Vignaud J, Claude C, Mink J: Roentgen anatomy of the orbit. In Arger PH (ed): *Orbital Roentgenology.* New York, John Wiley, pp 2–27.

Computed Tomography and Magnetic Resonance Imaging

Albert A, Lee BCP, Saint Louis L, Deck MDF: MRI of optic chiasm and optic pathways. *AJNR* 7:255, 1986.
Armington WG, Zimmerman RA, Bilaniuk LT: Imaging of the visual pathways. In Som PM, Bergeron RT (eds): *Head and Neck Imaging.* St Louis, Mosby Year Book, 1991, pp 829–874.
Atlas SW, Bilaniuk LT, Zimmerman RA, et al: Orbit. Initial experience with surface coil spin echo MR imaging at 1.5 T. *Radiology* 164:501, 1987.
Brodsky MC, Glasier CM, Pollock SC, Angtuago EJC: Optic nerve hypoplasia. Identification by magnetic resonance imaging. *Arch Ophthalmol* 108:1562, 1990.
Chambers RB, Davidorf FH, McAdoo JF, Chakeres DW: Magnetic resonance imaging of uveal melanomas. *Arch Ophthalmol* 105:917, 1987.
Char DH, Hedges TR, Norman D: Retinoblastoma. *Ophthalmology* 91:1347, 1984.
Char DH, Unsold R, Sobel DF, Salvolini U, Newton TH: Ocular and orbital pathology. In Newton TH, Hasso AN, Dillon WP (eds): *Computed Tomography of the Head and Neck.* New York, Raven Press, 1988, pp 9.1–9.64.
Consensus conference. Magnetic resonance imaging. *JAMA* 259:2132, 1988.
Council on Scientific Affairs. Fundamentals of magnetic resonance imaging. *JAMA* 258:3417, 1987.
Council on Scientific Affairs. Panel on Magnetic Resonance Imaging: Magnetic resonance imaging of the central nervous system. *JAMA* 259:1211, 1988.
Daniels DL, Pech P, Mark L, et al: Magnetic resonance imaging of the cavernous sinus. *AJNR* 6:187, 1985.
de Keizer RJW, Vielvoye GJ, de Wolff-Rouendaal D: Nuclear magnetic resonance imaging of intraocular tumors. *Am J Ophthalmol* 102:438, 1986.
Edwards MK, Farlow MR, Stevens JC: Multiple sclerosis: MRI and clinical correlation. *AJR* 147:571, 1986.
Giangiacomo J, Khan J, Levine C, Thompson VM: Sequential cranial computed tomography in infants with retinal hemorrhages. *Ophthalmology* 95:295, 1988.
Green BF, Kraft SP, Carter KD, et al: Intraorbital wood. Detection by magnetic resonance imaging. *Ophthalmology* 97:608, 1990.
Gross JG, Hesselink JR, Press GA, et al: Magnetic resonance imaging in the evaluation of vitreoretinal disease in eyes with intraocular silicon oil. *Am J Ophthalmol* 110:366, 1990.
Grossman RI: Radiation risks in CT scans. *Arch Ophthalmol* 109:30, 1991.
Grossman RI, Braffman BH, Brorson JR, et al: Multiple sclerosis: Serial study of gadolinium-enhanced MR imaging. *Radiology* 169:117, 1987.
Grove AS Jr: Computed tomography in the management of orbital trauma. *Ophthalmology* 89:433, 1982.
Guy J, Mancuso A, Quisling RG, et al: Gadolinium-DTPA-enhanced magnetic resonance imaging in optic neuropathies. *Ophthalmology* 97:592, 1990.
Haik BG, Saint Louis L, Bierly J: Magnetic resonance imaging in the evaluation of optic nerve gliomas. *Ophthalmology* 94:709, 1987.
Haik BG, Saint Louis L, Smith ME, et al: Magnetic resonance imaging in the evaluation of leukocoria. *Ophthalmology* 92:1143, 1985.
Healy ME, Hesselink JR, Press GA, Middleton MS: Increased detection of intracranial metastases with Gd-DPTA. *Radiology* 165:619, 1987.

Imes RK, Hoyt WF: Magnetic resonance imaging signs of optic nerve gliomas in neurofibromatosis I. *Am J Ophthalmol* 111:729, 1991.
Jacobs L, Kinkel WR, Polachini I, Kinkel RP: Correlations of nuclear magnetic resonance imaging, computerized tomography, and clinical profiles in multiple sclerosis. *Neurology* 36:27, 1986.
Jay WM: Advances in magnetic resonance imaging. *Am J Ophthalmol* 108:592, 1989.
Kanal E, Kemp S, Latchaw RE, Wolf GL: Gadolinium-DTPA-enhanced MR imaging of meningeal pathology at 1.5 Tesla. *AJNR* 9:1012, 1988.
Kline LB, Acker JD, Post MJD: Computed tomographic evaluation of the cavernous sinus. *Ophthalmology* 89:374, 1982.
Kolodny NH, Gragoudas ES, D'Amico DJ, Albert DM: Magnetic resonance imaging and spectroscopy of intraocular tumors. *Surv Ophthalmol* 33:502, 1989.
Lagouros PA, Langer BG, Peyman GA, et al: Magnetic resonance imaging and intraocular foreign bodies. *Arch Ophthalmol* 105:551, 1987.
LoBue TD, Deutsch TA, Lobick J, Turner DA: Detection and localization of nonmetallic foreign bodies by magnetic resonance imaging. *Arch Ophthalmol* 106:260, 1988.
Mafee MF (ed): *Imaging in Ophthalmology, Part I: The Radiology Clinics of North America*, vol 25, no 3. Philadelphia, WB Saunders, 1987.
Mafee MF (ed): *Imaging in Ophthalmology, Part II: The Radiology Clinics of North America*, vol 25, no 4. Philadelphia, WB Saunders, 1987.
Mafee MF, Goldberg MF, Cohen SB, et al: Magnetic resonance imaging versus computed tomography of leukocoric eyes and uses of in vitro proton magnetic resonance spectroscopy of retinoblastoma. *Ophthalmology* 96:965, 1989.
Mafee MF, Schatz CJ: The orbit. In Som PM, Bergeron RT (eds): *Head and Neck Imaging*. St Louis, Mosby Year Book, 1991, pp 693–828.
Miller DH, Newton MR, van der Poel JC, et al: Magnetic resonance imaging of the optic nerve in optic neuritis. *Neurology* 38:175, 1988.
Patrinely JR, Osborn AG, Anderson RL, Whiting AS: Computed tomographic features of nonthyroid extraocular muscle enlargement. *Ophthalmology* 96:1038, 1989.
Peyman GA, Mafee MF: Uveal melanoma and similar lesions: The role of magnetic resonance imaging and computed tomography. In Mafee MF (ed): *Imaging in Ophthalmology, Part II: The Radiology Clinics of North America*, vol 25, no 4. Philadelphia, WB Saunders, 1987, pp 471–486.
Sartor K, Karnaze MG, Winthrop JD, et al: MR imaging in infra-, para-, and retrosellar mass lesions. *Neuroradiology* 29:19, 1987.
Schroth G, Kretzschmar K, Gawehn J, Voight K: Advantage of magnetic resonance imaging in the diagnosis of cerebral infections. *Neuroradiology* 29:120, 1987.
Schulman JA, Peyman GA, Mafee MF, et al: The use of magnetic resonance imaging in the evaluation of retinoblastoma. *J Pediatr Ophthalmol Strabismus* 23:144, 1987.
Shellock FG: Biologic effects and safety aspects of magnetic resonance imaging. *Magn Reson Q* 5:243, 1989.
Shellock FG, Crues JV: Temperature, heart rate, and blood pressure changes associated with clinical MR imaging at 1.5 T. *Radiology* 163:259, 1987.
Slamovits TL, Gardner TA: Neuroimaging in neuro-ophthalmology. *Ophthalmology* 96:555, 1989.
Wilberger JE Jr, Deeb Z, Rothfus W: Magnetic resonance imaging in cases of severe head injury. *Neurosurgery* 20:571, 1987.
Wilson WB, Dreisbach JN, Lattin DE, Stears JC: Magnetic resonance imaging of nonmetallic foreign bodies. *Am J Ophthalmol* 105:612, 1988.
Zimmerman CF, Schatz NJ, Glaser JS: Magnetic resonance imaging of optic nerve meningiomas. Enhancement with gadolinium-DTPA. *Ophthalmology* 97:585, 1990a.
Zimmerman CF, Schatz NJ, Glaser JS: Magnetic resonance imaging of radiation optic neuropathy. *Am J Ophthalmol* 110:389, 1990b.

Cerebral Angiography

Chilcote WA, Modic MT, Pavlicek WA, et al: Digital subtraction angiography of the carotid arteries: A comparative study in 100 patients. *Radiology* 139:287, 1981.
Grossman RI, Sergott RC, Goldberg HI, et al: Dural malformations with ophthalmic manifestations: Results of particulate embolization in seven patients. *AJNR* 6:809, 1985.

Hanneken AM, Miller NR, Debrun GM, Nauta H: Treatment of carotid cavernous fistulas using a detachable balloon catheter through the superior ophthalmic vein. *Arch Ophthalmol* 107:87, 1989.

Lund G, Rysavy J, Kotula F, et al: Detachable steel spring coils for vessel occlusion. *Radiology* 155:530, 1985.

Manelfe C, Lasjaunias P, Ruscalleda J: Preoperative embolization of intracranial meningiomas. *AJNR* 7:963, 1986.

Fluorescein Angiography

Chamberlin JA, Bressler NM, Bressler SB: The use of fundus photographs and fluorescein angiograms in the identification and treatment of choroidal neovascularization in the macular photocoagulation study. *Ophthalmology* 96:1526, 1989.

Greenberg F, Lewis RA: Safety of fluorescein angiography during pregnancy. *Am J Ophthalmol* 110:323, 1990.

Halperin L, Olk RJ, Soubrane G, Coscas G: Safety of fluorescein angiography during pregnancy. *Am J Ophthalmol* 109:563, 1990.

Lipson BK, Yannuzzi LA: Complications of intravenous fluorescein injections. *Int Ophthalmol Clin* 29:200, 1989.

Weaver DT, Herman DC: A contraindication to injection of intravenous fluorescein. *Am J Ophthalmol* 109:490, 1990.

Wolfe DR: Fluorescein angiography basic science and engineering. *Ophthalmology* 93:1617, 1986.

Yannuzzi LA, Rohre KT, Tindel LJ, et al: Flurorescein angiography complication survey. *Ophthalmology* 93:611, 1986.

Laboratory Studies

Auran JD, Starr MB, Jakobiec FA: Acanthamoeba keratitis: A review of the literature. *Cornea* 6(1):2, 1987.

Brinser JH, Burd EM: Principles of diagnostic ocular microbiology. In Tabbara KF, Hyndiuk RA (eds): *Infections of the Eye*. Boston, Little, Brown, 1986, pp 73–92.

Brinser JH, Weiss A: Laboratory diagnosis in ocular disease. In Duane TD, Jaeger EA (eds): *Clinical Ophthalmology*. Philadelphia, Harper & Row, 1990, 4:Chap 1.

Dunkel EC, Pavan-Langston D, Fitzpatrick K, et al: Rapid detection of *Herpes simplex* (HSV) antigen in human ocular infections. *Curr Eye Res* 7:661, 1988.

External disease and cornea. In Basic and Clinical Science Course, sec 7. San Francisco, American Academy of Ophthalmology, 1988, pp 61–72.

Fedukowicz HB, Stetson S: *External Infections of the Eye*. Norwalk, CT, Appleton-Century-Crofts, 1985, pp 246–260.

Jones DB, Liesegang TJ, Robinson NM: *Laboratory Diagnosis of Ocular Infections, Cumulative Techniques and Procedures in Clinical Microbiology*. Washington, DC, Cumitech 13, American Society for Microbiology, 1981.

Wiley L, Springer D, Kowalski R, et al: Rapid diagnosis for ocular adenovirus. *Ophthalmology* 95:431, 1988.

Laboratory Studies in Uveitis

Nozik RA: Laboratory testing in uveitis. Focal points: Clinical Modules for Ophthalmologists. San Francisco, American Academy of Ophthalmology, 1983.

O'Connor GR: Tests in uveitis. In Duane TD, Jaeger EA (eds): *Clinical Ophthalmology*. Philadelphia, J.B. Lippincott, 1981, 4:Chap 34.

Pavesio CE, Nozik RA: Anterior and intermediate uveitis. *Int Ophthalmol Clin* 30(4):244, 1990.

Rosenbaum JT, Wernick R: Selection and interpretation of laboratory tests for patients with uveitis. *Int Ophthalmol Clin* 30:238, 1990.

Smith RE, Nozik RA: *Uveitis, A Clinical Approach to Diagnosis and Management*, ed 2. Baltimore, Williams and Wilkins, 1989.

3

Special Considerations in the Pediatric Patient

Robert A. Catalano

SPECIAL CONSIDERATIONS IN THE OCULAR EXAMINATION

As in adults, obtaining a visual acuity is the first step in the ocular examination of children, something often forgotten in infants and toddlers. Illiterate eye charts, with tumbling "E," Allen picture (Figure 3-1), or Landolt C optotypes are available for use in cooperative preschool children. In younger children, the ability to fixate and follow objects is tested.

A papoose board may be helpful in restraining infants for examination and minor treatments (Figure 3-2). To restrain toddlers, the parent sits facing the physician's assistant. Both are at the same level, with their knees close or touching. The child lies supine in the parent's and assistant's laps with legs wrapped around the parent's waist and head in the assistant's lap. The parent holds the child's hands folded across the child's waist. The physician's assistant, using both hands, immobilizes the child's head (Figure 3-3). In this position, corneal abrasions can be easily detected with the ultraviolet illumination of a hand-held Wood's lamp, after the installation of fluorescein dye (Figure 3-4). A portable slit lamp can also be brought close to the child for examination of the external eye and eyelids (Figure 3-5).

In cooperative infants, the intraocular pressure can be measured with a hand-held Perkin's applanation tonometer (Figure 3-6). Older children can often be coaxed into sitting behind a slit lamp (Figure 3-7).

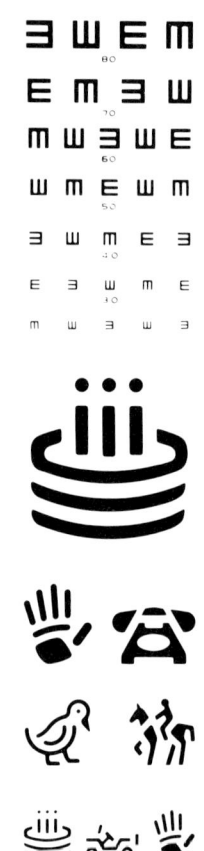

FIGURE 3–1. Illiterate "E" and Allen picture eye charts for use in preschool-aged children.

If at any time during the examination, suspicion of a ruptured globe develops, no further diagnostic examinations should be performed. A protective eye shield that fits entirely over the bony orbit, completely encasing the eye (without a pressure patch), should be taped to the face. Further examination and treatment should be carried out only under general anesthesia.

PEDIATRIC OCULAR TRAUMA, SPORTS-RELATED OCULAR INJURIES, AND CHILD ABUSE

Several studies have confirmed that young people account for a disproportionate share of ocular trauma. Reviews have shown that children and adolescents comprise approximately 50% of hospital admissions for ocular injuries

Text continues on page 96

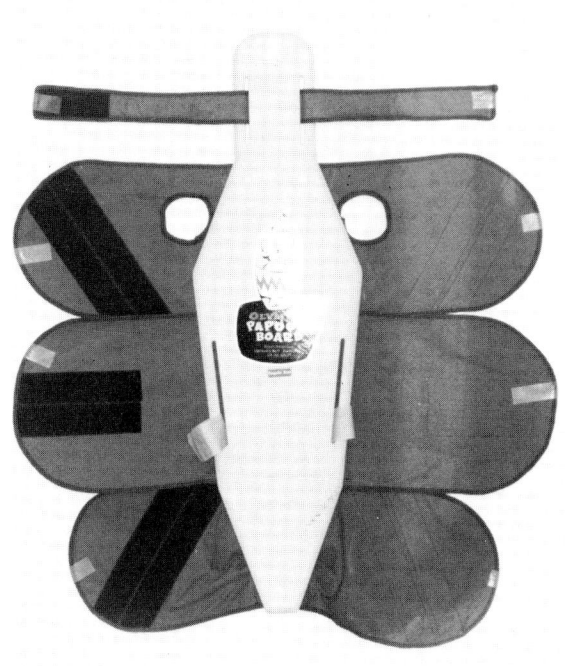

FIGURE 3–2. Papoose board useful in restraining infants.

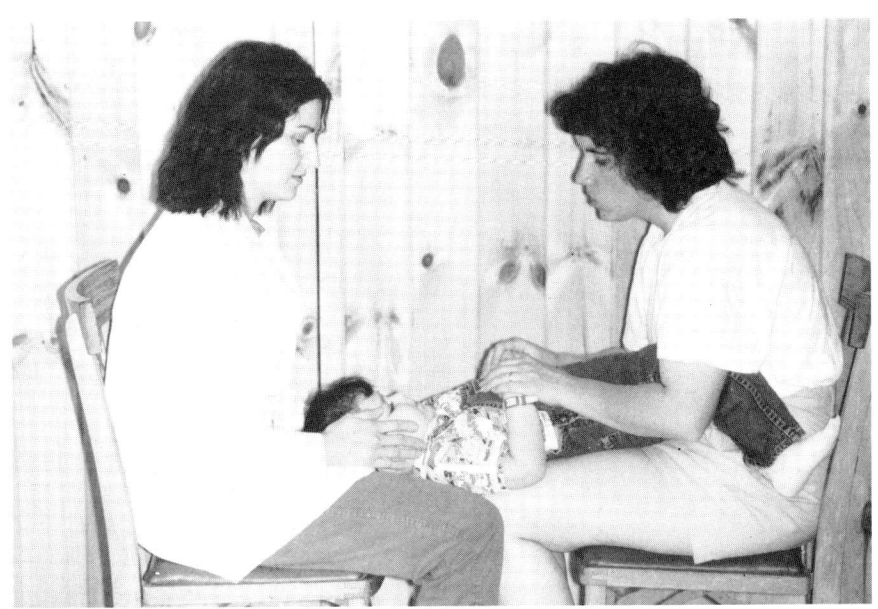

FIGURE 3–3. Positioning useful in restraining a toddler.

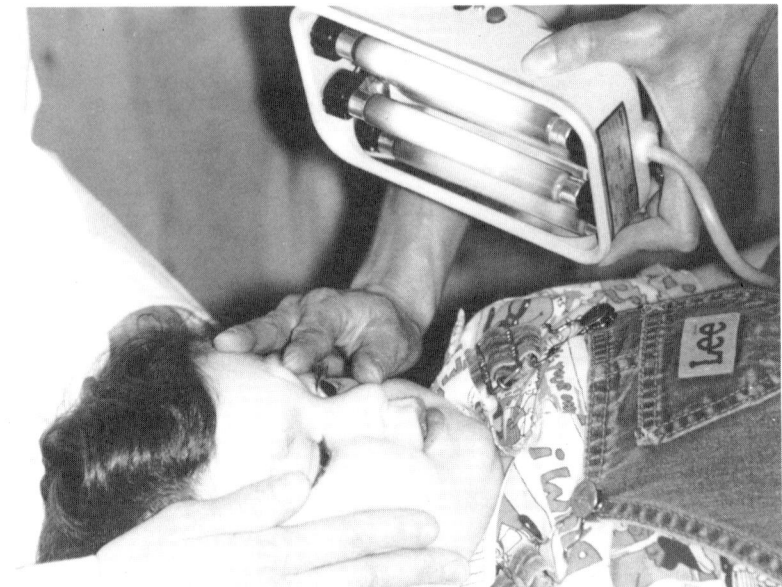

FIGURE 3–4. Ultraviolet Wood's lamp being used to detect a corneal abrasion or a herpetic corneal lesion after the instillation of fluorescein dye.

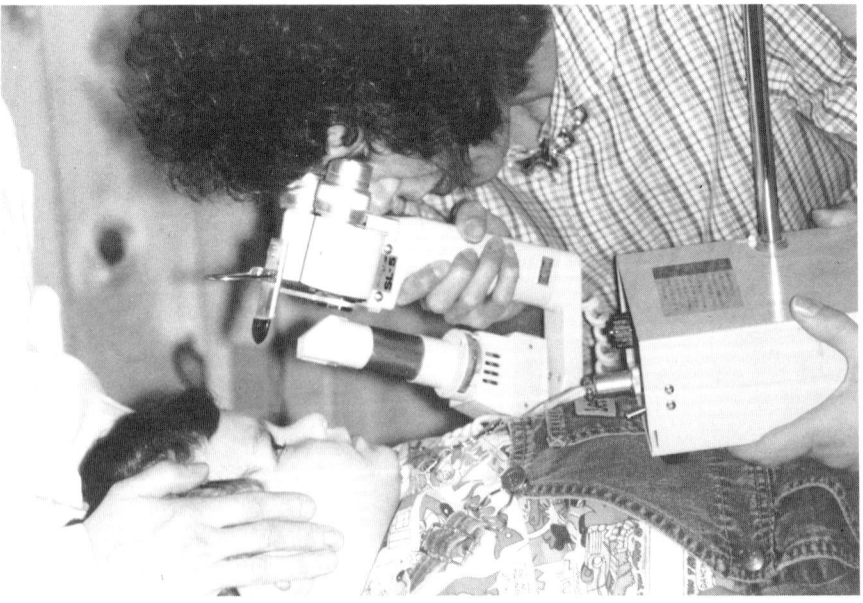

FIGURE 3–5. Portable slit lamp being used to examine the external eye and eyelids.

3—Special Considerations in the Pediatric Patient 95

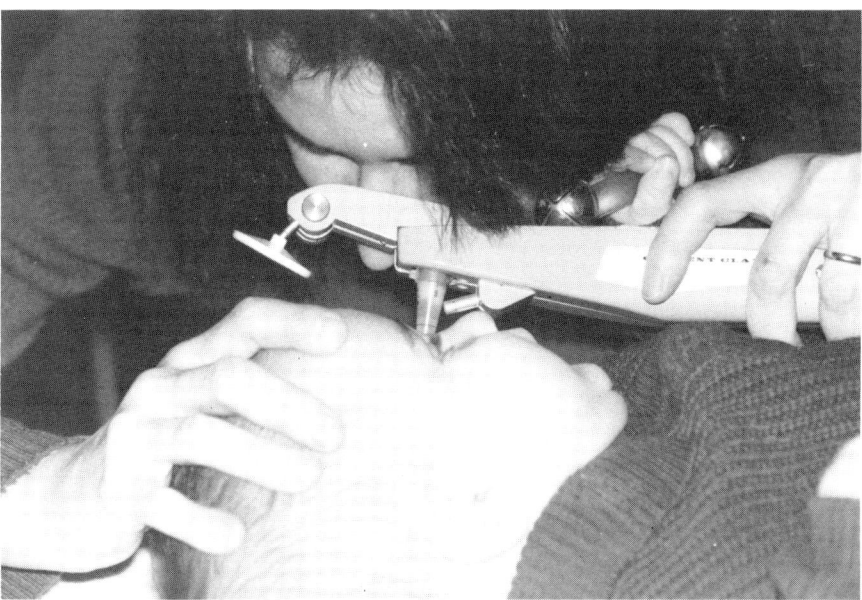

FIGURE 3–6. Intraocular pressure being measured in a cooperative infant with a hand-held Perkin's applanation tonometer. (From Stern JH, Catalano RA: Current status of diagnostic and therapeutic measures in infantile glaucoma. *Seminars of Ophthalmology* 5, no. 4, 1990. Reprinted with permission.)

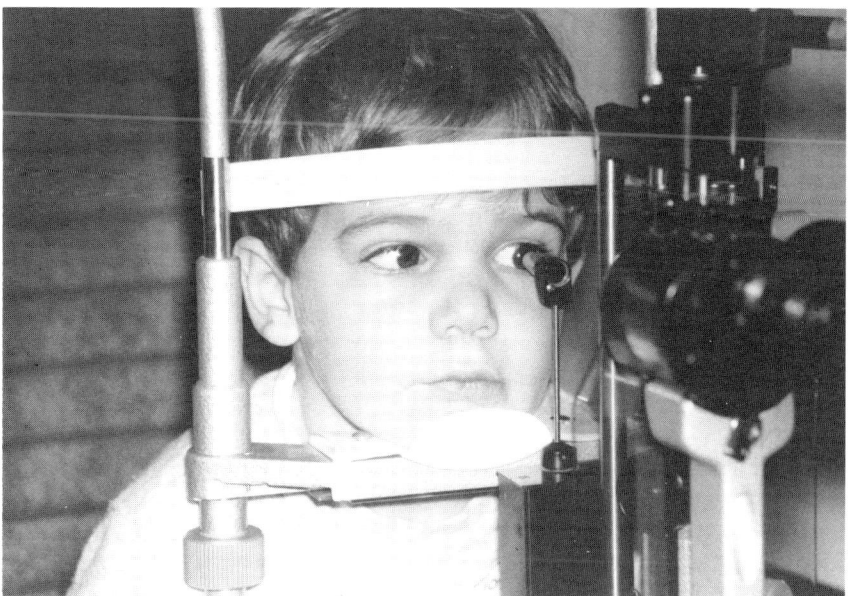

FIGURE 3–7. Older child having intraocular pressure checked at a slit lamp.

and that a similar proportion of penetrating ocular injuries occurs in this age group. Boys age 11 to 15 years are the most vulnerable; their injuries outnumber those in girls by a ratio of about 4:1. The majority of injuries are related to accidental blows, sports, toy darts or other projectiles, sticks, stones, and air-powered BB guns. BB guns cause particularly devastating ocular and orbital damage. In most studies, BB injuries are the most common cause of significant traumatic visual loss in children. Recently many states have reclassified all compressed carbon dioxide guns (including "toy" paint pellet guns) as firearms, removing them from toy stores and restricting their purchase to adults. These injuries will remain common, however, due to inadequate adult supervision.

As important as it is to obtain a detailed and accurate history of the mechanism of injury, the physician should be aware that there are various reasons why both the child and the guardian may give an inaccurate or misleading history. The child may fear punishment for performing a forbidden activity that resulted in injury; the parent may try to conceal or deny improper or inadequate supervision. Parental guilt and denial is particularly common when the child was assisting the parent perform a chore, such as splitting wood or lawn mowing, without adequate eye protection. Additionally, adults guilty of child abuse may fabricate or misrepresent the history. Occasionally abusing parents will not be aware that their action may have caused injury; this is most commonly seen in parents who shake their babies.

Sports-Related Ocular Injuries

In the early twentieth century, most ocular injuries occurred in the workplace. More recently, violent and sports-related activities have contributed to the majority of eye injuries. Although sports injuries occur in all age groups, far more children and adolescents participate in high-risk sports than adults. The greater number of participating children, their athletic immaturity, and the increased likelihood of their using inadequate or improper eye protection account for their disproportionate share of sports-related eye injuries.

The sports with the highest risk of eye injury are those in which no eye protection can be worn: boxing, wrestling, and the martial arts. High-risk sports include those that use a rapidly moving ball or puck, bat, stick, racket, or arrow (baseball, hockey, lacrosse, racquet sports, and archery) or involve aggressive body contact (football and basketball). Low-risk sports include swimming, track and field, and gymnastics. Related to both risk and frequency of participation, the highest percentage of eye injuries are seen in basketball and baseball. The latter are more severe and most commonly occur to the batter. Individual risk factors are past retinal detachment, corneal transplant, radial keratotomy, aphakia, amblyopia, previous severe ocular injury, and high myopia.

Protective eyewear, designed for a specific activity, is available for most sports. For basketball, racquet sports, and other recreational activities that do not require a helmet or face mask, molded polycarbonate sports goggles, secured to the head by an elastic strap, are suggested (Figure 3–8). For hockey (goalie), football, lacrosse, and baseball (batter), specific helmets with polycarbonate faceshields and guards are available (Figure 3–9). Children should also wear sports goggles under the helmets. For baseball, goggles and helmets should be worn for batting, catching, and base running; goggles alone are usually sufficient for other positions. For hockey, the goalie, forwards, and defensemen should wear goggles and a helmet; other players should wear goggles. The appropriate helmet for hockey is shown in Figure 3–9; the molded "Jason"-style hockey mask does not provide adequate ocular or orbital protection. For football, the helmet should have an attached polycarbonate face guard. Other sports for which a helmet and eye protection are advisable are horseback riding, ski racing, cycling, motorcycling, fencing, and snowmobiling. Finally, orthodonic headgear should never be worn while playing sports. The typical metallic bow, strapped to the head and anchored in the mouth, can slip with an impacting force, penetrating the eye.

Many optical and sporting good stores sell sports goggles and helmets. Table 3–1 lists the names and addresses of firms that manufacture sports eyewear.

Ophthalmologists are often asked to suggest guidelines for sports participation by amblyopic children. Jeffers (1990) defines a functionally one-eyed ath-

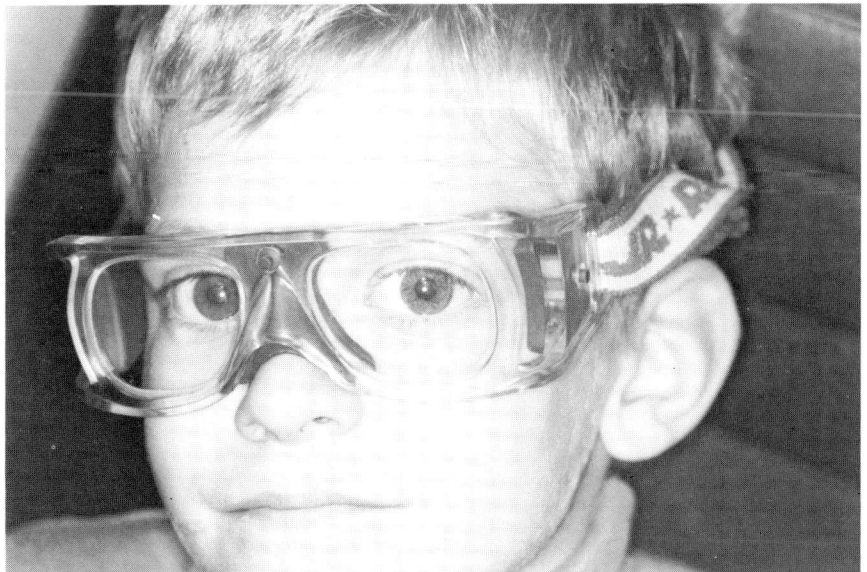

FIGURE 3–8.   Polycarbonate sports goggles with elastic head straps.

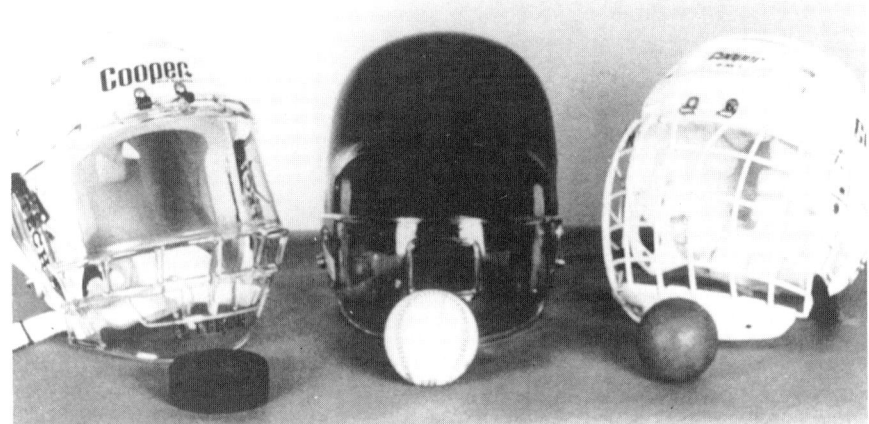

FIGURE 3-9. Sport-specific helmets for hockey (left), baseball (center), and lacrosse (right). (From: Jeffers JB: An on going tragedy: Pediatric sports-related eye injuries. *Sem Ophthalmol* 5:216, 1990, with permission.)

lete as one who has less than 20/50 vision in one eye and 20/20 best corrected vision in the other eye. He suggests that with appropriate eye protection these children can participate in most sports. But under no circumstances should they participate in boxing, wrestling, and martial arts or any other sport without eye protection. Even for everyday street wear, these children should be fitted with polycarbonate lenses with a minimum center thickness of 3 mm and sturdy frames. Informed parental consent is especially important in functionally one-eyed children. The parents, physician, athlete, coach, school administration, and legal counsel should all be involved in the decision.

TABLE 3-1. MANUFACTURERS OF SPORTS EYEWEAR

Liberty Optical	*LST Leader Sports*	*Viking Sports*
380 Verona Avenue	P.O. Box 591	5355 Sierra Road
Newark, NJ 07014	Essex, NY 12936	San Jose, CA 95132
800-879-9992	800-847-2001	800-535-3300
Ektelon	*Herslof Optical*	*Face Guard Inc.*
8929 Aero Drive	12000 W Carmen Avenue	P.O. Box 8425
San Diego, CA 92123	Milwaukee, WI 53225	Roanoke, VA 24014
800-854-2958	800-558-7073	800-336-9683
Cabot Safety Co.	*Titmus Optical*	
141 Broadway	P.O. Box 191	
Norwich, CT 06360	Petersburg, VA 23804	
800-982-2828	800-446-1802	

Child Abuse

Child abuse is a consideration whenever the history is incompatible with the findings, especially in infants. The most common precipitating factors are inconsolable crying, toileting incidents, whining, or refusing to eat.

Ophthalmologists are often asked to examine children suspected of being abused because of the frequency of ocular involvement in child abuse. The most striking and common ocular finding is intraocular hemorrhage. Prior to the use of magnetic resonance imaging, ophthalmologic examination was especially important in diagnosing abuse because retinal, preretinal, and vitreous hemorrhage often precede computed tomography and clinical findings of subdural hematoma. The detection of hemosiderin in the optic nerve or retina, on autopsy, is also useful forensically. Medicolegally, however, the presence of hemosiderin by itself is not sufficient to indicate repeated trauma. Hemosiderin first appears 3 days after injury and may remain in tissues for 20 years. The observation of independent hemorrhages of different ages is more important in the consideration of child abuse. Table 3–2 lists additional historical, social, and physical findings in the abused child.

The shaken baby syndrome represents an important subset of abused children. This syndrome is usually seen in infants under age 12 months; children over age 3 years are unlikely to be shaken. The child often has no other signs of abuse and is brought to the emergency room in a depressed state of consciousness or in status epilepticus. The perpetrator is usually a parent, babysitter, or boyfriend of a babysitter. Anatomical features increase the vulnerability of the infant to whiplash-type cerebral injuries from shaking. The infant brain is softer, due to immature myelinization, and more mobile, due to a greater proportion of cerebrospinal fluid, than the adult brain. The most telling intracranial manifestation of shaking is bilateral subdural hematomas, especially when the interhemispheric fissure in the parieto-occipital region, and the potential space overlying the cerebral convexities is involved (Figure 3–10). Diffuse cerebral swelling is also common. Subarachnoid hemorrhage is uncommon and intracerebral bleeding rare. Blindness, spastic hemiplegia or quadriplegia, mental retardation, and death can occur from this whiplash type of injury.

Ocular findings in the shaken baby syndrome include scattered round, almost confluent retinal and nerve fiber layer hemorrhages (some with white centers, depending on the hemorrhage's age). Preretinal hemorrhages, often with domelike elevations of the internal limiting membrane, are almost pathognomonic of a shaking injury. Involvement of the posterior pole, especially the macula, is most typical (Figure 3–11). Vitreous hemorrhage may occur initially but is often seen several days after the episode, following breakthrough of blood from preretinal loculations. Vitrectomy should be considered if bright flash retinography demonstrates preservation of the B-wave, and amblyopia from prolonged vitreous hemorrhage is suspected.

TABLE 3-2. HISTORICAL, SOCIAL, AND PHYSICAL FINDINGS IN THE ABUSED CHILD

Historical Findings
Nature of injury incompatible with history
Inconsistency between mechanism of injury and child's developmental stage
Male sex; age less than 1 year
History of spontaneously stopping breathing, choking, minor fall, or head getting caught in crib slats
Caretaker offering no explanation
Prior episodes of loss of appetite, irritability, seizures
Previously suspected failure to thrive
Multiple previous hospital admissions, for this child or siblings, at different institutions
Young child pleading affection to parent
Deterioration of older child's academic performance
Social withdrawal or history of running away in older child
Unusually high tolerance for pain in older child

Social findings
Perpetrator immaturity or inclination toward violent behavior
Perpetrator history of being an abused child
Perpetrator history of drug or alcohol abuse or mental illness
Familial financial or marital difficulties
Unwed mother
Cessation of new injuries during hospitalization
Parental failure to visit child during hospitalization

Systemic findings
Fractures of different ages of long bones and ribs
Fractures involving metaphysis or epiphyseal plates
Linear skull fractures in the frontal or parietal region
Hematoma involving the cervical spinal cord
Dislocated joints
Disproportionate soft tissue injuries
Bruises on the trunk with the imprint of an adult hand
Hot water burns or burns in the pattern of a hot plate, heating grate, or cigarette
Burns of the buttocks or genitalia
A burn of a single hand or foot above the wrist or ankle
Vomiting, abdominal distension, absent bowel sounds, and abdominal tenderness (ruptured liver, spleen, intestinal perforation)

Ocular findings
Subconjunctival hemorrhages
Intraocular hemorrhages: retinal and preretinal, vitreous, hyphema
Lid lacerations, ecchymosis, proptosis
Gonococcal and chlamydial conjunctivitis
Corneal laceration, abrasion, ulcer, opacification
Traumatic mydriasis, sphincter tear, iris disinsertion
Subluxated lens, cataract
Purtscher retinopathy with fat emboli from long bone fractures
Retinal detachment, retinodialysis, retinal folds, retinoschisis
Chorioretinal scarring
Optic disc edema, optic atrophy, optic nerve avulsion
Nystagmus, strabismus, cranial nerve palsy
Complete loss of eye movements and pupillary function
Cortical blindness

3—Special Considerations in the Pediatric Patient   101

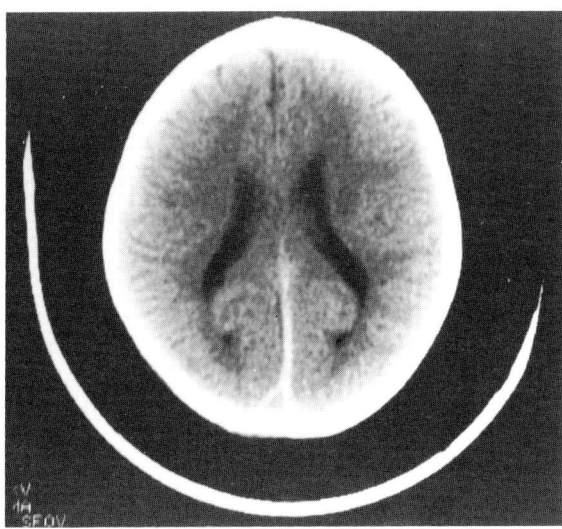

FIGURE 3-10. CT image showing acute subdural hematoma in the posterior interhemispheric fissure and over the cerebral convexity, in a shaken baby.

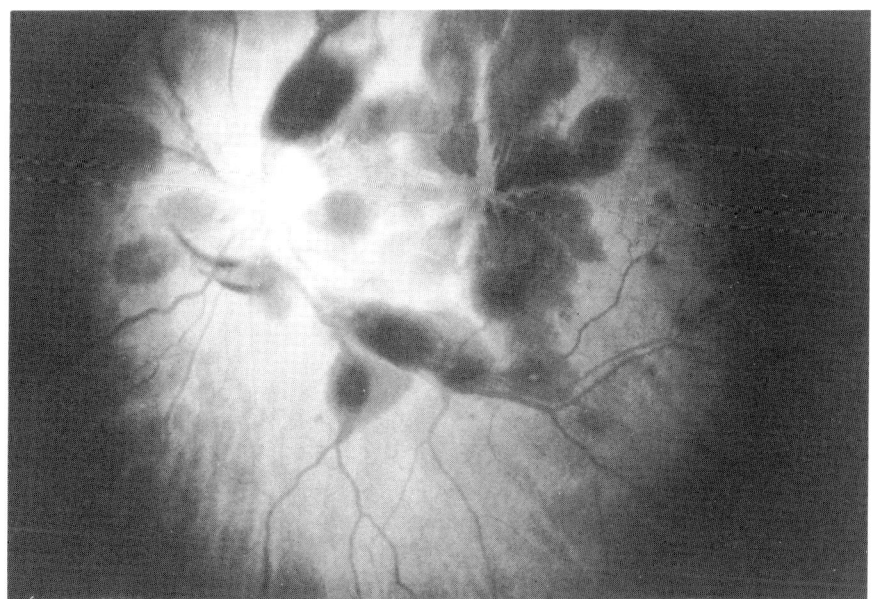

FIGURE 3-11. Very extensive, almost confluent preretinal and retinal hemorrhages, principally involving the macular area, in the shaken baby syndrome.

The differential diagnosis of retinal hemorrhages in a child includes leukemia, blood dyscrasia or anemia, cardiopulmonary resuscitation, retinal vasculitis, bacterial endocarditis, severe arterial hypertension, and birth trauma. With the exception of physical abuse, however, head trauma rarely causes massive retinal hemorrhage. The latter suggests shaking and dates the incident to within several weeks. The finding of migration of blood into the vitreous, after an initial observation of only preretinal hemorrhage, further suggests that the episode occurred a few days earlier. Eventually the fundus may appear normal, but pigment epithelial disturbances, retinal gliosis, and vascular attenuation may occur as late findings. Optic nerve injury is seen initially as disc edema and subsequently as optic atrophy. In general, preservation of the pupillary light reflex is a favorable prognostic sign.

It is the law in every state (and the District of Columbia) that physicians report child abuse to the county's child protective service agency. Personnel should be available in every hospital to assist the physician in the proper procedure. If the protocols are carried out in accordance with the law, physicians should be protected from civil or criminal liability, even when child abuse is not confirmed.

USE OF SEDATION IN EXAMINATION AND TREATMENT

The injured child may be anxious and uncooperative in the physician's office or emergency room. Sedation or general anesthesia may be necessary to complete an examination that would be routine in an adult. Several options for sedation exist (Table 3–3), but no drug has all of the desired characteristics of rapid onset, short duration, reversibility, and absolute safety. Infant death (presumably from respiratory depression) has been reported with even chloral hydrate (Jastak and Pallasch, 1988). At a minimum, the radial pulse rate and the respiratory rate should be monitored every 15 minutes with a stethoscope until a sedated child is fully awake.

The greatest experience with sedation has been with chloral hydrate, which has been used for over 30 years. Although the manufacturer (E. R. Squibb & Sons) recommends a dose of 50 mg/kg, three groups of investigators (Judisch, Anderson, and Bell, 1980; Whitacre and Ellis, 1984; Fox et al., 1990) have suggested using a higher dose of 80 mg/kg to 100 mg/kg. These investigators found this dose to be both safe and effective. Supplemental administration, when required, should be one-half the original dose, and the total dosage should not exceed 3 g. Vomiting is a common side effect, and idiosyncratic reactions of excitement or delirium are occasionally encountered.

Patients should fast for 4 hours prior to the administration of chloral hydrate to reduce the chance of aspiration should they vomit. In infants, the medication can be given by slow injection into the mouth with a needleless syringe. The drug should not be diluted with fruit juice or water. The onset of sedation

TABLE 3-3. ALTERNATIVES FOR SEDATION IN CHILDREN

DRUG	DOSE	ROUTE	COMMENT
Chloral hydrate	80–100 mg/kg; maximum 3 g	Oral	Safest, onset 30–60 minutes, no reversal, no analgesia
DPT "cocktail": Demerol, 25 mg/mL; phenergan 6.25 mg/mL; thorazine 6.35 mg/mL	1 mL of cocktail per 15 kgs; maximum 2 mL	IM	Onset 30–60 minutes, no reversal
Analgesic/narcotic Meperidine (Demerol)	1 mg/kg	IM/IV	Can give every 2–4 hours, reversible with naloxone (Narcan) 0.01 mg/kg
Morphine	0.1 mg/kg	IM/IV/SC	
Fentanyl	5–10 μgm/kg	IV	
	5–40 μgm/kg/hour	IV drip	
Valium	0.05–.2 mg/kg	IV	Rapid onset, no analgesia
Methohexital (Brevital)	1–2 mg/kg	IV	Rapid onset, duration 5–10 minutes
	10–15 mg/kg	Rectal	Onset 5–10 minutes, duration 30 minutes, may cause apnea

occurs variably between 30 minutes to 60 minutes after administration. Even using the maximum dose of 3 g, there is a higher risk of undersedation in heavier children. Undersedation results in arousal and unmanageability as soon as manipulations occur, requiring eventual conversion to another agent or general anesthesia. In practicality, using 100 mg/kg as a guideline, the maximum dose of 3 g is exceeded in most children over 5 years of age. For this reason, another anesthetic agent is usually required in uncooperative children older than 5 years of age.

Alternate options for sedation are listed in Table 3-3. At many institutions, the DPT, or "Pedi cocktail" of demerol, phenergan, and thorazine, has lost favor to reversible agents such as morphine, demerol, and fentanyl, although these require intravenous administration. Valium and brevital have a rapid onset, but valium provides no analgesia and may require large doses, and brevital may cause apnea. Chloral hydrate also does not provide analgesia. Uncomfortable procedures generally require an alternate agent or general anesthesia. Occasionally, however, a local anesthetic (lidocaine 1%) can be used concomitantly with chloral hydrate for minor lid procedures.

A few rudimentary general anesthetic measures that apply to both children and adults are discussed in Chapter 4. The physician should be aware of conditions that place the child at a higher general anesthetic risk (Table 3-4). Most of these are related to cardiovascular abnormalities, but children with neuromuscular disorders, including strabismus and congenital ptosis, have a higher risk of malignant hyperthermia.

TABLE 3-4. CONDITIONS WITH INCREASED ANESTHETIC RISK

Ophthalmologic
Strabismus
Congenital ptosis

Syndromes
Down's
Sturge-Weber
Marfan's
Homocystinuria
Craniofacial syndromes

Hemoglobinopathies
Sickle cell disease
Sickle thalassemia

Neuromuscular
Muscular dystrophy
Myotonic dystrophy

REFERENCES

Childhood and Sports-Related Eye Injuries

Bowen DI, Magauran DM: Ocular injuries caused by airgun pellets: An analysis of 105 cases. *Br Med J* 1:333, 1973.
Burke MJ, Sanitato JJ, Vinger PF, et al: Soccerball-induced eye injuries. *JAMA* 249:2682, 1983.
Caveness LS: Ocular and facial injuries in baseball. *Int Ophthalmol Clin* 28:238, 1988.
Committee on Accident and Poison Prevention. American Academy of Pediatrics: Ocular hazards. In *Injury Control for Children and Youth.* Elk Grove Village, IL, American Academy of Pediatrics, 1987, pp 226-234.
Committee on Sports Medicine. American Academy of Pediatrics: Eye injuries. In *Sports Medicine: Health Care for Young Athletes.* Evanston, IL, American Academy of Pediatrics, 1983, pp 282-296.
DeRespinis P, Caputo A, Fiore P, Wagner R: A survey of severe eye injuries in children. *AJDC* 143:711, 1989.
Elman M: Racket-sports ocular injuries. *Arch Ophthalmol* 104:1453, 1986.
Grin TR, Nelson LB, Jeffers JB: Eye injuries in childhood. *Pediatrics* 80:13, 1987.
Guyer B, Gallagher SS: An approach to the epidemiology of childhood injuries. *Pediatr Clin North Am* 32:5, 1985.
Jeffers JB: An on going tragedy: Pediatric sports-related eye injuries. *Sem Ophthalmol* 5:216, 1990.
LaRoche GR, McIntyre L, Schertzer RM: Epidemiology of severe eye injuries in childhood. *Ophthalmology* 95:1603, 1988.
Liggett PE, Pince KJ, Barlow W, et al: Ocular trauma in an urban population: Review of 1132 cases. *Ophthalmology* 97:581, 1990.
Nelson LB, Wilson TW, Jeffers JB: Eye injuries in childhood: Demography, etiology and prevention. *Pediatrics* 84:438, 1989.
Pashby T: Eye injuries in Canadian amateur hockey. *Can J Ophthalmol* 20:2, 1985.
Rapoport I, Romen M, Kinek M, et al: Eye injuries in children in Israel: A nationwide collaborative study. *Arch Ophthalmol* 108:376, 1990.
Simmons S, Krohel G, Hay P: Prevention of ocular gunshot injuries using polycarbonate lenses. *Ophthalmology* 91:977, 1984.
Sternberg P, de Juan E Jr, Green WR, et al: Ocular BB injuries. *Ophthalmology* 91:1269, 1984.
Strahlman E, Elman M, Daub E, Baker S: Causes of pediatric eye injuries: A population based study. *Arch Ophthalmol* 108:603, 1990.
Vinger PF: The eye in sports medicine. In Duane TD (ed): *Clinical Ophthalmology.* Philadelphia, Harper & Row, 1986, 5:chap 45.
Young DW, Little JM: Pellet-gun eye injuries. *Can J Ophthalmol* 20:9, 1985.

Child Abuse

Alexander RC, Crabbe L, Sato Y, et al: Serial abuse in children who are shaken. *Am J Dis Child* 144:58, 1990.

Alexander RC, Schor DP, Smith WL: Magnetic resonance imaging of intracranial injuries from child abuse. *J Pediatr* 109:975, 1986.
Caffey J: The whiplash shaken infant syndrome: Manual shaking by the extremities with whiplash-induced intracranial and intraocular bleedings, linked with residual permanent brain damage and mental retardation. *Pediatrics* 54:396, 1974.
Elner SG, Elner VM, Arnall M, Albert DM: Ocular and associated systemic findings in suspected child abuse. *Arch Ophthalmol* 108:1094, 1990.
Friendly DS: Ocular manifestations of physical child abuse. *Trans Am Acad Ophthalmol Otolaryngol* 75:318, 1971.
Gaynon MW, Koh H, Marmor MF, Frankel LR: Retinal folds in the shaken baby syndrome. *Am J Ophthalmol* 106:423, 1988.
Giangiacomo J, Barkett KJ: Ophthalmoscopic findings in occult child abuse. *J Pediatr Ophthalmol Strabismus* 22:234, 1985.
Gilliland MGF, Luckenbach MW, Massicotte SJ, Folberg R: The medicolegal implications of detecting hemosiderin in the eyes of children who are suspected of being abused. *Arch Ophthalmol* 109:321, 1991.
Greenwald MJ: The shaken baby syndrome. *Sem Ophthalmol* 5:202, 1990.
Jensen AD, Smith RE, Olson MI: Ocular clues to child abuse. *J Pediatr Ophthalmol Strabismus* 8:270, 1971.
Levin AV: Ocular manifestations of child abuse. *Ophthalmol Clin North Am* 3:249, 1990.
Levin AV, Magnusson MR, Rafto SE, Zimmerman RA: Shaken baby syndrome diagnosed by magnetic resonance imaging. *Pediatr Emerg Care* 5:181, 1989.
Levy I, Wysenbeek YS, Nitzan M, et al: Occult ocular damage as the leading sign in the battered child syndrome. *Metabol Pediatr Systemic Ophthalmol* 13:20, 1990.
Ludwig S, Warman M: Shaken baby syndrome: A review of 20 cases. *Ann Emerg Med* 13:104, 1984.
Merten DF, Carpenter BLM: Radiologic imaging of inflicted injury in the child abuse syndrome. *Pediatr Clin North Am* 37:815, 1990.
Newton RW: Intracranial hemorrhage and non-accidental injury. *Arch Dis Child* 64:188, 1989.
Rao N, Smith RE, Choi JH, et al: Autopsy findings in the eyes of fourteen fatally abused children. *Forensic Sci Int* 39:293, 1988.
Reece RM, Grodin MA: Recognition of nonaccidental injury. *Pediatr Clin North Am* 32:41, 1985.
Spaide RF, Swengel RM, Scharre DW, Mein CE: Shaken baby syndrome. *Am Fam Physician* 41:1145, 1990.
Tomasi LG, Rosman NP: Purtscher retinopathy in the battered child syndrome. *Am J Dis Child* 129:1335, 1975.
Wilkinson WS, Han DP, Rappley MD, Owings CL: Retinal hemorrhage predicts neurological injury in the shaken baby syndrome. *Arch Ophthalmol* 107:1472, 1989.
Williams DF, Meiler WF, Williams GA: Posterior segment manifestations of ocular trauma. *Retina* 10 (suppl):S35, 1990.

Anesthesia

Alpert CC, Salazar FG: Chloral hydrate sedation in children. *Am J Ophthalmol* 90:877, 1980.
Carabelle RW: Chloral hydrate. A useful pediatric sedative. *Am J Ophthalmol* 51:834, 1961.
Fox BES, O'Brien CO, Kangas KJ, Murphree AL, Wright KW: Use of high dose chloral hydrate for ophthalmic exams in children: A retrospective review of 302 cases. *J Pediatr Ophthalmol Strabismus* 27:242, 1990.
Jastak JT, Pallasch T: Death after chloral hydrate sedation: Report of a case. *J Am Dent Assoc* 116:345, 1988.
Judisch GF, Anderson S, Bell WE: Chloral hydrate sedation as a substitute for examination under anesthesia in pediatric ophthalmology. *Am J Ophthalmol* 89:560, 1980.
Nathan JE: Management of the refractory young child with chloral hydrate: Dosage selection. *J Dent Child* 54:93, 1987.
O'Malley PJ: Approach to the emergency pediatric patient. In Wilkins EW Jr (ed): *Emergency Medicine*. Baltimore, Williams and Wilkins, 1989, pp 495–486.
Whitacre MM, Ellis PP: Outpatient sedation for ocular examination. *Surv Ophthalmol* 28:643, 1984.

II

Ocular and Orbital Trauma

4

Eyelid Injuries

Robert A. Catalano

HISTORY

All patients with eyelid injuries should be questioned regarding the method, nature, and time of their injury. If a repair under general anesthesia is contemplated, the nature and time of their last meal is also important information. With children, more accurate information can occasionally be obtained in the absence of parents. Children who perceive parental disapproval often give erroneous or false histories.

General guidelines for history taking are noted in Chapter 1. For injuries to the eyelids and orbit, careful attention should be given to the possibility of foreign bodies or organic contamination. A history of an animal bite should be reported to the local or state health department and consideration given for rabies prophylaxis. The history should ascertain whether the patient is taking any anticoagulants, including aspirin, or has sickle cell disease. Epinephrine should not be used in the local anesthetic in sicklers. The status of tetanus immunization should be ascertained. Alcohol and recreational drug use are often associated with eyelid and orbital trauma. Any evidence of their use should be noted on the patient's record, and unless the injury is vision threatening, necessary surgery should be temporized until informed consent can be obtained. Finally, photographs should be taken or sketches drawn to document the injury.

PREPARATION OF THE PATIENT

The patient, or a responsible other, should be psychologically prepared with a frank discussion of the extent of injury and the preoperative functional and visual status. Realistic goals of the initial treatment, and anticipated or potential future treatments, should be clearly described and documented. Systemic conditions that can compromise treatment should be stabilized prior to treatment.

ECCHYMOSIS OF THE EYELID

Most orbital contusions due to blunt injuries cause soft tissue damage with little or no disability. Blunt trauma, however, can be associated with blowout or other orbital fractures, hyphema, angle recession, iridodialysis, retinal edema, and retinal breaks. Deep orbital bleeding can cause compression of the optic nerve or ophthalmic artery. Therefore, evaluation of orbital contusions includes a complete ocular examination. Examination of the peripheral retina, using scleral depression, may have to wait until orbital edema subsides. The examination should not be delayed, however, in patients symptomatic for a retinal break.

The distribution of hemorrhage can occasionally foretell a serious orbital injury. Blood under the superior conjunctiva suggests an orbital roof fracture. Basilar skull fractures are sometimes associated with a ringlike distribution of periorbital blood. Hemorrhage in the lower lid and inferior orbit may signal an orbital floor fracture.

Blunt trauma can also result in ptosis (droopy eyelid) secondary to a hematoma of the eyelid or levator palpebrae muscle (Figure 4–1). A permanent ptosis can result if the aponeurosis is stretched or torn. Fingers or hooks caught under the upper eyelid often result in this type of injury.

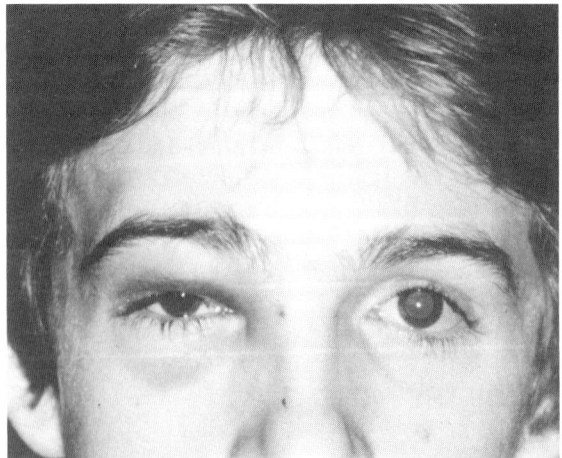

FIGURE 4–1. Eyelid ecchymosis and traumatic ptosis.

Treatment of lid ecchymoses consists of cold compresses for the initial 24-hour period followed by warm compresses as needed.

EYELID LACERATIONS

Evaluation and Initial Considerations

The particularities of the management of eyelid lacerations can be stated as six A's (assessment, anticoagulants, antitetanus, antirabies, antibiotics, anesthesia) and repair.

Assessment

A severe underlying injury to the eye may be associated with even the most negligible eyelid injury. The initial evaluation of any injury in the region of the eye must include a carefully documented (preferably photographically) ocular examination, with an assessment of visual acuity unless the patient is unconscious. Vision-threatening injuries to the globe always take precedence over eyelid injuries.

The overriding concern in evaluating an eyelid injury is to avoid aggravating a coexisting injury to the globe or compromise its repair. A protective eye shield will ensure that pressure is not transmitted to the eyeball, even if one is very certain that the eye is uninvolved, until the treatment is complete (Figure 4–2). Trained personnel should accompany the patient during diagnostic imaging or other studies where dressings may be disturbed.

If the integrity of the globe is certain, the eyelids and orbital region are evaluated in a stepwise fashion, from the eyelashes to the orbital septum, documenting any anatomic abnormalities, infection, or hemorrhage. Using sterile gloves, the physician can palpate the facial bones for crepitation, foreign bodies, or fragments of loose bones. Wounds should never be extended except when necessary to explore for an organic foreign body at the time of repair. Copious irrigation may be helpful in assessing the structures involved and the depth of involvement. Between the initial evaluation and subsequent treatment, moistened dressings should be placed on skin lacerations.

Visual acuity should be monitored frequently for the first 24 hours in patients sustaining lacerations deep to the orbital septum. An accumulating hematoma may compromise the optic nerve or its blood supply.

Anticoagulant Status

In emergency situations vitamin K (10 mg to 25 mg intramuscularly [IM] or subcutaneously [SC], repeated every 4 hours as necessary) can reverse a prolonged prothrombin time in 6 hours to 8 hours in patients taking direct and

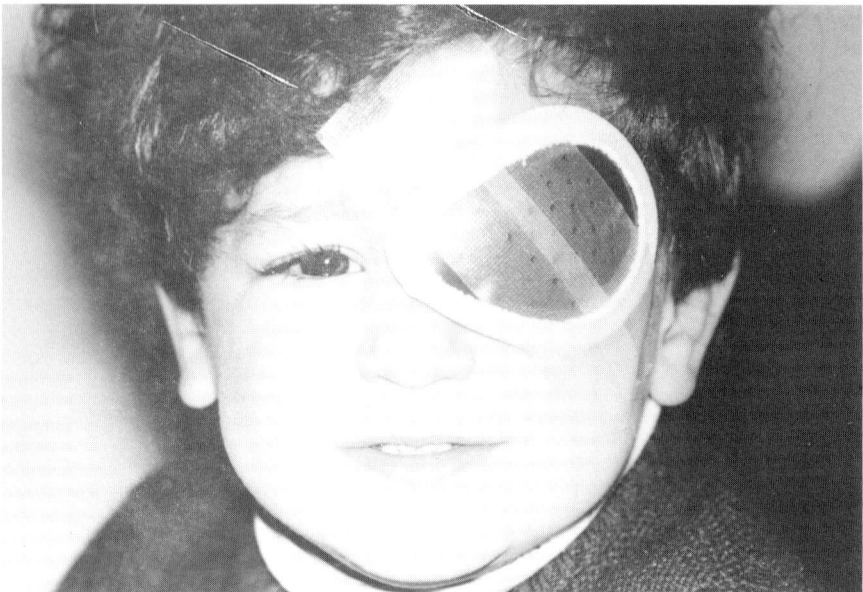

FIGURE 4–2. Eye shield used during transportation and while awaiting treatment.

indirect anticoagulants such as coumadin and warfarin. Transfusion with platelets, cryoprecipitates, or plasma may be needed in other instances.

Antitetanus Prophylaxis

The guidelines for tetanus prophylaxis are presented in Table 4–1 (and reviewed in Chapter 17). The dosage of tetanus toxoid booster is 0.5 mL IM or SC; that of human tetanus immune globulin is 250 IU intramuscularly.

TABLE 4–1. TETANUS PROPHYLAXIS IN EYELID AND ORBITAL TRAUMA

IMMUNIZATION HISTORY (DOSES)	CLEAN/NONPUNCTURE WOUNDS		ALL OTHER WOUNDS	
	Tetanus Toxoid	Human Immune Globulin	Tetanus Toxoid	Human Immune Globulin
≥ 3	No*	No	No†	No
2	Yes	No	Yes	No‡
0 to 1	Yes	No	Yes	Yes
Unknown	Yes	No	Yes	Yes

(Modified with permission from: Deutsch TA, Feller DB: *Paton and Goldberg's Management of Ocular Injuries*, 2nd ed. Philadelphia, WB Saunders Co., 1985, p 145.)
*Unless greater than 10 years since last booster.
†Unless greater than 5 years since last booster.
‡Unless wound is more than 24 hours old.

Irrigation and debridement of wounds is essential for tetanus (and rabies) prophylaxis.

Antirabies Prophylaxis

A culpable pet should be observed for 10 days for signs of illness; a wild animal should be killed and its brain tested for the presence of rabies using an available fluorescent antibody test. If prophylaxis is necessary, both passively administered antibody (human rabies immune globulin 20 IU/kg to 40 IU/kg) and vaccine (human diploid cell rabies vaccine) should be administered at the time of surgical repair. For most bites, it is recommended that one-half of the immune globulin be infiltrated at the site of the bite and the other half given intramuscularly. It may be difficult and even dangerous, however, to infiltrate this much volume in the eyelid. One milliliter of the vaccine is given on days 0, 3, 7, 14, and 28. Any questions regarding rabies protocol can be addressed to the Center for Disease Control, Viral Diseases Section, U.S. Public Health Service, Atlanta, Georgia 30333.

Antibiotics

There is no consensus on the use of antibiotics for elective eyelid surgery. Topical and systemic antibiotics, however, are usually used for trauma or infection. Debridement and irrigation with saline are helpful in reducing bacterial counts, and some surgeons irrigate wounds with ophthalmic neosporin-polymixin-gramicidin solutions at the time of repair. If contamination is suspected, a systemic antibiotic such as dicloxacillin 250 mg to 500 mg by mouth 4 times per day (for children 25 mg/kg/day to 50 mg/kg/day divided in 4 doses) covers most susceptible organisms. Cephalexin may be substituted, and penicillin should be considered for dog bites. Topical bacitracin is often used postoperatively. Additional information regarding antiobiotic use is presented in Chapters 16 and 17.

Anesthesia

The choice between general and local anesthesia is based on the severity of the ocular injury, the presence of associated neurologic or other injuries, the stability of chronic systemic conditions, the time of the patient's last meal, the ability of the patient to cooperate, and, when appropriate, the desire of the patient.

General anesthesia is mandatory to avoid orbital pressure on the globe from the infiltration of local anesthetics if the eye is lacerated. In this situation, however, depolarizing agents, such as succinylcholine, are avoided because they can cause an initial contraction of the extraocular muscles, with possible extrusion of intraocular contents. General anesthesia is also preferable to reduce orbital fractures, perform major reconstruction, or alleviate apprehension in children and some adults.

Common choices of local anesthetics are listed in Table 4-2. Even when general anesthesia is used, the operative field can be infiltrated with 0.5% to 1.0% lidocaine with epinephrine 1:100,000 to augment hemostasis. Epinephrine slows the absorption of the local anesthetic, prolonging its action and decreasing its toxicity. Hyaluronidase can be added to the local anesthetic mixture but should not be used in the absence of epinephrine. Topical ophthalmic anesthetics, proparacaine hydrochloride 0.5%, tetracaine 1.0%, and cocaine 4% can augment anesthesia if conjunctival or corneal abrasions are concomitant.

Regional Anesthesia Techniques

The van Lint technique involves local infiltration into the deep subcutaneous tissue at the orbital margin. Starting at the lateral canthal angle, the infiltration is extended superiorly and inferiorly. Up to 10 mL can usually be infiltrated.

To achieve anesthesia in the upper eyelid, the supraorbital and supratrochlear nerves can be infiltrated at the supraorbital notch. This notch can be palpated superiorly and nasally on the orbital rim. Additional anesthetic is usually infiltrated temporally in the area of the lacrimal nerve.

To achieve anesthesia of the lower eyelid, the infraorbital nerve can be infiltrated by injecting 1 mL of anesthetic into the infraorbital foramen, located 7 mm below the infraorbital rim, in line with the supraorbital notch. Additional anesthetic is usually infiltrated at the inferior temporal orbital margin.

The O'Brien technique involves infiltration of the facial nerve just anterior to the condyloid process of the mandible. The area just below and anterior to the tragus of the ear is used as a landmark to find the condyloid process. The

TABLE 4-2. LOCAL ANESTHETIC AGENTS

GENERIC NAME	MAXIMUM SAFE DOSE*	DURATION OF ACTION (Min)	REMARKS
Procaine 0.5%	1000 mg	60–90	Lowest potency and shortest duration
Xylocaine 0.5% to 2.0%	500 mg	90–200	Intermediate potency, rapid onset
Mepivacaine 0.5% to 1.0%	500 mg	120–240	Similar to Xylocaine
Bupivacaine 0.25% to 0.75%	200 mg	180–400	Longer duration, slowest onset

*Maximum safe doses include the use of epinephrine 1:100,000. When epinephrine is not used, the maximum safe dose listed must be reduced (e.g., without epinephrine, the maximum safe dose of xylocaine is 300 mg). The dose should also be reduced for children, elderly, and debilitated patients.

condyloid process can be felt to move as the patient opens his or her mouth. Two milliliters to 3 mL is injected just anterior to the joint, with the patient's mouth closed. This technique avoids lid swelling. Control of hemostasis, achieved by infiltrating epinephrine at the wound site, however, is sacrificed.

The retrobulbar technique is useful when the bulbar conjunctiva needs to be manipulated or when ocular motility is undesirable. A no. 23 35 mm Atkinson retrobulbar needle with a sharp but rounded tip is used. One common technique directs the patient to look upward and medially as the needle is introduced just above the inferior orbital rim at the junction of its middle and lateral thirds. The needle is directed upward and slightly inward toward the orbital apex, behind the globe. The plunger is retracted to ensure that a vessel has not been penetrated, and 1 mL to 3 mL of anesthetic is infiltrated.

Tarsal anesthesia is occasionally necessary for eyelid repairs. Injection is made from the conjunctival side, at the supratarsal border in the upper eyelid, and the infratarsal border in the lower eyelid.

Figure 4–3 illustrates most of these techniques.

Operative Techniques

To protect the cornea from abrasion, a plastic corneal shell is used during the repair (Figure 4–4). Topical anesthetic is used prior to installation, and for further protection, the shell can be coated with an antibiotic ointment.

The surrounding skin is cleaned with surgical soaps and/or betadine. Because betadine can devitalize tissue, it is not used on the wound itself. Rather, copious irrigation with saline or antibiotic solution is performed. Tissue separation during irrigation helps wash away foreign matter. Necrotic tissue is debrided. The eyelashes may be trimmed if necessary (they regrow within 4 to 6 weeks), but eyebrows should not be shaved because they may grow back irregularly or not at all. Draping of the skin should always include a head drape; cotton in the ear protects the patient from the annoyance of blood or irrigating solutions entering the ear canal. If oxygen is used under the drapes, the surgeon should request that it be turned off during cautery. Numerous reports exist of flash burns to the face from the use of cautery in the presence of cannulated oxygen.

A description of intricate skin and muscle transposition and graft techniques is beyond the scope of this book, but specific notes on the repair of minor injuries follow Table 4–3.

Small losses of eyelid skin without involvement of the eyelid margin can be repaired with slight undermining of the surrounding tissue. Small areas can be allowed to epithelialize spontaneously.

For lid margin lacerations with minimal loss of tissue, primary closure can usually be accomplished if one-fourth or less of the eyelid margin has been lost. Ragged edges are excised to give straight surgical margins to suture. The three-

FACIAL AND ORBITAL ANESTHESIA

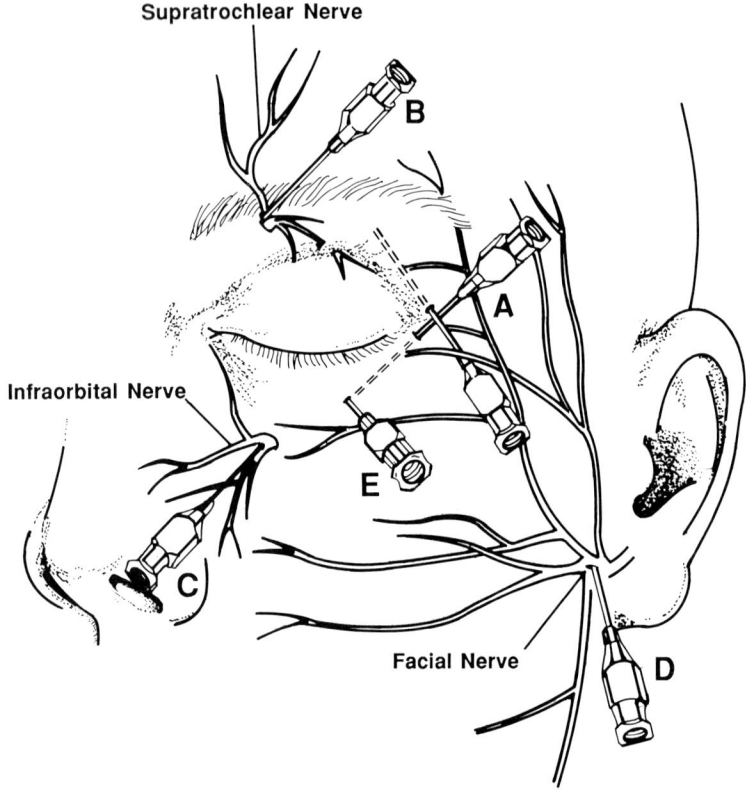

FIGURE 4–3. Regional anesthetic blocks: (A) van Lint, (B) supraorbital, (C) infraorbital, (D) O'Brien, (E) retrobulbar. (Modified with permission from Paton D, Goldberg MF: *Management of Ocular Injuries.* Philadelphia, WB Saunders Co, 1976, p 28.)

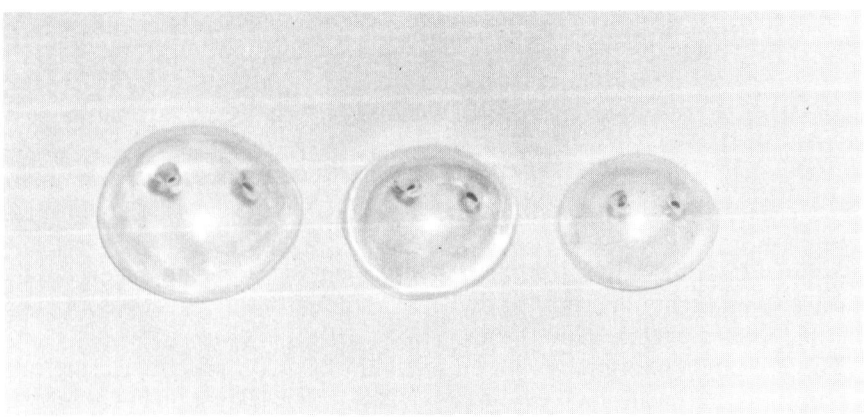

FIGURE 4–4. Adult and pediatric eye shields used to protect the globe during eyelid repairs.

TABLE 4-3. BASIC TENETS REGARDING THE REPAIR OF EYELID LACERATIONS

A delay of 48 to 72 hours, until optimum patient and operative conditions can be obtained, will not compromise the outcome of most eyelid lacerations.

Tissue should be conserved for later reconstruction. The eyelid is very vascular. Even tissue suspended by a narrow pedicle and "free grafts" can often be salvaged.

Identifiable landmarks, such as the eyelid margin and right angle corners, should be sutured first to anatomically align the lid most effectively. The eyelashes are the most important landmark in aligning the eyelid borders.

The eyelid is composed of three layers: the skin, the orbicularis muscle, and the tarsus/palpebral conjunctiva. In lacerations that transect the tarsus, each layer should be closed separately.

6-0 or 7-0 nonabsorbable sutures are used for skin closure and removed after 4 days to 5 days to decrease scarring. Steri-strips can be applied for 3 days after removal of sutures.

The tarsus should always be closed as a separate layer, with the knots tied away from the conjunctival surface using interrupted, longer-acting, absorbable 5-0 to 6-0 sutures.

A continuous strip of tarsus, 2 mm to 3 mm wide, must be present at the lid margin to prevent dimpling. Tarsus is not absolutely necessary for lacerations that start 2 mm to 3 mm away from the lid margin.

Only parallel, preferably vertical, incisions should be made through the tarsus in fashioning sliding flaps. V-shaped incisions should never be made.

If a lid laceration contains fat, the orbital septum has been lacerated. These lacerations are associated with a higher incidence of occult globe penetration. A lacerated superior orbital septum usually should not be sutured, as this can lead to lagophthalmos. An attempt at suturing should be made only if the septum is cut vertically, opposite the direction of the orbicularis fibers. In this situation 5-0 to 6-0 absorbable (e.g., Vicryl) sutures are used.

Infected or severely burned eyelids should be managed by allowing epithelialization and formation of granulation tissue.

Postauricular skin is the best donor site for full-thickness skin grafts to the eyelid. The upper lid can be used for lower lid reconstruction, but the opposite is not true.

Except when symptomatic corneal exposure exists, it is best to delay major reconstruction of ptosis, lid retraction, or cicatricial ectropion for 6 months to 9 months.

A temporary tarsorrhaphy can effectively hold both eyelids in a healing position but should not be used if there is an underlying injury to the globe.

(Modified with permission from: Deutsch TA, Feller DB: *Paton and Goldberg's Management of Ocular Injuries,* 2d ed. Philadelphia, WB Saunders Co., 1985, p 26.)

suture technique for eyelid margin repair uses three 6-0 silk sutures to close the laceration (Figure 4–5). In children chromic catgut can be substituted to avoid the need for suture removal.

Starting at the eyelid margin, the first suture is directed 3 mm into the eyelid at the level of the tarsus. The second suture is similarly directed, just posterior to the lash line. The third suture is placed between the first two sutures at the level of the gray line. The posterior two sutures are then incorporated in the knot of the lash line suture, keeping these sutures away from the cornea. Any

LID MARGIN REPAIR

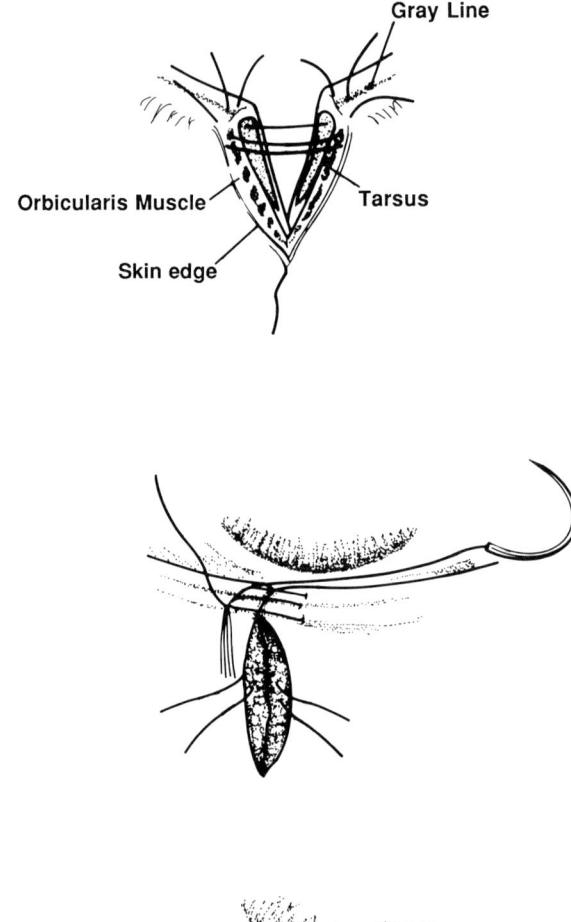

FIGURE 4–5. Three-suture technique to repair eyelid margin laceration with minimal loss of tissue.

remaining distal defect in the tarsus is closed with interrupted 5-0 or 6-0 absorbable sutures, directed through two-thirds of its thickness. The skin is closed with 6-0 silk sutures. Conjunctival sutures are not necessary because the conjunctiva will heal spontaneously if the tarsus is approximated. Skin sutures are removed in 4 days to 5 days but eyelid margin sutures are left for 10 days to 14 days.

A defect involving more than one-fourth but less than one-half of the eyelid margin can usually be closed by sliding tarsal flaps and/or a lateral canthotomy and cantholysis (Figure 4–6). A lateral canthotomy is performed using a Stevens scissors. This incision is made from the lateral canthal angle horizontally toward the orbital rim, without antecedent clamping of tissue. If this alone is not sufficient, an additional 3 mm to 5 mm of relaxation can be obtained by performing a cantholysis of the upper or lower segments of the lateral canthal tendon. The skin and conjunctiva at the canthotomy site can be closed with 6-0 silk sutures. Larger eyelid margin defects require tissue transfer techniques, such as the Tenzel semicircular flap or full thickness skin grafts.

Lacerated canaliculi are most easily repaired using the magnification of the operating microscope. A Bowman probe, placed through the punctum, can identify the proximal end of the torn canaliculus. Using the probe as a pointer and under magnification, the medial end of the canaliculus is sought. Irrigating

TECHNIQUE OF CANTHOLYSIS

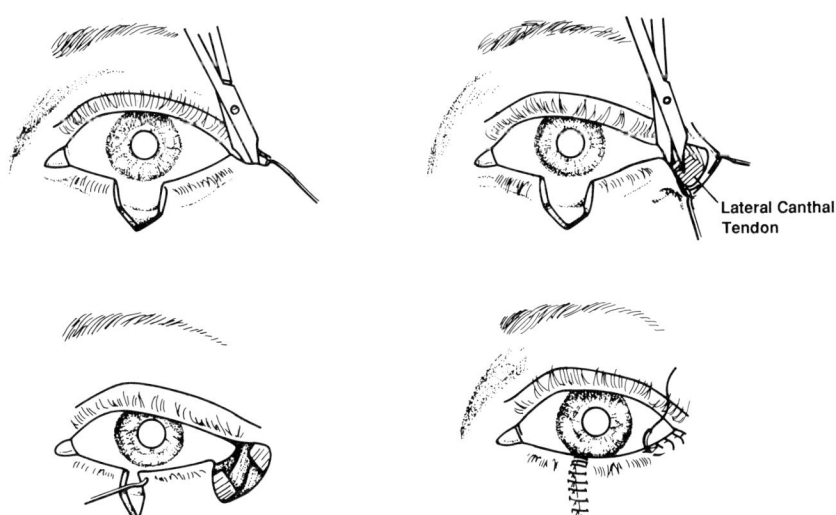

FIGURE 4–6. Technique of cantholysis to repair full thickness eyelid laceration with loss of one-fourth to one-half of the eyelid margin.

the other punctum and canaliculus can also be helpful in locating the medial end of the severed canaliculus. If both ends can be found, a silicone stent is placed through the punctum and across the wound. Depending on the tube used, the silicone can either be directed into the nose and tied under the inferior turbinate or simply through the lacrimal sac and tied at the medial canthal angle (Figure 4–7). The stent should be left in place 6 weeks to 2 months.

SPECIAL CONSIDERATIONS IN ANIMAL AND HUMAN BITES OR SCRATCHES OF THE EYELID

In the evaluation of any animal bite, a search for additional puncture wounds to the hand, occult facial fractures or cranial penetration should be made, as these commonly occur with animal bites. The latter is more prevalent in children under 2 years of age.

CANALICULAR REPAIR

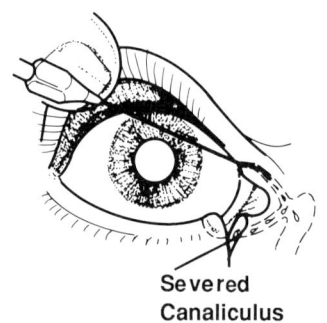

Severed Canaliculus

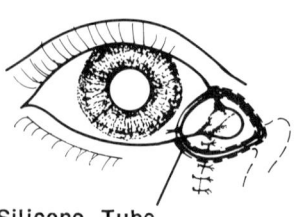

Silicone Tube

FIGURE 4–7. A method of identifying and repairing a severed canaliculus. (Modified with permission from Paton D, Goldberg MF: *Management of Ocular Injuries*. Philadelphia, WB Saunders Co, 1976, p 55.)

In addition to rabies, contamination with anaerobic and aerobic organisms is possible. Immunocompromised patients or those who have undergone a prior splenectomy are at increased risk of developing a fulminant dysgonic fermenter-2 (DF2) infection within 48 hours of a bite from a dog. This gram-negative rod is believed to be the most common bacteria in the dog mouth. Infections are heralded by a black eschar at the site of the bite and followed by septicemia and cardiovascular collapse.

The role of prophylactic antibiotics following dog bites is controversial. Complicating the management is the lack of correlation between preinfected wound cultures and Gram's stain findings, as well as the great diversity in microbes cultured from frankly infected dog bites. In patients at risk for dysgonic fermenter-2 infection, intravenous penicillin G (2 million to 4 million units every 4 hours in adults, and 75,000 U/kg per day divided every 4 hours to 6 hours in children) appears to be the antibiotic of choice. Amoxicillin/clavulanic acid (Augmentin) 40/mg/kg in three divided doses (up to 500 mg/dose) should be considered for all other bites involving the orbit. (See also Chapter 17.)

Early and effective wound decontamination is the most important principle in treating dog bites. Forceful irrigation with normal saline using a 19 gauge needle on a 35 mL syringe assists early decontamination. Surgical repair within 6 hours to 8 hours of a facial dog bite is generally recommended to prevent infection and loss of function, which can result from a delayed primary repair. Animal lacerations that present beyond this window are usually best managed by debridement and irrigation, and healing by secondary intention, due to the possibility of infection.

Periorbital cat scratches can become secondarily infected with *Pasturella multocida*. Penicillin G is the antibiotic of choice, followed by tetracycline and erythromycin in allergic individuals. *Cat scratch disease (fever)* (CSD) is a second disorder that can result from a cat scratch. The probable etiologic agent is a small, pleomorphic gram-negative bacillus. This disorder is heralded by a painless papule at the site of the scratch 1 week to 2 weeks following the injury, followed by regional lymphadenopathy (Figure 4-8). Low-grade fever, malaise, fatigue, and anorexia may last for 2 months to 3 months, and the lymph glands may become secondarily infected. When it involves the conjunctiva, granulomatous nodules develop on the affected side, with chemosis, injection, and a watery discharge (Figure 4-9). A CSD skin test is available and may be helpful in diagnosis. Treatment is generally reserved for secondary infections of the lymph glands. Ciprofloxacin 500 mg, by mouth, twice daily, has recently been reported as efficacious in adults with CSD (Holley, 1991).

Human bites may cause serious aerobic and anaerobic infections. Broad-spectrum prophylaxis with penicillin G and a penicillinase-resistant penicillin or cephalosporin is generally recommended. Two distinct types of *"rat bite fever"* have also been described. The first, Haverhill fever, consists of fever, malaise, and a migratory polyarticular arthritis. The etiologic organism is

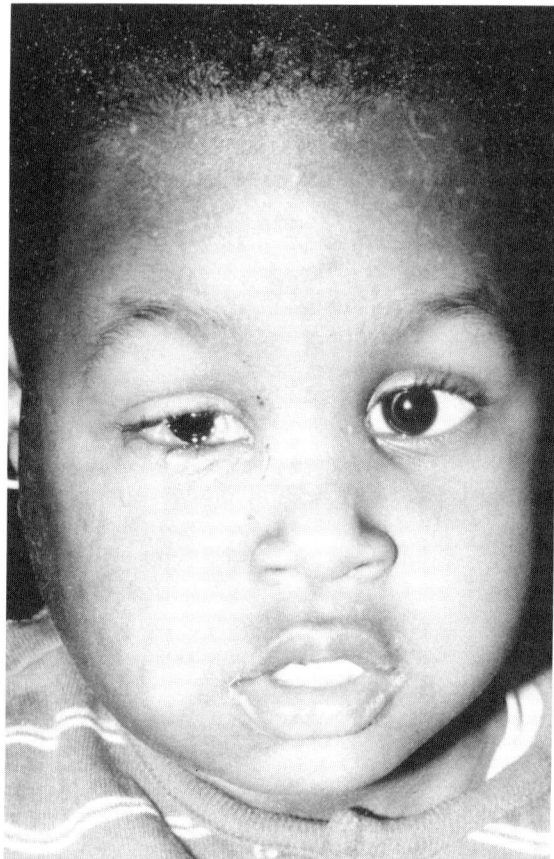

FIGURE 4–8. Massive hemifacial lymphadenopathy in cat scratch fever.

Streptobacillus moniliformis. The second, Sodoku, consists of erythema and eschar formation at the site of the injury, followed by a rash. Both are treated with penicillin; recurrences and relapses can occur in untreated cases.

FOREIGN BODIES EMBEDDED IN THE EYELID AND ORBIT

Irrigation and scraping of tissue is usually sufficient to remove superficial foreign bodies from the eyelid. (See also Chapters 8 and 17.) The treatment of deeper foreign bodies is based on any associated infectious or ocular problems. Some metallic and plastic orbital foreign bodies, such as small lead particles and methyl-methacrylate, are essentially inert. They need to be removed only

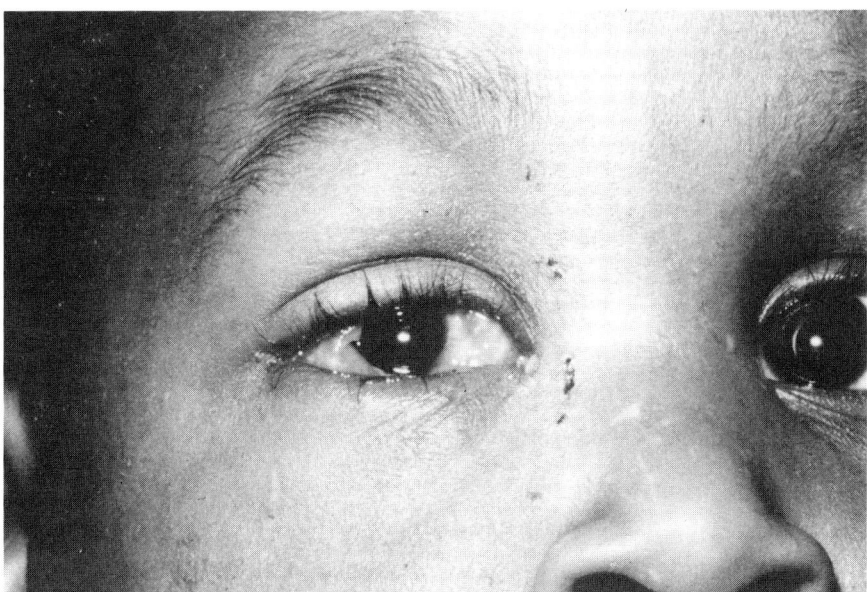

FIGURE 4-9. Nodular, granulomatous reaction with chemosis and erythema in cat scratch fever.

if they interfere with ocular motility or cause diplopia or a secondary reactive edema in the sclera and retina. Wood is a particularly difficult foreign body to remove effectively. If all wood fragments are not completely removed, chronic suppuration and further extrusion of retained foreign material may ensue for months.

Deep metallic foreign bodies can be visualized on plain film radiography (Figure 4-10). Axial and coronal computed tomography, performed with attenuation of the beam to allow only bone visualization, is helpful in localizing most other orbital foreign bodies (Figure 4-11). Magnetic resonance imaging (MRI) scanning may be better in localizing wooden foreign bodies.

Prophylactic antibiotic coverage for intraorbital foreign bodies and orbital cellulitis is reviewed in Chapters 8 and 16. The status of the patient's tetanus immunization should also be assessed and updated as necessary.

TRAUMATIC PTOSIS

A hemorrhage in the levator muscle can occur with a contusion injury to the upper eyelid, causing traumatic ptosis (Figure 4-12). This generally resolves within 6 months to 9 months, and surgical correction is therefore initially temporized. Any accompanying ocular motility disturbance should be corrected before surgical repair of the ptosis.

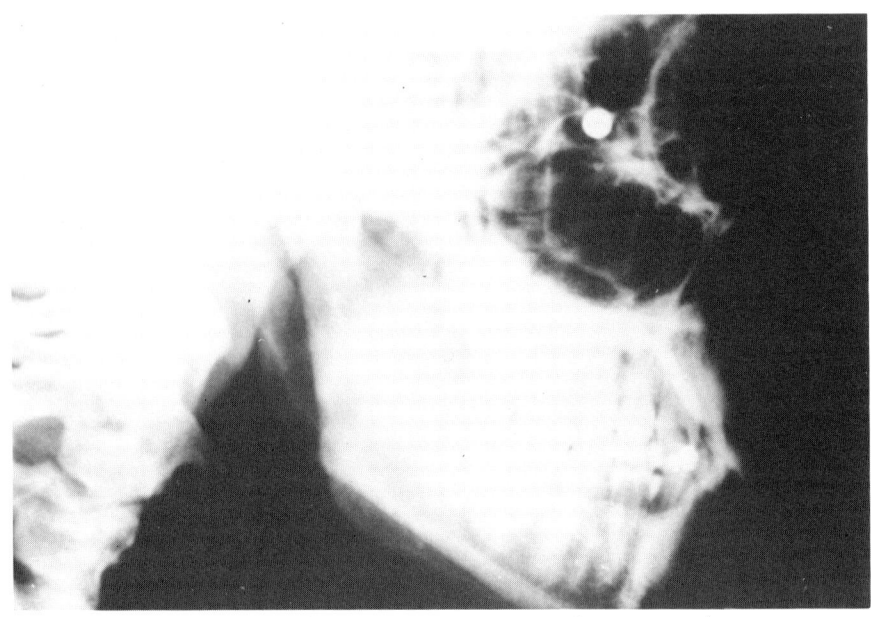

FIGURE 4–10. Lateral radiograph demonstrating intraorbital BB pellet.

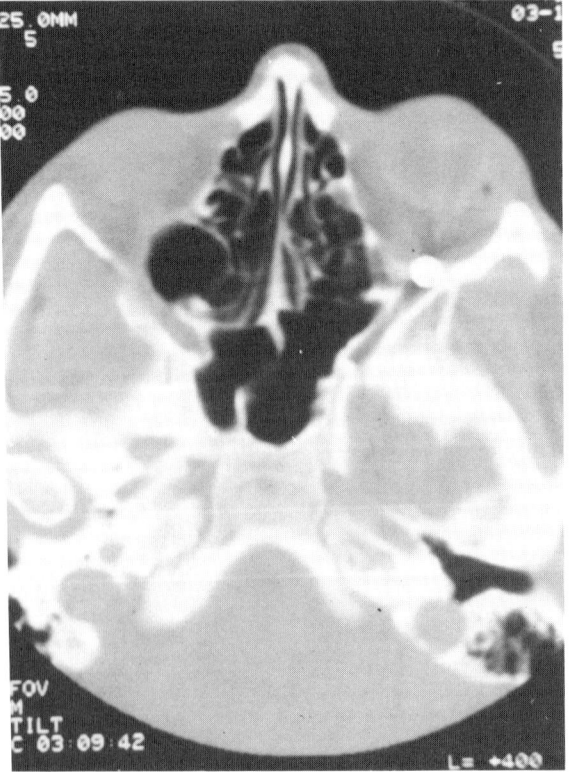

FIGURE 4–11. Computed axial tomograph demonstrating BB pellet in posterior orbit.

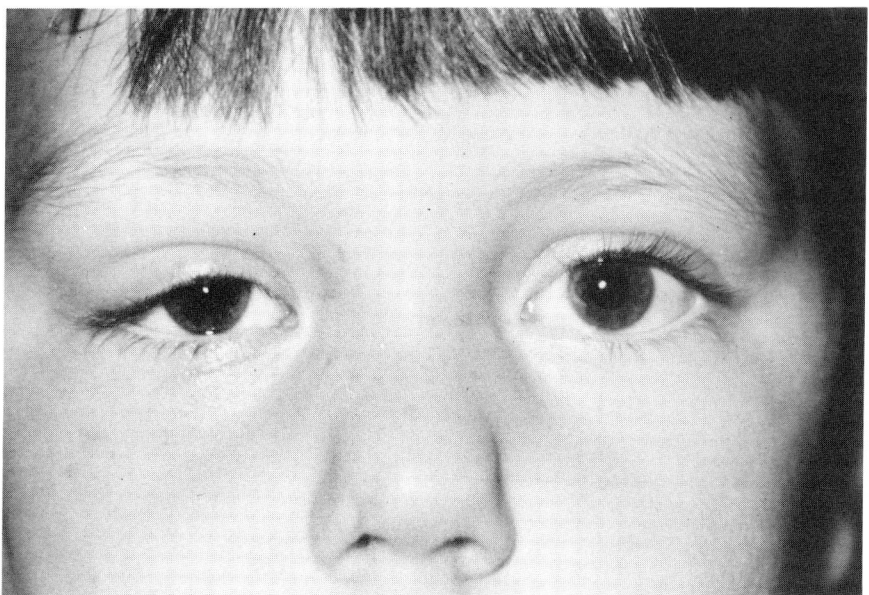

FIGURE 4-12. Traumatic ptosis following dog bite.

A readily apparent traumatic disinsertion, or laceration, of the levator aponeurosis should be repaired at the time of eyelid suturing. A completely severed levator muscle can often be found by isolating the superior rectus muscle and exploring its dorsal border. Lacerations should be sutured with 5-0 or 6-0 nonabsorbable sutures. The technique illustrated in Figure 4-13 is useful if the aponeurosis has been disinserted from the tarsus. Three 5-0 double-armed, nonabsorbable sutures are placed through the tarsus, 3 mm to 4 mm above the eyelid margin. Both arms of each suture are then placed through the aponeurosis. Adjustment of lid position is possible in the awake patient by having the patient look upward. Eyelid creases can be recreated by placing two to three sutures from the skin layer through the superficial aponeurosis.

TRAUMATIC RETROBULBAR HEMORRHAGE

During the first 24 hours of blunt or penetrating orbital injuries (especially if the orbital septum is penetrated), a retrobulbar hematoma can accumulate. (See also Chapter 5.) This is suggested by dissection of the conjunctiva anteriorly by hemorrhage and tension and proptosis of orbital tissues (Figure 4-14). The intraocular pressure can be secondarily increased and the optic nerve or

LEVATOR REPAIR

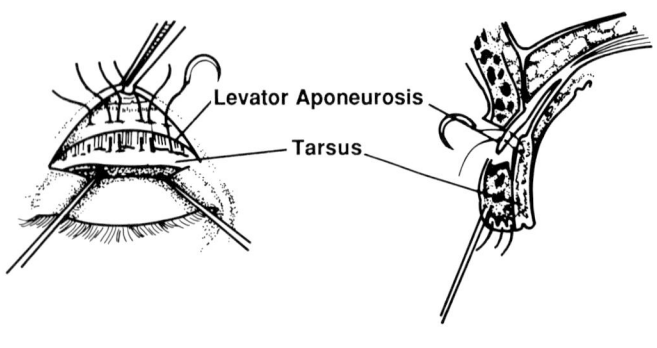

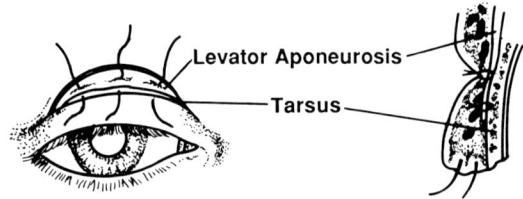

FIGURE 4–13. Technique to repair a disinserted levator aponeurosis.

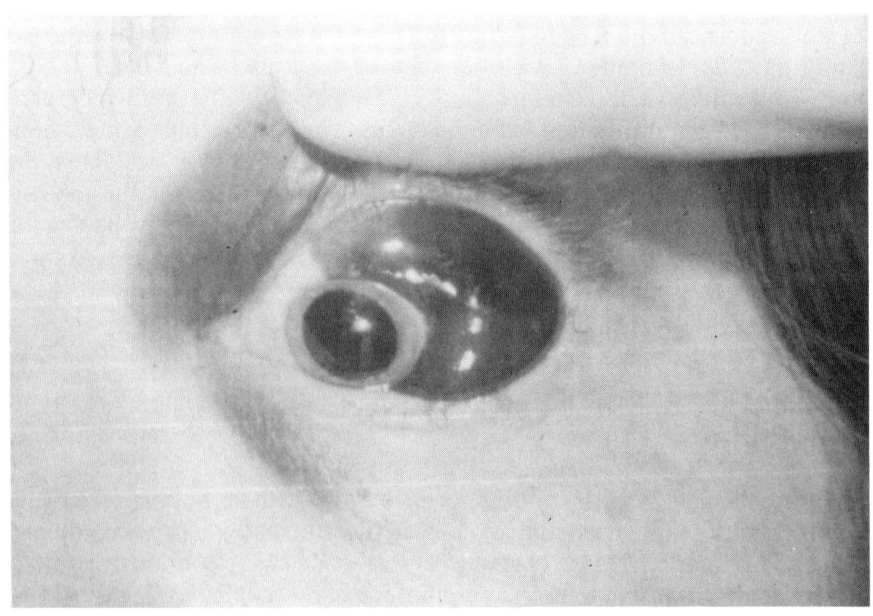

FIGURE 4–14. Traumatic retrobulbar hemorrhage dissecting anteriorly.

its blood supply compressed. If this occurs, any previously sutured wounds should be opened and clots evacuated. If this technique is unsuccessful, a canthotomy and cantholysis of both limbs of the canthal tendon should be performed. Through the same incision, the lateral attachments of the orbital septum can also be divided. Finally, the orbital septum can be opened widely. Ocular massage, systemic acetazolamide, topical beta-blockers, or paracentesis can be combined to lower the intraocular pressure further.

THERMAL AND CHEMICAL BURNS OF THE EYELIDS

With most thermal burns, the globe is protected because of reflex closure of the eyelids. (See also Chapter 7.) In house fires, individuals reflexively cover their face with their hands. A first-degree skin burn is very superficial, involving only the epidermis; a sunburn is an example. Signs are erythema, edema, pain to touch, and warmth. A second-degree burn involves the epidermis and part of the dermis. Pain and blisters are usually present, but the skin heals with minimal scarring. A third-degree burn involves the full thickness of the dermis, with charring of the skin. Pain and blisters are absent because the nerves and vascular supply are destroyed.

The ophthalmologic examination should be performed as early as feasible because the eyelids become very edematous within 24 hours to 48 hours of most burns. Unnecessary delay may result in the need for painful lid retraction to examine the eye. Edema also prevents blinking and increases the susceptibility of ocular infection. As the edema resolves, an ectropion can develop, resulting in corneal exposure. Damage to the meibomian glands or the conjunctiva can result in corneal drying.

Unlike thermal burns, chemical burns usually injure the eye as well as the adnexa. Emergency treatment consists of copious, immediate irrigation with water or saline. Local debridement and removal of foreign particles should be performed while still irrigating. Irrigation should generally be continued for at least 30 minutes and can be continued for 48 hours with some alkali burns (see Chapter 7).

After lavage, silver sulfadiazine or bacitracin ointment is applied to the eyelid. Some studies have suggested that prophylactic ocular treatment may lead to conjunctival colonization with virulent gram-negative bacteria. Initially, therefore, ocular lubricants alone should be used. Repeated cultures of the burned area and conjunctiva indicate whether an antibiotic preparation should be used. Elevation of the head may reduce swelling. Treatment of corneal exposure is best performed using lubricating ointments and a "Saran wrap" moisture chamber (Figure 4–15). Tarsorrhaphy can cause further distortion of the eyelid and is generally avoided. Burns involving the medial eyelid can cause closure of the puncta and canaliculi. Daily dilation of the puncta or silicone intubation may be necessary.

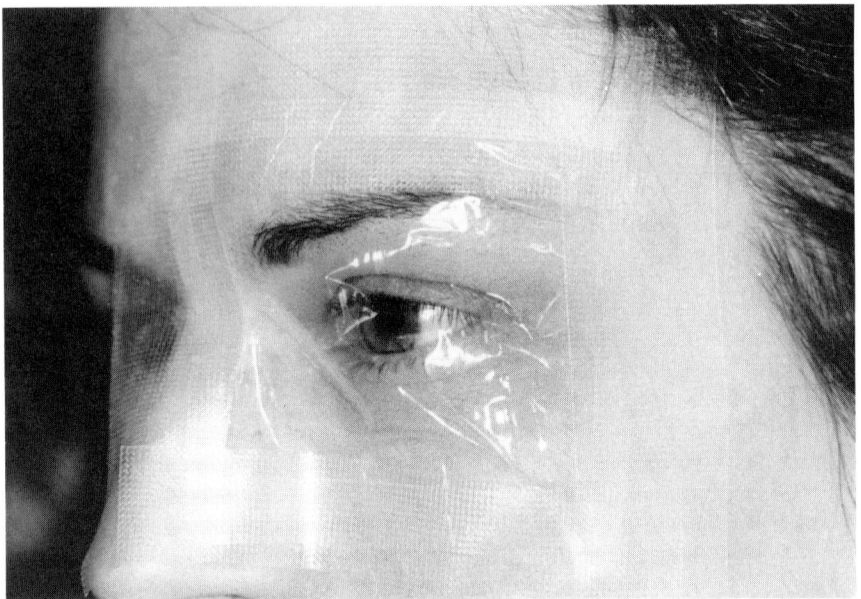

FIGURE 4-15. "Saran wrap" moisture chamber used to protect against corneal exposure.

TOXIC AND ALLERGIC EYELID REACTIONS

Certain individuals develop a *contact dermatitis* to topical medications, particularly atropine and neomycin (Figure 4-16). Often the lower eyelid skin and cheek are preferentially involved, suggesting a local hypersensitivity. The affected skin becomes erythematous and boggy; itching and irritation may be profound. Following removal of the allergan or irritant, cool saline compresses should be applied. Topical fluorinated corticosteroid lotions can be used in severe cases.

Hereditary angioedema (angioneurotic edema) is characterized by repeated attacks of eyelid and facial skin edema; the respiratory and intestinal tracts may also be involved. In contrast to contact dermatitis, urticaria does not occur, but skin involvement may be well demarcated. The disorder is due to an inherited deficiency of C-1 esterase inhibitor, a protein that inactivates the first component of the complement pathway. The pathway becomes uncontrollably activated by trauma, physical exertion, infections, rapid changes in temperature, emotional stress, menstruation, and other poorly understood stimuli. Three groups of medications have been found helpful: antifibrinolytic agents (tranexamic acid 3 g/day in adults), anabolic steroids (methyltestosterone, danazol, or oxymethalone), and fresh frozen plasma. In rare instances, orbital edema can threaten the optic nerve and globe, requiring surgical decompression.

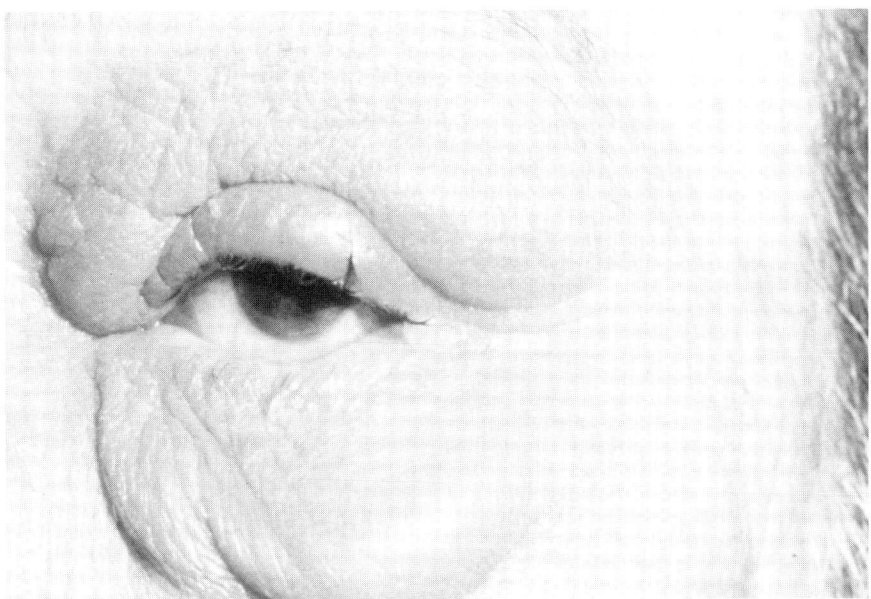

FIGURE 4-16. Contact dermatitis secondary to topical atropine use.

INDICATIONS FOR OPHTHALMOLOGIC REFERRAL

Consideration for referral should be given for any eyelid laceration requiring a complicated or microsurgical repair: lacerations involving the lacrimal drainage apparatus, the levator aponeurosis, the medial or lateral canthal tendon, and those with extensive tissue loss or intraorbital foreign bodies.

A complete ocular examination should be performed prior to the surgical repair of any eyelid lacerations and as an immediate step in patients with thermal or chemical burns of the eyelid.

REFERENCES

Beyer-Machule CK, Shapiro A: Skin wound repair in orbital and periorbital trauma. In Hornblass A (ed): *Oculoplastic, Orbital and Reconstructive Surgery.* Baltimore, Williams and Wilkins, 1988, 1:415–421.

Bruce RA Jr, McGoldrick K, Oppenheimer P: *Anesthesia for Ophthalmology.* Birmingham, AL, Aesculapius, 1982.

Callaham M: Controversies in antibiotic choices for bite wounds. *Ann Emerg Med* 9:79, 1988.

Deutsch TA, Feller DB: *Paton and Goldberg's Management of Ocular Injuries.* 2nd ed. Philadelphia, WB Saunders Co, 1985, pp 9–36, 93–103, 145.

Dortzbach RK, Angrist RA: Silicone intubation for lacerated lacrimal canaliculi. *Ophthalmic Surg* 16:639, 1985.

Edlich RF, Spengler MD, Rodeheaver GT, et al: Emergency department management of mammalian bites. *Emerg Med Clin North Am* 4:595, 1986.
Engrav LH, Heimbach DM, Walkinshaw MD, et al: Excision of burns of the face. *Plast Reconstr Surg* 77:774, 1986.
Frank A, Wachtel T: The early treatment and reconstruction of eyelid burns. *J Trauma* 23:874, 1983.
Friedlaender MH: Contact allergy and toxicity in the eye. *Int Ophthalmol Clin* 28:317, 1988.
Garber PF, Macdonald D, Beyer-Machule CK: Management of trauma to the eyelids. In Smith BC (ed): *Ophthalmic Plastic and Reconstructive Surgery.* St. Louis, CV Mosby Co, 1987, 1:437–469.
Gonnering RS: Orbital and periorbital dog bites. In Bosniak SL, Smith BC (eds): *Advances in Ophthalmic Plastic and Reconstructive Surgery.* Elmsford, NY, Pergamon Press, 1988, 7:171–180.
Gonnering RS: Eyebrow reconstruction. In Hornblass A (ed): *Oculoplastic, Orbital and Reconstructive Surgery.* Baltimore, Williams and Wilkins, 1988, 1:291–297.
Green BF, Kraft SP, Carter KD, et al: Intraorbital wood: Detection by magnetic resonance imaging. *Ophthalmol* 97:608, 1990.
Hawes MJ: Canalicular lacerations. In Linberg JV (ed): *Oculoplastic and Orbital Emergencies.* Norwalk, CT, Appleton and Lange, 1990, pp 15–27.
Herman DC, Bartley GB, Walker RC: The treatment of animal bite injuries of the eye and ocular adnexa. *Ophthalmol Plast Reconstr Surg* 3:237, 1987.
Holley HP Jr: Successful treatment of cat-scratch disease with ciprofloxacin. *JAMA* 265:1563, 1991.
Kalb R, Kaplan MH, Tenebaum MJ, et al: Cutaneous infection at dog bite wounds associated with fulminant DF-2 septicemia. *Am J Med* 78:687, 1985.
Kaplan AP: The pathogenesis of urticaria and angioedema: Recent advances. *Am J Med* 70:755, 1981.
Konovitch B: Anesthesia. In Smith BC (ed): *Ophthalmic Plastic and Reconstructive Surgery.* St. Louis, CV Mosby Co, 1987, 1:405–414.
Kulwin DR, Kersten RC: Acute eyelid and periocular burns. In Linberg JV (ed): *Oculoplastic and Orbital Emergencies.* Norwalk, CT, Appleton and Lange, 1990, pp 77–85.
McNab AA, Collin JRO: Eyelid and canthal lacerations. 13. In Linberg JV (ed): *Oculoplastic and Orbital Emergencies.* Norwalk, CT, Appleton and Lange, 1990, pp 1–13.
Marrone AC: Thermal eyelid burns. In Hornblass A (ed): *Oculoplastic, Orbital and Reconstructive Surgery.* Baltimore, Williams and Wilkins, 1988, 1:433–447.
Mindlin AM, Nesi FA, Silver B, Lisman RD: Basic concepts in eyelid repair. In Smith BC (ed): *Ophthalmic Plastic and Reconstructive Surgery.* St. Louis, CV Mosby Co, 1987, 1:417–436.
Montandon D, Maillard GF, Morax S, Garey LJ: *Plastic and Reconstructive Surgery of the Orbital Region.* New York, Churchill Livingstone, 1991.
Mustardé JC (ed): *Repair and Reconstruction in the Orbital Region.* 3d ed. New York, Churchill Livingstone, 1991.
Ordog GJ, Balasubramanium S, Wassaberger J: Rat bites: Fifty cases. *Ann Emerg Med* 14:126, 1985.
Roen JL, Della Rocca RC: Basic principles of ophthalmic plastic surgery. In Smith BC (ed): *Ophthalmic Plastic and Reconstructive Surgery.* St. Louis, CV Mosby Co, 1987, 1:345–356.
Spoor TCV, Nesi FA: *Management of Ocular, Orbital and Adnexal Trauma.* New York, Raven Press, 1988.
Tsur H: Eyelid burns: A general plastic surgeon's approach. In Hornblass A (ed): *Oculoplastic, Orbital and Reconstructive Surgery.* Baltimore, Williams and Wilkins, 1988, 1:448–454.
Zolli CL: Microsurgical repair of lacrimal canaliculus in medial canthal trauma. In Hornblass A (ed): *Oculoplastic, Orbital and Reconstructive Surgery.* Baltimore, Williams and Wilkins, 1988, 1:426–432.
Zook EG, Miller M, Van Beek AL, et al: Successful treatment protocol for canine fang injuries. *J Trauma* 20:243, 1980.

5

Blunt Injuries and Fractures of the Orbit

Robert A. Catalano

ANATOMY OF THE ORBIT AND OCULAR ADNEXA

The orbit is an anteriorly opening concavity comprised of seven bones (Figure 5-1). Described as being pear, pyramid, or cone shaped, it contains, or is associated with, seven muscles, six cranial nerves, five major foramen, four paraorbital sinuses, three different types of glands, two eyelids, and one eye.

The superior rim of the orbit is formed by the frontal bone. Along its medial border can be palpated the *supraorbital notch,* from which the supraorbital nerve and vessels emanate. Deep to the upper lateral corner of the orbit is the *lacrimal gland fossa,* within which lies the orbital portion of the lacrimal gland. Deep to the upper medial corner of the orbit lies the *trochlea.* The superior oblique muscle passes through this pulleylike structure and is reflected posteriorly to insert on the globe.

The medial orbital rim is formed by the frontal and maxillary bones. Along its inferior border a discontinuity, formed by the anterior and posterior lacrimal crests, can be palpated. The *lacrimal sac* begins within this space.

The inferior rim is formed by the maxillary and zygomatic bones. The *infraorbital foramen,* from which emanates the inferior orbital nerve and vessels, is located approximately 7 mm below the inferior orbital margin.

The lateral rim is formed by the zygoma and frontal bones. Below and deep to their suture, the lateral orbital *tubercle of Whitnall* can be palpated. Attaching to this tubercle is the lateral retinaculum.

BONES OF THE ORBIT

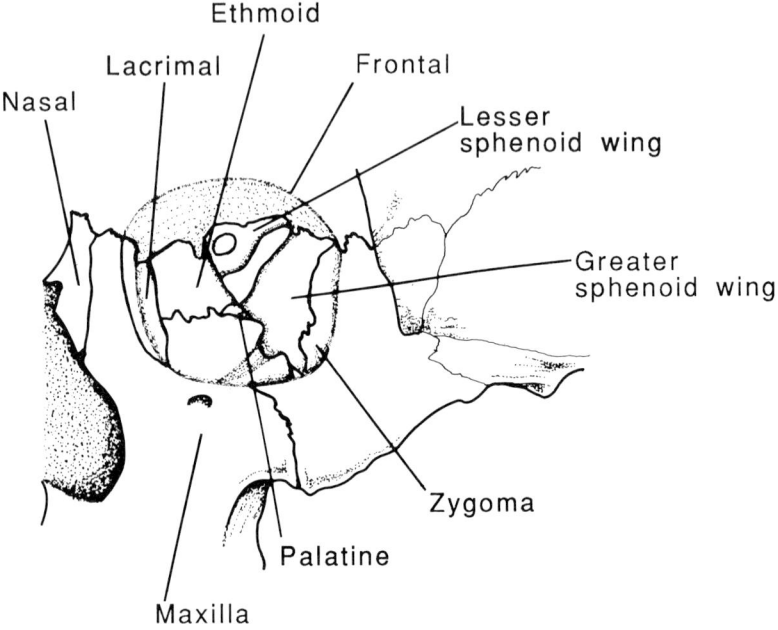

FIGURE 5-1. Bones of the orbit.

With the exception of the medial wall, which is rectangular, each of the orbital walls is triangular, tapering posteriorly to the orbital apex. The medial walls are nearly parallel, but if the lateral walls were to be extended posteriorly, they would form an approximate 90° angle with each other. The bones that contribute to each wall are listed in Table 5-1. The superior and lateral walls are composed of relatively thicker bone than the paper-thin inferior and medial walls. As a result, the inferior and medial walls are much more commonly injured in blunt orbital trauma. The orbital width (40 mm) is slightly greater than the height (35 mm). The volume of the orbit is approximately 35 cc in the adult.

The posterior orbit is primarily composed of the sphenoid bone. The greater wing forms the posterior lateral wall, and the lesser wing forms the posterior orbital roof (orbital apex). The *superior orbital fissure* is formed between the roof and lateral wall. This fissure passes laterally and upward from the orbital apex, and through it the third, fourth, and sixth cranial nerves and branches of the ophthalmic division of the fifth cranial nerve are transmitted. Because the orbital apex is one of few sites (along with the brain stem and cavernous sinus)

TABLE 5-1. BONY CONTRIBUTIONS TO THE ORBITAL WALLS

Superior
Anteriorly: Orbital plate of the frontal bone
Posteriorly: Lesser wing of the sphenoid bone

Medial
Anteriorly: Frontal process of the maxillary bone; lacrimal bone
Posteriorly: Orbital plate of the ethmoid bone; lesser wing of the sphenoid bone

Inferior
Anteriorly: Orbital plate of the maxillary bone
Posteriorly: Palatine bone
Laterally: Zygoma

Lateral
Anteriorly: Zygoma; zygomatic process of the frontal bone
Posteriorly: Greater wing of the sphenoid bone

---

where multiple cranial nerves lie together, injuries or inflammations that involve multiple cranial nerves are often localized to this area. The *inferior orbital fissure* similarly forms between the floor and the lateral wall but passes laterally and downward from the orbital apex. This fissure transmits the maxillary nerve and artery, which become the infraorbital nerve and artery at the infraorbital foramen. This nerve is often injured in orbital floor fractures, resulting in localized numbness of the cheek and upper lip. At the orbital apex, within the lesser wing of the sphenoid, lies the *optic canal*. The optic nerve, ophthalmic artery, and sympathetic nerves to the eye and orbit pass through this canal. The relative strength of the superior and lateral walls protects the optic nerve from traumatic injury.

Six extraocular muscles insert on the eye; a seventh muscle (the levator palpebrae) inserts in the upper eyelid. The muscles that insert on the eye are named according to their location and the direction they traverse to insert on the globe. Four muscles follow a straight course from the apex of the orbit to the eye and are called *rectus muscles* (Figure 5-2). Two oblique muscles also insert on the eye. The *superior oblique muscle* becomes tendinous before passing through the trochlea, where it is reflected inferiorly and posteriorly to insert in the superior temporal quadrant of the eye. The *inferior oblique muscle* arises from the anterior margin of the floor of the orbit, just lateral to the nasolacrimal groove. It passes posteriorly, laterally, and superiorly to insert in the inferior temporal quadrant of the eye.

Except for the inferior oblique, all of the extraocular muscles, and the levator palpebrae, originate in a tendinous ring that surrounds the optic canal and the medial part of the superior orbital fissure. This ring is called the *annulus of Zinn*. The third cranial, or ocular motor (CN III) nerve, innervates most of the extraocular muscles and all of the intraocular muscles. It passes in two divisions through the annulus of Zinn into the *muscle cone* to innervate the superior,

ORBITAL NERVES

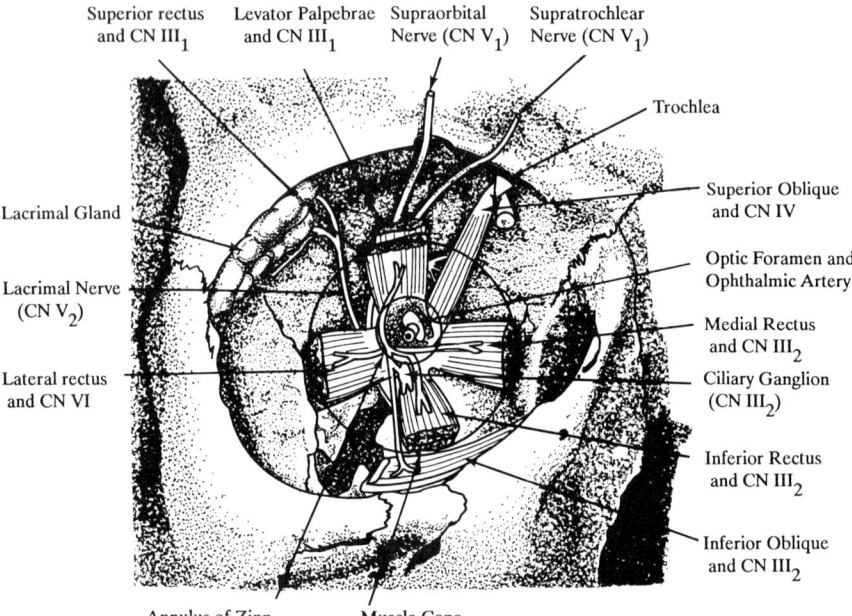

FIGURE 5-2. Extraocular muscles and orbital nerves. (Adapted from Warwick R: *Eugene Wollf's Anatomy of the Eye and Orbit, 8th ed.* London: Chapman and Hall, 1992, forthcoming.)

medial, and inferior rectus muscles; the inferior oblique and levator palpebrae muscles; the ciliary body muscles (which act to accommodate the lens in focusing near objects); and the sphincter muscle of the iris. The sixth cranial nerve innervates only the lateral rectus muscle; disorders resulting in an inability to abduct (turn out) the eye can be localized to this muscle or nerve. The fourth cranial nerve innervates only the superior oblique muscle. Unlike the nerves to the other extraocular muscles, it does not pass through the muscle cone and therefore often is not anesthetized by retrobulbar blocks into the muscle cone.

For each extraocular muscle, there is a singular position of the eye for which it is the primary mover. Because of this, the action of each muscle can be individually tested. There are six extraocular muscles; therefore six positions, called the *cardinal positions of gaze,* exist (Figure 5-3). Table 5-2 lists the cardinal position of gaze and the respectively acting extraocular muscles for the right eye.

The lacrimal excretory system has its origins in the inferior medial orbit. The system begins with the upper and lower *lacrimal puncta,* which are located on

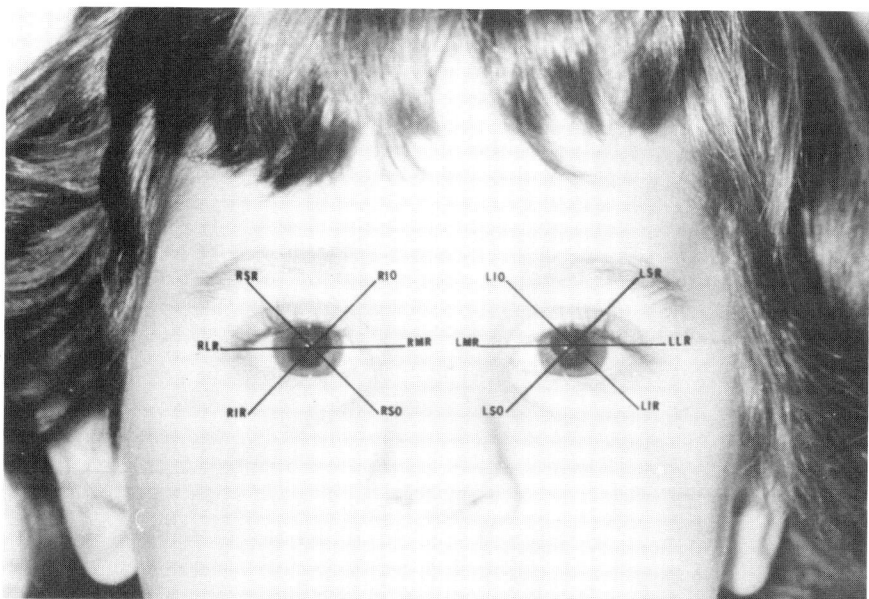

FIGURE 5-3. Cardinal positions of gaze. RSR, right superior rectus; RLR, right lateral rectus; RIR, right inferior rectus; RSO, right superior oblique; RMR, right medial rectus, RIO, right inferior oblique; LIO, left inferior oblique; LMR, left medial rectus; LSO, left superior oblique; LIR, left inferior rectus; LLR, left lateral rectus; LSR, left superior rectus. (From Nelson LB and Catalano RA: *Atlas of Ocular Motility*. Philadelphia: WB Saunders Co, 1989.)

the eyelid margins, 5 mm to 7 mm from the medial canthal angle (see Figure 9-1). The upper punctum is usually 1 mm to 2 mm more medial than the lower punctum. The puncta should be opposed to the globe; if they are visible on external examination, by definition an ectropion (turning out) of the eyelid is present. The puncta open into the *canaliculi*. These extend approximately 2 mm in a vertical direction and then turn horizontally to fuse as the *common canaliculus,* which opens into the *lacrimal sac*. The lacrimal sac begins in the

TABLE 5-2. CARDINAL POSITIONS OF GAZE USED TO TEST EXTRAOCULAR MUSCLE ACTIONS (RIGHT EYE)

EXTRAOCULAR MUSCLE	MOVEMENT
Right superior rectus	Up and to the right
Right lateral rectus	Straight right
Right inferior rectus	Down and to the right
Right superior oblique	Down and to the left
Right medial rectus	Straight left
Right inferior oblique	Up and to the left

lacrimal fossa, located between the anterior and posterior lacrimal crests in the inferiomedial orbital wall. The lacrimal sac extends 3 mm to 5 mm above the site where the common canaliculus enters and approximately 10 mm to 15 mm inferiorly to empty into the *nasolacrimal duct.* This duct extends an additional 10 mm to 15 mm and enters the nose below the inferior meatus at the *valve of Hasner.* The most common site of nasolacrimal obstruction in infants is at this valve.

Four paranasal sinuses surround the orbit. Their mucous membranes are continuous with the nasal cavity, accounting for their common infectious involvement. The largest paranasal sinus is the maxillary *sinus,* located beneath the orbital floor (Figure 5-4). Orbital blowout fractures expand into this sinus. The maxillary sinus opens onto the middle meatus, near the opening of the frontal sinus, which lies above and medial to the orbit, in the frontal bone. The *ethmoid sinus* is located medial to the orbit, from which it is separated by only a thin plate of bone. Comprised of 15 or more thin-walled air cells, the ethmoid is the most common focus of infection in orbital cellulitis. The *sphenoid sinus* is located posteriorly, in the body of the sphenoid bone. Its

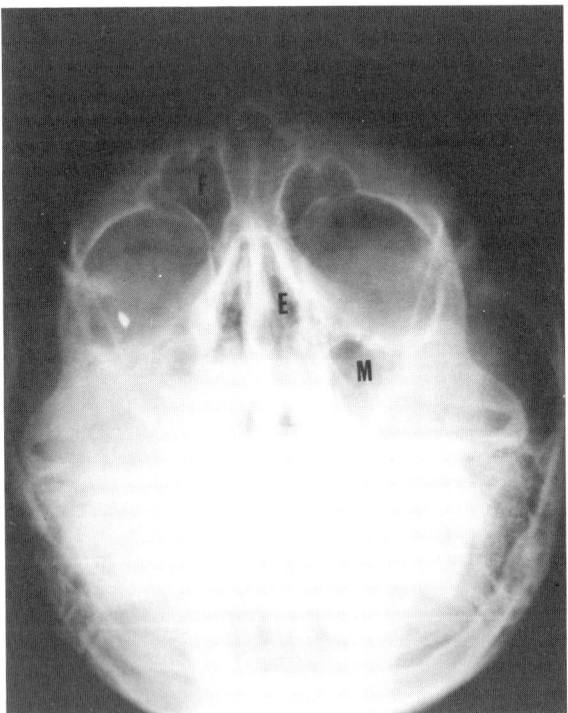

FIGURE 5-4. Plain film X ray demonstrating the paranasal sinuses. F, frontal sinus; E, ethmoid sinus; M, maxillary sinus.

important relations include the optic chiasm above and the cavernous sinus and internal carotid artery laterally. All of the paranasal sinuses are small at birth and increase in size with the eruption of secondary dentition. The frontal sinuses expand throughout adolescence.

THE EVALUATION OF BLUNT INJURIES AND FRACTURES OF THE ORBIT

The evaluation of any ocular injury should follow the 10-step sequence outlined in Chapter 1. The following points are especially useful in evaluating blunt orbital injuries and orbital fractures. As with all other traumatic injuries, photographic documentation is suggested.

The *history* details the mechanism and time of injury. A penetrating, rather than blunt, injury should be suspected if a projectile or pointed object was involved. Any symptoms, such as diplopia, decreased vision, visual floaters, or flashing lights, are recorded, and any treatment already given and any other injuries sustained are noted. The past ocular history includes the need for spectacles, previous ocular injuries, inflammation, or poor vision in an eye. The medical history records current medications, drug allergies, and the patient's tetanus immunization status.

The *visual acuity* is always recorded, even if only a gross estimate of vision (e.g., able to detect hand motion at a distance of 5 feet) is possible. Profound loss of vision from avulsion of the optic nerve is more likely to occur with lateral wall fracture.

The *external examination* notes any lid lacerations, with particular attention directed to potential injury of the lacrimal drainage system (see Chapter 4). Palpation of the orbital rim can detect any interruptions, step-offs, or depressions suggesting an orbital rim fracture. Because much greater forces are necessary to fracture the orbital rim than the medial wall or orbital floor, an orbital wall fracture should be suspected if the orbital rim is discontinuous. Displacement of a globe to one side is suggestive of an orbital wall fracture at the side of the displacement. In the average adult, the interpupillary distance is more than twice the intercanthal distance. An increased intercanthal distance suggests a medial canthal tendon injury or nasal fracture. Exophthalmometry can detect enophthalmos (suggestive of orbital fracture with herniation of tissue into either the maxillary or ethmoid sinus) or exophthalmos (suggestive of orbital emphysema or hemorrhage). Skin elevation and crepitus (orbital emphysema) suggest fracture of the ethmoid or orbital floor. Hypesthesia in the region of the infraorbital or supraorbital nerve suggests orbital floor or roof fracture, respectively. The presence of rhinorrhea and hemorrhage into the upper eyelid and lateral conjunctiva is indicative of an orbital roof fracture. Rhinorrhea can also result from basilar skull fractures.

Ocular motility is assessed to detect ophthalmoplegia. Ocular rotations are examined in each of the cardinal positions of gaze (Figure 5-3), as well as straight up and down. Limitation of movement suggests either entrapment of an extraocular muscle or ocular motor paresis. Forced duction testing can help differentiate the two but may be positive due to orbital edema or hemorrhage. Laceration or disinsertion of an extraocular muscle is extremely rare. When reported, it is usually associated with either a high-impact motor vehicle accident or an atypical penetrating orbital injury.

SOFT TISSUE INJURIES

Eyelid Abrasions and Avulsed Skin

Eyelid abrasions should be cleaned of foreign and necrotic debris to reduce the risk of infection and skin tattooing. This is often best accomplished with vigorous irrigation. A prophylactic topical antibiotic (bacitracin, erythromycin, or neomycin-bacitracin-polysporin ointment 4 times daily) is indicated because of the increased incidence of periorbital cellulitis due to staphylococci or streptococci. Tetanus immunization should be updated if devitalized tissue or deep wounds are present (see Chapter 17). Large abrasions should be kept moist with antibiotic ointment, and if dressings are necessary, they should be changed wet to avoid denuding the healing epithelium. Alternatively, Telfa strips can be used.

Glancing blows can avulse the skin. Unless frankly necrotic, skin should not be removed, and wound edges should never be surgically sharpened. The periorbital skin, especially on the eyelid, is richly vascularized. Even partially avulsed skin, rolled upon itself and attached by only a pedicle, may survive if unrolled and reattached in its anatomic position. Complete avulsions deeper than the dermis, however, may require skin grafting.

Eyelid Ecchymosis

If the force of impact crushes the subcutaneous tissue, hemorrhage and edema result (Figure 5-5). An eyelid ecchymosis, commonly referred to as a *black eye,* is treated with ice packs for the initial 48 hours, followed by warm compresses to reduce swelling and relieve discomfort. Infected hematomas require surgical incision and drainage to reduce the spread of infection. Occasionally it is necessary to evacuate surgically a large, noninfected hematoma of the eyelid to reduce the risks of skin necrosis or scar tissue formation.

Orbital Hemorrhage

Orbital hemorrhage is defined as bleeding into the orbital space behind the globe and orbital septum. Blunt and penetrating trauma are the most common

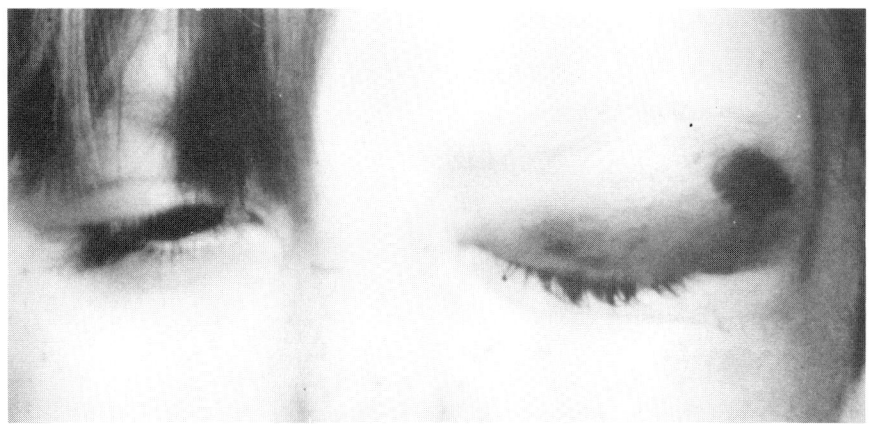

FIGURE 5-5. Eyelid ecchymosis (black eye).

causes, but orbital hemorrhage can also result from a surgical procedure. Rarely, orbital hemorrhage can occur spontaneously following a Valsalva maneuver, rupture of an ophthalmic artery aneurysm, or in association with a coagulopathy (see Chapter 12). Conditions in which orbital hemorrhage occurs following minor trauma are listed in Table 5-3. When it occurs, the bleeding time—prothrombin and partial thromboplastin time—as well as platelet count, should be investigated.

Symptoms of orbital hemorrhage include pain, nausea and vomiting, and diplopia. Signs include proptosis, globe displacement, dissection of blood anteriorly under the conjunctiva (Figure 5-6), elevated intraocular pressure, restriction of ocular motility, increased resistance to globe retropulsion, conjunctival vascular congestion, and reduced visual acuity. Typically, localized hemorrhage dissects between tissues and gives the appearance of spreading during the initial 24 hours to 48 hours. Unless there is optic nerve compression or elevated intraocular pressure, orbital hemorrhages are treated conservatively with head elevation, ice to the orbit, and avoidance of aspirin.

The presence of retinal artery pulsation or nonperfusion or intraocular pressure elevation of greater than 30 mm Hg (20 mm Hg in an eye with glaucoma) requires emergent treatment. A lateral canthotomy and cantholysis should be

TABLE 5-3. SYSTEMIC CONDITIONS ASSOCIATED WITH ORBITAL HEMORRHAGE FOLLOWING MINOR TRAUMA

Hemophilia or other platelet abnormality	Orbital lymphangioma
Anticoagulant therapy	Ophthalmic artery aneurysm
Vitamen deficiency (scurvy)	Metastatic neuroblastoma
Alcoholism	

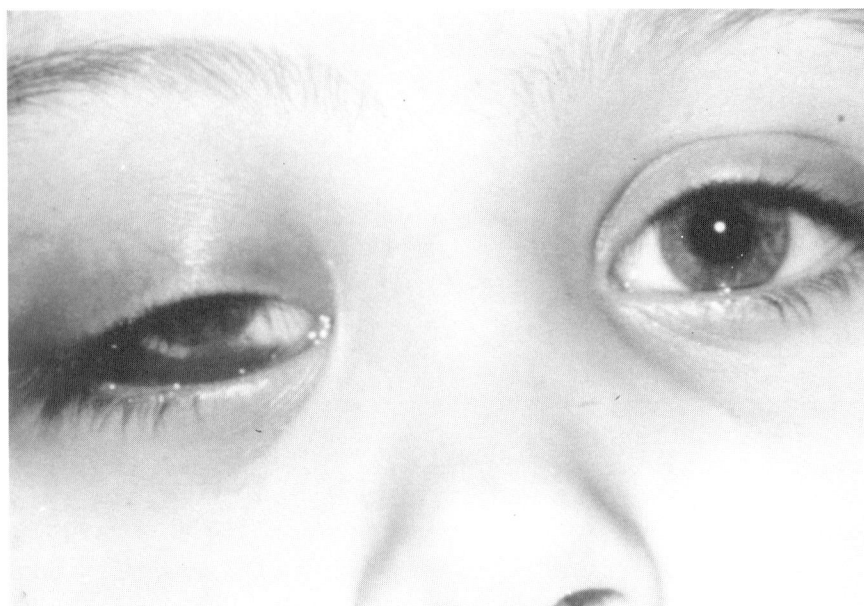

FIGURE 5-6. Orbital hemorrhage. Note dissection of blood anteriorly under the conjunctiva.

performed (see Chapter 4). If orbital hemorrhage follows a surgical procedure, the sutures are removed and any subcutaneous clots evacuated. If the hemorrhage is dissecting anteriorly, a conjunctival peritomy may allow sufficient egress of blood to lower the intraorbital and intraocular pressure. Sharp dissection with Wescott scissors at the site of the subconjunctival clot, under topical anesthesia, is recommended. Reduction of intraocular pressure using acetazolamide 250 mg intravenously (or 250 mg to 500 mg by mouth), a topical beta-blocker (repeated once in 30 minutes), mannitol 20% (1.5 g/kg, intravenously over 45 minutes), and even paracentesis may be necessary if retinal vascular perfusion is compromised. After adequate reduction of pressure, a computed tomography (CT) scan is indicated to rule out an orbital fracture or ruptured globe. Rarely, two-wall orbital decompression is indicated, and reports of visual recovery after delayed decompression exist. Orbital hemorrhages resorb over the course of weeks. As they resorb, ocular motility improves, and proptosis resolves.

Ophthalmoplegia

Ophthalmoplegia is defined as paralysis of extraocular muscle movement. Unless visual acuity is reduced in one eye, ophthalmoplegia is accompanied by diplopia in at least one position of gaze. The differential diagnosis of restricted ocular motility following blunt orbital trauma is presented in Table 5–4. Axial and coronal 2 mm CT scanning (see Chapter 2) and forced duction testing help differentiate extraocular muscle entrapment or other restriction from ocular motor nerve palsy. Ocular restriction due to only orbital edema or hemorrhage resolves in a few weeks. Paresis due to an extraocular muscle hematoma may take several months to resolve. Traumatic ocular motor nerve palsies can take 6 months to 9 months to resolve, and full recovery occurs in less than 50% of cases.

In the absence of extraocular muscle entrapment, the treatment of ophthalmoplegia consists of observation and alleviation of diplopia. Occasionally the latter can be achieved with ocular prisms, but more commonly occlusion of one eye is necessary. If prolonged occlusion is necessary in children (greater than 1 week per year of age), the eyes should be alternately occluded to prevent the development of amblyopia. Botulinum injection of the affected muscle's antagonist can be considered to reduce its unopposed action, as can systemic corticosteroids when the ocular restriction is secondary to orbital edema.

ORBITAL FRACTURES

Orbital Emphysema

Orbital fractures involving the ethmoid bone or orbital floor can result in the expulsion of air from the ethmoid or maxillary sinus into the orbit. Orbital emphysema can be grossly apparent clinically (Figure 5–7) or evident only on imaging studies (see Figure 2–19). Additional signs are subcutaneous crepitus, subconjunctival air, and proptosis.

Orbital emphysema can dramatically increase with sneezing, coughing, or blowing the nose, all of which cause a sudden rise in paranasal sinus pressure. It is not unusual for this finding to occur several hours after injury. Patients with orbital fractures should be forewarned against blowing their nose, and coughing episodes should be vigorously treated with antitussives (including codeine phosphate 10 mg to 20 mg every 4 hours to 6 hours if necessary).

The treatment of orbital emphysema is conservative except when visual loss,

TABLE 5–4. CAUSES OF OPHTHALMOPLEGIA FOLLOWING ORBITAL TRAUMA

ORBITAL	EXTRAOCULAR MUSCLE	OTHER
Edema	Entrapment	Brain stem injury
Hemorrhage	Avulsion	Carotid-cavernous fistula
Emphysema	Contusion/hematoma	Decompensated phoria

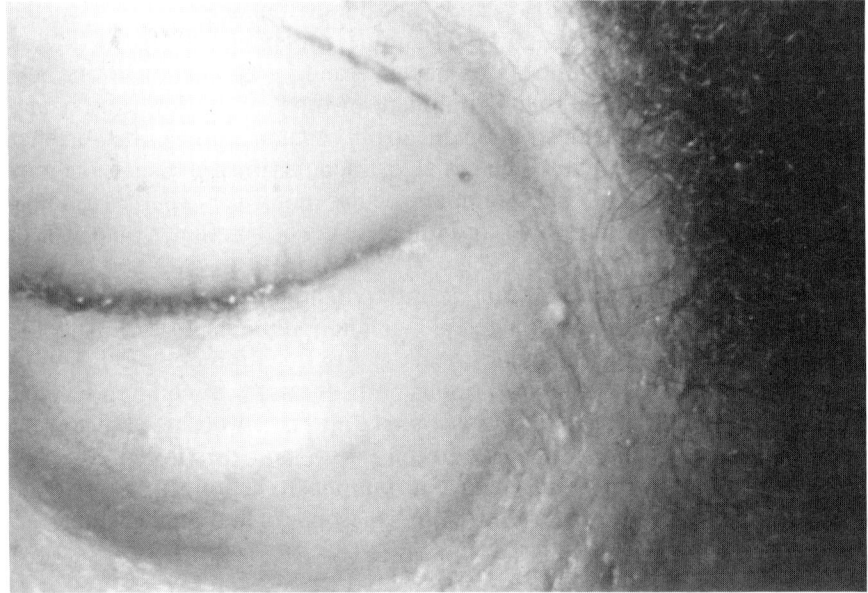

FIGURE 5-7. Orbital emphysema in a patient with an ethmoid fracture who sneezed.

afferent pupillary defect, or central retinal artery occlusion occurs from secondary optic nerve compression. This is more likely to occur when a bone fragment acts as a one-way valve, preventing the release of air from the orbit. Referred to as the *orbital compartment syndrome,* emergent decompression is indicated. Because the orbital space has been potentially seeded by sinus pathogens, prophylactic antibiotic therapy is indicated. A broad-spectrum oral antibiotic (cephalexin 250 mg to 500 mg or erythromycin 250 mg to 500 mg four times a day; or cefaclor 40 mg/kg/day divided every 8 hours) for 10 days to 14 days is appropriate. If preseptal or orbital cellulitis develops, appropriate cultures and directed antibiotic therapy are instituted (see Chapter 17). Additional measures include ice packs for the initial 48 hours and Afrin 0.05% nasal spray twice a day for 10 days to 14 days.

Blowout Fracture of the Orbital Floor

The term *direct orbital floor fracture* describes a floor fracture associated with an orbital rim fracture. Much greater forces are needed to fracture the orbital rim than the orbital floor. The term *indirect orbital floor fracture* describes an isolated floor fracture and is more commonly known as a *blowout fracture.* Two theories have been developed to explain the pathogenic mechanism of a blowout fracture. The first maintains that these fractures result when the intraorbital pressure is suddenly elevated by a nonpenetrating blunt force. The orbital tissues are compressed, and the weakest part of the orbit, the 0.5 mm thick orbital floor, becomes the avenue of decompression (Figure 5–8). A more recent theory suggests that a blunt force applied to the inferior orbital rim compresses the bone and causes a buckling of the orbital floor. Floor fractures are common when objects larger than the orbital opening, such as a ball, a fist, or the dashboard of an automobile, impact the orbit, particularly the inferior lateral orbit. *Macaca* monkey experiments have suggested that forces greater than 2 *Joules* are needed to produce a floor fracture and that orbital wall fractures fail to protect the globe from rupture.

The most apparent clinical sign of an orbital floor fracture is a limitation of upward gaze (Figure 5–9). A concomitant limitation of downward gaze, however, is a more certain indication of inferior rectus or oblique muscle entrapment. Entrapment is more likely to occur when an articulated bone fragment acts like a trapdoor, restricting the movement of the inferior rectus or oblique muscle. This occurs most frequently with small, indirect floor fractures, and most commonly the inferior rectus muscle, posterior to its adventitial connection to the inferior oblique muscle, is involved. Additional signs are lid ecchymosis, nosebleed, orbital emphysema, and hypesthesia of the ipsilateral cheek

ORBITAL FLOOR FRACTURE

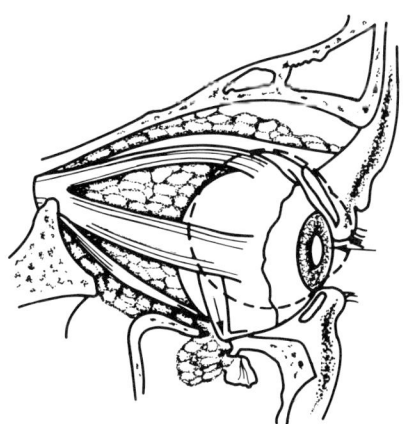

FIGURE 5–8. Schematic to demonstrate a blowout fracture of the orbital floor. The dotted line indicates the normal position of the globe. The small opening into the maxillary sinus entraps the inferior rectus and oblique muscles. (Adapted from: Paton D, Goldberg MF: *Management of Ocular Injuries.* Philadelphia, WB Saunders Co, 1976.)

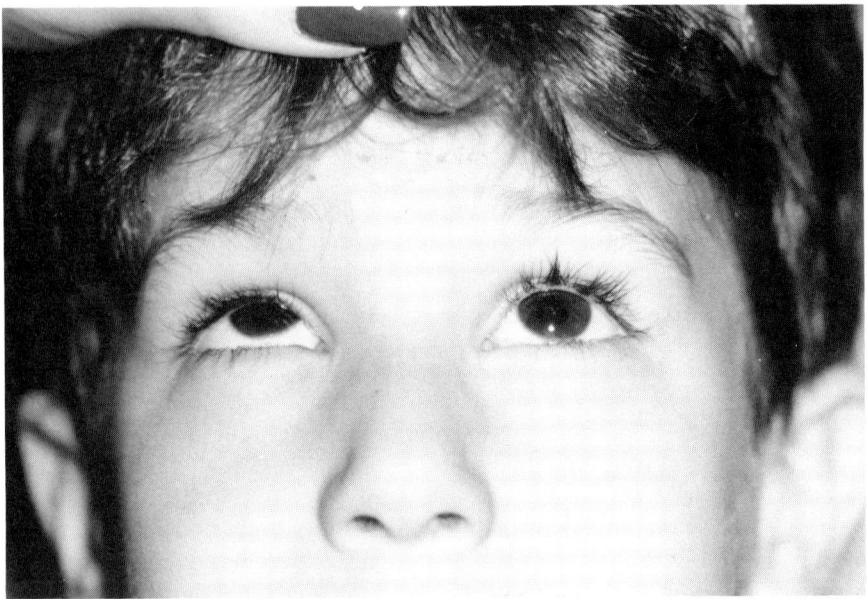

FIGURE 5-9. Limitation of upward gaze of the left eye following longstanding blowout fracture of the orbital floor.

and upper lip, which results from disruption of the infraorbital nerve as it traverses the orbital floor. Enophthalmos results from expansion of the orbital volume and is an overt sign of orbital floor fracture. It occurs more commonly with direct orbital floor fractures, but it may not become apparent until orbital edema resolves. Exophthalmos from orbital edema, hematoma, or inflammation is more likely to be present acutely.

The best imaging techniques to visualize an orbital floor fracture are plain film radiography and CT scanning. The optimal plain film projection is the Waters view, because it best demonstrates the orbital floor and maxillary sinus (Figure 5-10). A floor fracture is suggested by the prolapse of orbital contents into the maxillary sinus, an air-fluid level in the sinus, or orbital emphysema. Whereas the Waters view is suggested for screening, direct, coronal 1.5 mm to 2.0 mm CT scanning should be obtained if surgical repair is contemplated because it provides more soft tissue and bone fragment detail.

The indications for surgical repair of a blowout fracture are controversial. The radiographic presence of fracture is not an indication for surgery, nor is the sole finding of infraorbital hypesthesia. Generally accepted indications for repair include a motility disturbance due to extraocular muscle entrapment (within 30° of the primary position) or enophthalmos. Surgical intervention for a limitation of motility is based on true mechanical restriction, suggested by

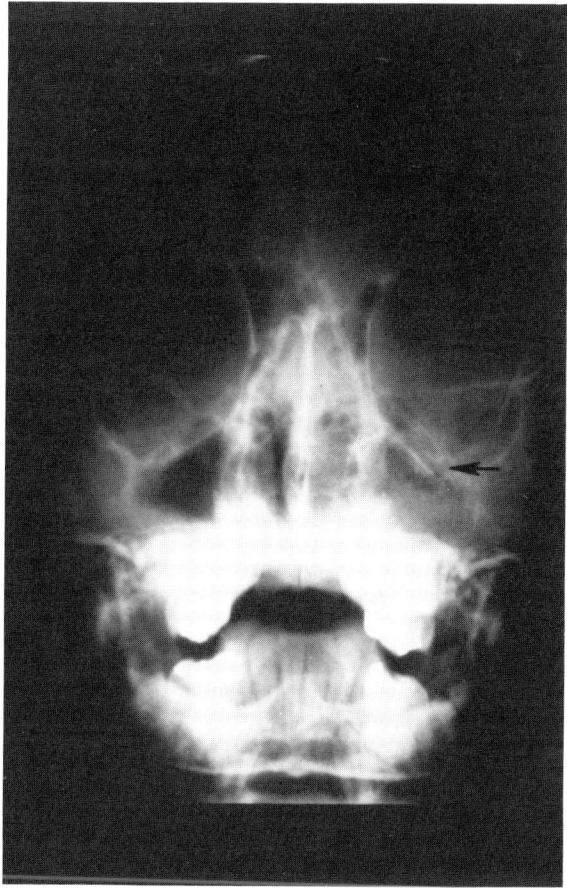

FIGURE 5-10. Waters view demonstrating blowout fracture of the orbital floor.

persistent positive forced traction testing and confirmed radiographically. It should be remembered, however, that techniques other than floor fracture repair (prisms, strabismus surgery) may be effective in relieving diplopia. Enophthalmos of greater than 2 mm generally requires repair as it is usually cosmetically unacceptable. Because the necessary exposure of an orbital floor fracture places pressure on the globe, the presence of a penetrating ocular injury is an absolute contraindication to orbital floor repair.

The timing of surgical repair is also controversial. A blowout fracture never needs emergent treatment. Most ophthalmologists agree that surgery can be safely delayed for 10 days to 14 days without risking the development of scarring or fibrosis. The passage of several days is usually needed to allow orbital swelling to subside enough to perform an adequate clinical examination. An indication for early surgical repair may be the presence of enophthalmos in the acute stage of an orbital floor fracture. Orbital edema and hematoma usually mask the early appearance of enophthalmos; its acute presence indicates a substantial extrusion of orbital contents into the maxillary sinus.

Additional therapeutic measures in the acute setting are antibiotic prophylaxis, nasal decongestants, and ice packs.

Fracture of the Medial Wall of the Orbit

The thin, lateral wall of the ethmoid sinus, the *lamina papyracea,* can be fractured by the same forces that cause orbital floor fractures. Additionally, medial wall fractures can occur with blows to the bridge of the nose that result in complex naso-orbital fractures.

Signs of a medial wall fracture are orbital emphysema, epistaxis, a depressed bridge of the nose, and enophthalmos. If the nasal septum is also fractured, the nose will be deviated and nasal breathing impaired. Medial canthal tendon injuries are commonly associated with medial wall fractures and should be suspected if the intercanthal distance is increased. The nasolacrimal drainage system can also be disrupted, resulting in epiphora, lacrimal sac mucocele, or dacryostenosis.

Entrapment of the medial rectus muscle is a rare consequence of medial wall fracture. Entrapment is difficult to demonstrate on plain film radiography because of the multitude of overlying structures. CT scanning is recommended if there is suspicion of entrapment (Figure 5-11). Clinically, both adduction and abduction of the affected eye are restricted, but the limitation of abduction is usually more profound. Surgical exploration and repair is difficult but should be attempted within 10 days to 14 days, beyond which time fibrosis and scarring occur. In the absence of entrapment, patients are managed conservatively with ice packs, antibiotics, and nasal decongestants. Medial wall fractures without entrapment usually heal without significant sequelae. Surgical repair, when necessary, usually involves reduction of any nasal fractures and wiring of the medial canthus.

Fracture of the Superior Wall of the Orbit

Superior wall (orbital roof) fractures are less common than inferior or medial wall fractures but more life threatening. They more commonly occur in association with penetrating injuries, and the possibility of central nervous system injury, pneumocephalus, and/or an intracranial foreign body should be considered. Late complications include brain abscess and infectious meningitis. For these reasons, neurosurgical evaluation and management is recommended.

Signs of an orbital roof fracture include cerebrospinal fluid leakage (rhinor-

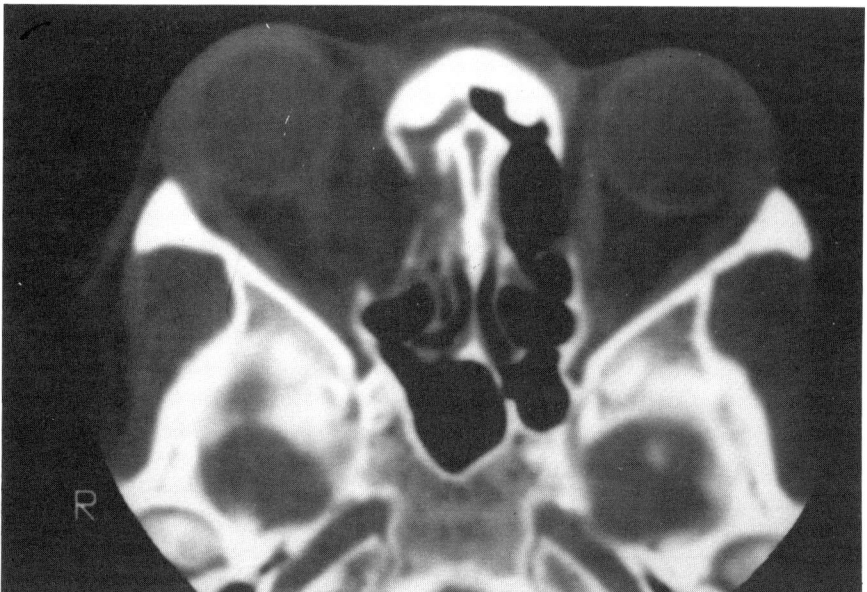

FIGURE 5-11. Medial wall fracture with entrapment of the medial rectus muscle.

rhea) and superior and lateral subconjunctival hemorrhage. Rhinorrhea is usually transient because dural tears are usually self-sealing. Entrapment of the superior rectus or oblique muscles is rare, but hemorrhage into these muscles may limit their action. A hematoma in the levator palpebrae muscle is more common and results in a traumatic ptosis. An additional complication is disruption of the frontonasal duct that drains the frontal sinus, resulting in the development of a frontal sinus mucocele. An optic nerve injury can also occur. The orbital roof and frontal sinuses can be visualized on the Waters view, but CT scanning is recommended to define bony fragments more completely.

Depending on the extent of injury, orbital roof fractures often require surgical repair. Some advocate obliterating the frontal sinus at the time of repair to prevent the subsequent development of a mucocele. Treatment of a superior rectus or levator palpebrae muscle dysfunction (ptosis) is usually temporized for at least 6 months to allow edema, hemorrhage, and neurogenic dysfunction to resolve (see Chapter 4).

Tripod Fracture

A *tripod (trimalar) fracture* is a three-part zygomatic fracture; it involves the zygomatic arch and its lateral and inferior orbital rim articulations. These articulations form the frontozygomatic and zygomaticomaxillary sutures, respectively (Figure 5-12). Radiographically, a submental vertex or bucket handle view allows the most complete view of a tripod fracture.

Because fractures of the inferior orbital rim often extend into the orbital floor, signs similar to a blowout fracture are common. If the zygoma is displaced inferiorly, there may be increased scleral show laterally, but usually edema obscures this finding in the acute setting. Of greater importance is limitation of mandibular movement and the inability to open the mouth (trismus).

If the zygoma is not displaced, no reduction or fixation is necessary. Open or closed reduction may be necessary, however, with displaced fractures to allow full mandibular excursion. The zygoma is also responsible for the prominence of the cheek, and unreduced, depressed, or rotated tripod fractures are cosmetically disfiguring. Wiring of the orbital margin within 2 weeks of the injury is usually necessary in the latter cases.

TRIPOD FRACTURE

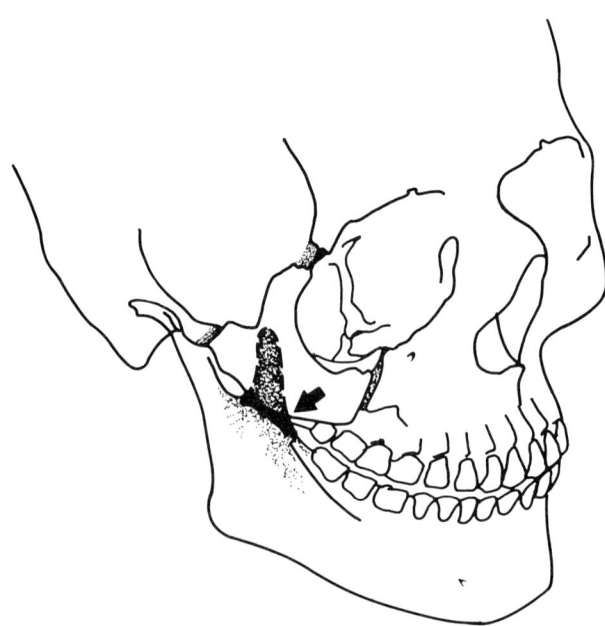

FIGURE 5-12. Tripod fracture of the zygoma. Note the articulation of the zygoma with the coronoid process of the mandible (shaded). Inferior displacement of the zygoma may result in an inability to open the mouth. (Adapted from: Converse JM (ed): *Reconstructive Plastic Surgery,* vol 2. Philadelphia, WB Saunders Co, 1977.)

Le Fort Fractures

Midfacial fractures result from severe blunt trauma that separates facial structures. Le Fort classified these into three categories (Figure 5-13), but asymmetry, overlap, and variations are common. In addition to the signs listed below, plain film radiography, particularly the Waters and frontal views, and CT scanning are diagnostic.

Le Fort I: A horizontal fracture across the maxilla, separating the teeth from the rest of the maxilla but not involving the orbit. Signs include epistaxis, pharyngeal bleeding, and a mobile alveolar segment of the maxilla.

LE FORT FRACTURES

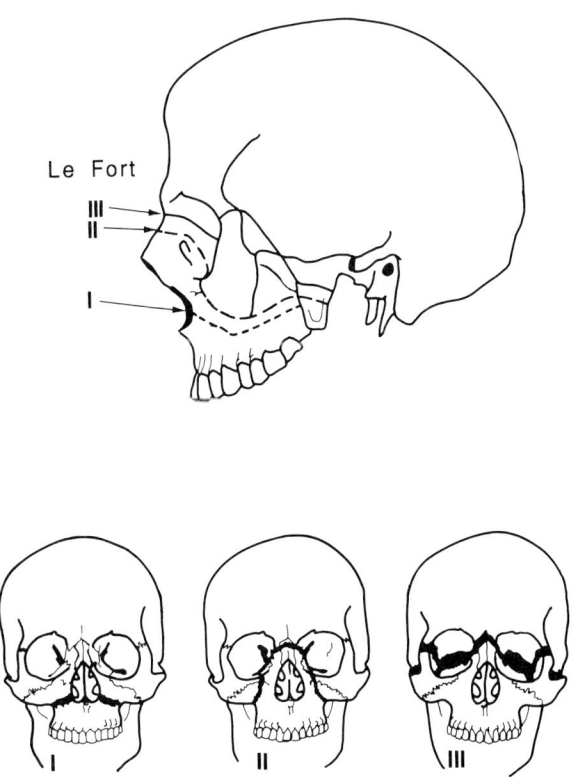

FIGURE 5-13. Le Fort classification of midfacial fractures. Top, lateral view; bottom, frontal view. (Adapted from Kazanjian VH, Converse JM: *The Surgical Treatment of Facial Injuries.* Baltimore: Williams & Wilkins, 1974.)

Le Fort II: A pyramidal fracture involving the nasal, lacrimal, and maxillary bones. Its apex is the nasal bridge, and it extends posteriorly to involve both medial orbital walls and inferiorly to involve both orbital floors and maxillary sinuses. It is the most common of the Le Fort fractures and results in a separation of the maxilla and nose from the rest of the facial skeleton. Signs include those of orbital floor and medial wall fractures, dental malocclusion, and trismus. In addition, there may be optic nerve injury and cerebrospinal fluid leakage. Orbital reconstruction and open internal fixation are usually indicated.

Le Fort III: A complete disjunction of the facial skeleton from the base of the skull. Beginning at the nasal bridge, the fracture extends laterally through the lateral orbital wall and zygomatic arch. The medial, inferior, and lateral walls are involved. Because of its posterior extension, optic nerve injury is more likely. Surgical management includes orbital reconstruction and open internal fixation as with Le Fort II fractures.

REFERENCES

Beyer CK, Fabian RL, Smith B: Naso-orbital fractures: Complications and treatment. *Ophthalmology* 89:456, 1982.

Chole RA, Yee J: Antibiotic prophylaxis for facial fractures: A randomized clinical trial. *Arch Otolaryngol Head Neck Surg* 113:1055, 1987.

Cruse CW, Blevins PH, Luce ES: Naso-ethmoid-orbital fractures. *J Trauma* 20:551, 1980.

Dutton J, Slamovits T: Management of blowout fractures of the orbital floor. *Surv Ophthalmol* 35:279, 1991.

Fujino T, Makino K: Entrapment mechanism and ocular injury in orbital blowout fracture. *Plast Reconstr Surg* 65:571, 1980.

Goldfarb MS, Hoffman DS, Rosenberg S: Orbital cellulitis and orbital fractures. *Ann Ophthalmol* 19:97, 1987.

Green RP Jr, Peters DR, Shore JW, et al: Force necessary to fracture the orbital floor. *Ophthalmic Plast Reconstr Surg* 6:211, 1990.

Greenwald HS, Keeny AH, Shannon GM: A review of 128 patients with orbital fractures. *Am J Ophthalmol* 78:655, 1974.

Grover AS Jr: Computed tomography in the management of orbital trauma. *Ophthalmology* 89:433, 1982.

Grove AS Jr, McCord C: Acute orbital trauma, diagnosis and management. In McCord C, Tanenbaum M (eds): *Oculoplastic Surgery.* New York, Raven Press, 1987.

Hawes MJ, Dortzbach RK: Surgery on orbital floor fractures: Influence of time of repair and fracture size. *Ophthalmology* 90:1066, 1983.

Healy JF: Computed tomography of orbital trauma. *CT* 6:1, 1984.

Jones SEP, Evans JNG: Blowout fractures of the orbit: Investigation into their anatomical basis. *J Laryngol* 81:109, 1967.

Jordan DR, et al: Orbital emphysema: A potentially blinding complication following orbital fractures. *Ann Emerg Med* 17:853, 1988.

Kersten RC, Rice CD: Subperiosteal orbital hematoma: Visual recovery following delayed drainage. *Ophthalmic Surg* 18:423, 1987.

Krohel GB, Wright JE: Orbital hemorrhage. *Am J Ophthalmol* 88:254, 1979.

Lindberg JV: Orbital compartment syndromes following trauma. *Adv Ophthalmic Plast Reconstr Surg* 6:51, 1987.

McLachan DL, Flanagan JC, Shannon GM: Complications of orbital roof fractures. *Ophthalmology* 89:1274, 1982.

Millman AL, et al: Steroids and orbital blowout fractures: A new systematic concept in medical management and surgical decision-making. *Adv Ophthalmic Plast Reconstr Surg* 6:291, 1987.

Nelson LB, Catalano RA: *Atlas of Ocular Motility*. Philadelphia, WB Saunders Co, 1989, pp 2–23.
Pfeiffer RL: Traumatic enophthalmos. *Adv Ophthalmic Plast Reconstr Surg* 6:301, 1987.
Putterman AM, Stevens T, Urist M: Non-surgical management of blowout fractures of the orbital floor. *Am J Ophthalmol* 77:233, 1974.
Silkiss RZ, Baylis HI: Management of traumatic ptosis. *Adv Ophthalmic Plast Reconstr Surg* 7:149, 1987.
Smith BC (ed): *Ophthalmic Plastic and Reconstructive Surgery*, vol 1. St Louis, CV Mosby, 1987.
Waring GO III, Flanagan JC: Pneumocephalus: A sign of intracranial involvement in orbital fracture. *Arch Ophthalmol* 98:847, 1975.
Wilkins RB, Havins WE: Current treatment of blowout fractures. *Ophthalmology* 89:464, 1982.
Zismor J, Noyek A: Radiologic diagnosis of orbital fractures. In Aston SJ, Meltzer MA, Rees TD (eds): *Third International Symposium of Plastic and Reconstructive Surgery of the Eye and Adnexa*. Baltimore, Williams and Wilkins, 1982.

6

Blunt Ocular Injuries

Robert A. Catalano

Each ocular tissue can be injured by concussive and compressive forces. These forces horizontally displace the volume of the eye, stretching and tearing fixed structures as the eye expands in this dimension. Potential injuries are traumatic hyphema, recession of the anterior chamber angle, avulsion of the vitreous base, retinodialysis, retinal tear, and choroidal rupture.

The full extent of injury is not always apparent at presentation, particularly if hemorrhage is present under the conjunctiva or within the eye. Patients should never be given an optimistic prognosis until visual function, particularly visual acuity, can be assessed. Sequential examinations and diagnostic tests (e.g., ultrasound) may be necessary. Signs that portend a poor prognosis are listed in Table 6-1.

Permanent loss of vision from blunt trauma usually results from an injury involving the posterior segment of the eye (vitreous, choroid, and retina). Table 6-2 lists factors associated with a favorable prognosis in eyes with vitreoretinal and choroidal damage requiring vitrectomy (Hutton and Fuller, 1984). The visual evoked potential was the most accurate predictor of the final visual acuity in this study.

Although this chapter reviews blunt ocular injuries by structure, it is important to remember that more than one structure can be damaged when the eye is compressed by a blunt force.

INJURIES TO THE CONJUNCTIVA AND SCLERA

A *subconjunctival hemorrhage* commonly accompanies blunt trauma (Figure 6-1). In the absence of other injury, an affected patient is treated with

TABLE 6-1. FACTORS PORTENDING A SIGNIFICANT OCULAR INJURY

Markedly reduced visual acuity

A relative afferent pupillary defect (see Chapter 1)

Relative shallowing of the anterior chamber

Irregularity of the pupil

Conjunctival chemosis (clear fluid under the conjunctiva)

Blood in the anterior eye (hyphema) or posterior eye (vitreous hemorrhage)

Markedly reduced intraocular pressure

TABLE 6-2. FACTORS ASSOCIATED WITH A FAVORABLE VISUAL OUTCOME IN SEVERELY INJURED EYES

Preoperative visual acuity > 5/200

Foreign body injuries > blunt injuries > ocular lacerations

Penetrating injuries > blunt injuries > perforating injuries

Normal or reduced amplitude electroretinography > absent response

Normal visual evoked potential > reduced amplitude response > absent response

(From: Hutton WL, Fuller DG: Factors influencing final visual results in severely injured eyes. *Am J Ophthalmol* 97:715, 1984.)

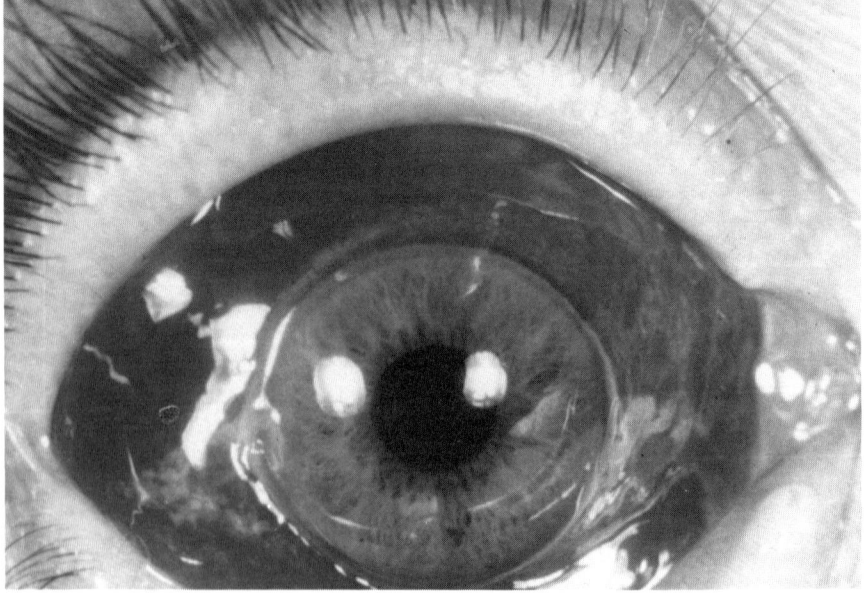

FIGURE 6-1. Traumatic subconjunctival hemorrhage.

reassurance alone. The patient is told that the hemorrhage may appear to become larger over the first several days as gravity and the weight of the eyelid smooth out blood clots, which can dissect under normal conjunctiva. Rarely, if ever, does a subconjunctival hemorrhage rebleed. The blood gradually resorbs over 2 weeks to 3 weeks.

Conjunctival edema (chemosis) can accompany a minor injury, but whenever it is present, it raises the suspicion of scleral rupture or a retained foreign body. Air under the conjunctiva *(emphysema)* suggests fracture through the ethmoid or maxillary sinus. Emphysema appears cystic and causes crepitus on palpation.

A *laceration of the conjunctiva* is especially common when a sharp object, such as a fingernail or glass, strikes the eye. In addition to conjunctival hemorrhage, prolapse of whitish-appearing Tenon's tissue or orbital fat may be evident. A complete examination to rule out an occult scleral laceration or retained foreign body is necessary. If sliding the conjunctiva does not allow adequate visualization, blunt dissection and inspection of the sclera are performed. Dilated ophthalmoscopy and ultrasound are used to rule out an intraocular foreign body. These measures are usually sufficient to exclude a more serious injury, but the physician should not hesitate to conduct an examination under anesthesia or obtain imaging studies if uncertainty exists. Small conjunctival lacerations do not need suturing, but lacerations greater than 6 mm should be closed with absorbable suture (e.g., 7-0 plain gut), taking care not to incorporate Tenon's tissue in the wound (see Chapter 8). One should also respect the normal anatomic relationship of the caruncle and semilunar fold in the repair. The conjunctival defect heals within 2 weeks to 3 weeks.

Occult scleral rupture can occur with blunt trauma. In addition to a bullous conjunctival hemorrhage and chemosis, signs of rupture include an asymmetric reduction in intraocular pressure, shallowing or deepening of the anterior chamber, irregularity or peaking of the pupil, hyphema, decreased visual acuity, and subconjunctival pigmentation. The last is due to prolapsed uveal tissue at the site of rupture. In suspected cases, as much as a 360° conjunctival peritomy should be performed (incising the conjunctiva at the limbus and retracting it posteriorly to expose the underlying sclera), with particular attention directed to the area under the rectus muscle insertions, where the sclera is thinnest (see also Chapter 8).

INJURIES TO THE CORNEA

Blunt ocular trauma from any cause can damage endothelial cells. The forceful impact of a small particle (e.g., a BB) can induce a stress wave in the cornea. Endothelial cells directly beneath the impact are relatively uniformly displaced and not damaged, but cells at the edge of the wave are distended and disrupted. The result is a ring-shaped endothelial opacity *(traumatic posterior annular keratopathy)* that presents within hours of injury and resolves within days. Endothelial cells can also be diffusely damaged from blunt trauma. One study suggested that the degree of endothelial cell loss was related to the intensity of the contusion and the degree of intraocular pressure elevation. The presence of blood in the anterior chamber did not appear to be related to cell loss (Slingsby and Forstot, 1981). Another type of corneal injury can result from being struck with a gelatin pellet fired during a recreational sport war game. Depressed circular bull's eye lesions, corneal edema, radiating folds in Descemet's membrane, angle recession, and hyphema are common with this type of injury.

More severe corneal contusion can rupture Descemet's membrane and disrupt the corneal endothelium. This results in massive corneal edema *(acute hydrops)*, characterized by cloudiness of the cornea and breaks in Descemet's membrane. These are distinguished from the Haab striae of congenital glaucoma by their vertical orientation and absence of an enlarged globe (buphthalmos). They heal in 2 months to 3 months with retraction of the disrupted Descemet's membrane and enlargement and sliding of the endothelium over the defect to restore corneal deturgescence. Numerous treatments have been advocated for this type of injury, including patching, soft contact lenses, hypertonic eye drops, and topical intraocular pressure–reducing medications, but none has been proved to hasten corneal repair. Obstetrical forceps injuries cause such an injury (Figure 6–2). Physicians should be aware that a forceps injury

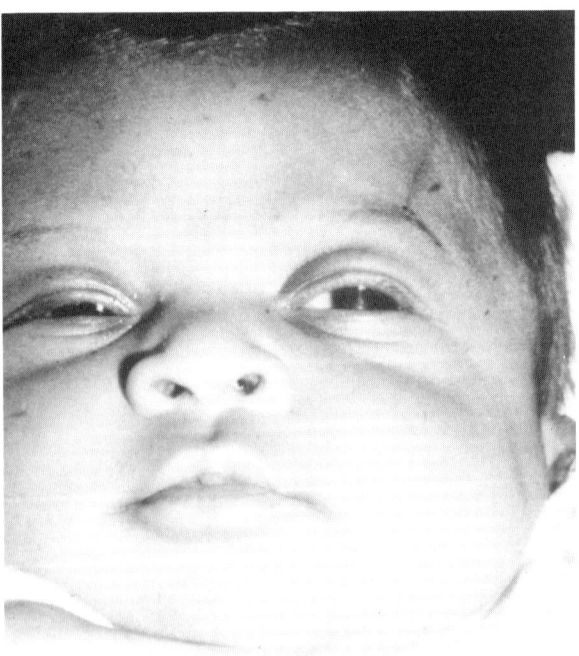

FIGURE 6–2. Corneal forceps injury of the left eye. Note the linear, vertical mark on the cornea extending onto the forehead.

can create a large, irregular astigmatism, which can be amblyogenic in this age group.

Traumatic rupture of the cornea is rare; it is more common in eyes predisposed by previous corneal surgery or a stromal thinning disorder. Trauma to an eye following radial keratotomy can have variable results. In this procedure, 90% to 95% of the depth of the cornea is incised. It appears that the remaining 5% to 10% of nonincised corneal stroma and Descemet's membrane afford a relatively strong barrier to trauma. Most reported cases have not resulted in serious injury, despite the occurrence of hyphema or other ocular injury. In a few cases, however, trauma opened radial incisions. Most of these patients were successfully treated with a bandage contact lens and did not sustain a permanent reduction in visual acuity. A few cases sustained more severe corneal rupture along keratotomy scars. Histologic and ultrastructural studies in some of these eyes demonstrated incomplete wound healing 1 year to 2 years after surgery. The full thickness incision of a penetrating keratoplasty (corneal transplant) is much more vulnerable than the radial keratotomy incision. Even with radial keratotomy, however, the tensile strength of the wound appears never to equal that of the normal cornea (Binder et al., 1988). Individuals who undergo these procedures should be fully informed of the increased risk of corneal rupture with direct ocular trauma.

INJURIES TO THE IRIS

Blunt ocular contusion can injure the iris sphincter muscle, resulting in pupillary constriction *(traumatic miosis)* during the first several hours, followed by dilation *(traumatic mydriasis)*. Patients present with pain, photophobia, perilimbal conjunctival injection, and anisocoria (asymmetry in pupil size). An accommodative spasm or paralysis may be associated, resulting in blurred vision and difficulty with near tasks. Signs include inflammatory or pigment cells in the anterior chamber *(traumatic iritis)* and iris sphincter tears, both of which are recognizable on slit lamp examination. Additionally, the pupil does not constrict to light stimulation as briskly as the unaffected eye or dilate as rapidly when the illumination is reduced. Pharmacologic testing with pilocarpine 1% usually demonstrates reduced sensitivity, which is useful in distinguishing traumatic mydriasis from parasympathetic denervation (e.g., Adie's pupil), in which the iris is suprasensitive.

In addition to direct contusion injury to the iris, mydriasis can be caused by traumatic injury to the ciliary ganglion (this is a rare complication of orbital floor fractures). Miosis can be a component of traumatic Horner's syndrome, due to injury of the carotid plexus, cervical ganglion, cervical spine, or brain stem. Accompanying features of this syndrome are ipsilateral ptosis (lid droop), anhidrosis (decreased sweating), and relative enophthalmos (recession of the eye within the orbit) (see Figure 13–9).

It may be difficult to distinguish traumatic iritis from traumatic microhyphema. A hyphema is characterized by red blood cells in the anterior chamber, as opposed to the white blood cells of iritis. Allowing the patient to sit quietly for several minutes allows red blood cells, which were dispersed with patient movement, to layer, confirming the diagnosis of hyphema. The diagnosis is always hyphema when both red and white blood cells are present in the anterior chamber. The presence of both is actually characteristic of hyphema. Other disorders in the differential of traumatic iritis include long-standing, untreated corneal abrasions and traumatic retinal detachments, both of which can result in a secondary anterior chamber reaction. Pigment in the anterior vitreous (tobacco dust) is also seen in detachments.

The treatment of traumatic mydriasis or miosis is supportive. Cycloplegia alone (e.g., scopolamine ¼% 3 times a day or cyclogel 1% to 2% 4 times a day) may be sufficient in relieving spasm and pain. More severe iritis should also be treated with a topical corticosteroid (e.g., prednisolone acetate ⅛% to 1% three or four times a day). Corticosteroids reduce the formation of anterior and posterior synechiae (abnormal adhesions of the iris to the cornea and lens, respectively). Both medications are tapered over several days.

Disinsertion of the iris at its root *(iridodialysis)* is characterized by polycoria (the appearance of multiple pupils) and a D-shaped pupillary aperture (Figure 6–3). Its occurrence is usually accompanied by hyphema. Rare iris injuries include iris atrophy and iridoschisis (a split within the iris stroma). Patients with an iris injury often experience glare and photophobia and may have di-

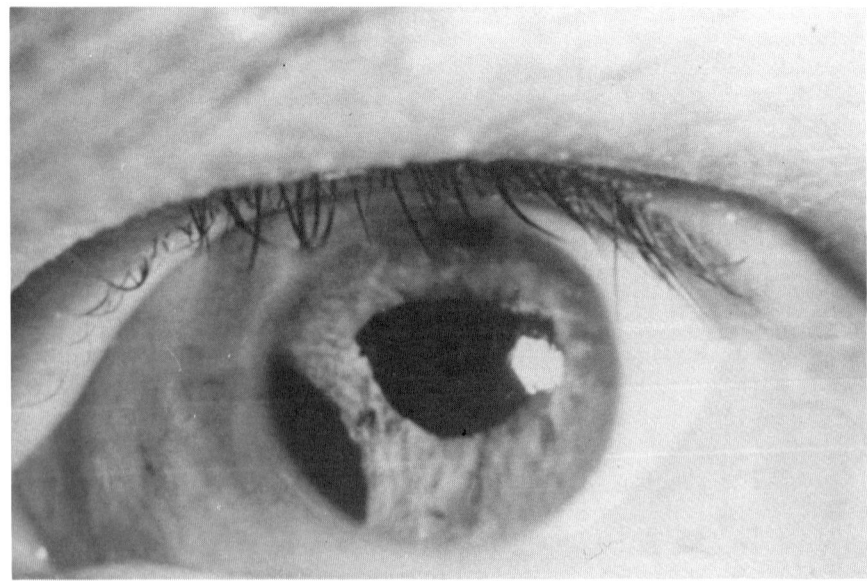

FIGURE 6–3. Iridodialysis.

plopia. A tinted contact lens or a dyed lens with an artificial pupil (available through Narcissus Medical Foundation, 66 San Pedro Road, Daly City, California 94015) can reduce these symptoms and conceal the cosmetic deformity. Sphincterotomy with the neodymium:YAG laser (in aphakic and pseudophakic eyes) or argon laser (phakic eyes) may clear the central visual axis and improve visual acuity in patients with an eccentric pupil. Surgical repair of sphincter lacerations and tears can be accomplished using the suture technique described by McCannel (1976).

Any iris abnormality should be clearly documented because other physicians may mistake pupillary asymmetry or irregularity as a sign of third nerve dysfunction, related to uncal herniation.

TRAUMATIC HYPHEMA

Blunt ocular injury causing a tear in the face of the anterior ciliary body is the most common cause of *hyphema* (bleeding into the anterior chamber) (Figure 6-4). If a history of trauma is not elicited in a child with hyphema, one should suspect leukemia, hemophilia, juvenile xanthogranuloma, retinoblastoma, a fictitious history by the child, or child abuse. Spontaneous hyphema in an adult is consistent with neovascularization of the iris, leukemia, malignant

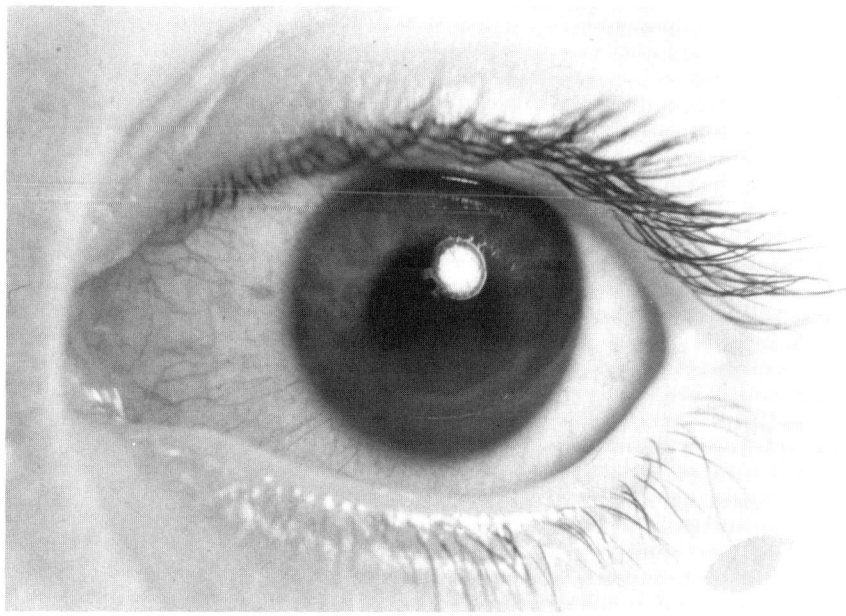

FIGURE 6-4. Hyphema.

lymphoma, intraocular tumor, hypertension, the use of anticoagulants (warfarin, heparin, aspirin, alcohol), and scurvy. Hyphemas that occur following intraocular surgery usually resorb within days without sequelae, but the physician should be cognizant of a consequent rise in intraocular pressure.

Most patients with hyphema present with pain, and children may be somnolent. The history should elicit the mechanism of injury and any complicating factors, such as a bleeding disorder, anticoagulant therapy, kidney or liver disease, or sickle cell disease or trait. Hyphemas are graded at presentation based on the amount of blood present in the anterior chamber (Table 6–3). This can be documented as the height (in mm) of layered blood. Gonioscopy in the early stages may reveal the site of bleeding and can confirm the presence of angle recession.

The management of traumatic hyphema is variable and controversial. There is no consensus as to whether patients should be at strict bed rest or allowed limited ambulation and whether they can watch television or read. Nor is there agreement as to the efficacy of hospitalization, occlusion of one or both eyes, patching of the traumatized eye, cycloplegics, topical corticosteroids, and antifibrinolytic agents. Community standards often dictate hospitalization policies. Considerations for which hospitalization may be prudent include the patient's age (children and elderly), probability of noncompliance (immature patients or those without assistance at home), and likelihood of developing complications (patients with sickle cell disease or trait or with elevated intraocular pressure at presentation). Patients with a rebleed are more likely to develop complications and should be hospitalized.

Antifibrinolytic agents (aminocaproic acid, tranexamic acid) should be used in populations with high rebleed rates (lower socioeconomic status, urban, younger age, delayed time from injury to admission). The side effects of nausea, vomiting, postural hypotension, tinnitus, lethargy, and hematuria should also be considered when making this decision. Contraindications include pregnancy and cardiac, hepatic, renal, or intravascular clotting disorder. Relative contraindications include sickle cell disease or trait and total hyphema, because these agents reduce the rate of resorption of blood. Suggested treatment of traumatic hyphema is presented in Table 6–4, and indications for surgical evacuation of the clot are reviewed in Table 6–5.

TABLE 6–3. GRADING OF HYPHEMA

GRADE	PERCENTAGE OF ANTERIOR CHAMBER FILLED WITH BLOOD
Microscopic	Circulation of red blood cells only, no layering
I	< 33%
II	33% to 50%
III	50% to 95%
IV	100% (total or "eight ball" hyphema)

TABLE 6-4. TREATMENT OF HYPHEMA

SUGGESTED ORDERS	COMMENT
Hospitalization	Young children and elderly; all patients with rebleeds. Reliable adults with microhyphema may be treated with bed rest at home if community standards allow. They should be examined daily for 5 additional days, refrain from any activity, and return immediately if any pain or decrease in vision occurs.
Bed rest	With the head of the bed elevated 30°; bathroom privileges with assistance.
Sedation as needed	Adults: Lorazepam (Ativan) 2 mg/day to 3 mg/day every 8 hours to 12 hours by mouth; children: chloral hydrate 50 mg/kg 3 to 4 times daily (see also Table 3-3). Sleeping pill at night for adults (e.g., flurazepam [Dalmane] 30 mg by mouth).
Laxative of choice	Adults only.
Shield involved eye	Patch only if there is an associated corneal abrasion.
Eye rest	May watch television at a distance, no prolonged reading or near visual tasks.
Cycloplegia	Atropine 1% topically, three to four times per day.
Topical steroids	Prednisolone acetate 1% every 2 hours to 6 hours if a fibrinous anterior chamber reaction develops.
No aspirin products	Use acetaminophen with or without codeine for analgesia.
Antiemetic as needed	Prochloroperazine (Compazine): Adults: 10 mg intramuscularly every 8 hours or 25 mg suppository every 12 hours; children: 0.06 per pound body weight intramuscularly, or 2.5 mg suppository two to three times per day. Promethazine hydrochloride (Phenergan): Adults: 25 mg intramuscularly or suppository every 4 hours to 6 hours; children: 0.5 mg/lb body weight (maximum dose 25 mg). The safety of these medications in children less than 20 pounds in weight or 2 years in age has not been established.
Antiglaucoma medications	For elevations of intraocular pressure > 40 mm Hg at presentation, or > 30 mm Hg for 2 weeks or more subsequently (20 mm Hg in those with sickle cell trait or disease): *First line:* Topical beta-blocker (e.g., levobunolol or timolol ¼% two times per day) *Second line:* Acetazolamide 250 mg by mouth four times daily. (In sickle cell use Neptazane 50 mg 2 to 3 times per day.) *Third line:* Mannitol 1–2 g/kg intravenously over 45 minutes once every 24 hours.
Aminocaproic acid (Amicar)	Use based on community standards and patient presentation (see text); dose is 50 mg/kg by mouth every 4 hours (maximum 30 g per day). *If no rebleeding occurs:* halve dose on day 3 and discontinue on day 4. Be cognizant that intraocular pressure may rise suddenly upon cessation of use. *If rebleeding occurs:* continue Amicar for 5 additional days, check clotting studies, bleeding time, platelet count.

TABLE 6-4. TREATMENT OF HYPHEMA (continued)

SUGGESTED ORDERS	COMMENT
Laboratory studies	Complete blood count; clotting studies, platelet count, and liver function tests if history of bleeding disorder. Baseline creatinine and blood urea nitrogen (BUN) if aminocaproic acid is to be used. Sickle cell prep, hemoglobin electrophoresis in black patients.
Surgical evacuation of clot	See Table 6-5 for indications.

Rebleeding of a hyphema usually occurs from the second to the fifth day following injury. Rebleeds are frequently of greater magnitude than the original hemorrhage and more likely to be associated with elevated intraocular pressure. An increase in size of the hyphema, particularly the presence of bright red blood over darker, clotted blood confirms this occurrence. If rebleeding does not occur, cycloplegic agents and steroids are tapered beginning on the sixth day after injury, with the rapidity of tapering based on the presence of anterior chamber inflammation. Antiglaucoma medication may have to be continued indefinitely. The patient should continue to refrain from strenuous exercise and wear an eye shield at night for an additional 2 weeks. Normal activities can resume 1 month after injury, but the patient should be instructed to use polycarbonate eye protection for sports or hazardous labor for the rest of his or her life. A dilated fundus examination with scleral depression and gonioscopy should be performed 1 month after injury. Patients with *recession of the anterior chamber angle* should be informed of the necessity of yearly eye examinations, to detect the onset of glaucoma, which can occur years after the injury.

TABLE 6-5. INDICATIONS FOR SURGICAL EVACUATION OF CLOT IN HYPHEMA

INDICATION	COMMENT
Elevated intraocular pressure (IOP) unresponsive to medical therapy	IOP > 50 mm Hg for 5 days IOP > 35 mm Hg for 7 days IOP > 25 mm Hg for 1 day in patients with sickle cell disease or trait or preexisting glaucoma
Corneal bloodstaining	At the first sign of bloodstaining, regardless of IOP or grade of hyphema. If IOP > 25 mm Hg and total hyphema to prevent bloodstaining
Prolonged clot duration	Persistent total hyphema > 5 days Persistent small hyphema > 10 days

INJURIES TO THE LENS

Trauma is the most common cause of *dislocation of the ocular lens* (Figure 6-5). Other causes include congenital dislocation, systemic syndrome (e.g., Marfan's, homocystinuria), inflammation, and buphthalmos (see Chapter 10).

Traumatic dislocation results when contusion-induced equatorial expansion of the eye disrupts the zonule. A complete rupture results in a free-floating ("luxated") lens; partial severance results in a "subluxated" lens. Symptoms of dislocation are fluctuating vision, glare, monocular diplopia, and decreased vision, the last resulting from functional aphakia or induced astigmatism.

A partial dislocation is occasionally difficult to diagnose. The pupil should be dilated and the lens examined using retroillumination at the slit lamp. The zonules can often be seen with a gonioscopy lens. Visualization of vitreous between broken zonules or the edge of the lens within the pupil confirms the diagnosis. Additional signs are shallowing (or deepening) of the anterior chamber, iridodonesis (movement of the iris with ocular movement) and phacodonesis (fine movement of the lens on ocular movement). Patients with a dislocated lens are always evaluated for other signs of ocular injury.

Complications of dislocated lenses include refractive disorders, pupillary block glaucoma, and lenticular-corneal touch. Incomplete rupture of the zonule causes the lens to be drawn to the side of the intact zonular fibers. If the lens is dislocated out of the visual axis, functional aphakia results. If the edge of the

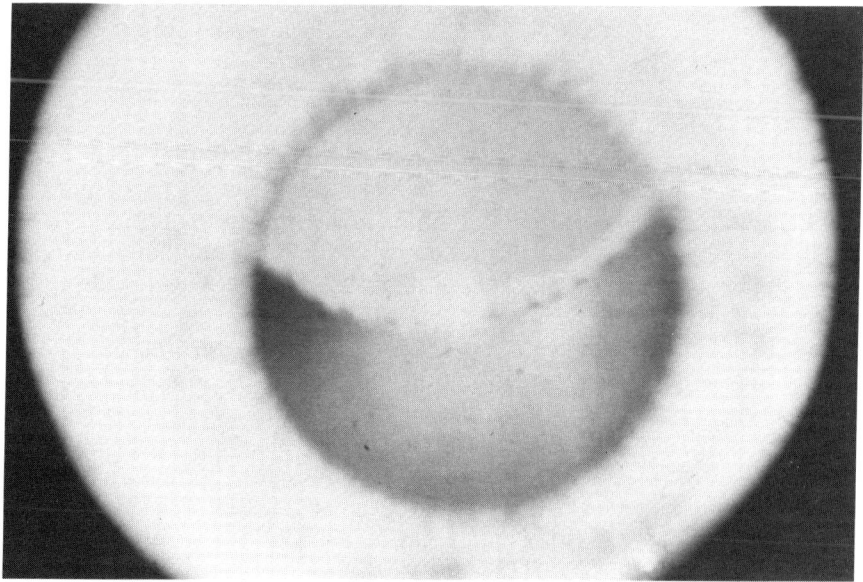

FIGURE 6-5. Traumatic dislocation of the ocular lens.

lens lies on this axis, astigmatism and monocular diplopia can result. Pupillary block occurs when the pupillary aperture is occluded by the dislocated lens. An anteriorly dislocated lens can also touch the posterior cornea, damaging the endothelial cells. Rarely, nonpupillary block glaucoma can result from misdirection of aqueous humor or anterior displacement of the lens-iris diaphragm. This is suggested by shallowing of the central anterior chamber, absence of lens movement, and myopic shift in refraction. Nonpupillary block is treated with cycloplegic-mydriatic agents to relax the ciliary body and allow for posterior movement of the lens-iris diaphragm. As with any "malignant glaucoma" simulating disorder, iridectomy and miotics may worsen this condition.

A noncataractous, dislocated lens may be stable and asymptomatic for years. The patient, however, should be forewarned of the symptoms of pupillary block glaucoma and advised to wear eye protection for sports and hazardous labor. Contact lenses can be used to correct an induced aphakic or astigmatic refractive error. These are preferable to spectacles because they produce less image size disparity with the normal eye (aniseikonia). Pupillary dilation or constriction occasionally improves visual acuity. Patients treated with miotics should be informed of the possibility of pupillary block glaucoma, and those treated with mydriatics warned of possible dislocation of the lens into the anterior chamber and corneal decompensation. In some cases, the neodymium:YAG laser can be used to lyse the remaining zonules, achieving a clear aphakic visual axis. The surgical considerations for removal of a dislocated lens are reviewed in Chapter 10. Indications include pupillary block, corneal touch, inflammation, and decreased vision.

A *contusion cataract* results when the lens capsule is ruptured by a direct or contrecoup injury. In addition to lenticular opacification (Figure 6–6), affected patients present with decreased vision, elevated intraocular pressure, and/or intraocular inflammation. The rapidity of cataract formation depends on whether the lens capsule was ruptured. In the absence of rupture, a cataract may not develop for months; with rupture, the lens can become hydrated and cataractous within hours. Not every cataract is progressive; a small rent may self-seal with the development of a fibrous plaque at the site of the injury. When the visual acuity is not appreciably reduced and glaucoma or inflammation not induced, the preferred management is observation. Miotics may be helpful in reducing glare and diplopia induced by focal opacities.

As with subluxated lenses, the evaluation should include an assessment of associated injuries, as well as the location and extent of lens injury. The status of the posterior capsule and presence of any zonular rupture (dislocation of the lens) are the two most important factors in surgical planning. The lens capsule can usually be assessed at the slit lamp, but occasionally a fibrinous reaction in the anterior chamber, or opacification of the lens, will prevent an adequate assessment. A water bath ultrasound may be helpful in these instances. If the posterior capsule is ruptured, a pars plana approach may be prudent to minimize the risk of nuclear dislocation into the vitreous.

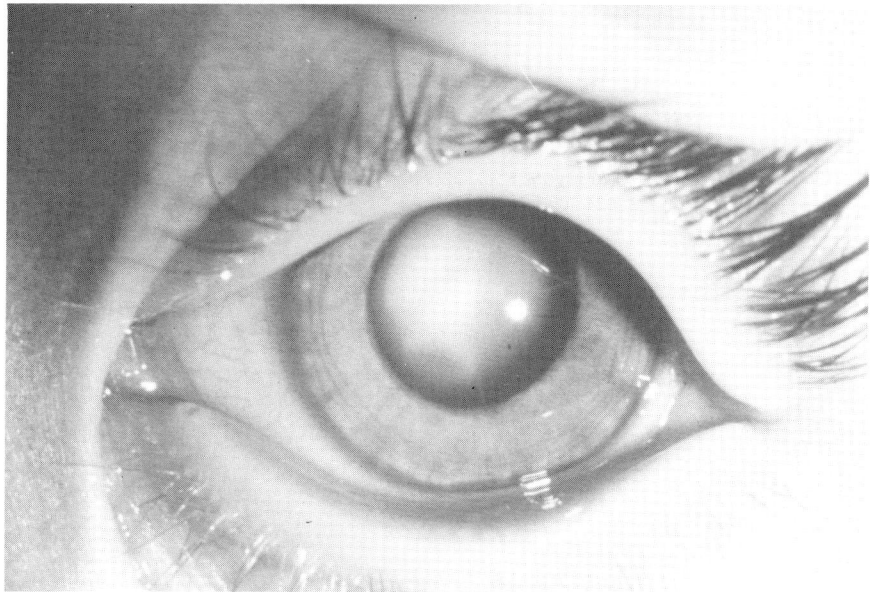

FIGURE 6-6. Contusion cataract.

Lens-induced glaucoma can result from two mechanisms other than pupillary block. The trabecular meshwork can be blocked by high-molecular-weight lens proteins liberated by trauma *(lens-particle glaucoma)*. Additionally, denatured lens material from a cataractous lens can leak through an intact lens capsule and be engulfed by macrophages that clog the anterior chamber angle *(phacolytic glaucoma)*. Lens-induced glaucoma is suspected when a break in the lens capsule and fluffy white particles in the anterior chamber and chamber angle are seen on slit lamp examination. Phacolytic glaucoma is suspected by the presence of iridescent particles, cells, and protein flare. Similar particles may be present on the surface of the lens capsule and in the gonioscopically open anterior chamber angle. Phacolytic glaucoma can be confirmed by the presence of macrophages filled with lens material on microscopic examination of aqueous humor obtained by paracentesis. Both problems are treated with corticosteroids (e.g., prednisolone acetate 1% every 6 hours in lens induced and as frequently as every hour in phacolytic glaucoma); antiglaucoma medications (e.g., timolol or levobunolol ½% every 12 hours, acetazolamide 500 mg initially followed by 250 mg every 6 hours, or mannitol 1 g/kg to 2 g/kg intravenously over 45 minutes); and topical cycloplegia (e.g., cyclogel 1% every 8 hours). Cataract extraction is performed after the intraocular pressure has been brought under control (usually within 24 hours to 36 hours).

VITREOUS HEMORRHAGE

Vitreous hemorrhage following blunt ocular trauma suggests a retinal tear, choroidal rupture, avulsion of the optic nerve head, and/or an occult foreign body. If the hemorrhage prevents adequate examination, an ultrasound should be performed. Retinal examination with scleral depression to examine the anterior retina for dialyses and tears should be performed as soon as it is evident that an occult scleral laceration is not present.

Vitrectomy may be necessary if there is an associated retinal detachment. A retinal detachment that threatens the macula should be treated as soon as feasible. The ideal time to perform vitrectomy if the macula is not threatened is debatable. Surgical evacuation of vitreous hemorrhage is easier after dissolution of clotted blood, which occurs 10 or more days after injury. A posterior vitreous detachment also often occurs by this time, making vitrectomy technically easier. Proliferative vitreoretinopathy, an important cause of failure to reattach the retina anatomically, however, may be lessened by early removal of intraocular blood.

INJURIES TO THE CHOROID

The choroid is susceptible to concussive injury because it lacks the strength of the sclera and the elasticity of the retina. The horizontal expansion of the posterior eye that accompanies anteroposterior compression tears the relatively inelastic Bruch's membrane of the choroid, creating a *choroidal rupture,* which is usually accompanied by disruption of the underlying vascular layer of the choroid (choriocapillaris) and the overlying retinal pigment epithelium.

Choroidal ruptures can occur with direct trauma, in which case they are located anteriorly and parallel to the ora serrata. More frequently, the rupture occurs due to a contrecoup injury, in which case it is posterior, crescent shaped, and usually concentric with the optic disk (Figure 6-7). The macular region is often involved, but ruptures can occur anywhere; rarely are they multiple or radially oriented. At presentation, hemorrhage may obscure the eventual finding of a yellow-white curvilinear streak.

Visual dysfunction occurs immediately upon injury, with visual acuity often reduced below 20/200 in posterior ruptures. Transection through the foveal area, and extensive pigmentary changes in the macular area, are poor prognostic indicators for visual acuity. A multitude of visual field abnormalities can also occur depending on the site of rupture but often fail to correlate with the ophthalmoscopic findings. Late complications of choroidal rupture include the development of a subretinal neovascular membrane (SRNM) and atrophy of the overlying retina.

Fluorescein angiography can confirm the presence of a choroidal rupture or a subretinal neovascular membrane, unless overlying hemorrhage blocks flu-

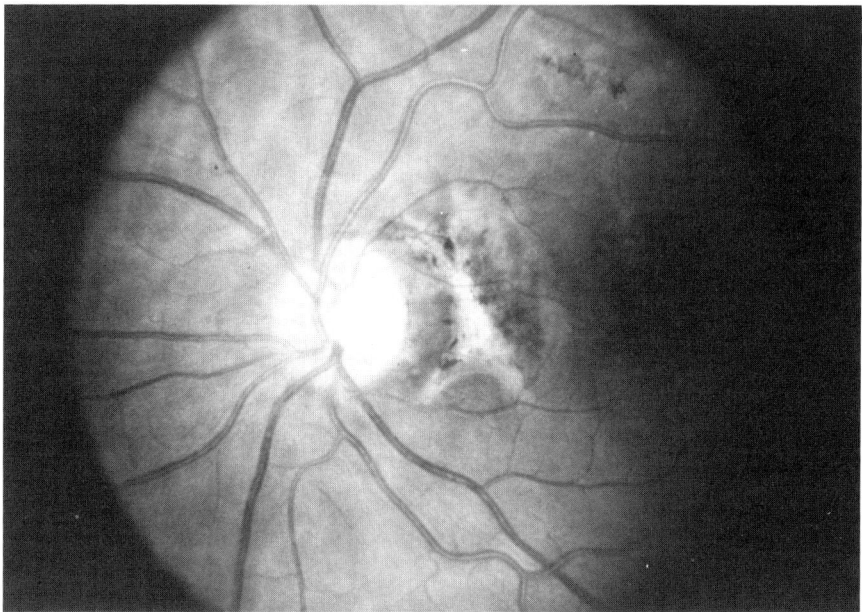

FIGURE 6-7. Choroidal rupture.

orescence. Patients should be followed every 1 week to 2 weeks until the choroid can be visualized. Confirmation of a rupture mandates daily use of an Amsler grid by the patient for the early detection of a SRNM (see Chapter 1) and fundus examinations every 3 months to 6 months. No treatment for the choroidal rupture exists, but laser photocoagulation may be of benefit if an SRNM develops within the macular area. Indications for treatment include a membrane more than 200 microns from the center of the fovea and the absence of foveolar hemorrhage or exudate.

INJURIES TO THE RETINA

Commotio retinae (retinal edema, concussion edema, Berlin's edema) typically involves the retina opposite the side of an anterior segment impact (contrecoup injury). Minutes to hours after the impact, edematous swelling of the involved outer retina becomes manifest. It is recognized as a white opacification with ill-defined borders. A geographic pattern of involvement is common; the peripheral retina, macula, peripapillary area, or any combination of areas may be affected (Figure 6-8). If the entire posterior pole is involved, a pseudo–cherry red macular spot may be present. Normal blood flow through the inner retinal vessels easily differentiates this from a central retinal artery occlusion.

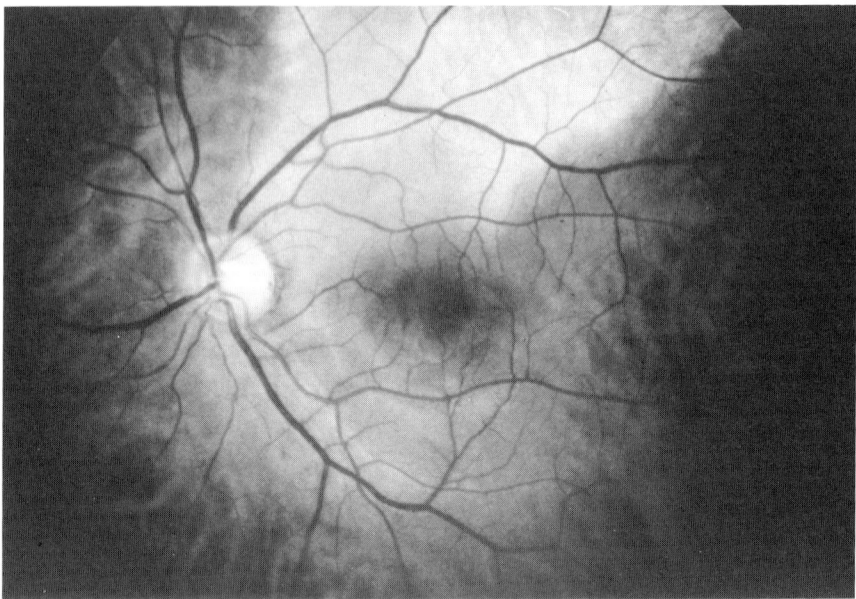

FIGURE 6-8. Commotio retinae.

Macular involvement is manifest by an acute loss of central vision with a potential reduction in acuity of up to 20/400. Peripheral commotio retinae may be asymptomatic, but the ophthalmoscopic appearance, especially several days after the episode, does not correlate with the level of acuity. The histologic findings are controversial but likely involve disorganization and degeneration of the photoreceptors, with or without intracellular edema of the retinal pigment epithelium (RPE).

The appearance of retinal opacification subsides over several weeks, and visual function usually gradually returns to its pretrauma level. A permanent loss of vision, however, is not unusual and can be associated with RPE mottling, hyperplasia, or atrophy. Rarely, microcystic areas can develop in the macula, coalesce to form a large cyst, and rupture to form a full or partial thickness macular hole. Associated injuries, such as choroidal rupture and retinal hemorrhages, contribute to a poor prognosis.

No treatment for commotio retinae is efficacious, and generally the prognosis is favorable. Fluorescein angiography during the acute period may be of some prognostic benefit. Abnormalities such as hyperfluorescent staining at the level of the RPE suggests RPE necrosis and potential long-term visual dysfunction.

Retinitis sclopetaria (chorioretinitis sclopetaria, chorioretinitis proliferans) is a concussive injury to the posterior eye resulting from shock waves produced by orbital penetration of a high-velocity missile (often a BB pellet). The missile does not penetrate the eye but ruptures the choroid and retina in the area adjacent to its path. Extension into the macula and concussive optic nerve injury is frequent. Initially, extensive intraocular hemorrhage is seen, and retinal destruction and proliferation become apparent with resorption. Fibrous proliferation reduces the likelihood of subsequent retinal detachment, but visual acuity is almost always poor.

Traumatic macular holes can follow commotio retinae, choroidal ruptures, and subretinal hemorrhages. They can also occur with whiplash-type injuries of the eye, subsequent to the firm adherence of the vitreous to the retina in the macular area. Sudden deceleration creates traction, causing the vitreous and the adherent inner retina to detach from the outer retina.

Similar to idiopathic macular holes (Chapter 14), those due to trauma have sharp, well-demarcated margins (Figure 6–9). The hole may be partial (lamellar) or full thickness. Visual function is more severely affected with full thickness holes, which are associated with acuities of 20/80 to 20/200. In addition to better acuity, lamellar holes can be differentiated by biomicroscopic examination of the retina and fluorescein angiography. The presence of an intact outer retinal layer and the absence of subretinal fluid are characteristic of a lamellar hole. A retinal pigment epithelial window defect on fluorescein angiography is more characteristic of a full thickness hole.

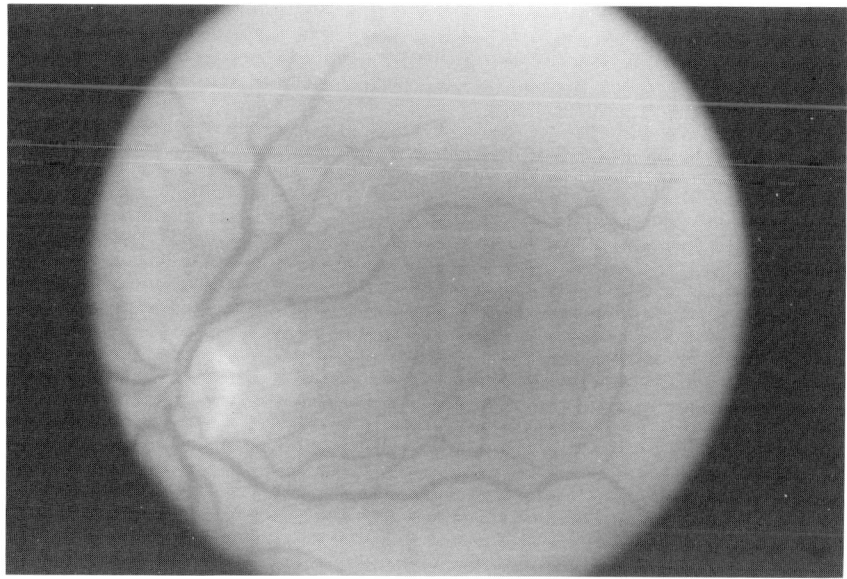

FIGURE 6–9. Traumatic macular hole.

Traumatic retinal holes subsequent to commotio retinae or subretinal hemorrhage may take months to years to develop and are preceded by cystic changes in the macula. Once a macular hole develops, progressive detachment of the posterior retina is not typical but is more likely to occur in highly myopic eyes. Prophylactic laser photocoagulation to the margin of macular holes has been tried but has not been proved to reduce the incidence of subsequent detachment. The majority of affected patients should be followed conservatively unless and until progressive detachment occurs. Vitrectomy, scleral buckle, and laser photocoagulation can then be performed in an attempt to preserve peripheral vision.

Traumatic retinal breaks and detachments result from the same forces that cause choroidal ruptures. Anteroposterior compression of the eye expands the equatorial diameter of the globe, creating traction at the vitreous base. This traction is transmitted to the peripheral retina, which is firmly adherent to the vitreous. Consequent injuries include avulsion of the vitreous base, dialysis of the retina, peripheral retinal tears, and irregular retinal holes with ragged edges in the equatorial zone of the retina. The most frequent locations of pathology are the inferotemporal and superonasal quadrants, but retinal breaks can occur in any quadrant, especially at sites of strong vitreoretinal attachment such as lattice degeneration. Large, irregular tears can occur from direct shearing forces. Usually these occur in the temporal retina and are associated with intraretinal hemorrhages and edema.

Avulsion of the vitreous base may be asymptomatic, or the patient may note flashes (photopsia) and/or a few floaters. Vitreous base avulsion does not need to be treated, but the patient should be warned of the signs of retinal detachment (the onset of a shower of new floaters, photopsia, and/or a progressive loss of visual field similar to a curtain being drawn over the eye).

A *retinal dialysis* is a disinsertion of the peripheral retina from its anteriormost attachments at the ora serrata (Figure 6-10). The dialysis usually occurs on impact, but the patient may note only photopsia, floaters, or mildly disturbed vision at this time. A small dialysis is recognized as a slitlike separation of the retina at the ora and is best appreciated using indirect ophthalmoscopy with scleral depression. Not all dialyses lead to retinal detachment; spontaneous chorioretinal readhesion, usually manifest by marked pigmentary changes, can occur. In the absence of retinal detachment, a dialysis should be treated prophylactically with laser photocoagulation or cryopexy. A retinal detachment may progress slowly, and one or more demarcation lines may develop at successive stages of detachment. Associated floaters and photopsia may go unheeded until the detachment progresses posterior to the equator, and a visual field loss is noted. Treatment consists of cryopexy and the placement of a circumferential scleral buckle; the visual results from surgery are excellent if the macula has not detached.

Retinal tears due to blunt trauma include small peripheral holes without apparent vitreoretinal traction, larger irregular-shaped holes (usually at the

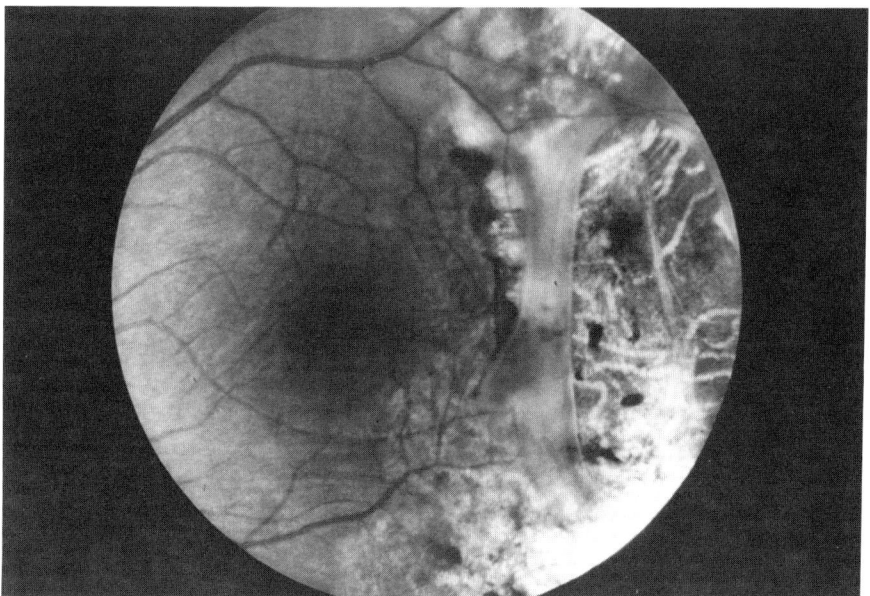

FIGURE 6-10. Retinal dialysis.

direct site of impact), macular holes (see above), and tractional horseshoe tears. Retinal tears usually produce symptoms of floaters and photopsia and may be accompanied by vitreous and retinal hemorrhage. With the exception of macular holes, tears are more likely than dialysis to progress to retinal detachment. The time interval between ocular contusion and retinal detachment is variable. Nearly half of all traumatic retinal detachments are apparent within 1 month of injury, and the majority occur within 2 years of injury. Prophylactic treatment includes laser photocoagulation and cryopexy. Once a detachment has occurred, a scleral buckle and cryopexy are usually indicated. Small detachments can be managed occasionally using laser photocoagulation or cryopexy alone, and eyes with large areas of retinal necrosis may need vitrectomy and the placement of an intraocular gas bubble. The prognosis for small tears, without involvement of the macula and without a large area of retinal necrosis, is excellent. Retinal detachments with substantial subretinal hemorrhage carry a more guarded visual prognosis. Surgical drainage of subretinal blood combined with pars plana vitrectomy can result in anatomic reattachment, but the prognosis for visual acuity is poor if blood has dissected under the macula.

A giant retinal tear is one that extends more than 90° of the circumference of the globe (involves more than one quadrant). Giant tears occur especially in traumatized myopic eyes. They are usually circumferentially located at the border of the vitreous base and may be associated with retinal necrosis at the site of impact. Signs are acute and dramatic and include floaters, photopsia, and decreased vision. Prophylactic laser photocoagulation or cryopexy is indicated in the absence of retinal detachment, and a prophylactic scleral buckle should be placed if there is any evidence of vitreous traction. The presence of a retinal detachment necessitates vitrectomy with fluid-gas or silicone oil exchange. Retinal sutures, tacks, and cyanoacrylate tissue adhesive have also been used. Proliferative vitreoretinopathy (PVR) is a not infrequent complication of a giant retinal tear. Tears greater than 180° and those with PVR have a reduced visual prognosis.

OPTIC NERVE INJURY

Optic nerve lacerations or avulsions usually result from direct penetrating orbital injuries. Rarely, a blunt orbital injury can fracture the optic canal, and the resultant bony fragments can lacerate the optic nerve. A definitive fracture of the optic canal, however, is often not found with blunt injuries. In these cases, it is presumed that the optic nerve or its vascular supply has been torn, thrombosed, or compressed. Rarely, optic nerve compression from orbital emphysema has been implicated. The most common site of impact for blunt injuries causing optic nerve injury is the brow or slightly above it.

It is essential when obtaining the history to note whether the loss of vision was immediate, suggesting an avulsion or laceration of the optic nerve, or whether it occurred after a brief period of vision, suggesting optic nerve contusion or central retinal vein compression. In addition to the immediate decrease in vision, intraocular hemorrhage emanating from the optic nerve suggests laceration or avulsion (Figure 6–11). These can usually be confirmed by computed tomography or magnetic resonance imaging. No treatment exists for completely avulsed nerves.

Traumatic optic neuropathy, associated with optic disc swelling and the retinal appearance of a central retinal vein occlusion, may show dramatic improvement with optic nerve sheath fenestration. In this disorder, neuroimaging will demonstrate an enlarged optic nerve due to blood in the subarachnoid space. Without treatment, vision rarely improves.

The treatment of patients with suspected traumatic optic neuropathy with a normal-appearing optic disc is more controversial. Without treatment, vision can spontaneously improve in 20% to 35% of affected patients (Seiff, 1991). Vision has been reported to return spontaneously, albeit with some residual defects, even in patients with no light perception at presentation (Wolin and Lavin, 1990). Optic nerve decompression and systemic corticosteroid therapy have been advocated by many to improve the prognosis. A number of surgical approaches to the optic canal have been described, but a transethmoid-sphenoid approach with removal of the medial wall of the optic canal may be as effective as, and possibly safer than, other approaches (Joseph et al, 1991).

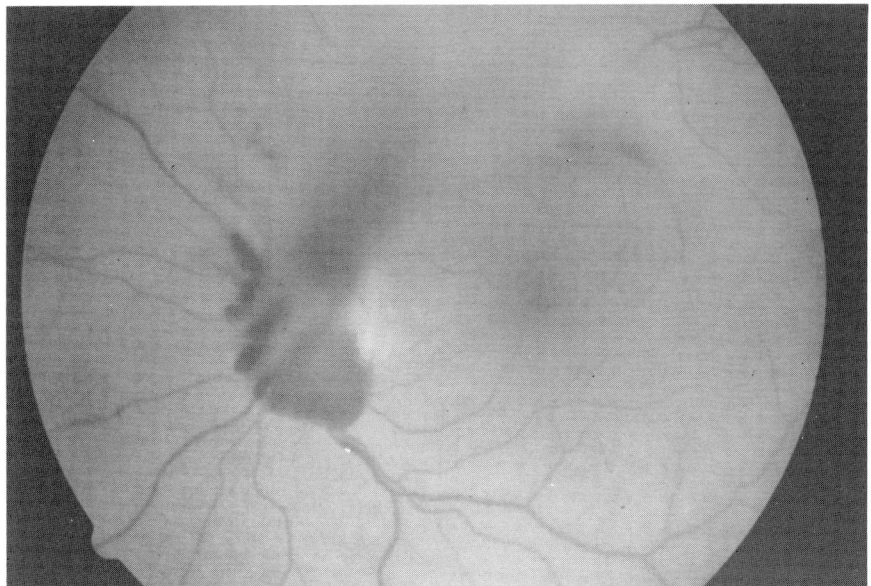

FIGURE 6-11. Acute optic nerve avulsion.

Among others, Anderson, Panje, and Gross (1982) reported corticosteroid use as an alternative or adjunct to optic canal decompression. They recommended 0.75 mg/kg dexamethasone sodium phosphate as a loading dose, followed by 0.33 mg/kg every 6 hours for the initial 24 hours. Steroids are then reduced to 1 mg/kg per day of dexamethasone for the subsequent 24-hour to 48-hour period. If a response occurs within the first 48 hours, steroids are slowly tapered over 5 days to 7 days; if no response occurs, steroids are rapidly tapered. Optic nerve decompression is recommended when visual loss following frontal head trauma is delayed or when an initial return of vision with megadose steroids is followed by subsequent visual decrease while on or with tapering of steroids. Megadose steroids are never recommended for the routine treatment of orbital fractures. When used, one should consider the concomitant use of an H_2 blocker (oral ranitidine hydrochloride [Zantac] 150 mg every 12 hours) to reduce gastrointestinal bleeding.

REFERENCES

Corneal and Scleral Injuries

Binder PS, Waring GO III, Arrowsmith PN, Wang C: Histopathology of traumatic corneal rupture after radial keratotomy. *Arch Ophthalmol* 106:1584, 1988.
Cherry PMH: Indirect traumatic rupture of the globe. *Arch Ophthalmol* 96:252, 1978.

Cibis GW, Weigeist TA, Krachmer JH: Traumatic corneal endothelial rings. *Arch Ophthalmol* 96:485, 1978.
Deg JK, Zavala EY, Binder PS: Delayed corneal wound healing following radial keratotomy. *Ophthalmology* 92:734, 1985.
Farley MK, Pettit TH: Traumatic wound dehiscence after penetrating keratoplasty. *Am J Ophthalmol* 104:44, 1987.
Forstot SL, Damiano RE: Trauma after radial keratotomy. *Ophthalmology* 95:833, 1988.
Maloney WF, Colvard M, Bourne WM, Gardon R: Specular microscopy of traumatic posterior annular keratopathy. *Arch Ophthalmol* 97:1647, 1979.
Raber IM, Arentsen JJ, Laibson PR: Traumatic wound rupture following successful penetrating keratoplasty. *Arch Ophthalmol* 98:1407, 1980.
Russell SR, Olsen KR, Folk JC: Predictors of scleral rupture and the role of vitrectomy in severe blunt ocular trauma. *Am J Ophthalmol* 105:253, 1988.
Simmons KB, Linsalata RP: Ruptured globe following blunt trauma after radial keratotomy: A case report. *J Refract Surg* 4:132, 1988.
Slingsby JG, Forstot SL: Effect of blunt trauma on the corneal endothelium. *Arch Ophthalmol* 99:1041, 1981.
Wellington DP, Johnstone MA, Hopkins RJ: Bull's eye corneal lesion resulting from war game injury. *Arch Ophthalmol* 107:1727, 1989.

Choroidal and Iris Injuries

Aguilar JP, Green WR: Choroidal rupture: A histopathologic study of 47 cases. *Retina* 4:269, 1984.
Hilton GF: Late serosanguinous detachment of the macula after traumatic choroidal rupture. *Am J Ophthalmol* 79:997, 1975.
Hornblass A: Pupillary dilation in fractures of the floor of the orbit. *Ophthalmic Surg* 10:44, 1979.
Maberley AL, Carvounis EP: The visual field in indirect traumatic rupture of the choroid. *Can J Ophthalmol* 12:147, 1977.
McCannel MA: A retrievable suture idea for anterior uveal problems. *Ophthalmic Surg* 7:98, 1976.
Paton D, Craig J: Management of iridodialysis. *Ophthalmic Surg* 4:38, 1973.
Peli E: Functional difficulties resulting from traumatic anisocoria. *Am J Optom Physiol Opt* 61:548, 1984.
Smith RE, Kelly JS, Harbin TS: Late macular complications of choroidal ruptures. *Am J Ophthalmol* 77:650, 1974.

Traumatic Hyphema

Agapitos PJ, Noel LP, Clarke WN: Traumatic hyphema in children. *Ophthalmol* 94:1238, 1987.
Belcher CD, Brown SVL, Simmons RJ: Anterior chamber washout for traumatic hyphema. *Ophthalmic Surg* 16:475, 1985.
Cassel GH, Jeffers JB, Jaeger EA: Wills Eye Hospital traumatic hyphema study. *Ophthalmic Surg* 16:441, 1984.
Collet BI: Traumatic hyphema: A review. *Ann Ophthalmol* 14:52, 1982.
Crouch ER, Frenkel M: Aminocaproic acid in the treatment of traumatic hyphema. *Am J Ophthalmol* 81:355, 1976.
Deutsch TA, Weinreb RN, Goldberg MF: Indications for surgical management of hyphema in patients with sickle cell trait. *Arch Ophthalmol* 102:566, 1984.
Dieste MC, Hersh PS, Kylstra JA, et al: Intraocular pressure increase associated with epsilon-aminocaproic acid therapy for traumatic hyphema. *Am J Ophthalmol* 106:383, 1988.
Edwards WC, Layden WF: Traumatic hyphema. *Am J Ophthalmol* 75:110, 1973.
Farber MD, Fiscella R, Goldberg MF: Aminocaproic acid versus prednisone for the treatment of traumatic hyphema: A randomized clinical trial. *Ophthalmology* 98:279, 1991.
Ganley JP, Geiger JM, Clement JR, et al: Aspirin and recurrent hyphema after blunt ocular trauma. *Am J Ophthalmol* 96:797, 1983.
Gilbert HD, Jensen AD: Atropine in the treatment of traumatic hyphema. *Ann Ophthalmol* 5:1297, 1973.
Goldberg MF: Sickled erythrocytes, hyphema, and secondary glaucoma. *Ophthalmic Surg* 10:17, 1979.

Goldberg MF: Antifibrinolytic agents in the management of traumatic hyphema. *Arch Ophthalmol* 101:1029, 1983.
Howard GM: Spontaneous hyphema in infancy and childhood. *Arch Ophthalmol* 68:615, 1962.
Kennedy RH, Brubaker RF: Traumatic hyphema in a defined population. *Am J Ophthalmol* 106:123, 1988.
Kraft SP, Christianson MD, Crawford JS, et al: Traumatic hyphema in children: Treatment with epsilon-aminocaproic acid. *Ophthalmology* 94:1232, 1987.
Kutner B, Fourman S, Brein K, et al: Aminocaproic acid reduces the risk of secondary hemorrhage in patients with traumatic hyphema. *Arch Ophthalmol* 105:206, 1987.
Loewy DM, Williams PB, Crouch ER Jr, Cooke WJ: Systemic aminocaproic acid reduces fibrinolysis in the aqueous humor. *Arch Ophthalmol* 105:272, 1987.
McGetrick JJ, Jampol LM, Goldberg MF, et al: Aminocaproic acid decreases secondary hemorrhage after traumatic hyphema. *Arch Ophthalmol* 101:1031, 1983.
Palmer DJ, Goldberg MF, Frenkel M, et al: A comparison of two dose regimens of epsilon aminocaproic acid in the prevention and management of secondary traumatic hyphemas. *Ophthalmology* 93:102, 1986.
Pilger IS: Medical treatment of traumatic hyphema. *Surv Ophthalmol* 20:28, 1975.
Read J, Goldberg MF: Comparison of medical treatment for traumatic hyphema. *Trans Am Acad Ophthalmol Otolaryngol* 78:799, 1974.
Rynne MV, Romano PE: Systemic corticosteroids in the treatment of traumatic hyphema. *J Pediatr Ophthalmol Strabismus* 17:141, 1980.
Spoor TC, Hammer M, Belloso H: Traumatic hyphema: Failure of steroids to alter its course: A double blind prospective study. *Arch Ophthalmol* 98:116, 1988.
Spoor TC, Kwitko GM, O'Grady JM, Ramocki JM: Traumatic hyphema in an urban population. *Am J Ophthalmol* 109:23, 1990.
Thomas MA, Parrish RK, Feuer WJ: Rebleeding after traumatic hyphema. *Arch Ophthalmol* 104:206, 1986.
Uusitalo RJ, Ranta-Kemppainen L, Tarkkanen A: Management of traumatic hyphema in children. *Arch Ophthalmol* 106:1207, 1988.
Vangsted P, Nielsen PJ: Tranexamic acid and traumatic hyphema. *Acta Ophthalmol* 618:447, 1983.
Weiss JS, Parrish RK, Anderson DR: Surgical therapy of traumatic hyphema. *Ophthalmic Surg* 14:343, 1983.
Williams DF, Han DP, Abrams GW: Rebleeding in experimental traumatic hyphema treated with intraocular tissue plasminogen activator. *Arch Ophthalmol* 108:264, 1990.
Wilson FM: Traumatic hyphema: Pathogenesis and management. *Ophthalmology* 87:910, 1980.
Wright KW, Sunal PM, Urrea P: Bed rest versus activity ad lib in the treatment of small hyphemas. *Ann Ophthalmol* 20:143, 1988.
Yasuna E: Management of traumatic hyphema. *Arch Ophthalmol* 91:190, 1974.

Traumatic Lens Injuries

Chandler PA, Grant WM: Mydriatic-cycloplegic treatment in malignant glaucoma. *Arch Ophthalmol* 68:353, 1962.
Epstein DL, Jedziniak JA, Grant WM: Obstruction of aqueous outflow by lens particles and heavy-molecular weight soluble proteins. *Invest Ophthalmol Vis Sci* 17:272, 1978.
Hemo Y, Ben Ezra D: Traumatic cataracts in young children: correction of aphakia by intraocular lens implantation. *Ophthalmic Pediatr Genet* 8:203, 1987.
Illiff CE, Kramer P: A working guide for the management of dislocated lenses. *Ophthalmic Surg* 2:251, 1971.
Jarrett WH: Dislocation of the lens: A study of 166 hospitalized cases. *Arch Ophthalmol* 78:289, 1967.
Kutner BN: Acute angle closure glaucoma in nonperforating blunt trauma. *Arch Ophthalmol* 106:19, 1988.
Nelson LB, Maumenee IH: Ectopia lentis. *Surv Ophthalmol* 27:143, 1982.
Nelson LB, Szmyd SM: Aphakic correction in ectopia lentis. *Ann Ophthalmol* 17:445, 1985.
Sellyei LF Jr, Barraquer J: Surgery of the ectopic lens. *Ann Ophthalmol* 5:1127, 1973.
Tchah H, Larson RS, Nichols BD, Lindstrom RL: Neodymium: YAG laser zonulysis for treatment of lens subluxation. *Ophthalmology* 96:230, 1989.

Optic Nerve Injuries

Anderson RL, Panje WR, Gross CE: Optic nerve blindness following blunt forehead trauma. *Ophthalmology* 89:445, 1982.
Giovinazzo VJ: The ocular sequelae of blunt trauma. *Adv Ophthalmic Plast Reconstr Surg* 6:107, 1987.
Guy J, Sherwood M, Day AL: Surgical treatment of progressive visual loss in traumatic optic neuropathy. *J Neurosurg* 70:799, 1989.
Joseph MP, Lessell S, Rizzo J, Momose J: Extracranial optic nerve decompression for traumatic optic neuropathy. *Arch Ophthalmol* 108:1091, 1990.
Joseph MP, Lessell S, Rizzo J, Momose J: Therapy for traumatic optic neuropathy: In reply. *Arch Ophthalmol* 109:610, 1991.
Lessell S: Indirect optic nerve trauma. *Arch Ophthalmol* 107:382, 1989.
Miller N: The management of traumatic optic neuropathy. *Arch Ophthalmol* 108:1086, 1990.
Petro J, Tooze FM, Bales CR, et al: Ocular injuries associated with periorbital fractures. *J Trauma* 19:730, 1979.
Seiff SR: High dose corticosteroids for treatment of vision loss due to indirect injury to the optic nerve. *Ophthalmic Surg* 21:389, 1990.
Seiff SR: Therapy for traumatic optic neuropathy. *Arch Ophthalmol* 109:610, 1991.
Wolin MJ, Lavin PJM: Spontaneous visual recovery from traumatic optic neuropathy after blunt head injury. *Am J Ophthalmol* 109:430, 1990.

Retinal and Vitreous Injuries

Aaberg TM, Blair CJ, Gass JDM: Macular holes. *Am J Ophthalmol* 69:555, 1970.
Assaf A: Traumatic retinal detachment. *J Trauma* 25:1085, 1985.
Appiah AP, Hirose T: Secondary causes of premacular fibrosis. *Ophthalmology* 96:389, 1989.
Blight R, Hart JCD: Structural changes in the outer retinal layers following blunt mechanical non-perforating trauma to the globe: An experimental study. *Br J Ophthalmol* 6:573, 1977.
Chang S, Reppucci V, Zimmerman N, et al: Perfluorocarbon liquids in the management of traumatic retinal detachments. *Ophthalmology* 96:785, 1989.
Cox MS, Freeman HM: Traumatic retinal detachment. In Freeman HM (ed): *Ocular Trauma*. New York, Appleton-Century-Crofts, 1979, pp 285–293.
Cox MS, Schepens CL, Freeman HM: Retinal detachment due to ocular contusion. *Arch Ophthalmol* 76:678, 1966.
de Juan E Jr, Hickingbotham D, Machemer R: Retinal tacks. *Am J Ophthalmol* 99:272, 1985.
Delori F, Pomerantzeff O, Cox MS: Deformation of the globe under high-speed impact: Its relation to contusion injuries. *Invest Ophthalmol* 8:290, 1969.
Dumass JJ: Retinal detachment following contusion of the eye. *Int Ophthalmol Clin* 7:19, 1967.
Federman JL, Shakin JL, Lanning RC: The microsurgical management of giant retinal tears with trans-scleral retinal sutures. *Ophthalmology* 89:832, 1982.
Fuller B, Gitter KA: Traumatic choroidal rupture with late serous detachment of macula: Report of successful argon laser treatment. *Arch Ophthalmol* 89:354, 1973.
Glaser BM: Treatment of giant retinal tears combined with proliferative vitreoretinopathy. *Ophthalmology* 93:1193, 1986.
Glaser BM, Cardin A, Biscoe B: Proliferative vitreoretinopathy: The mechanism of development of vitreoretinal traction. *Ophthalmology* 94:327, 1987.
Goffstein R, Burton TC: Differentiating traumatic from nontraumatic retinal detachment. *Ophthalmology* 89:361, 1982.
Han DP, Mieler WF, Schwartz DM, Abrams GW: Management of traumatic hemorrhagic retinal detachment with pars plana vitrectomy. *Arch Ophthalmol* 108:1281, 1990.
Hart JCD, Frank HJ: Retinal opacification after blunt nonperforating concussional injuries to the globe. *Trans Ophthalmol Soc UK* 95:94, 1975.
Hutton WL, Fuller DG: Factors influencing final visual results in severely injured eyes. *Am J Ophthalmol* 97:715, 1984.
Kelly JS, Hoover RE, George T: Whiplash maculopathy. *Arch Ophthalmol* 96:834, 1978.
McCuen BW II, Hida T, Sheta SM: Transvitreal cyanoacrylate retinopexy in the management of complicated retinal detachment. *Am J Ophthalmol* 104:127, 1987.

Michels RG, Rice TA, Blakenship G: Surgical techniques for selected giant retinal tears. *Retina* 3:139, 1983.
Richards RD, West CE, Meisels AA: Chorioretinitis sclopetaria. *Am J Ophthalmol* 66:852, 1968.
Ross WH: Traumatic retinal dialysis. *Arch Ophthalmol* 99:1371, 1981.
Sipperley JO, Quigley HA, Gass JDM: Traumatic retinopathy in primates: The explanation of commotio retinae. *Arch Ophthalmol* 96:2267, 1978.
Zion VM, Burton TC: Retinal dialysis. *Arch Ophthalmol* 98:1971, 1980.

7

Burns of the Eye

Michael W. Belin
Robert A. Catalano
James L. Scott

CHEMICAL BURNS

Chemical burns of the cornea and adnexal tissue are among the most urgent of ocular emergencies. They occur frequently because strong alkalies and acids are found in many common household and industrial products (Table 7–1). Intentional injury with chemicals is also seen in some urban areas, with black males age 30 years to 49 years at greatest risk. Although the majority of chemical burns are minor, strong alkalies and acids can have a devastating effect on ocular tissues.

Alkali burns are usually more destructive than acid burns. Alkalies react with fats to form soaps, which damage cell membranes, allowing further penetration of the alkali into the eye. The severity of the injury is related to the volume and concentration of the chemical and how rapidly it diffuses through the cornea. The following alkalies are listed in order of their speed of penetration from slowest to fastest: calcium hydroxide (mortar and plaster), potassium hydroxide (drain cleaner), sodium hydroxide (drain and oven cleaners), and ammonium hydroxide (ammonia). Calcium hydroxide does not penetrate well since the calcium soaps formed upon saponification are relatively insoluble and precipitate out, forming a barrier to further penetration.

Acids generally cause less severe, more localized tissue damage. The corneal epithelium offers moderate protection against weak acids, and little damage is seen unless the pH is 2.5 or less. Most stronger acids precipitate tissue proteins, creating a physical barrier against their further penetration. Buffering by sur-

TABLE 7-1. COMMON ACIDS AND ALKALI

PRODUCT	CHEMICAL	pH
Acids		
Toilet cleaner	Sulfuric acid (80%)	1.0
Battery fluid	Sulfuric acid (30%)	1.0
Pool cleaners	Sodium or calcium hypochlorite (70%)	1.0
Bleaches	Sodium hypochlorite (3%)	1.0
Alkalies		
Drain cleaner	Sodium or potassium hydroxide	14
Ammonia	Ammonium hydroxide (9%)	12.5
Dishwasher detergent	Sodium tripolyphosphate	12.0
Oven cleaners	Sodium hydroxide	14

rounding tissue proteins also helps localize the damage to the initial area of contact. Exceptions include burns from hydrofluoric acid and from acids containing heavy metals, which rapidly penetrate the cornea.

Clinical Manifestations

Mild acid or alkali burns are characterized by conjunctival hyperemia, diffuse chemosis, and mild corneal clouding or epithelial erosions (Figure 7–1). The stroma may be mildly edematous, and the anterior chamber may have mild to moderate cell and flare. More severe alkali burns are characterized by corneal opacification and limbal ischemia. They are classified according to the damage they cause to the limbus, the most important factor in determining the prognosis for recovery (Table 7–2). The two most important processes for repair of the chemically burned eye are vascularization and reepithelization. Injury to the deep structures at the limbus destroys the principal area for initiation of these processes.

Grading schemes for alkali burns are useful in predicting prognosis. Treatment modalities, however, are based more on the interval since injury. For severe alkali burns, three stages in the temporal sequence of events are distinguished. The immediate, or acute, phase begins at the time of injury and lasts approximately 3 days. During this stage, the corneal and conjunctival epithelium necrose, and the alkali rapidly penetrates into the anterior chamber, ciliary body, and iris. The intraocular pressure rises, probably due to the immediate shrinkage of collagen fibers, and conjunctival chemosis, injection, and limbal blanching occur. The cornea becomes opaque, the epithelium may slough, and there is widespread stromal edema.

The intermediate, or subacute, phase begins from 3 days to 7 days after injury and is characterized by a prolonged period of active inflammatory destruction of the eye. During this stage, new blood vessels begin to invade the

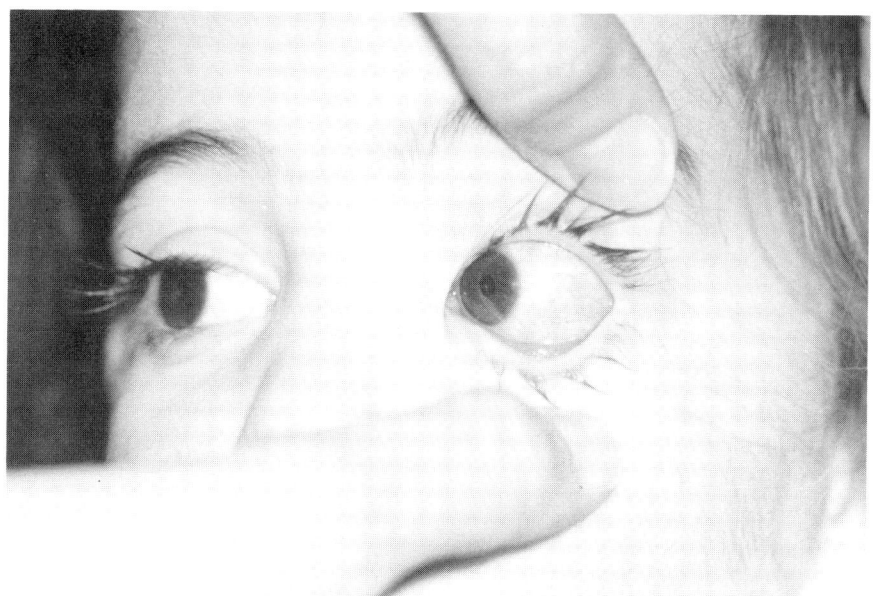

FIGURE 7-1. Mild ocular acid burn. The conjunctiva is diffusely hyperemic and chemotic.

corneal stroma. Polymorphonuclear leukocytes (PMNs), liberating destructive enzymes, advance ahead of the vascularization, while fibroblasts parallel the vessel ingrowth. Stromal ulceration and possible perforation can occur in severe cases (grades 3 and 4). The conjunctival fornices can also become obliterated by symblepharon formation.

The late, or chronic, phase usually occurs only with severe burns. Cicatrix formation limits both globe and eyelid movement, and vision is reduced due to corneal vascularization and opacification. These eyes have a propensity to ulcerate secondary to any insult.

In burns caused by strong acids, the cornea and conjunctiva rapidly become white and opaque (nitric and chromic acids, however, turn tissue yellow-

TABLE 7-2. CLASSIFICATION OF ALKALI BURNS

Grade 1	Grade 3
Corneal epithelial damage	Total epithelial loss with stromal haze, iris detail seen
No conjunctival ischemia	One-third to one-half of limbus ischemic
Good prognosis	Vision reduced, perforation rare
Grade 2	**Grade 4**
Hazy cornea, iris details seen	Cornea opaque, no details of iris seen
Less than one-third of limbus ischemic	More than one-half of limbus ischemic
Good prognosis	Poor prognosis, chronic course

brown). The epithelium may slough, leaving a relatively clear stroma; this appearance may initially mask the severity of the burn. Eventually, however, the cornea opacifies. Very severe acid burns also cause complete corneal anesthesia, limbal pallor, and uveitis.

Control of Ulceration via Chemical Mediators

One of the most serious complications of alkali-burned corneas is corneal ulceration, which can occur within weeks of the initial injury and progress to corneal perforation, commonly causing irreversible blindness. To prevent ulceration, a multitude of medications are used to promote collagen synthesis, inhibit the enzyme collagenase, and enhance epithelization.

Corneal ulceration occurs when collagenolytic activity is greater than fibrillogenesis. These two events proceed simultaneously in the repair process. The corneal periphery usually remains intact because of the favorable balance between collagen production by incoming fibroblasts and collagenase-induced destruction by PMNs. Centrally, however, there are no fibroblasts, and without collagen synthesis, the balance is in favor of destruction, ulceration, and eventual perforation (Figure 7–2).

PATHOGENESIS OF ULCERATION IN THE ALKALI BURNED CORNEA

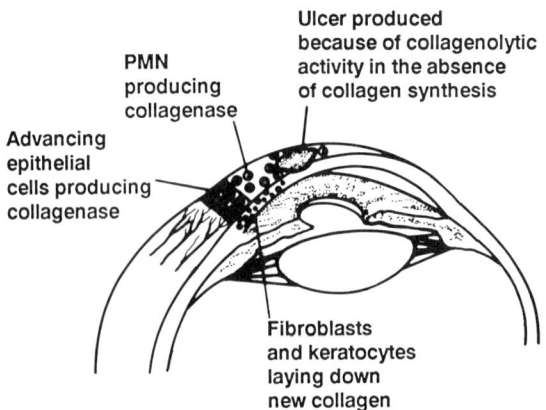

FIGURE 7–2. Pathogenesis of ulceration in the alkali-burned cornea. Ulceration occurs when there is collagenase production in areas devoid of adequate collagen synthesis.

Both L-cysteine and N-acetyl-L-cysteine (acetylcysteine) have been shown to have in vivo activity against collagenase (Ralph, 1989). Acetylcysteine has the advantage of being more stable and readily available (Mucomyst, available in both 10% and 20% concentrations, in 4 mL, 10 mL, and 30 mL dropper bottles). The tetracyclines (doxycycline, minocycline, and tetracycline) have also been shown to have in vivo activity against collagenase (Seedor, Perry, McNamara, et al., 1987). Tetracycline inactivates collagenase by binding to the enzyme via a calcium bridge. More recently, synthetic thiol peptides have been shown to be efficacious in preventing experimentally induced corneal ulceration and perforation (Burns, Gray, and Paterson, 1990).

Steroids can also decrease the ability of tissue to produce collagenase. It has been our clinical experience, however, that local corticosteroid application enhances corneal melting. Corticosteroids inhibit fibroblasts from repopulating the acellular stroma and thereby potentiate collagenolytic activity by a general antianabolic effect, even in the face of decreased collagenase production. Corticosteroids should therefore be avoided during the second and third weeks after an alkali burn. During the first week, collagenase activity has not peaked, and after 4 weeks to 5 weeks, the inhibition of collagen synthesis is less deleterious.

Ascorbic acid is involved in the biosynthesis and maintenance of collagen. Specifically, it is required for the hydroxylation of proline and lysine. Ascorbate is actively transported by the ciliary body into the aqueous. In severe alkali burns, damage to the ciliary body results in a decrease in the active transport of ascorbate and a relative scorbutic state of the anterior segment. In this state, impaired hydroxylation results in the formation of unstable collagen, which is very vulnerable to the action of proteolytic enzymes. It follows that exogenous supplementation by ascorbic acid may reverse the relative ascorbate deficiency and prevent corneal ulceration. Animal experiments have confirmed this (Levison, Paterson, and Pfister, 1976). Ascorbic acid given subcutaneously, parenterally, or topically raised aqueous ascorbate levels and decreased the incidence of corneal ulceration in alkali-burned rabbit corneas. Topical sodium citrate has also been effective in preventing ulceration in severely burned rabbit corneas (Pfister, Nicolaro, and Paterson, 1981).

It has long been known that an intact epithelium is an effective barrier against corneal ulceration. While earlier investigators focused on the inhibition of proteolytic enzymes, more recent investigators have focused on promoting epithelization. Fibronectin and epidermal growth factor are two agents currently being investigated. Fibronectin is a naturally occurring adhesive glycoprotein that promotes cellular attachment to the underlying stroma. Epidermal growth factor is a polypeptide isolated from mouse submaxillary glands that increases the rate of epithelial migration. While both of these substances alone or in combination have had a positive effect on promoting epithelization, most experimental corneas have ulcerated upon cessation of therapy.

While there are few data supporting the usefulness of chemical mediators in controlled human studies, their clinical use appears justified based on experimental animal studies and the uniformly poor prognosis of severe alkali burns once ulceration begins.

Intraocular Pressure Response

Substantial changes in intraocular pressure have been demonstrated following chemical burns. The ocular pressure response varies according to the severity, elapsed time from injury, and the pH of the offending agent. From experimental studies, it is likely that there is an acute rise in intraocular pressure due to collagen shrinkage in alkali burns of pH 11 or higher. A second pressure elevation occurs within the first few hours, most likely due to the intraocular release of prostaglandins. A similar subsequent pressure response can also be seen after moderate and severe acid burns.

After the first few hours, the pressure can be elevated or depressed. Eyes that have been more severely burned, as demonstrated by vascular changes in the deep sclera, trabeculum, iris, and ciliary body, tend to be hypotensive. More mildly burned eyes show persistent pressure elevation, possibly the result of continued formation of aqueous by the ciliary body in the presence of a blocked outflow channel. The latter occurs initially as a result of mechanical obstruction of the trabecular meshwork and later due to fibrous proliferation in the angle.

Treatment of Chemical Burns

The therapy for chemical burns is directed toward preventing further damage and preserving ocular function. Recognizing that there is overlap, three phases can be defined: (1) the acute phase, beginning at the time of injury and lasting approximately 1 week, (2) the intermediate stage, beginning from 3 to 7 days after injury and representing the period of inflammatory destruction of the eye, and (3) the chronic or cicatricial stage. Table 7–3 outlines the management by stages.

Acute Phase

Copious irrigation should be the initial treatment for every chemical eye burn regardless of the etiologic agent. Topical anesthetic (0.5% proparacaine) and lid retractors or a lid speculum facilitate continuous irrigation. At times, severe orbicularis spasm may require a lid block in order to accomplish adequate irrigation (see Chapter 4). If needed, systemic analgesics are preferable to repeated use of topical anesthetics. If the nature of the chemical injury is unknown, the use of pH paper is helpful in determining whether the agent was

TABLE 7-3. TREATMENT SUMMARY OF CHEMICAL BURNS TO THE EYE

Acute
1. Copious irrigation with saline or water for at least 30 min or 2 L of irrigant. Analgesics, anesthetics, and a lid speculum may be necessary. Continue until the pH is normal (7.3–7.7). Recheck in 30 minutes.
2. Debridement of any retained particles.
3. Atropine 1% or scopolamine 0.25% topically 1 to 3 times daily for cycloplegia.
4. Topical corticosteroids as needed in the first 5–7 days to control the inflammatory response.
5. Acetazolamide 250 mg every 6 hours or methazolamide 50 mg every 8 hours, and/or a topical beta-blocker (e.g., Timoptic, Betagan, Betoptic) as needed to control elevated intraocular pressure.
6. Antibiotic ointment and a semipressure patch to prevent infection and promote epithelization. Mild cases should require only a daily application of a cycloplegic, antibiotic, and steroid with continuous patching.
7. Ascorbic acid (5–10 g) and doxycycline (100 mg twice daily) may be given orally.
8. Daily evaluation of inflammatory response, intraocular pressure, and epithelization.
9. Severe cases are started on 10% topical sodium citrate hourly.

Intermediate
1. Ascorbic acid, doxycycline, and topical sodium citrate are continued. Topical steroids should be discontinued by the end of the first week.
2. N-acetyl-L-cysteine (Mucomyst) 20% should be started hourly in any case that shows progressive ulceration and/or cessation of epithelization.
3. If epithelization stops, a soft bandage lens might promote epithelial healing and protect the ocular surface.
4. Daily lysis of adhesions with a lubricated glass rod.
5. Corneal thinning may be treated with a soft bandage lens or lamellar keratoplasty.
6. Small corneal perforations may heal with a soft bandage lens or sealed with cyanoacrylate adhesive.
7. Larger perforations require either a blowout patch or penetrating keratoplasty.

Late
1. Frequent tear supplementation is necessary to combat severe dry eye. Lacriserts or a thin, low-water-content bandage lens may help.
2. Lid and conjunctival anatomy should be restored if possible by surgical intervention.
3. Corneal transplantation should be attempted only by those very familiar with the technique. Care should be taken to protect donor epithelium.
4. Careful postoperative management is needed to control inflammation, vascularization, and intraocular pressure and to promote epithelial healing.
5. In eyes with persistent epithelial defects, conjunctival transplantation may be helpful.
6. Keratoprosthesis surgery might be successful in cases where penetrating keratoplasty has repeatedly failed.

basic or acidic. Irrigation should continue for at least 30 minutes or 2 L of irrigant in mild cases, and 2 hours to 4 hours or 10 L of irrigant in severe cases. At the end of irrigation, the pH should be within a normal range (7.3–7.7). The pH should be checked again approximately 30 minutes after irrigation to ensure that it has not changed. This is particularly important in alkali burns because particulate matter can slowly dissolve and cause a persistent elevation in the pH. Prolonged irrigation can be accomplished with the use of a polymethylmethacrylate scleral lens with an attached perfusion tube (Medi-Flow or Morgan Therapeutic Lens), by a perforated silicone tube designed to fit into the conjunctival fornices (Oklahoma Eye Irrigating Tube), or by placement of an Angiocath inserted percutaneously into the conjunctival fornix. Due to the extremely rapid penetration of alkali through the cornea and into the anterior chamber, the irrigant of choice remains the one most readily available (tapwater or saline). Because most chemical burns occur outside the physician's office, the initial therapy is usually carried out by nonmedical personnel.

In calcium hydroxide burns (fresh lime, mortar, and plaster) there may be some benefit to irrigating with 0.024 M disodium EDTA (0.5 M Endrate with 20 parts normal saline), which chelates the calcium and helps loosen particles lodged in the fornices. Anterior chamber paracentesis remains controversial. Its use is suggested in moderate to severe burns if performed within 1 hour from the time of accident.

Once irrigation is complete, a careful search must be made for any retained particles. A topical anesthetic should be utilized and the lids should be doubly everted and the fornices swabbed with a cotton applicator moistened with ointment or EDTA (see Figure 8-3). Larger particles can be removed with smooth forceps. Any redundant conjunctiva should be unfolded, as these areas are likely to hide particulate matter.

All but the mildest chemical burns are associated with a significant uveitis. For relief of pain and prevention of posterior synechiae, adequate cycloplegia is essential. Atropine 1% or scopolamine 0.25% 2 or 3 times daily are the drugs of choice. The mydriatic phenylephrine is contraindicated because its vasoconstricting properties can worsen preexisting perilimbal ischemia.

Intraocular pressure responses after chemical burns may vary. Elevated pressure in the initial postburn period can be managed with carbonic anhydrase inhibitors and/or beta-blockers. Acetazolamide 250 mg every 6 hours or methazolamide 50 mg every 8 hours can be used, though smaller doses may be effective.

Following adequate irrigation, antibiotic ointment (tetracycline may have a theoretic advantage) and a semipressure patch are applied. The goal is to promote epithelization as rapidly as possible. The eyes are examined daily and the fluorescein staining pattern drawn. In moderate to severe inflammation, corticosteroid drops are applied (e.g., prednisolone acetate or phosphate, or dexamethasone). In all but the mildest cases, we usually begin ascorbic acid orally. Exact dosages are not defined, but pharmacologic doses (5 g to 10 g daily) are recommended. Tetracycline (doxycycline 100 mg twice daily) is also started. The number of drops given in the acute phase is limited in order to keep the semipressure patch in place to promote epithelization (Figure 7-3). Early in severe cases (grade 3 and 4), where the likelihood of complete early epithelization is low, the chemical mediators outlined in the intermediate phase may be started.

FIGURE 7-3. Progressive epithelization in a mild alkali burned cornea over a period of 1 week treated with atropine, antibiotic-steroid ointment, and semipressure patches.

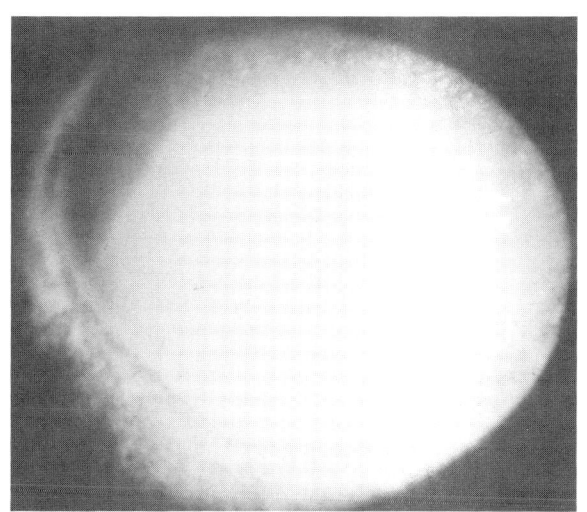
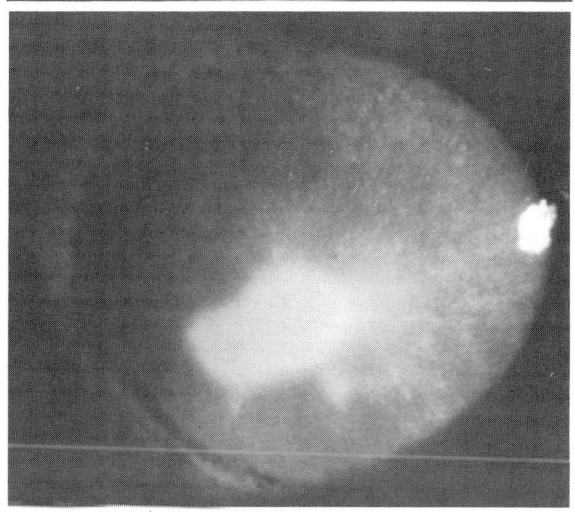
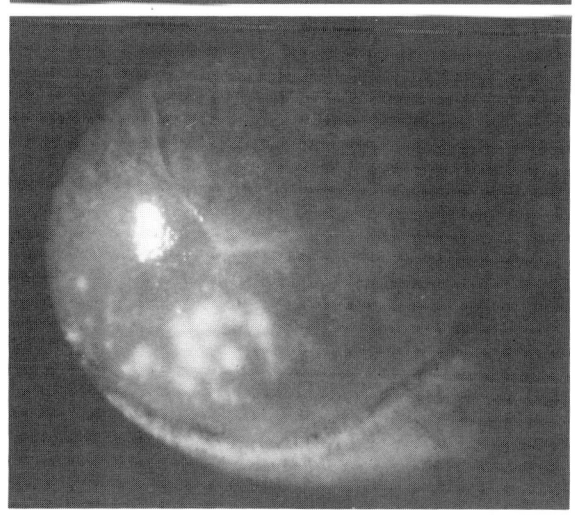

Intermediate Phase

The goal of therapy in the intermediate phase is the prevention of ulceration and/or perforation and the limitation of symblepharon formation. The final goal in severe cases is the retention of an intact globe that will maximize the chance of a successful corneal transplant in the future.

Chemical mediators are initiated if epithelization stops despite patching. Topical 10% sodium citrate is given hourly. Of the collagenase inhibitors discussed, Mucomyst (N-acetyl-L-cysteine) has the advantage of being readily available, easy to administer, and relatively nontoxic. Mucomyst 20% can be given by dropper as often as every hour. It should be kept refrigerated and has an offensive odor, similar to rotten eggs. Ascorbic acid seems to reduce ulceration by promoting collagen synthesis. Dosages outlined in the acute phase should be continued. On the basis of experimental data, anticollagenase agents should be used until the epithelium has healed or for a minimum of 6 weeks. Close observation is needed upon cessation of therapy because ulceration can supervene.

Therapy needs to be directed toward promoting corneal epithelial healing. In mild cases, all that might be needed is continuation of an effective semipressure patch or bandage lens. Some clinicians advocate almost immediate mucosal grafting to replace necrotic conjunctiva. The most severe cases, those that would benefit most from mucosal grafting, are, however, associated with extensive scleral necrosis, which limits the viability of the graft.

Soft bandage lenses also aid in epithelization, and numerous bandage lenses are available. The lens should be large enough to cover the entire limbus at all times. It should also move approximately 1 mm to 2 mm during a blink. Because severe alkali burns are associated with destruction of the tear-producing elements of the eye, an ultrathin, low-to-moderate water-content lens may be more beneficial than a high-water-content lens.

Within a few days following a severe chemical burn, fibrin formation begins to obliterate the conjunctival fornices. Areas of the bulbar and palpebral conjunctiva that are denuded of epithelium form adhesions. The fibrinous bands are then replaced by fibrovascular tissue. A glass rod lubricated with ointment can be used to sweep the fornices and lyse adhesions once or twice daily. The use of scleral shells to prevent apposition of tissue has met with only minimal success. Whether these procedures result in less symblepharon formation when active inflammation begins to wane is debatable.

Small perforations can be treated with a bandage lens (Figure 7–4) or the application of tissue adhesive (cyanoacrylate). Histo-acryl-Blau (butyl-2-cyanoacrylate, B. Brown Melsungen A.G.) is not available in the United States but can be obtained in Canada. The area to be sealed needs to be debrided of necrotic tissue and dried. A small amount of glue is applied via a polyethylene disc or thin tube and allowed to polymerize. The cornea is then covered with a hydrophilic bandage lens. Perforations too large to be sealed with tissue adhesive require either penetrating keratoplasty or a patch graft (blowout patch).

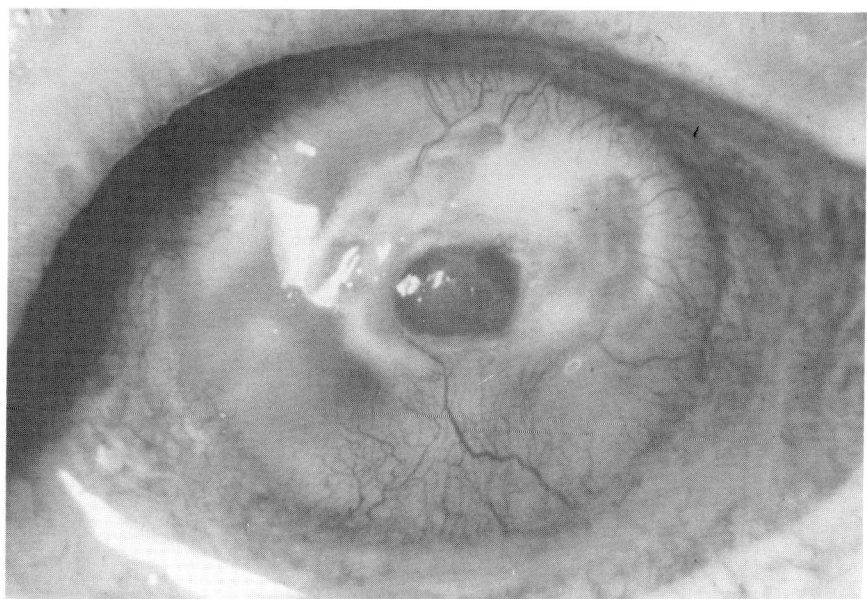

FIGURE 7-4. Central perforation sealed with the application of a soft bandage lens.

Postoperatively steroids should be avoided but collagenase inhibitors continued.

Late or Chronic Phase

The treatment of the late stage begins when the inflammatory destruction of the intermediate stage ends. The major goals of therapy are supplementation of a deficient tear film, reestablishment of normal lid anatomy, and restoration of a clear visual axis.

Extensive involvement of the conjunctiva in advanced alkali burns results in the development of a severe dry eye. The aqueous component is decreased by obstruction of the main and accessory lacrimal glands, and the mucin component is decreased or altered by widespread injury to the limbal conjunctiva. Frequent tear supplementation with some of the newer mucomimetic tear replacements is helpful. Nonpreserved drops offer an advantage to an already compromised corneal surface (e.g., Celluvisc). Lacriserts may offer relief in patients whose fornices are not obliterated, but often these are poorly retained. A thin, low-water-content bandage lens may also be of assistance.

Another prerequisite for maintaining the precorneal tear film is periodic blinking. Symblepharon that restricts lid movements, cicatricial entropion, trichiasis, and obliteration of the fornices all make proper corneal wetting impossible (Figure 7-5). Before penetrating keratoplasty can be performed, normal lid and conjunctival anatomy need to be restored, if possible.

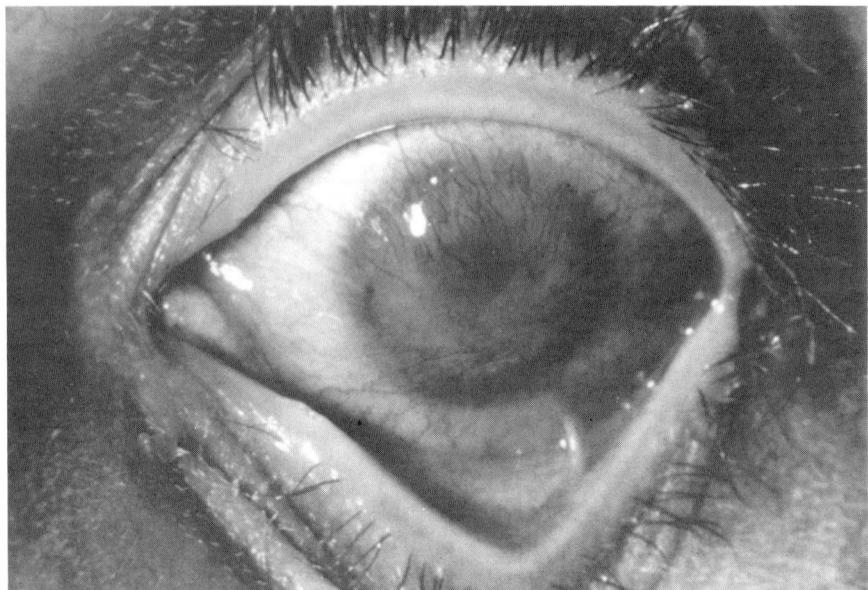

FIGURE 7–5. The late stage of an alkali-burned eye showing corneal opacification, severe vascularization, and symblepharon.

Corneal transplantation in the severely burned eye has been fraught with difficulties. Immunologic rejection, ulcer formation, vascularization, and lingering epithelial defects are the rule rather than the exception. In addition, an inflammatory reaction that had been quiet for months or years may suddenly be reactivated. Both tissue typing and the use of topical immunodilators (cyclosporine) are being investigated in an attempt to improve the universally poor prognosis.

Thoft developed two techniques for the treatment of severe alkali burns with conjunctival involvement. The first was autotransplantation of healthy conjunctival tissue from the uninjured fellow eye (Thoft, 1977), and the second was keratoepithelioplasty (Thoft, 1984). In this latter procedure, limbal tissue from a fresh donor eye is transplanted to serve as a source of new epithelium. In severe bilateral cases (those with markedly altered conjunctiva and lids), penetrating keratoplasty has an extremely poor prognosis. Keratoprosthesis surgery may offer the only chance for vision.

THERMAL BURNS

Although thermal burns of the face and periorbital structures are common, direct thermal injury of the eye itself is relatively rare. Because of the rapidity of the lid reflex, the majority of thermal injuries affect the eyelids, lashes, eyebrows, and surrounding skin only. Exceptions are flying sparks, which may enter the eye, or flame or flash burns, which may reach the cornea. Because of the lid reflex, even these injuries result in short exposure and therefore usually only superficial corneal injuries. Although the eye must be examined for deeper injuries or penetration of a flying particle, most of these burns can be managed with analgesics and topical care.

The eyelid in a thermal burn usually presents a greater problem. The eyelid response to burns is similar to skin on other parts of the body, but because the subcutaneous tissue is areolar, there may be marked swelling after a burn. A first-degree burn consists of injury to the epidermis only and is marked by a moderate amount of edema, erythema, and associated pain. Second-degree burns involve the epidermis and dermis and result in blistering in addition to erythema and pain. Third-degree burns involve the full thickness of the epidermis and dermis and progress to, or through, the subcutaneous tissue. They are characterized by a black or white eschar and, because the subcutaneous nerve endings have been destroyed, dysasthesia or anesthesia of the area. First- and second-degree burns have marked swelling, and this should be viewed as a positive prognostic sign. Swelling indicates that the subcutaneous structures are intact and responding to the injury appropriately. The swelling associated with first- and second-degree burns also serves to close the lid and protect the globe. Because this may result in decreased motility and tear production, frequent application of artificial tears or ointments may be necessary to maintain adequate lubrication of the cornea. Because of extensive subcutaneous destruction, third-degree burns may have little swelling.

The first priority in treating a thermal burn is to remove the person from the heat source and cool the tissues as rapidly as possible. This is best accomplished with cool compresses, such as sterile towels soaked in an ice bath. Cooling serves to decrease further injury and increase patient comfort. Analgesics, including parental narcotics, may be necessary to relieve pain. Vision must be assessed and the eye evaluated for evidence of superficial or deep corneal injuries.

First-degree lid burns require an antibiotic ointment and follow-up only. Second-degree burns should be dressed with an antibiotic ointment (silver sulfadiazine or bacitracin) and a nonocclusive dressing, such as Telfa. It is important to keep the skin moist to reduce subsequent scarring. Any dressings should be changed wet to prevent denuding the healing epithelium. Third-degree burns require admission and consideration of early grafting and reconstruction (see also Chapter 4).

Burns of the lids are often colonized with bacteria, especially *Pseudomonas* species, and may become infected. Only true infections need systemic treatment, and a biopsy of the tissue may be necessary to document the infection. The date of the most recent tetanus immunization must be determined, and if this was more than 5 years prior to the injury, tetanus prophylaxis should be updated (see Chapter 17).

Over several days, the edema will decrease, and the wounds may need to be debrided. The amount of lid retraction should be assessed at this time and repeatedly as the healing continues. If there is significant retraction, the lids should be temporarily sutured shut to protect the cornea and minimize further lid contraction. A long process of skin grafting and reconstruction is then begun to approximate normal anatomy as much as possible.

ELECTRICAL INJURIES

Direct electrical injuries to the eyes are rare, but current passing across the face or through the head is not. The most common complication of this injury is the development of cataracts (Figure 7-6). Cataracts may occur in up to 9% of patients with significant electrical injuries involving the head. They often take 6 months to 12 months to develop and are usually bilateral. Careful slit lamp examination of the lens 2 weeks after an electric shock can identify vacuolization of the lens and early cataract formation. No specific treatment or prevention is available, and surgical correction is often necessary.

RADIATION INJURIES

The most common type of radiation to cause injury to the eye is ultraviolet (UV) radiation. Sunshine and welding arcs routinely account for these expo-

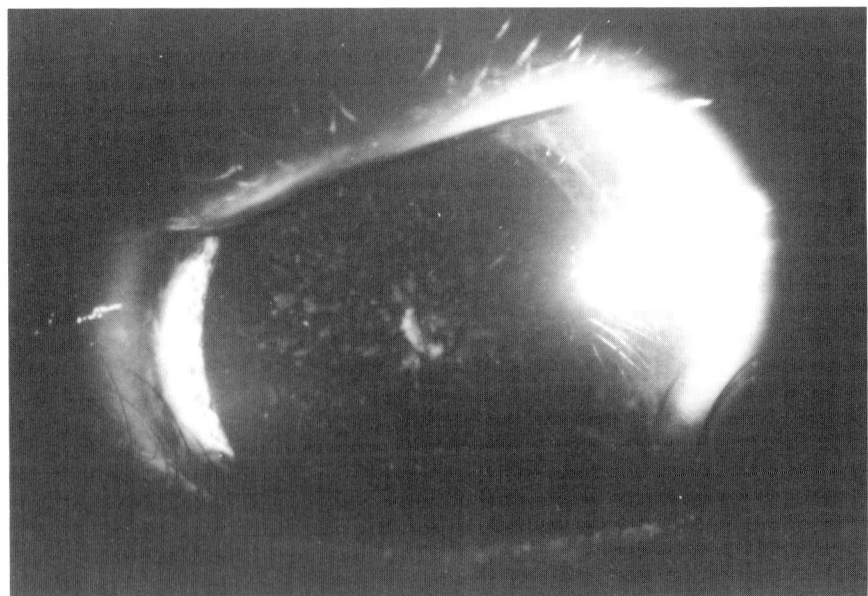

FIGURE 7-6. Electrical cataract.

sures. UV radiation results in punctate keratitis over the entire corneal surface, which will stain positively with fluorescein. A diffuse corneal haze will be evident in severe cases, and the conjunctiva will be chemotic and hyperemic. Severe pain, photophobia, and corneal irregularity usually begin 6 hours to 10 hours after the initial injury (Figure 7–7). Slightly decreased visual acuity is the rule; a significant reduction in vision is a harbinger of more serious injury. Ultraviolet burns may be the most painful condition seen in ophthalmology. The pain can be relieved by topical anesthetics for a short period of time, but a short-acting cycloplegic should be used to relieve the pain of a secondary iritis. A systemic analgesic may be necessary. A topical antibiotic ointment should also be administered and the eye pressure patched for 24 hours. The prognosis for this type of injury is excellent, and the cornea is usually completely healed within 24 hours. Following resolution, however, affected eyes are often light sensitive for many months.

Infrared radiation is now a rare cause of keratitis. "Glassblower cataract," or true exfoliation of the lens capsule due to prolonged exposure to infrared radiation, was common in industries where workers were exposed to severe heat before the development of protective eyewear (Figure 7–8).

Serious visual loss also results from prolonged staring at the sun. This loss of vision is not due to a corneal injury but secondary to retinal damage. It can develop after prolonged welding exposure or secondary to eclipse viewing, but more commonly occurs in sunbathers, sailors, and patients with an altered

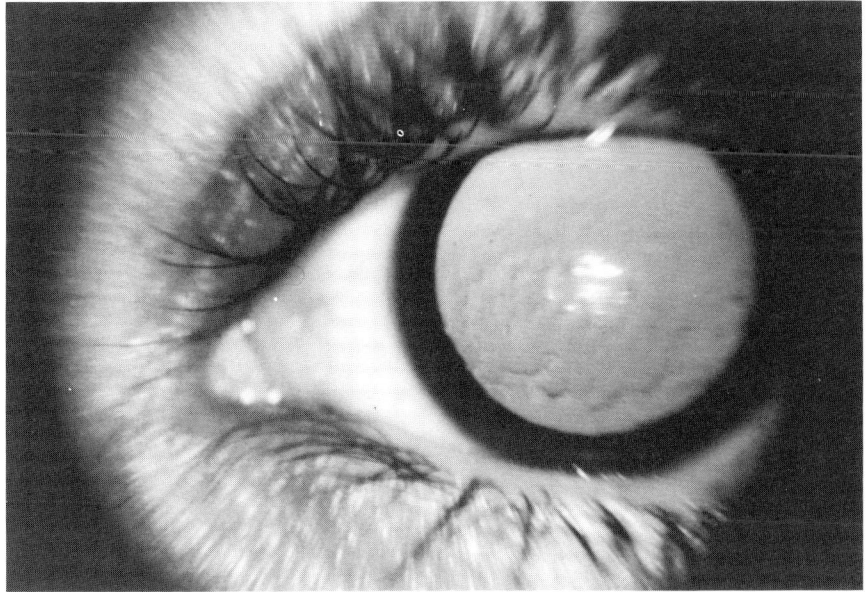

FIGURE 7–7. Corneal irregularity 12 hours after exposure to UV light (welding arc burn).

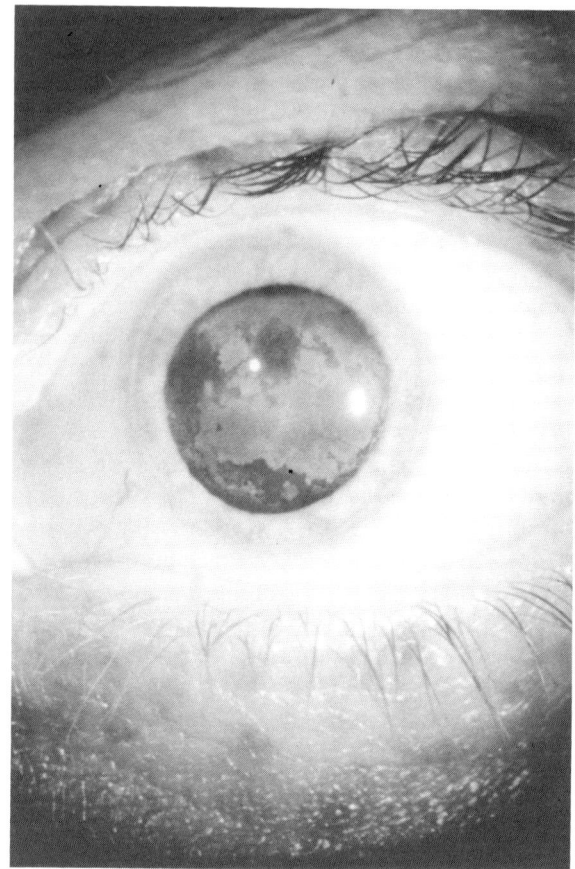

FIGURE 7-8. Glassblower cataract (true exfoliation of lens capsule).

mental status. It may be more common in military recruits seeking discharge. In these cases, it is often unilateral.

The mechanism of injury from extended exposure to UV light is thought to be a delayed photochemical reaction. It is noteworthy that staring at the sun may not be as painful as is usually presumed. Furthermore, it usually takes 1 day to 2 days for the visual disturbance to be noted. Within this time, a yellow-white dome-shaped lesion develops in the fovea (Figure 7-9). Histologically this has been found to be a bullous detachment of the retinal pigment epithelium. An abnormally prolonged photostress test and fluorescein leakage from the underlying choroid confirm the diagnosis.

There is no specific therapy for this injury. Patients should be referred to an ophthalmologist for documentation and follow-up. Significant healing and regeneration may occur within 4 months to 6 months and is typical after solar eclipse viewing. Permanent reduction in visual acuity, however, is not unusual.

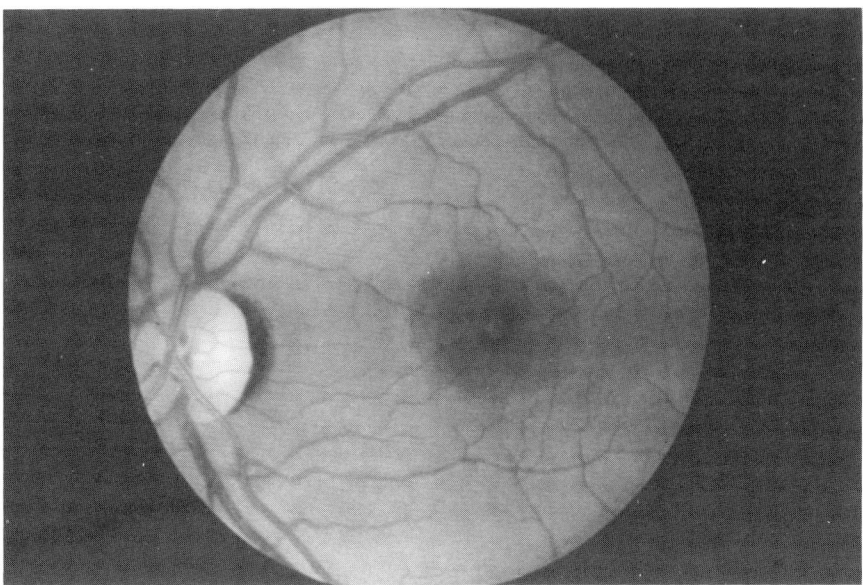

FIGURE 7-9. Dome-shaped, yellow-white, retinal pigment degeneration secondary to sun gazing.

REFERENCES

Chemical Burns

Belin MW, Krachmer JH: Chemical burns of the cornea. In Easty DL, Smolin G (eds): *External Eye Disease*. London, Butterworth, 1985, pp 304–305.
Burns FR, Gray RD, Paterson CA: Inhibition of alkali-induced corneal ulceration by a thiol peptide. *Invest Ophthalmol Vis Sci* 31:197, 1990.
Burns FR, Stack MS, Gray RD, Paterson CA: Inhibition of purified collagenase from alkali-burned rabbit corneas. *Invest Ophthalmol Vis Sci* 30:1569, 1989.
Levison RA, Paterson CA, Pfister RR: Ascorbic acid prevents corneal ulceration and perforation following experimental alkali burns. *Invest Ophthalmol Vis Sci* 15:986, 1976.
Perry HD, Kenyon KR, Lamberts DW, et al: Systemic tetracycline hydrochloride as adjunctive therapy in the treatment of persistent epithelial defects. *Ophthalmology* 93:1320, 1986.
Pfister RR: Chemical injuries of the eye. *Ophthalmology* 90:1246, 1983.
Pfister RR, Nicolaro ML, Paterson CA: Sodium citrate reduces the incidence of ulcerations and perforations in extreme alkali burned eyes. *Invest Ophthalmol Vis Sci* 21:486, 1981.
Purdue GF, Hunt JL: Adult assault as a mechanism of burn injury. *Arch Surg* 125:268, 1990.
Ralph RA: Chemical burns of the eye. In Tasman W (ed): *Duane's Clinical Ophthalmology*. Philadelphia, Harper & Row, 1989, pp 1–25.
Ralph RA, Slansky HH: Therapy of chemical burns. *Int Ophthalmol Clin* 4:171, 1974.
Seedor JA, Perry HD, McNamara TF, et al: Systemic tetracycline treatment of alkali-induced corneal ulceration in rabbits. *Arch Ophthalmol* 105:268, 1987.
Stone M. Assault by burning and its relationship to social circumstances. *Burns* 14:461, 1988.
Tenn PF, Fujikawa LS, Dweck MD, et al: Fibronectin in alkali-burned rabbit cornea: Enhancement of epithelial wound healing. *Invest Ophthalmol Vis Sci* (suppl) 29:92, 1988.
Thoft RA: Conjunctival transplantation. *Arch Ophthalmol* 95:1425, 1977.
Thoft RA: Keratoepithelioplasty. *Am J Ophthalmol* 97:1, 1984.

II—Ocular and Orbital Trauma

Thermal, Electrical, and Radiation Burns

Burns CL, Chylack LT: Thermal burns: The management of thermal burns of the lids and globes. *Ann Ophthalmol* 11:1358, 1979.
Gladstone GJ, Tasman W: Solar retinitis after minimal exposure. *Arch Ophthalmol* 96:1368, 1978.
Johnson EU, Kline LB, Skalka HW: Electrical cataracts: A case report and review of the literature. *Ophthalmic Surgery* 18:283, 1987.
Marrone AC: Thermal eyelid burns. In Hornblass A, Hanio CT (eds): *Oculoplastic, Orbital and Reconstructive Surgery. Eyelids*. Baltimore, Williams and Wilkins, 1988, 1:443–447.
Peterson HD: Eyelids. In Baswick JA Jr., (ed): *The Art and Science of Burn Care*. Rockville, MD, Aspen Publishers, 1987, pp 339–345.
Tso MM, LaPiana RG: The human fovea after sungazing. *Trans Am Acad Ophthalmol Otolaryngol* 79:788, 1975.

8

Foreign Bodies and Penetrating Injuries to the Eye

Michael W. Belin

The presence of an occult foreign body or a penetrating ocular injury should always be considered when examining a patient with a red eye. Corneal or scleral lacerations and intraocular or intraorbital foreign bodies can present as benign-looking conjunctivitis. Patients may have only mild complaints of decreased vision and give no history of trauma. The examiner is obligated to consider trauma and to perform a thorough exam to rule it out.

SUBCONJUNCTIVAL HEMORRHAGE

The conjunctiva, a loose vascular tissue, is the globe's outermost protective coating. It is fixed to the underlying eye where the cornea and sclera meet (the limbus) and is loosely applied to the remainder of the eye (bulbar conjunctiva). From the globe, it is reflected on to the posterior surface of the upper and lower eyelids, where it is firmly adherent to the underlying tarsus of the eyelids (palpebral conjunctiva).

Because the conjunctiva is freely mobile and extensible, blunt trauma usually results only in breakage of fragile conjunctival blood vessels. The resultant subconjunctival hemorrhage presents as a painless, bright red accumulation of blood, usually limited to one section or quadrant of the eye (Figure 8-1). A more severe underlying ocular injury may be present, however, and a complete

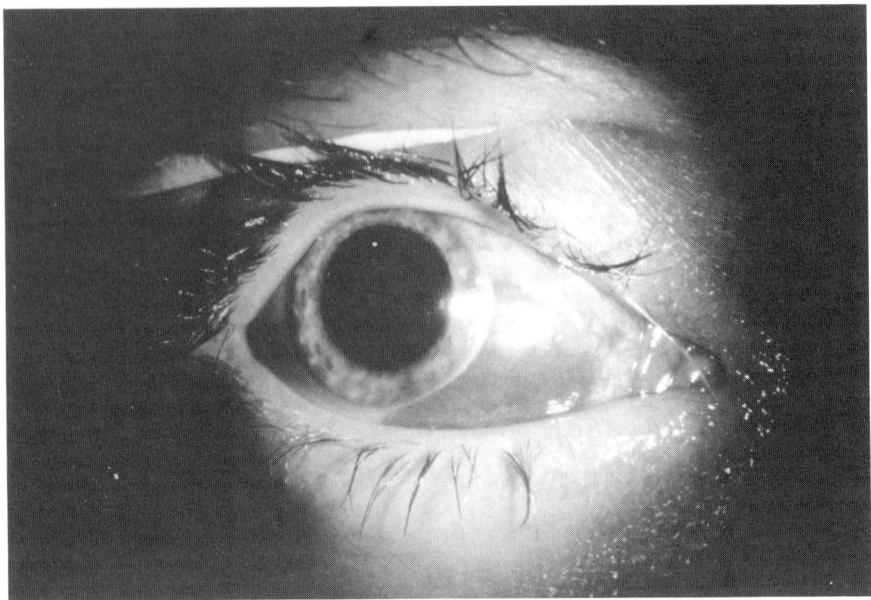

FIGURE 8-1. Subconjunctival hemorrhage.

ophthalmologic examination is warranted. Accumulated blood can hide a retained foreign body or an occult scleral laceration. In addition to blunt trauma, subconjunctival hemorrhage can result from eye rubbing, hypertension, or sneezing, or it can be idiopathic. Isolated subconjunctival hemorrhages require no treatment. Resorption of blood is generally complete within 10 days to 14 days.

CONJUNCTIVAL LACERATIONS

Small, isolated conjunctival lacerations rarely require treatment. Their identification is important, however, because they often indicate a deeper, more severe injury to the globe. It is imperative to examine the underlying sclera to rule out an accompanying scleral laceration. This may be difficult because these lacerations are usually accompanied by a subconjunctival hemorrhage, making examination of the deeper sclera more difficult. When it appears that the globe has been severely traumatized, it may be necessary to enlarge the conjunctival opening to increase exposure and explore the sclera better. The conjunctiva can be opened with a pair of dull scissors (Westcott) and a small conjunctival forceps (Bishop-Harmon forceps with cross-serrated tips).

Lacerations greater than 6 mm may require closure. The patient should be placed in the recumbent position and topical anesthesia applied. A wire lid speculum (Barraquer) is preferable to a larger heavier lid speculum and can usually be tolerated by the patient without the use of a lid block. When necessary, a lid block can be accomplished by local infiltration (see Chapter 4). The conjunctival edge should be grasped with a serrated forceps (Bishop-Harmon). Particular attention is necessary to identify the edge of the conjunctiva because loose conjunctiva has a tendency to roll upon itself. The opposing edges should be closed with interrupted sutures; 7-0 or 8-0 absorbable suture material is commonly used (vicryl, chromic, plain, etc.); 8-0 silk can also be used if tied tightly, as it will usually fall out in a number of days. Although the needle design is probably not critical, a tapered point lessens the chance of tearing the conjunctiva. Tapered points, however, are less stable to grasp with a needle holder and more likely to penetrate the globe inadvertently. Postoperatively, a semipressure patch may make the patient more comfortable but is optional. The routine use of topical antibiotics is probably not warranted, and ointments should be avoided.

CORNEAL AND CONJUNCTIVAL FOREIGN BODIES

Corneal and conjunctival foreign bodies are relatively common causes of acute ocular pain. A history of working under a car or at a construction site raises one's suspicion. After the history is obtained and the visual acuity recorded, the eyes should be examined under direct illumination with a penlight or at the slit lamp. Magnification can be obtained with a pair of loops, a magnifying glass, or the direct ophthalmoscope (using the plus lens settings). Low or no magnification, however, may be best.

The cornea and bulbar conjunctiva is examined directly. The palpebral conjunctiva of the lower eyelid and the inferior cul-de-sac can be examined by pulling down the lower eyelid and having the patient look upward. Examination of the palpebral conjunctiva of the upper eyelid and the upper cul-de-sac is more difficult. "Double" eversion of the upper eyelid may be required. A single eversion of the upper eyelid can be achieved by gently grasping the eyelid at the lash line and pulling it down while placing minimal counterpressure at the upper border of the eyelid with a cotton applicator. The patient should be instructed to look down during the procedure. Elevation of the lid margin, counterpressure at the upper board, and gentle lid rotation will usually evert the lid (Figure 8-2). "Double" eversion of the upper eyelid is accomplished by substituting a Desmarre retractor for the cotton applicator and pulling the eyelid forward as it is rolled around the retractor (Figure 8-3). A careful search is then made of both the palpebral conjunctiva and the cul-de-sac. Upper lid eversion is uncomfortable. Discomfort can be minimized by instructing the patient to look down continually.

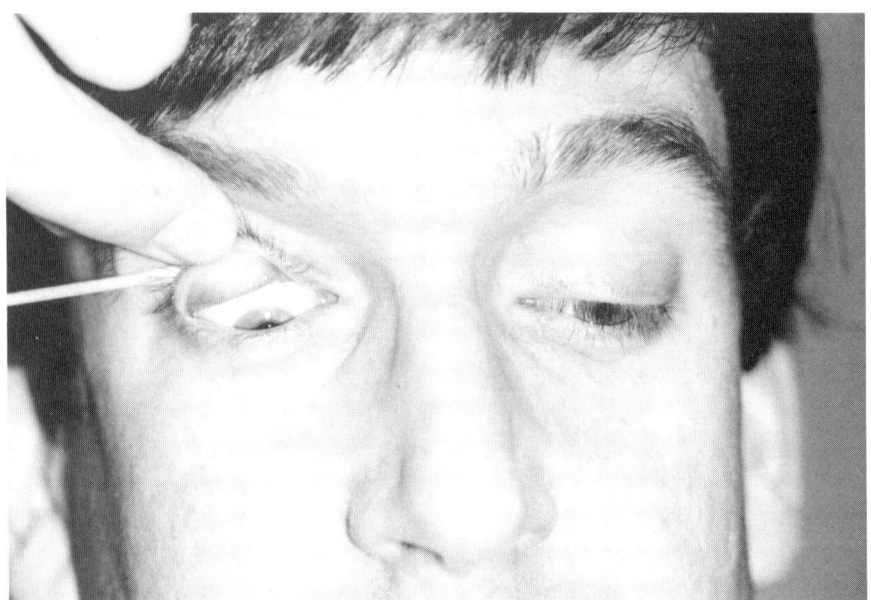

FIGURE 8-2. Eversion of upper eyelid with cotton applicator.

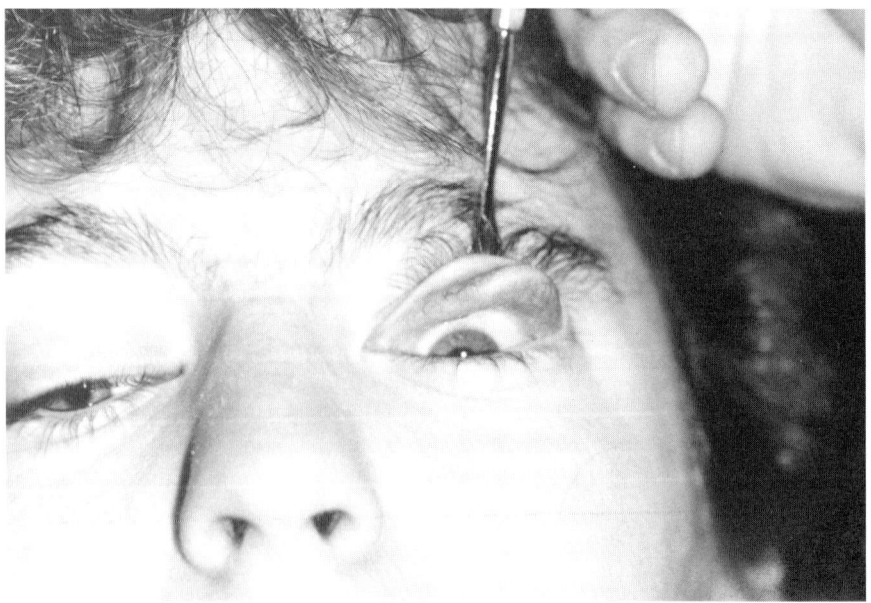

FIGURE 8-3. "Double" eversion of upper eyelid with Desmarre retractor.

If a foreign body is found, it can usually be easily removed. Adequate anesthesia is obtained with topical anesthetics (proparacaine 0.5% or tetracaine 0.5%). One drop is usually adequate, but additional applications at intervals of 3 minutes to 5 minutes may be necessary. Prior to removal of the conjunctival foreign body, the underlying sclera should be examined to rule out a penetrating injury. If the conjunctiva as well as the retained foreign body is not easily movable over the underlying sclera or if the foreign body appears fixed to deeper structures of the globe, an accompanying scleral injury should be suspected. Further manipulations and treatment should be carried out in the operating room, under the operating microscope.

If the foreign body appears to be adherent to only the cornea or conjunctiva, it can be removed with either foreign body spud, fine forceps (jewelers or tying forceps), or the edge of a large-bore needle (22 gauge). This is best done at the slit lamp with the physician's hand resting on the patient's cheekbone. This position lessens the chance of striking the globe with a sharp object; any movement of the patient is automatically followed by the physician's hand (Figure 8–4). Many foreign bodies can also be removed by applying a bland ophthalmic ointment (lacrilube, duratears) to the end of a cotton applicator and swabbing the foreign body, a safer approach to use when a slit lamp is not available. While this technique will remove loose and/or recent occurring foreign bodies, it is less effective with foreign bodies that have been present for a longer duration and have become more adherent. Once a conjunctival foreign body is removed, further treatment is usually not indicated. Once a corneal foreign body is removed, the treatment should follow the guidelines outlined below for corneal abrasions. Iron-containing corneal foreign bodies often leave a deposit of rust that may leech into the deeper layers of the cornea. The residual rust will often resolve with time but can cause persistent foreign body–like complaints. The rust ring can be scraped with a dull object, like a foreign body spud, or easily removed with a mechanical corneal burr (a battery-operated low-speed drill).

CORNEAL ABRASIONS

A corneal abrasion is one of the most common ocular complaints seen in an emergency setting. The corneal epithelium begins at the termination of the conjunctival epithelium and covers the cornea proper. The epithelium covering the cornea is distinct in morphology and function from the conjunctival epithelium. When the corneal epithelium is scratched, abraded, or denuded, it exposes the underlying basement layer and superficial corneal nerves. This is accompanied by pain, tearing, and photophobia. Extensive abrasions can also cause a significant drop in visual acuity because the underlying layers do not offer the same smooth, reflective surface as the normal corneal epithelium. The treatment of corneal abrasions is directed at promoting healing and relieving

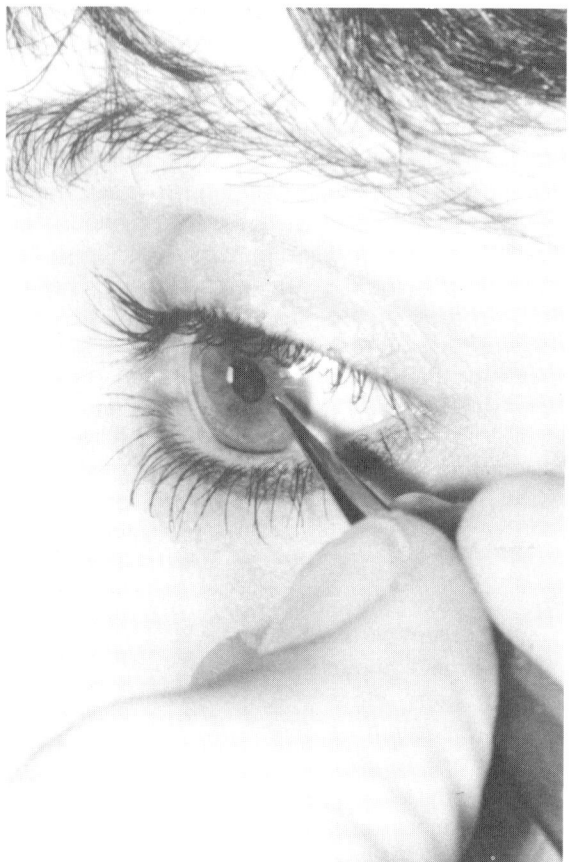

FIGURE 8-4. Method to remove foreign body at the slit lamp. The foreign body is approached obliquely from the side, lessening the chance of striking the globe with a sharp object.

pain. The corneal epithelium initially heals by sliding in existing epithelium in an attempt to cover the abrasion. This is later accompanied by true cellular division. Initially, the newly relocated cells have not developed normal adhesions to the underlying basement layer and are more susceptible to injury. Most physicians use semipressure patches to immobilize the lid and protect the newly migrated epithelium from the constant trauma of repeated blinking. Similar protection may be afforded by simply taping the lid closed. Ocular lubricants or ointment may also be effective with small abrasions.

The corneal epithelium serves as an effective barrier against the entrance of bacteria. Any abrasion compromises this barrier and should be treated with prophylactic antibiotics. One should select an antibiotic that possesses good gram-positive coverage and is not substantially toxic to the corneal epithelium (e.g., sulfacetamide drops and ointment, Polytrim drops, Polysporin ointment).

Small abrasions can be treated with frequent applications of topical antibacterials (drops or ointment 4 times a day) with or without immobilization of the lid. Larger abrasions usually require lid immobilization for comfort. Applying a small ribbon of 1-inch tape horizontally across the lash margin may be a simple, effective method of stabilizing the lid (Figure 8–5). Patients with larger abrasions should be followed until epithelial healing has occurred. Topical anesthetics result in almost immediate relief of pain, but all topical anesthetics are epithelial toxic. There is no indication for their prolonged use.

CORNEAL LACERATIONS

Corneal lacerations can be categorized as:

1. Partial thickness, without entrance into the anterior chamber.
2. Full thickness, self-sealing, with a deep anterior chamber, without active aqueous leakage and without involvement of uveal or lens material.
3. Full thickness, with aqueous leakage but without involvement of uveal or lens material.
4. Full thickness, with uveal and/or lens involvement (Figure 8–6).

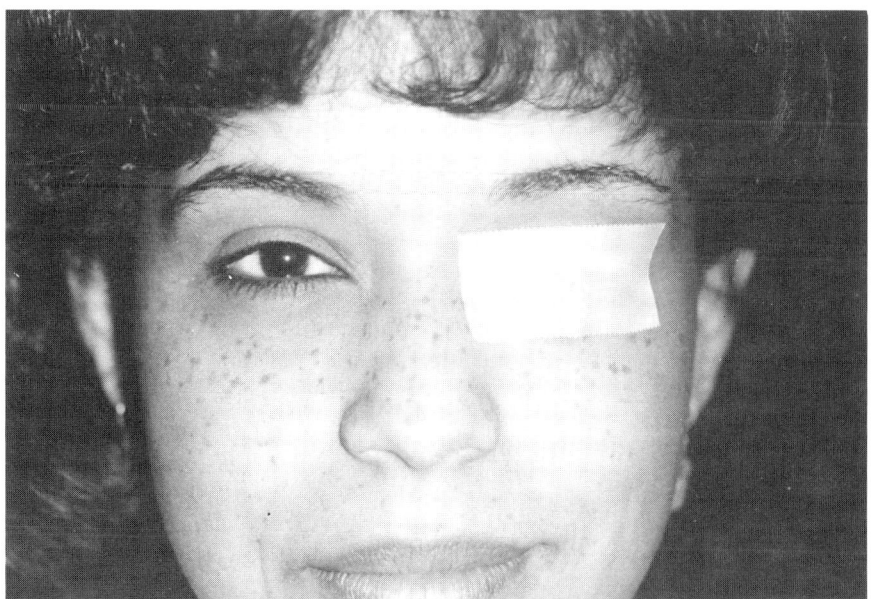

FIGURE 8–5. Immobilization of eyelids with 1-inch tape across eyelid margins.

CORNEAL LACERATIONS

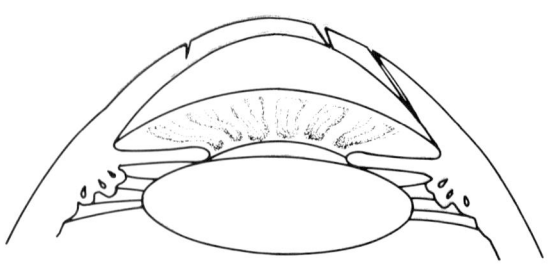

FULL THICKNESS LACERATION WITH UVEAL PROLAPSE

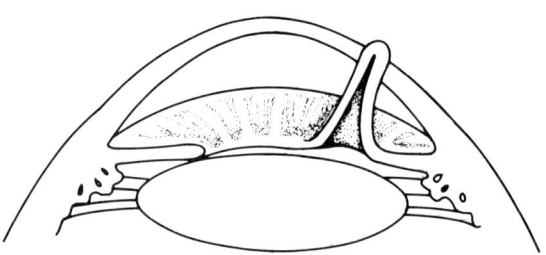

FIGURE 8-6. (a) Schematic showing partial thickness corneal laceration (left), full thickness laceration with aqueous leakage but without uveal prolapse (center), and full thickness, self-sealing laceration (right). (b) Schematic showing full thickness laceration with uveal prolapse.

Because the treatment of a partial thickness laceration differs from the treatment of a full thickness injury, the examiner needs to rule out a slow, intermittent leak. This is done by comparing the depths of the anterior chambers of the two eyes and by performing a Seidel test on the traumatized eye. A significant difference in the anterior chamber depth suggests a loss of chamber contents in the traumatized eye. A Seidel test is performed by applying a dry strip of fluorescein over the wound while observing the cornea at the slit lamp with the cobalt blue light. A slow leak is visible as dilution of the green fluorescein dye. If this test is negative, gentle pressure can be put on the globe to see if an active leak can be induced. At times the leakage can be intermittent, leaking only after enough fluid has accumulated to raise the intraocular pressure above a certain critical level. Gentle pressure on the globe similarly increases intraocular pressure. A negative Seidel test suggests no communication with the anterior chamber.

A small, partial thickness laceration can generally be treated as a corneal abrasion with topical prophylactic antibiotic drops. A larger or extremely shelved partial thickness laceration may require some support (a semipressure patch or lid taping) to prevent the loose corneal tissue from moving during blinking and to promote epithelization. In patients who object to monocular occlusion, a soft bandage contact lens can be used. Dissolvable collagen lenses (with dissolution rates of 24 hours to 72 hours) can serve in a similar fashion. Topical prophylactic antibiotics should be given until the wound is secure and epithelization is complete. Ocular ointments should not be used with bandage contact lenses. Only in extreme cases where the patient is uncooperative and the laceration is extensive and deep should suturing the wound be considered.

Small, full thickness lacerations without aqueous leakage can be treated with a semipressure patch, bandage contact lens, or collagen shield. Because the globe's integrity has been violated, endophthalmitis may develop. The possibility of an occult intraocular foreign body also needs to be considered.

Large, self-sealing wounds may be treated as noted in reliable and cooperative patients. In children and unreliable patients, it is prudent to close the wound surgically. The most important surgical principle in repairing a full thickness, self-sealing corneal wound is to maintain a formed anterior chamber to avoid the complications of uveal prolapse. Almost all penetrating ocular injuries require general anesthesia to eliminate the risk of expulsive hemorrhage. Occasionally small, self-sealing lacerations may be repaired with topical anesthesia in cooperative patients. After preparing the patient, a lightweight speculum (Barraquer or Jaffe) is used to retract the eyelids. In most cases, it is wise to perform an anterior chamber stab (paracentesis) incision first. This controlled surgical incision allows for the reformation of the anterior chamber should the wound leak during repair. Viscoelastic agents (Healon, Viscoat, Amvisc, Occucoat, and others) can be introduced into the anterior chamber through the paracentesis site to stabilize the chamber. Once the chamber has been stabilized, the wound should be repaired with minimal manipulation of the wound edges. The newer 4 mil needles (Ethicon CS or TG-160-4, Alcon CU-15) allow for corneal passage with no or minimal counterpressure. The suture of choice remains 10-0 nylon. Once secured, the suture knots should be buried just beneath the surface and the wound checked for leakage by applying slight pressure to the globe. Absorbable sutures promote vascularization, are less comfortable, and should be avoided in corneal repairs.

The treatment of a leaking, full thickness wound generally follows the surgical guidelines outlined above. Small wounds with minimal leakage and a formed chamber, however, may be observed after the application of a bandage soft contact lens in reliable patients. Dissolvable collagen lenses have no place in the acute management of leaking wounds. At times, the placement of a soft bandage lens will allow the epithelium to heal, stopping the flow of aqueous. If the chamber stays deep but the flow of aqueous continues beyond 48 hours to 72 hours, it is prudent to proceed surgically. Prolonged leakage, even in the presence of a formed chamber, increases the likelihood of infection, promotes the development of a choroidal effusion, and may lead to fistula formation.

Corneal wounds with uveal involvement (Figure 8–7) are surgically repaired. The necessity for anesthesia should be kept in mind when initially evaluating the patient. Patients should be given nothing by mouth, and appropriate antibiotic prophylaxis should be instituted (see Chapter 17). Particular care should be given to wounds that are obviously contaminated. The eye should be adequately shielded after the initial examination since it is likely that the patient will need a number of preoperative tests and may require other examinations if there is multisystem trauma. If there is any suspicion of a potential intraocular foreign body, X rays and/or computed tomography (CT) scanning is warranted (see Chapter 2). A complete ocular examination may have to wait until the patient is in the operating room, under anesthesia.

The goals of surgery remain the same: to secure the eye and retain all viable intraocular contents. It is not uncommon for the iris to act as a plug, sealing the wound and stopping the flow of aqueous. In these cases, the anterior chamber is partially formed. Prior to removing the incarcerated iris and repairing the corneal laceration, it is advisable to use the benefit of a formed or partially formed chamber and make a peripheral stab incision into the anterior chamber. The anterior chamber can then be gently reformed with a viscoelastic agent. The initial stab incision should be large enough to allow for easy

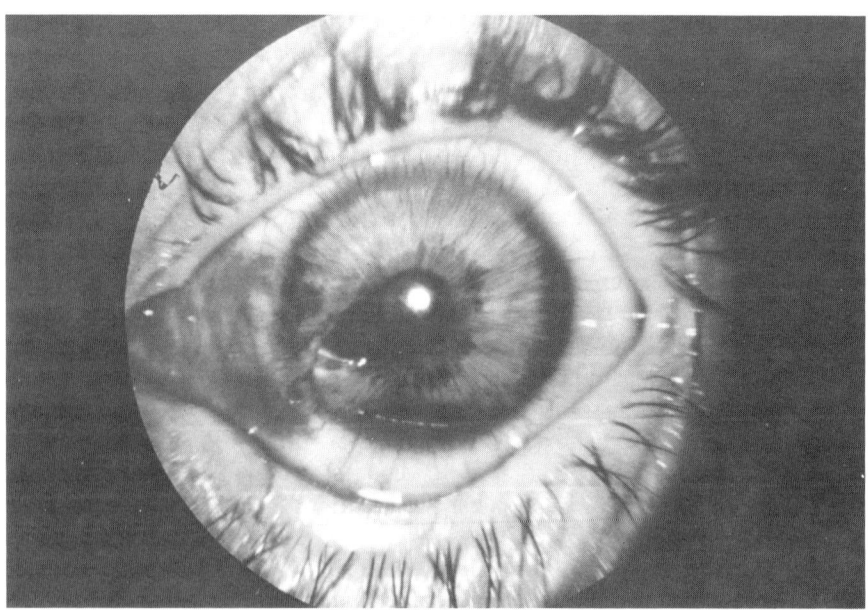

FIGURE 8–7. Full thickness corneal laceration with iris incarceration.

entrance of instruments. When reforming the chamber with viscoelastics, the wound of the stab incision should be slightly depressed to allow aqueous to egress; otherwise, the aqueous may be forced out the wound site, causing even greater iris incarceration. Once the chamber has been deepened, the part of the wound that does not have iris incarceration should be closed with interrupted 10-0 nylon. Again, small, thin-wire needles allow for easy corneal penetration with minimal wound manipulation. It should be anticipated that once the iris is removed from the wound, the chamber could be lost. This is the rationale behind establishing a peripheral entrance, deepening the chamber with viscoelastics, and closing as much of the wound as possible before addressing the portion of the wound with the incarcerated tissue. If the wound approaches or crosses the limbus, the conjunctiva should be opened and the sclera explored to be certain that the full extent of the wound has been found. Scleral lacerations can be closed with 9-0 or 10-0 interrupted nylon sutures. As long as the wound is in front of the pars plana (approximately 3.5 mm from the limbus), no additional treatment is required for the scleral extension.

Following the closure of all sites without iris incarceration, the incarcerated tissue can be approached. Unless the prolapsed tissue is obviously contaminated or necrotic, an attempt should be made to reposit the tissue. The chamber can be deepened with a pupillary constrictor (Miochol or Miostat), but this is rarely effective by itself. It is usually necessary to sweep the tissue out of the wound with a dull spatula placed through the stab incision. Foresight given to the initial placement of the peripheral stab incision will optimize the eventual iris manipulation. In general, placing the stab incision between 90° and 120° away from the iris incarceration simplifies this maneuver. Most surgeons prefer placing the stab incision at the temporal border of the cornea, when possible, for easier access. After the iris has been swept free from the wound, additional constricting agents (Miochol or Miostat) may be given. Closure of the wound is then completed.

PENETRATING INJURIES TO THE LENS

Any penetrating or perforating injury to the anterior segment may be complicated by damage to the crystalline lens. Lens damage can vary from a small rent in the anterior capsule, leading to a small localized cataract, to a total disruption with flocculent lens material filling the anterior chamber. There are three reasons that a damaged, cataractous lens should be primarily removed:

1. Preclusion of an adequate view and/or repair of posterior segment trauma.
2. Total disruption of the lens with flocculent material and vitreous in the anterior chamber.
3. Interference with primary corneal closure or reestablishment of the anterior chamber by a swollen or dislocated lens.

If none of these conditions exists, it is better to leave a damaged lens in place. Some anterior capsular rents will seal, and small traumatic cataracts may remain localized, interfering with vision only minimally. Additionally, if the eye can be stabilized without surgery on the lens, the option of a secondary procedure on the lens, under more controlled conditions, is retained. Postponing lens surgery allows the wound to heal, improving visualization and allowing for a closed chamber procedure. This may allow for a more complete lens removal or intraocular lens insertion, which may not have been contemplated or possible in the acute setting.

PENETRATING INJURIES TO THE RETINA

Posterior segment pathology is common in acute ocular trauma. While the posterior segment is physically more protected than the anterior segment, it can be involved in both penetrating and perforating injuries. In addition, severe blunt trauma may lead to a posterior scleral rupture. Part of the initial examination of any patient with acute anterior segment trauma is a careful examination of the posterior segment. If the ocular media is clear, indirect ophthalmoscopy is the most reliable method of examination. The status of the retina, the presence or absence of a vitreous hemorrhage, and the location of a retained intraocular foreign body can all be evaluated. An accurate evaluation of the posterior segment through a well-dilated pupil usually outweighs any potential disadvantage of dilating the pupil and subsequent pupillary management during surgical repair. When the optical media precludes an accurate assessment, orbital X rays, CT scanning, and ultrasound can be utilized. Ultrasound is an effective method for determining the presence of vitreous opacities, vitreous hemorrhage, and/or the presence of a retinal detachment, but it usually requires direct contact with the lid on the globe, and as such its use is limited in unrepaired traumatized eyes. Orbital X rays and soft tissue films are often helpful in identifying and localizing a radiopaque foreign body. CT scanning is particularly useful in localizing the foreign body in the globe (Figure 8–8). Magnetic resonance imaging (MRI) scanning should never be used when a metallic intraocular foreign body potentially exists. The magnetic pull may cause movement of the metallic foreign body, exacerbating an injury.

The majority of general ophthalmologists are uncomfortable and unfamiliar with the techniques needed for extensive posterior segment repair. If posterior segment injury is noted during the initial evaluation, an opportunity exists to discuss the case with a retina/vitreous specialist. More often, however, a complete evaluation of the posterior segment is not possible, and the extent and presence of posterior segment trauma are unknown until the patient is brought to the operating room. The dilemma of managing unexpected posterior segment trauma often arises intraoperatively. The main goal of acute management is the restoration of an intact globe. While it may seem preferable to do

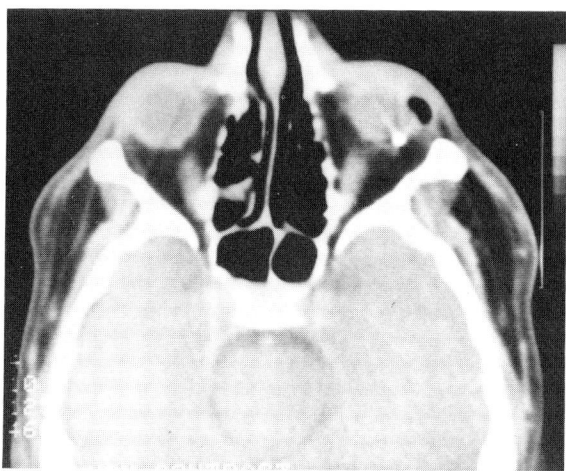

FIGURE 8-8. CT demonstrating metallic foreign body embedded in the posterior sclera.

a definitive procedure, it is often best to defer difficult and extensive intraocular repair until the eye has stabilized, the possibility of infection has been eliminated, and more extensive preoperative testing can be performed.

The use of mechanical vitrectors and the performance of a limited anterior vitrectomy are well within the scope of most ophthalmologists. When there is a totally disrupted lens intermixed with vitreous, the mechanical vitrector should be utilized to remove as much of the lens material as possible and any vitreous in the anterior segment. Vitreous hemorrhage and more posterior pathology are often best left untreated. Many retinal/vitreous surgeons prefer to work in a theoretical optimal window between 3 days and 10 days after the initial trauma. Deferring surgery reduces the chance of bleeding and allows time for the posterior vitreous to separate from the retina, resulting in a potentially easier and safer vitrectomy. Ultrasound can be utilized after the initial repair to determine the status of the retina and the posterior vitreous face prior to a second procedure. Finally, significant vitreous organization is uncommon prior to 10 days.

Another common difficulty that presents during surgical repair of corneoscleral lacerations is determining the full extent of retinal injury in scleral lacerations that extend beyond the pars plana. The scleral laceration should be repaired as discussed. When the media is cloudy and the underlying retina cannot be examined, a decision has to be made if "blind" cryotherapy should be applied to the area of injury. While this remains controversial, the pathophysiology and likelihood of a subsequent detachment is different with traumatic retinal holes than with acute idiopathic retinal holes. Our opinion is not to perform prophylactic cryotherapy unless direct observation is possible.

INTRAOCULAR FOREIGN BODY

The possibility of an intraocular foreign body should always be considered when evaluating a patient with ocular trauma. The degree of the evaluation and extent of the workup is often directed by the history and type of injury. Any patient who presents with ocular complaints after working on high-speed metal drills or presses or has a history of striking metal against metal should be carefully examined. If the examination reveals a local area of conjunctival injection, a hyphema, a localized cataract, and/or iris injury, the patient needs a thorough indirect ophthalmologic exam, X rays, and possibly a CT scan (Figure 8–9). The physician needs to convey to the radiologist that a small intraocular foreign body is possible and should request both axial and coronal views. While an X ray is suitable for screening for radiopaque material, the CT scanner is better at localizing the foreign body and determining whether the foreign material is intraocular or extraocular (orbital) (Figure 8–8). The history is also helpful in identifying the type of material. Many foreign bodies are relatively inert (glass, stone, high quality plastics, stainless steel and other quality alloys) and tolerated by the eye with minimal reaction. Organic material, iron and low-quality alloys, copper, magnesium, aluminum, and low-grade plastic, however, are poorly tolerated and potentially toxic to the eye. Iron and copper, left in place, can cause widespread ocular destruction. Copper, in particular, is

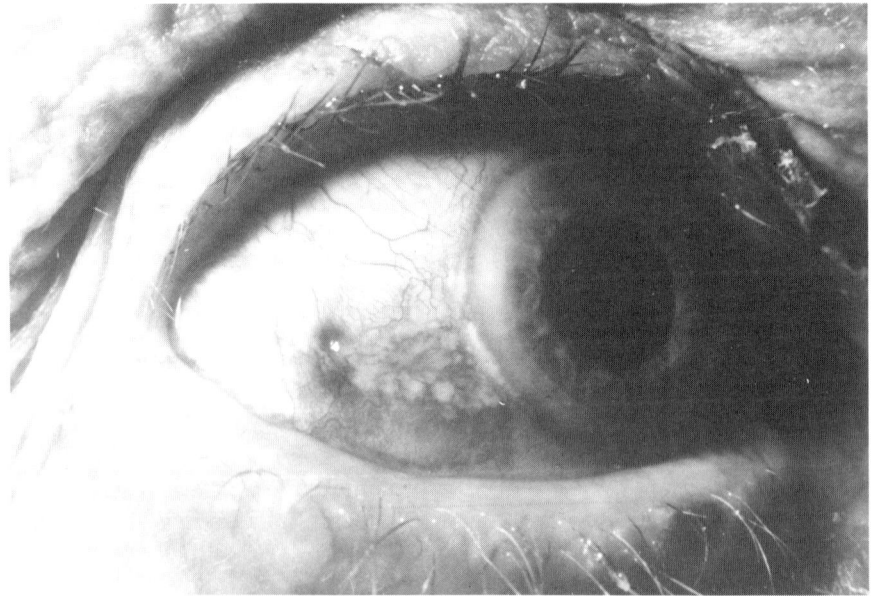

FIGURE 8–9. Small, almost innocuous-appearing penetration site of an intraocular foreign body.

extremely toxic and should be removed as soon as possible. If the material is metallic, it is important to determine whether it is magnetic. Iron and related compounds (magnetic) can often be removed with magnetic extraction. Other metals require intraocular forceps for delivery.

If the foreign body can be localized and the lens has been damaged to the degree that it needs to be removed, an intraocular foreign body may be best removed through a limbal-based corneal incision or through removal of a corneal button ("open sky" vitrectomy). Otherwise, it is preferential to deliver the foreign material through the pars plana. As long as visualization is adequate, a pars plana approach allows for better surgical control and allows for vitrectomy and/or endolaser to be performed as necessary. In contaminated or low-speed projectile injuries, intravitreal antibiotics should be given at the conclusion of the case (see Chapter 17). Many small metallic foreign bodies travel at high speed, generating a high temperature that sterilizes the foreign body and lessens the risk of endophthalmitis.

INTRAORBITAL FOREIGN BODY

Foreign bodies may be lodged in the orbit, causing no associated ocular problems (Figure 8–10). Large orbital foreign bodies, however, may have caused blunt injury to the globe, and small, sharp foreign bodies may have traversed (perforated) the globe and subsequently lodged in the orbit. The initial evaluation requires localization of the foreign body and examination of the eye for occult injury. Indirect ophthalmoscopy is mandatory. Any findings of vitreous hemorrhage, localized cataract, localized conjunctival and/or scleral injection, iris perforation, or hyphema suggest that the intraorbital foreign body may have traversed the globe. Particularly suggestive of a traversing injury is a finding of damage in the globe opposite to the side of a lodged intraorbital foreign body. In such cases, management of the globe takes precedence. Intraorbital foreign bodies can also be associated with intracranial extension.

Orbital X rays are useful in identifying and localizing radiopaque material. Repeat films taken with the eye in different fields of gaze assist in verifying the extraocular location, as orbital foreign bodies should not move. CT scanning offers better localization, and axial and coronal cuts should be obtained. Recently MRI scanning has proved useful in identifying non-metallic intraorbital foreign bodies not previously identified by X ray, CT scanning, or orbital ultrasound (see Chapter 2).

Inorganic materials, glass, stone, plastic, and metal, with the exception of copper, are well tolerated. Unless they are protruding from the skin, superficial, or causing optic nerve compression, they are probably best left undisturbed. Organic material is usually not well tolerated and may cause a chronic granulomatous, acutely exacerbating, inflammatory reaction. In addition, any foreign body, but particularly organic material, may seed the orbit and

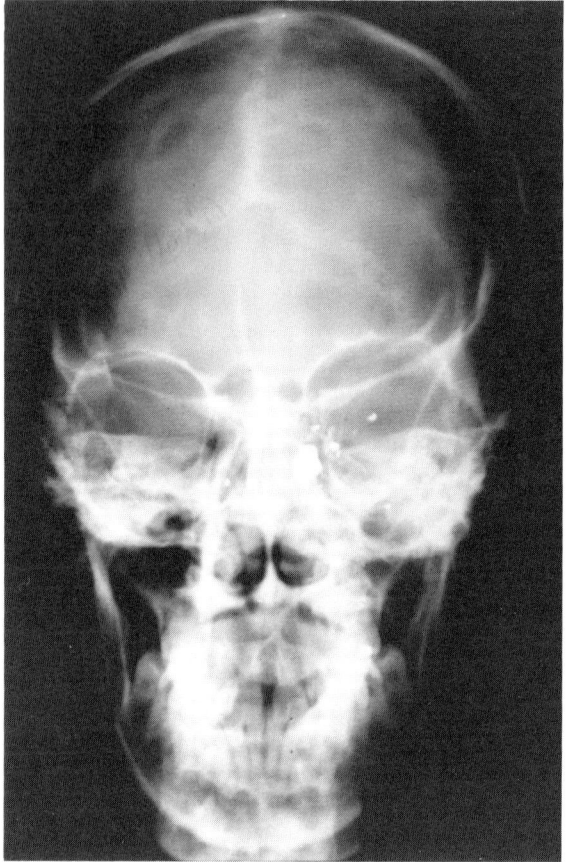

FIGURE 8-10. Multiple inert intraorbital foreign bodies secondary to gunshot wound, 30 years earlier. Both globes were uninjured.

cause an orbital cellulitis. It is therefore advisable to remove organic materials. When possible, removal should be attempted along the original site of entry to minimize further structural damage. Any discharge should be cultured.

Even if it is decided not to remove the intraorbital foreign body, the patient should be hospitalized and treated with intravenous antibiotics. A commonly used combination is gentamicin 1.75 mg/kg as a loading dose, followed by 1 mg/kg every 8 hours with cefazolin 1 g or clindamycin 600 mg every 8 hours. A 14-day course is recommended, but the patient can be switched to oral antibiotics and discharged on day 5 if no complications become apparent. Further suggestions regarding prophylaxis against orbital cellulitis are given in Chapter 17. Tetanus prophylaxis is given as needed (see Chapters 4 and 17).

REFERENCES

Abbott, RL (ed): *Surgical Intervention in Corneal and External Diseases.* Orlando, Grune & Stratton, 1970.
Eagling EM, Roper-Hall MJ: *Eye Injuries.* Philadelphia, JB Lippincott & Co., 1986.
Eastly DL, Smolin G: *External Eye Disease.* London, Butterworth, 1985.
Green BF, Kraft SP, Carter KD, et al: Intraorbital wood. Detection by magnetic resonance imaging. *Ophthalmology* 97:608, 1990.

III

Nontraumatic Ocular and Orbital Emergencies

9

Evaluation and Management of Nontraumatic Disorders of the Lacrimal Drainage System

Dale R. Meyer

The most common presenting symptom of a lacrimal drainage disorder is epiphora, or overflow of tears onto the cheeks. Epiphora results from an imbalance between tear production and drainage. Except when associated with a fulminant infection of the lacrimal sac (acute dacryocystitis) or conjunctivitis, it does not require urgent treatment. It is, nonetheless, a common and debilitating malady. This chapter focuses on the evaluation and treatment of the tearing patient with emphasis on obstructive disorders of the nasolacrimal drainage system. Conditions that present with similar signs and symptoms (particularly the "dry eye syndrome") and infections of the lacrimal system will also be discussed.

ANATOMY AND INITIAL CONSIDERATIONS

The lacrimal drainage system consists of three distinct portions: the puncta and canaliculi, the lacrimal sac, and the lacrimal duct (Figure 9–1). The puncta are small (0.33 mm) openings located on the medial one-third of the eyelids through which tears enter the lacrimal system. The canaliculi, measuring 10 mm in length, carry tears from the puncta to the lacrimal sac. Each is enveloped by orbicularis muscle and connective tissue. In most cases, the two canaliculi join to form a common canaliculus before entering the lacrimal sac. In approximately 10% of individuals, however, they enter the sac directly. A small fold of mucosa, known as the valve of Rosenmueller, is usually present at the junction of the common canaliculus with the lacrimal sac. This "valve" prevents reflux of fluid and air from the lacrimal sac, a 13-mm-long pouch that lies within the bony lacrimal fossa (see Chapter 5). Approximately two-thirds of the

THE LACRIMAL SYSTEM

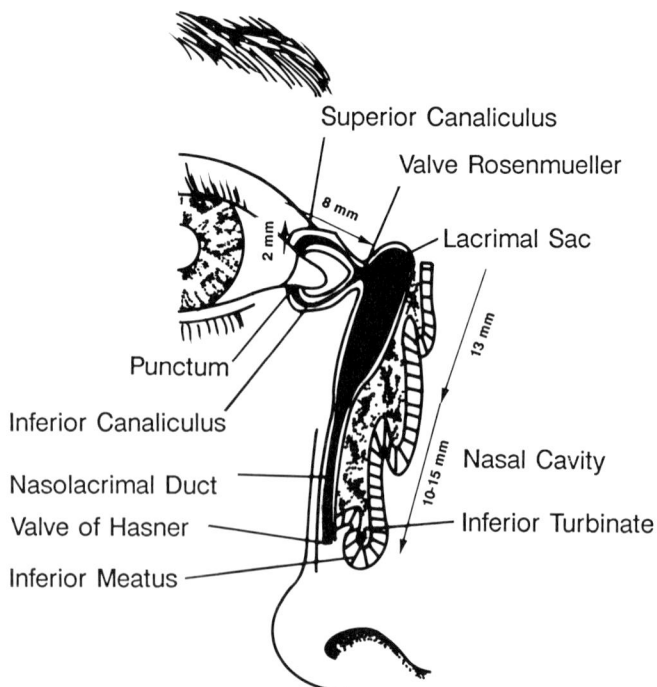

FIGURE 9–1. Anatomy of the nasolacrimal drainage system.

lacrimal sac is situated below the medial canthus, and one-third is above. Inferiorly, the lacrimal sac narrows to join the nasolacrimal duct, which passes within a bony canal to open into the nose, under the inferior turbinate. The course of the nasolacrimal duct is angled posteriorly and slightly laterally relative to the position of the medial canthus. Its length is approximately 10 mm to 15 mm in adults. A small flap of mucosa, known as the valve of Hasner, is normally present at the osteal opening; similar to the valve of Rosenmueller, it prevents reflux of fluid or air from the nose.

Tear flow obstruction can occur at any point from the puncta to the nasal cavity. In the vast majority of patients, it occurs in the distal portion of the nasolacrimal duct. In addition to anatomic patency of the nasolacrimal system, tear flow requires normal eyelid function and position. Lid malpositions such as an inward turning of the eyelid margin (entropion) or an outward turning of the eyelid (ectropion) interfere with lacrimal pump function. Disorders that lead to orbicularis weakness can also interfere with pump action. Facial nerve palsy (Bell's palsy) is particularly problematic.

The evaluation of the tearing patient begins with a directed history and proceeds with a determination of whether the etiology is obstructive or nonobstructive. Some clinicians reserve the term *epiphora* for tearing due to outflow obstruction and use the term *pseudoepiphora* for other causes (e.g., reflex tearing associated with corneal disease, misdirected eyelashes, lid malpositions, and dry eye syndrome). The assessment and treatment of tearing in children differs from adults and will be discussed separately. In both children and adults, however, tear flow obstruction can lead to tear stasis, potentiating infections of the conjunctiva or lacrimal sac.

CONGENITAL DISORDERS

Congenital nasolacrimal duct obstruction (NLDO) occurs in nearly 5% of otherwise healthy newborns. It is usually the result of a failure of the distal end of the lacrimal duct to canalize into the nose fully. In most cases, development proceeds, and canalization is completed within the first weeks of life. The rate of spontaneous opening of the lacrimal duct slows after 6 months of age, reaching a plateau around the first birthday. Beyond this age, spontaneous resolution is rare.

Infants with congenital NLDO present with unilateral or bilateral tearing and variable crusting of the lid margins on the affected side (Figure 9-2). A secondary conjunctivitis may also be present. Some patients present with a dilated lacrimal sac filled with mucoid material (lacrimal sac mucocele) or an indolent infection with mucopurulent discharge (chronic dacryocystitis). A small percentage of infants present with fulminant acute dacryocystitis, requiring urgent treatment.

The differential diagnosis of tearing in infancy includes infantile glaucoma,

220 III—Nontraumatic Ocular and Orbital Emergencies

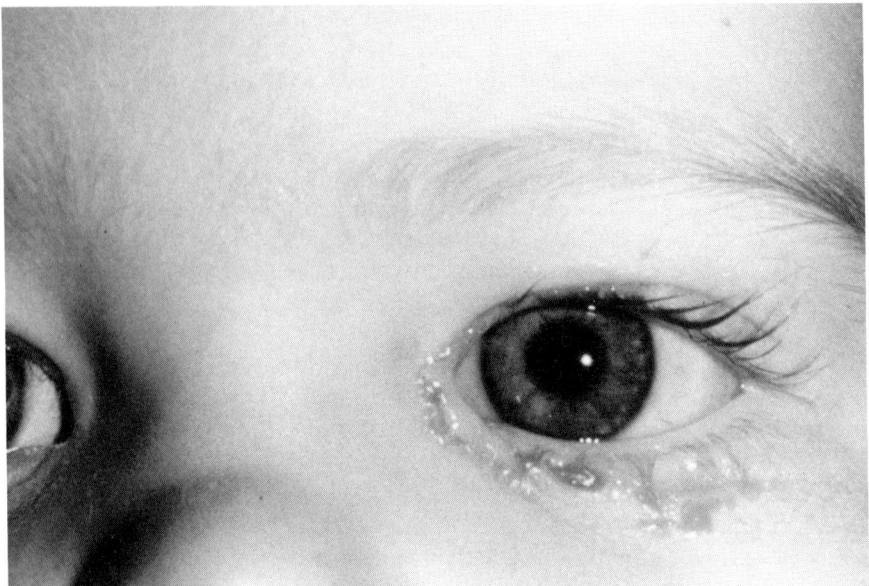

FIGURE 9-2. Congenital left nasolacrimal duct obstruction.

primary infectious conjunctivitis, keratitis (corneal inflammation or irritation), uveitis (intraocular inflammation), and eyelid anomalies. Infantile glaucoma is characterized by corneal edema or haze, increased corneal diameter, enlarged cup to disc ratio, and myopia (see Chapter 11). It also presents with photophobia (light sensitivity), as do keratitis and uveitis. Primary conjunctivitis is characterized by discharge rather than tearing. Older children with conjunctivitis also have follicles or papillae. In contrast, reflux of mucopurulent material from the puncta upon palpation ("massage") of the lacrimal sac is diagnostic of NLDO. Its absence, however, does not preclude this diagnosis. If lacrimal obstruction cannot be differentiated from chronic conjunctivitis, cultures should be obtained (see Chapter 16). Corneal irritation and reflex tearing from trichiasis (abnormally growing eyelashes), entropion, or other eyelid anomalies are usually easily recognized.

Most of the tests used to assess lacrimal drainage in adults cannot be performed on infants or children. A notable exception is the fluorescein dye disappearance test. This test is performed by placing one drop of fluorescein 2% ophthalmic solution in each eye. Normally the dye is not visible in the tear film after 5 minutes. A significant residual confirms lacrimal drainage impairment but does not localize the site of the obstruction. Alternatively, the examiner can inspect the nasal passage or throat for dye with a cobalt blue light or Wood's lamp. Its presence confirms patency of the nasolacrimal system, but its absence should not be taken as an absolute indication of lacrimal obstruction.

The definitive treatment of congenital NLDO is irrigation or probing of the nasolacrimal duct. This technique serves to "open" the distal obstruction. In one large series (Baker, 1985), a single probing of the nasolacrimal duct was curative in approximately 94% of infants, and with one repeat probing, the success rate exceeded 99%. The appropriate time to perform probing is controversial. Some clinicians advocate massage of the lacrimal sac until the child is 12 months of age, with the use of topical antibiotics (e.g., Polytrim, erythromycin, sulfacetamide) when conjunctivitis develops. These clinicians note that since most obstructions clear within the first year of life, a conservative course will spare many children a surgical procedure. Other clinicians believe that probing should be performed early to spare the patient and family an extended period of waiting. One advantage of early probing is that it can be done in the office under topical anesthesia. Older infants require sedation or general anesthesia. Beyond 13 months of age, the success rate of probing for congenital NLDO diminishes proportionally to age. Almost all authorities agree that probing should be performed by this age.

I recommend that probing be performed on any child who has developed acute dacryocystitis after appropriate systemic antibiotic therapy has been completed to avoid recurrence of this serious condition. Similarly, early probing of congenital lacrimal sac mucoceles is advised because they are associated with a high rate of secondary infection. In patients with chronic, copious mucopurulent discharge (which suggests ongoing inflammation of the lacrimal sac), probing at age 6 months is suggested. In the absence of chronic conjunctivitis, the infant can be managed conservatively up to 12 months of age. The parents should participate in this decision.

If the initial probing fails, it can be repeated one or more times. If the child is still symptomatic, the nasolacrimal system should be intubated with a silicone tube. This prevents closure of the nasolacrimal osteum during healing and is usually left in place for 6 weeks to 12 weeks. Infracture of the inferior turbinate is suggested if it is closely opposed to the lateral wall of the nose, possibly contributing to outflow obstruction. A very small percentage of patients with persistent obstruction or with a bony obstruction not amenable to probing require dacryocystorhinostomy to bypass the obstruction surgically.

Less common congenital anomalies of the lacrimal system include lacrimal sac mucocele (amniocele, amniotocele, dacryocystocele), lacrimal sac fistula, atresia of the lacrimal puncta or canaliculi, and supernumerary puncta or canaliculi. Mucoceles of the lacrimal sac usually present within the first few days of life as firm, bluish, cystic masses inferior to the medial canthal angle (Figure 9–3). They result from combined obstruction of the nasolacrimal system distal and proximal to the lacrimal sac. Mucous is unable to reflux onto the eye and continues to accumulate until pressure within the sac prevents its further production. The differential of a lacrimal sac mucocele includes encephalocele, ethmoid mucocele, hemangioma, and dermoid. These disorders should be considered when the mass extends above the medial canthal tendon. Radio-

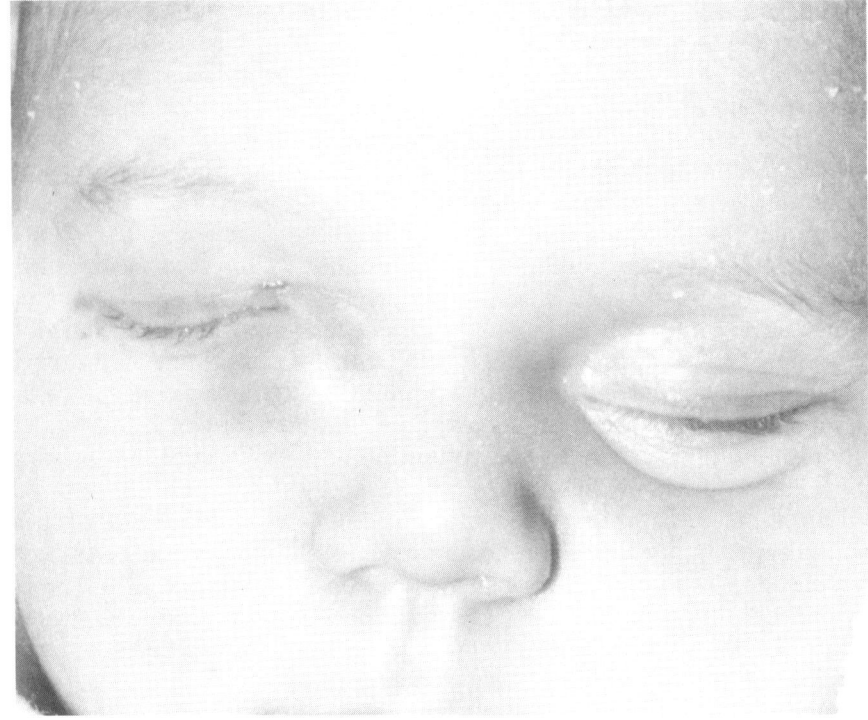

FIGURE 9-3. Mucocele of the right lacrimal sac.

logic imaging should be obtained if the diagnosis is uncertain, especially if an encephalocele is a possibility.

Warm compresses and gentle massage may relieve the obstruction in lacrimal sac mucoceles and should be tried as the initial therapy. If this treatment is unsuccessful after several days or if any sign of inflammation develops, probing of the lacrimal duct should be performed. Untreated mucoceles usually become infected, often with a fulminant course. The earliest manifestation is erythema of the skin overlying the mucocele; if acute dacryocystitis or cellulitis develops, intravenous antibiotics are required.

Occasionally, an infected dilated sac spontaneously decompresses with the development of a lacrimal sac fistula (Figure 9-4). Fistulas can also occur in the absence of dacryocystitis. They usually present below the medial canthal angle and act as the lacrimal drainage site. Treatment is directed toward relieving any distal obstruction by probing the lacrimal system. This usually results in closure, but occasionally a fistula has to be excised surgically.

Atresia of the lacrimal puncta is characterized by the persistence of an epithelial covering over the opening. Inspection of the medial inner eyelid will reveal a grayish dimple in the center of a slightly raised area (papilla) where the

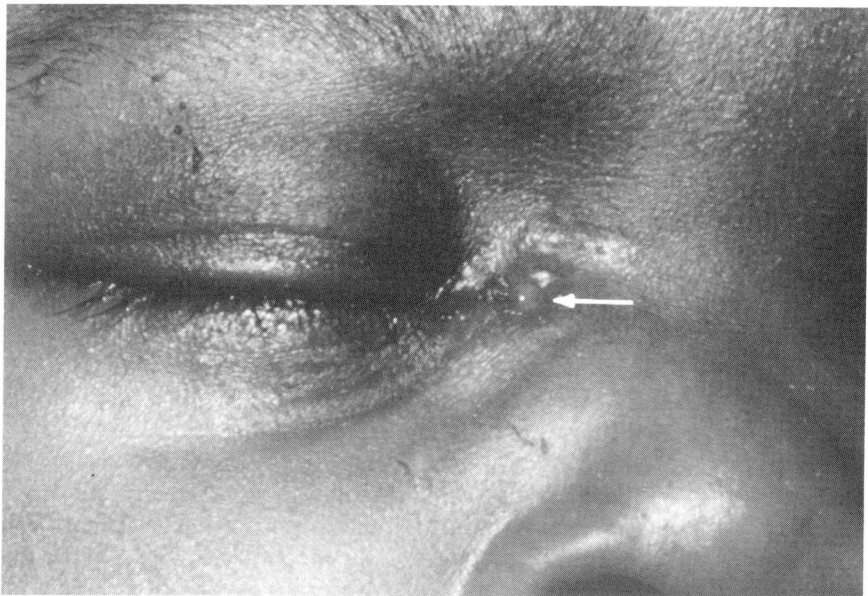

FIGURE 9-4. Lacrimal sac fistula (arrow).

puncta should be. Often this can be easily opened with a sharp pin. Atresia of the canaliculus presents greater difficulty. Surgical repair of complete canalicular atresia is difficult, and a conjunctivodacryocystorhinostomy with insertion of a Pyrex glass (Jones) tube is often necessary. Supernumerary puncta or canaliculi (also known as lacrimal anlage ducts or congenital lacrimal fistulae) are usually asymptomatic and do not require treatment.

ACQUIRED DISORDERS

Acquired obstruction of the lacrimal drainage system occurs predominantly in adults. The spectrum of causative disorders is more diverse than those of congenital obstructions, but the etiology can usually be established by methodical office evaluation. The goal of the evaluation is to differentiate nonobstructive etiologies of tearing from primary and secondary lacrimal obstruction.

Causes of Acquired Disorders

The most common lacrimal drainage disorder in adults is an acquired primary obstruction of the nasolacrimal duct, usually caused by chronic submucosal inflammation within the duct (Linberg and McCormick, 1986). This progresses to fibrosis, with eventual narrowing or total obstruction of the duct lumen. Obstruction of the lacrimal sac or proximal drainage apparatus (canaliculi) is relatively uncommon.

The most common cause of secondary nasolacrimal duct or sac obstruction is a neoplasm. Tumors can arise intrinsically or spread from the adjacent nasal cavity, sinuses, or orbit. Intrinsic epithelial neoplasms are rare, but they are often malignant and can be fatal (Figure 9-5). A wide surgical excision is required. Dacryoliths (also known as lacrimal stones) are another cause of secondary obstruction. They are the result of sluggish or stagnant tear flow and can form in any part of the lacrimal drainage system. Granulomatous processes, including sarcoidosis, Wegener's granulomatosis, and pseudotumor, may also involve the lacrimal sac and the nasolacrimal duct and cause a secondary obstruction. Finally, structural alterations of the nasolacrimal duct, the osseous nasolacrimal canal, or the lacrimal sac can result from trauma (e.g., midfacial fracture) or surgery on adjacent sinuses or the nose.

Obstruction of the canaliculi by intrinsic neoplasms is extremely rare. Direct extension from conjunctival or medial canthal skin malignancies, however, can occur. Punctal or canalicular stenosis is more commonly due to a cicatrizing process of the conjunctiva or the skin or a toxic effect of systemic antineoplastic agents (e.g., 5FU), topical eye medications (e.g., phospholine iodide), or primary herpetic ocular infections. Canaliculitis is an unusual inflammatory

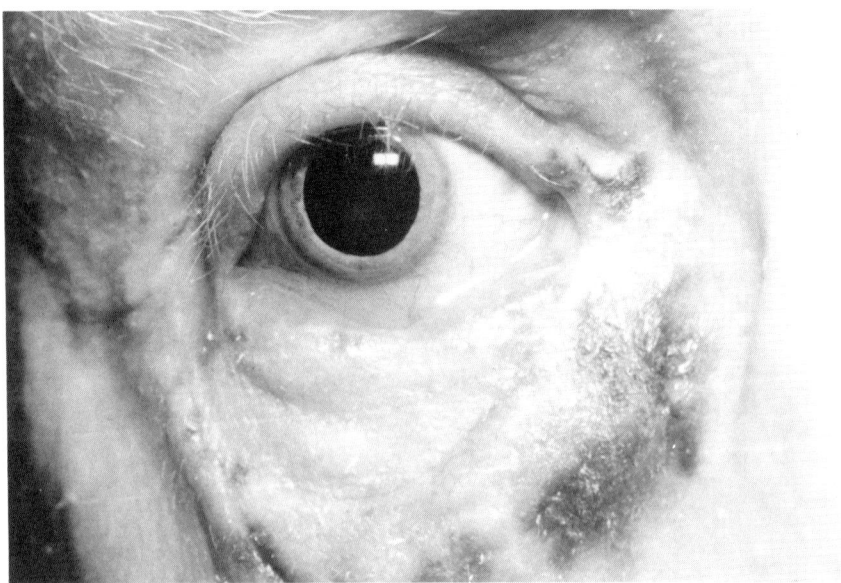

FIGURE 9-5. Carcinoma of the lacrimal sac extending into the upper and lower eyelids, causing secondary nasolacrimal duct obstruction.

cause of canalicular obstruction. It is caused by colonization by actinomycetes species and is accompanied by concretions of gram-positive filamentous rods within the canaliculi. These concretions can often be expressed by pressure on the canaliculi with cotton-tipped applicators.

Nonobstructive causes of epiphora in the adult include eyelid malpositions (Figures 9–6 and 9–7), trichiasis (Figure 9–8), ocular surface disease, and the dry eye syndrome. Each of these can lead to reflex tearing mediated by the trigeminal nerve. Tearing can also be associated with pain due to sinus or dental disease. Hypersecretion of tears may be idiopathic or associated with parasympathetic nervous system dysfunction (e.g., crocodile tears seen with regeneration of parasympathetic facial nerve fibers after Bell's palsy).

The Workup of the Adult with Epiphora

Practically and statistically, most cases of epiphora in the adult are due to reflex tearing (usually due to the dry eye syndrome) or nasolacrimal duct obstruction. If obstructive disease is present, it is important to know the level of the obstruction for surgical planning.

The physician should inquire about the duration and onset of tearing, as well as its severity, specifically asking whether tears overflow onto the cheek. The patient should be asked whether tearing is constant or intermittent and if any

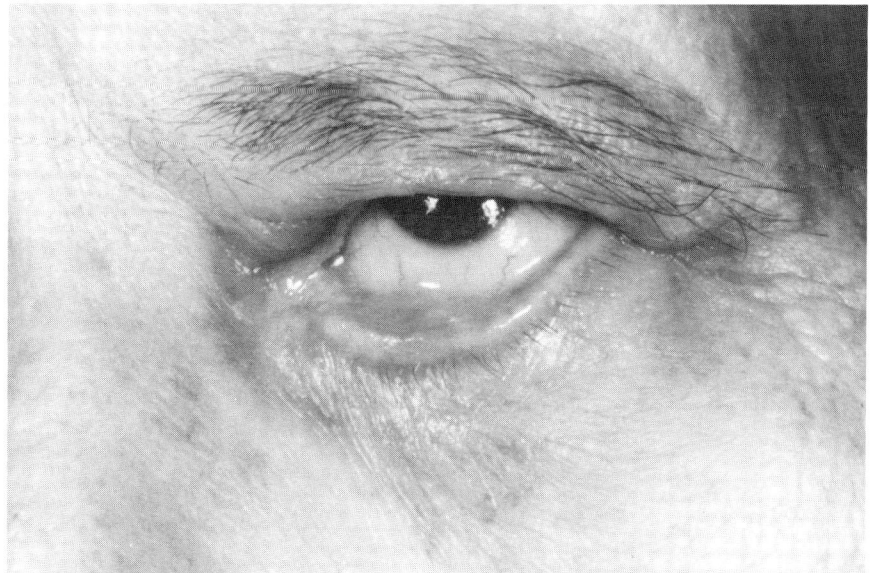

FIGURE 9–6. Ectropion, left lower eyelid.

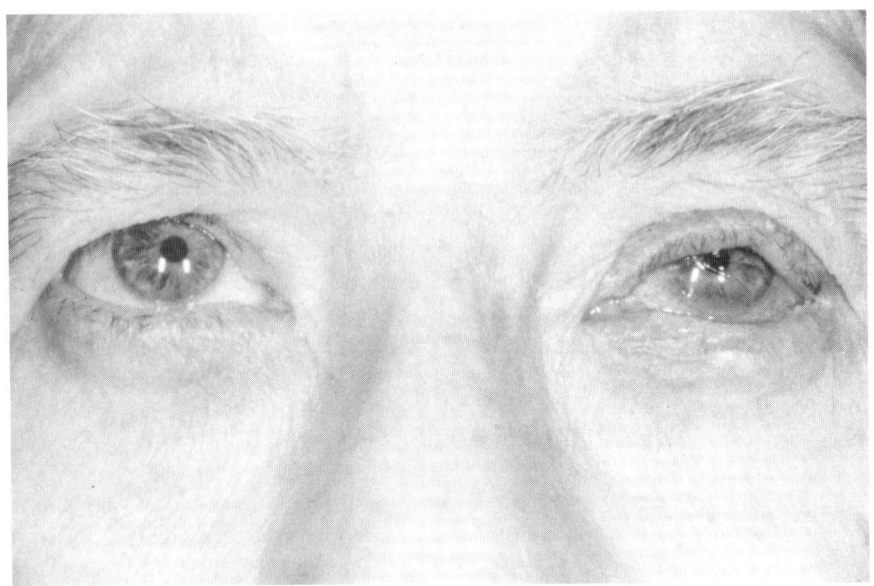

FIGURE 9-7. Entropion, left lower eyelid.

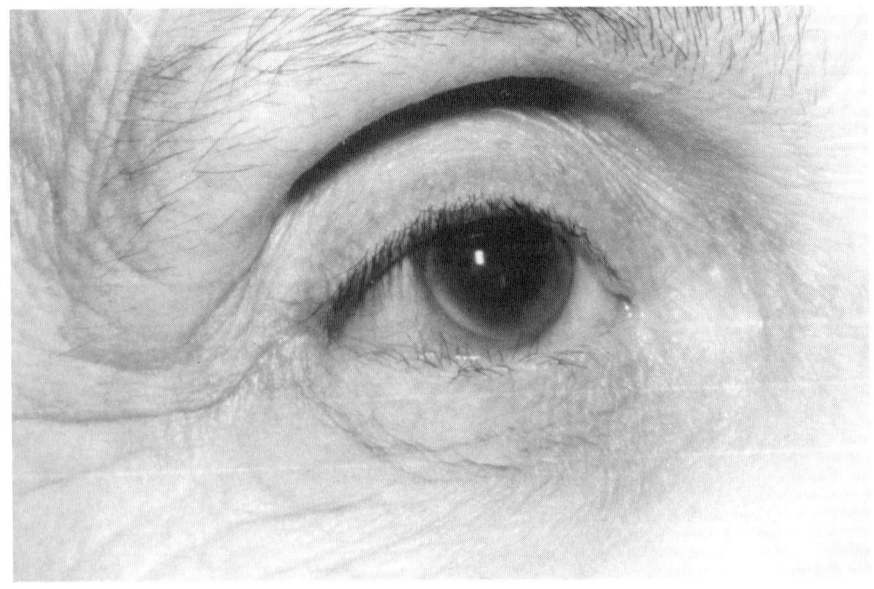

FIGURE 9-8. Trichiasis, right lower eyelid.

environmental factors (wind, sun, cold, allergies, or occupational exposure) are aggravating. The use of potentially sensitizing topical eye medications should be reviewed, as should the use of systemic medications that can decrease tear production (e.g., antihistamines or other drugs with anticholinergic activity). The patient should be asked if the tearing is associated with pain and, if so, the nature of the pain. Bloody tears and frequent epistaxis raise the suspicion of malignancy. When itching is a prominent complaint, allergy should be suspected.

The past medical history should detail any known ocular or sinus disease or surgery. A history of midfacial (fracture) or medial canthal (laceration) trauma should also be sought. Radiation therapy involving the midface can cause lacrimal obstruction, and recent or previous facial nerve dysfunction might contribute to tearing by limiting lacrimal pump function or causing an overproduction of tears from aberrant seventh nerve regeneration (crocodile tears).

After obtaining the medical history, a physical examination is performed. Many aspects of the lacrimal system evaluation are included in the routine ophthalmic examination (see Chapter 1). Other features must be specifically addressed. The eyelids are examined for evidence of lid malposition (ectropion or entropion) and trichiasis. The puncta are examined for signs of aversion, stenosis, or canaliculitis. Dynamic eyelid function, including the frequency of blinking and strength of forced closure, are assessed because these functions are essential for normal lacrimal pump action. Any lid retraction or lagophthalmos (incomplete closure) should be noted, as these can lead to corneal exposure and reflex tearing.

The medial canthus and lacrimal sac area are examined for the presence of any masses or signs of inflammation. A distended lacrimal sac usually feels fluctuant, and, as in infants, reflux of mucoid or mucopurulent discharge from the puncta with pressure over the sac is indicative of NLDO. A palpable hard mass is suggestive of tumor. Large tumors that extend into the orbit may also cause ocular dystopia (displacement of the eye), proptosis (protrusion of the eye, Figure 9–9), and/or limitation of ocular motility. The presence of a mass above the medial canthal tendon is suggestive of a neoplasm.

Slit lamp biomicroscopy is useful in evaluating eyelid margin disorders (e.g., blepharitis, malpositions), punctal abnormalities, and conjunctival cicatrizing processes and is essential for examination of the ocular surface. Tear film characteristics, including tear meniscus height, tear film distribution, and tear break-up time (usually greater than 10 seconds), should be noted. Because conjunctival or corneal epithelial defects can be associated with reflex tearing, examination using topical fluorescein and/or rose bengal stains may be indicated (see Chapter 1). Fluorescein should be used in conjunction with lacrimal drainage dye tests. Keratitis, iritis, and acute narrow angle glaucoma are potential ocular causes of reflex hypersecretion. These are usually readily diagnosed and not likely to be confused with other causes of epiphora in adult patients. Nasal examination is also important because inflammatory, neoplastic, and

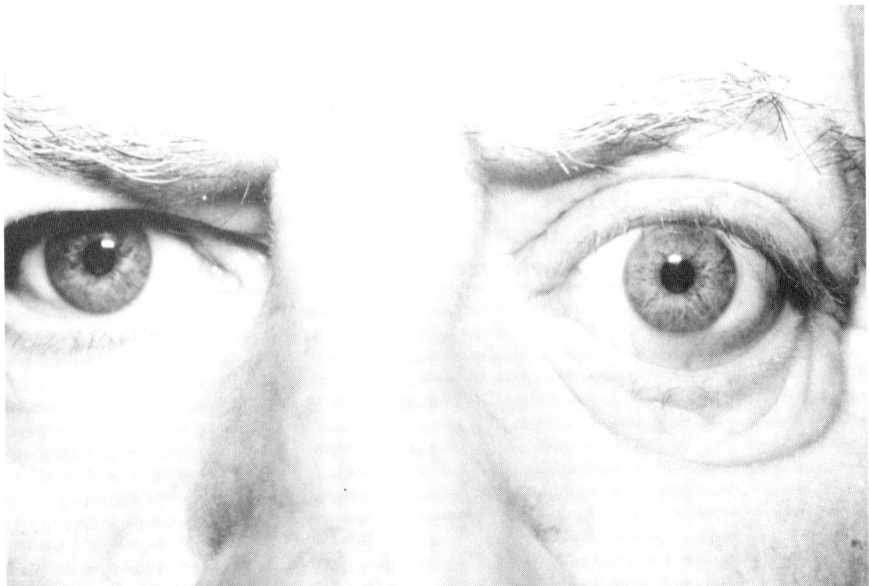

FIGURE 9-9. Proptosis of the left eye secondary to a lacrimal sac mass extending into the orbit.

structural disorders of the nasal passages are potential causes of tearing. A nasal speculum and the light of an indirect ophthalmoscope are convenient for this purpose. The nose is also examined in conjunction with lacrimal drainage tests.

Most nonobstructive etiologies of tearing will be detected by the evaluation already detailed. The dry eye syndrome is diagnosed by Schirmer testing, performed by placing a strip of filter paper in each conjunctival cul-de-sac after blotting the tear meniscus. The amount of wetting along the length of the filter paper strip is measured in millimeters after 5 minutes (see Figure 1-9). The Schirmer I test is performed without anesthesia. Less than 15 mm of wetting is suggestive of aqueous tear insufficiency. If the Schirmer I test is abnormal, a basic secretion test (frequently erroneously called a Schirmer II test) is performed. This test measures the "basal" tear secretion that remains after anesthetizing the ocular surface with a topical anesthetic to prevent reflex tearing. A normal result on this test is a wetting of 10 mm or more. The true Schirmer II test also stimulates the nasal mucosa mechanically (cotton-tipped applicator) or chemically (ammonium chloride) to determine "stressed" reflex tear secretion (see also Chapter 1).

The fluorescein dye disappearance and Jones dye tests, along with diagnostic lacrimal probing, are used to confirm an acquired lacrimal obstruction. When they are used in a logical, sequential manner, the anatomic location of the blockage can be determined.

The fluorescein dye disappearance test is most sensitive in detecting proximal obstructions (those involving the canaliculi). Dye disappearance may be normal or only minimally abnormal with a distal NLDO accompanied by a dilated lacrimal sac. The test will also be unreliable if the eyelids are strongly squeezed after instillation of the drop, and the dye overflows onto the cheeks.

The primary Jones dye test (Jones I) is a test of functional tear flow. It determines whether fluorescein instilled into the conjunctival cul-de-sac can pass through the lacrimal system into the nose. The test is usually performed 5 minutes or more after the fluorescein dye disappearance test. A thin cotton-tipped applicator is inserted under the inferior turbinate in the area near the osteum of the nasolacrimal duct. Gross patency of the lacrimal system is confirmed by the detection of dye in the nose; however, a partial obstruction cannot be completely ruled out. Inability to detect dye in the nose may be due to a physiologic or anatomic lacrimal outflow disorder or technical difficulty in performing the test. Approximately 20% of normal asymptomatic patients will have a falsely negative Jones I test.

When the primary Jones test suggests an obstruction, the Jones II test should be conducted. This test of anatomic patency is performed by irrigating clear saline into one canaliculus using a 3 cc syringe and a 23-gauge lacrimal cannula. The patient's head should be tilted forward to allow the irrigant to drain from the nose. Because pressure is used, the test is nonphysiologic, but if fluid can be irrigated into the nose, a complete obstruction of the lacrimal system is ruled out. The location of the obstruction can be determined based on the outcome of the test. In the presence of a negative Jones I test, clear fluid obtained from the nose with the Jones II test suggests partial blockage (stenosis) proximal to the common canaliculus. Dye-tinged effluent from the nose suggests that fluorescein pooled within the sac during the Jones I test and was flushed through the duct with irrigation. The inability to irrigate any fluid into the nose suggests a complete anatomic obstruction at the level of the nasolacrimal duct. This is usually accompanied by a palpable distention of the lacrimal sac with or without regurgitation of dye-tinged fluid from the opposite canaliculus. Regurgitation of clear fluid from the opposite canaliculus suggests obstruction at the common canaliculus, and regurgitation of clear fluid from the same canaliculus indicates obstruction proximal to the common canaliculus (or lacrimal sac). If a canalicular obstruction is suspected, diagnostic probing is indicated to determine the exact location of the obstruction. The distance of the obstruction from the lacrimal puncta (measured in millimeters) should be noted, as this has implications for surgical management.

In most cases, these office tests will determine the nature of lacrimal dysfunction and the level of obstruction. Sometimes additional tests may be required. These include dacryoscintigraphy, dacryocystography, computed tomography (CT), and magnetic resonance imaging (MRI). Dacryoscintigraphy is a radionucleotide scan used to assess physiologic tear flow. The remaining tests are used to define the lacrimal drainage anatomy and/or to detect mass lesions. Dacryocystography provides a radiographic image of the internal lumen of the lacrimal drainage apparatus after injection of radiopaque dye into the canaliculi. This test is especially useful in demonstrating masses within the passageway (Figure 9-10). CT is indicated when the history and physical examination suggest a neoplastic process. This modality provides greater bony detail than MRI (see Chapter 2). If it confirms the presence of a mass, an incisional or excisional biopsy is usually indicated.

Treatment of Acquired Disorders

While most lacrimal drainage disorders do not require emergent care, the physician evaluating an adult with tearing should be familiar with available treatments. Management of an obstructive disorder is based on the level of obstruction. Unlike congenital NLDO, primary acquired NLDO in adults is rarely responsive to nasolacrimal probing. If a lower nasolacrimal duct obstruction is present, the treatment of choice is a dacryocystorhinostomy. As the name suggests, this is a procedure to anastomose the tear sac with the nasal mucosa after removal of the intervening bone. A stent can be placed within the newly created osteum to prevent closure during healing; silicone tubing (intu-

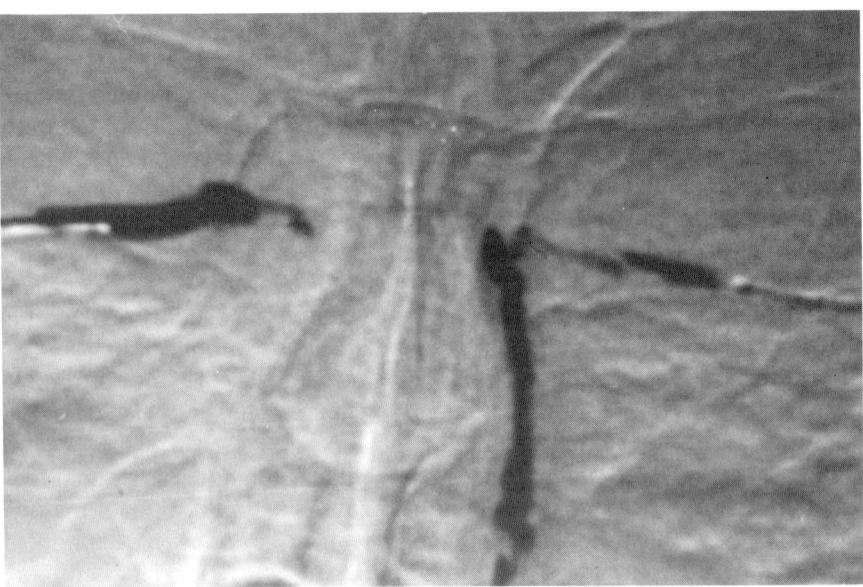

FIGURE 9-10. Dacryocystogram indicating right lacrimal obstruction near the common canaliculus (digital subtraction technique). The left system is patent.

bation) is convenient for this purpose. The success rate of this procedure is approximately 95% for primary acquired NLDO.

With the exception of punctal stenosis, which can usually be treated simply with a 2 mm vertical snip incision, proximal obstructions are more difficult to treat. Focal canalicular obstructions can be treated by dilation or localized excision, with reanastomosis of the canaliculi by silicone intubation. The tubing is left in place for a minimum of 3 months to prevent recurrent stenosis. Diffuse or total canalicular obstruction requires a conjunctivodacryocystorhinostomy with placement of a Jones Pyrex glass tube. This acts as a direct conduit for tear drainage from the medial aspect of the eye to the nose.

LACRIMAL DRAINAGE SYSTEM INFECTIONS

Acute dacryocystitis (a fulminant infection of the lacrimal sac) requires urgent treatment because it can rapidly progress to preseptal cellulitis, orbital cellulitis, or sepsis (Figure 9–11). This is especially true in neonates and immunocompromised patients.

The first step is to differentiate acute from chronic dacryocystitis. The latter results when exudate can reflux through the canaliculi. Its mild inflammation can smolder for months with minimal symptoms. In contrast, acute dacryocystitis results when pathologic organisms are trapped within the closed space of the lacrimal sac. Acute infection progresses over hours to days, with worsening lacrimal sac distention, erythema, and pain. Healthy adults are usually not systemically ill early on, but their while blood cell count may be elevated. Infants or immunocompromised patients, however, may rapidly develop sepsis with fever, chills, malaise, and tachycardia. Eventually the lacrimal sac swells and may burst, usually draining through the skin. Infrequently, infection can spread into the orbit or sinuses.

The organisms that most frequently cause acute dacryocystitis are *Staphylococcus* (*aureus* and *epidermidis* species), and less commonly *Streptococcus* (including *pneumococcus* and alpha and beta hemolytic species). *Haemophilus influenza,* though relatively uncommon, should be considered in infants and young children. Several other types of bacteria, and rarely fungi, have also been reported. Although they occur only rarely, they accentuate the importance of obtaining cultures with sensitivities.

The treatment of acute dacryocystitis involves the use of oral or intravenous systemic antibiotics based on the age, immunologic competence, and clinical status of the patient. The initial therapy is empiric; modifications are based on Gram's stain and culture/sensitivity testing. Immunocompetent patients without signs of orbital involvement can be managed on an outpatient basis with oral antibiotics such as dicloxicillin (adults: 500 mg every 6 hours; children: 50 mg/kg per day divided every 6 hours) or a cephalosporin such as cephalexin

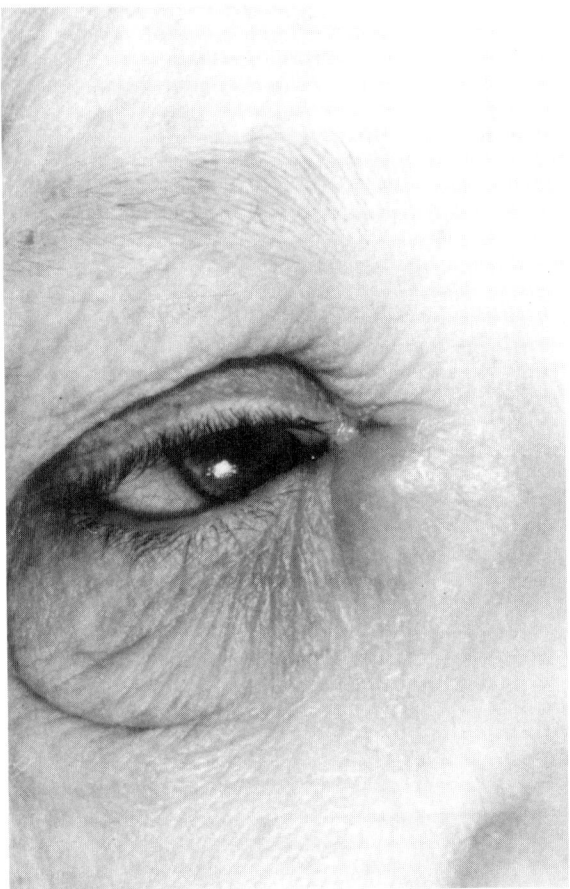

FIGURE 9-11. Acute dacryocystitis.

(Keflex, adults: 500 mg every 6 hours; children: 40 mg/kg per day divided every 6 hours) or cefaclor (Ceclor, adults: 500 mg every 8 hours; children: 40 mg/kg per day divided every 8 hours), which has better *H. influenza* coverage. Neonates and patients with signs of orbital involvement, sepsis, or immune deficiency should be admitted to the hospital and treated with intravenous antibiotics after obtaining cultures (usually by percutaneous aspiration or incision of the lacrimal sac). Although several antibiotics or combinations are appropriate, most of these patients can be successfully treated with intravenous cefuroxime (Zinacef), a second-generation cephalosporine that covers most of the pathogens causing acute dacryocystitis, including *H. influenza*. The dose in adults is 750 mg to 1.5 g every 8 hours; in children, the dose is 50 to 100 mg/kg per day divided every 8 hours (see also Chapters 16 and 17).

Percutaneous drainage is recommended when the lacrimal sac is markedly inflamed or distended to obtain material for Gram's stain and culture and to decrease the microbial load, as well as to relieve pain. Drainage can be accomplished by making a single incision with a number 11 Bard-Parker blade. The depth of the incision need not be more than 5 mm. A percutaneous incision of this type combined with antibiotic therapy rarely, if ever, creates a permanent fistula. Following resolution of acute dacryocystitis, evaluation of the lacrimal system usually confirms NLDO. Because of the risk of recurrence, lacrimal drainage surgery is indicated.

THE DRY EYE SYNDROME

A brief overview of the management of dry eye syndrome (keratoconjunctivitis sicca) is appropriate because epiphora is frequently due to reflex tear secretion secondary to aqueous tear insufficiency. The causes of dry eye are numerous and beyond the scope of this chapter. While keratoconjunctivitis sicca occurs with systemic autoimmune or collagen vascular diseases (e.g., Sjögren's syndrome), the vast majority of dry eye patients suffer from "essential" dry eye related to decreased tear production. Management of dry eye is based on the severity of the condition. Mild symptoms can be treated with topical lubricating artificial tears (e.g., Refresh, Hypotears, Tears Plus, Celluvisc). Preservative-free solutions (Refresh) are recommended for patients with known hypersensitivity to a preservative or those who require very frequent applications.

Severe dry eye syndrome may require more frequent artificial tears or lubricating ointment (Refresh PM) during the daytime and lubrication combined with patching at night. An artificial tear insert (Lacrisert) may be helpful, as may 10% to 20% acetylcysteine drops (Mucomyst) if mucous filaments are bothersome. If medical therapy alone is insufficient or unduly inconvenient, the puncta can be occluded to conserve available tears. Commercially available collagen inserts or silicone plugs can be used on a temporary basis. In this way, a patient's response to occlusion can be assessed to ensure that it will not result in a "too wet" state. Silicone plugs can be left in place indefinitely unless they begin to cause ocular irritation. The simplest and most effective method of permanent occlusion is thermal cautery using a hand-held unit. While some clinicians advocate the use of a laser for this purpose, this has not been shown to be more efficacious and is certainly not cost-effective. The majority of patients with mild to moderately severe dry eye can be managed with a combination of these methods.

SUMMARY

Tearing (epiphora) is a frequent ophthalmic complaint. Ophthalmologists, as well as primary care and emergency room physicians, should be aware of the variety of conditions causing this complaint. The history and physical examination will separate nonobstructive from obstructive lacrimal disorders, and appropriate treatment can then be recommended. Acute dacryocystitis or fulminant infection of the lacrimal sac is a true medical emergency requiring prompt treatment, particularly in neonates, immunocompromised patients, and patients with signs of orbital involvement or sepsis.

REFERENCES

Baker JD: Treatment of congenital nasolacrimal system obstruction. *J Pediatr Ophthalmol Strabismus* 22:34, 1985.
Busse H, Muller KM, Kroll P: Radiologic and histologic findings of the lacrimal passages of newborns. *Arch Ophthalmol* 9:528, 1980.
Carlin R, Henderson JW: Malignant lymphoma of the nasolacrimal sac. *Am J Ophthalmol* 78:511, 1974.
Chavis RM, Welham AN, Maisey MN: Quantitative lacrimal scintillography. *Arch Ophthalmol* 96:2066, 1978.
Cole JG, Brackup A, Hanley JS, Higgins GK: Pseudotumor of the lacrimal sac. *Am J Ophthalmol* 55:136, 1963.
Doane MG: Blinking and the mechanics of the lacrimal drainage system. *Ophthalmology* 88:844, 1981.
Dortzbach RK, France TD, Kushner BJ, Gonnering RS: Silicone intubation for obstruction of the nasolacrimal duct in children. *Am J Ophthalmol* 94:585, 1982.
Doxanas M, Anderson RL: *Clinical Orbital Anatomy.* Baltimore, Williams & Wilkins, 1984, pp 89–107.
Dressner SA, Klussman K, Meyer DR, Linberg JV: Outpatient dacryocystorhinostomy. *Ophthalmic Surg* 22:1–3, 1991.
Duke-Elder S: Normal and abnormal development. Part 2. Congenital deformities. In Duke-Elder S (ed): *System of Ophthalmology.* St. Louis, CV Mosby, 1963, 3:911–940.
Duke-Elder S, Cook C: Normal and abnormal development. Part 1. Embryology. In Duke-Elder S (ed): *System of Ophthalmology.* St. Louis, CV Mosby, 1963, 3:241–245.
Durso F, Hand SI Jr, Ellis FD, Helveston EM: Silicone intubation in children with nasolacrimal obstruction. *J Pediatr Ophthalmol Strabismus* 17:389, 1980.
Ghose S, Mahajan VM: Microbiology of congenital dacryocystitis—its clinical significance. *J Ocul Ther Surg* 4:54, 1985.
Harris GJ, Williams GA, Clarke GP: Sarcoidosis of the lacrimal sac. *Arch Ophthalmol* 99:1198, 1981.
Haynes BF, Fishman ML, Fauci AS, Wolff SM: The ocular manifestations of Wegener's granulomatosis: Fifteen years' experience and review of the literature. *Am J Med* 63:131, 1977.
Hurwitz JJ, Maisey MN, Welham RAN: Quantitative lacrimal scintillography. I. Method and physiologic application. *Br J Ophthalmol* 59:308, 1975.
Jones LT: An anatomical approach to problems of the eyelids and lacrimal apparatus. *Arch Ophthalmol* 66:111, 1961.
Jones LT: The lacrimal tear system and its treatment. *Am J Ophthalmol* 62:47, 1966.
Jones LT, Wobig JL: *Surgery of the Eyelids and Lacrimal System.* Birmingham, AL, Aesculapius, 1976.
Katowitz JA, Welsh MG: Timing of initial probing and irrigation in congenital nasolacrimal duct obstruction. *Ophthalmology* 94:698, 1987.
Linberg JV, McCormick SA: Primary acquired nasolacrimal duct obstruction: A clinicopathologic report and biopsy technique. *Ophthalmology* 93:1055, 1986.
McCormick SA, Linberg JV: The pathology of nasolacrimal duct obstruction: Clinicopathologic correlates of lacrimal excreting system disease. In Linberg JV (ed): *Lacrimal Surgery.* New York, Churchill Livingston, 1988.
Maurice DM: The dynamics and drainage of tears. *Int Ophthalmol Clin* 13:103, 1973.
Meyer DR, Antonello A, Linberg JV: Assessment of tear drainage after canalicular obstruction using fluorescein dye disappearance. *Ophthalmology* 97:1370, 1990.

Meyer DR, Linberg JV: Acute dacryocystitis: Diagnosis and management. In: Linberg JV (ed): *Oculoplastic and Orbital Emergencies.* Norwalk, CT, Appleton & Lange, 1989, pp 29–43.

Meyer DR, Wobig JL: Acute dacryocystitis due to *Pasteurella multocida. Am J Ophthalmol* 110:444, 1990.

Milder B, Weil, BA: *The Lacrimal System.* Norwalk, CT, Appleton-Century-Crofts, 1983.

Older SS: Congenital lacrimal disorders and management. In Linberg JV (ed): *Lacrimal Surgery.* New York, Churchill Livingston, 1988, pp 91–108.

Petersen RA, Robb RM: The natural course of congenital obstruction of the nasolacrimal duct. *J Pediatr Ophthalmol Strabismus* 15:246, 1978.

Ryan SJ, Font RL: Primay epithelial neoplasms of the lacrimal sac. *Am J Ophthalmol* 76:73, 1973.

Sood NN, Ratnaraj A, Balarman G, Madhavan HN: Chronic dacryocystitis—a clinico-bacteriological study. *All-India Ophthalmol Soc* 15:107, 1967.

Spaeth EB: Carcinomas and tumors of the lacrimal sac. *Arch Ophthalmol* 57:689, 1952.

Spira R, Mondshine R: Demonstration of nasolacrimal duct carcinoma by computed tomography. *Ophthalmic Plast Reconstr Surg* 2:159, 1986.

Stokes WH: Dacryocystitis in lymphatic leukemia. *Arch Ophthalmol* 20:85, 1938.

Stranc MF: The pattern of lacrimal injuries in nasoethmoid fractures. *Br J Plast Surg* 23:339, 1970.

Warwick R: *Eugene Wolff's Anatomy of the Eye and Orbit.* 7th ed. Philadelphia, WB Saunders, 1976.

Weinstein GS, Biglan AW, Patterson JH: Congenital lacrimal sac mucoceles. *Am J Ophthalmol* 94:106, 1982.

Whitaker LA, Katowitz JA, Randall P: The nasolacrimal apparatus in congenital facial anomalies. *J Maxillofac Surg* 2:59, 1974.

Whitnall SE: *The Anatomy of the Human Orbit and Accessory Organs of Vision.* 2d ed. London, Oxford University Press, 1932.

Zappia RJ, Milder B: Lacrimal drainage function. 1. The Jones fluorescein test. *Am J Ophthalmol* 74:154, 1972.

Zappia RJ, Milder B: Lacrimal drainage function. 2. The fluorescein dye disappearance test. *Am J Ophthalmol* 74:160, 1972.

10

Nonpenetrating, Noninfectious Emergencies of the Cornea and Ocular Lens

Michael W. Belin
Robert A. Catalano

NONPENETRATING, NONINFECTIOUS CORNEAL EMERGENCIES

Inflammatory (Noninfectious) Corneal Ulcers

Inflammatory corneal ulcers occur in a wide variety of settings (Table 10-1). They share a common clinical presentation of progressive stromal thinning associated with an epithelial defect (Figure 10-1). The pathogenesis of stromal ulceration was reviewed in the discussion of chemical burns (Chapter 7). As with burns, stromal ulceration due to inflammation rarely occurs when the epithelial layer is intact, and progressive ulceration usually arrests if the epithelial surface can be made contiguous. Therefore, reestablishment of the ocular surface is the primary goal in treating inflammatory corneal ulcers.

TABLE 10-1. DIFFERENTIAL OF NONINFECTED CORNEAL ULCERS

Chemical injuries
Collagen vascular disease (e.g., rheumatoid arthritis)
Dry eyes (keratitis sicca)
Exophthalmos (e.g., thyroid disorder)
Herpes zoster
Keratomalacia
Lid dysfunction (ectropion, entropion, seventh nerve palsy)
Mooren's ulcer
Neurotrophic cornea
Ocular cicatricial pemphigoid
Post–herpes simplex
Postsurgical, nonhealing epithelial defect
Radiation
Rosacea
Stevens-Johnson syndrome
Toxic

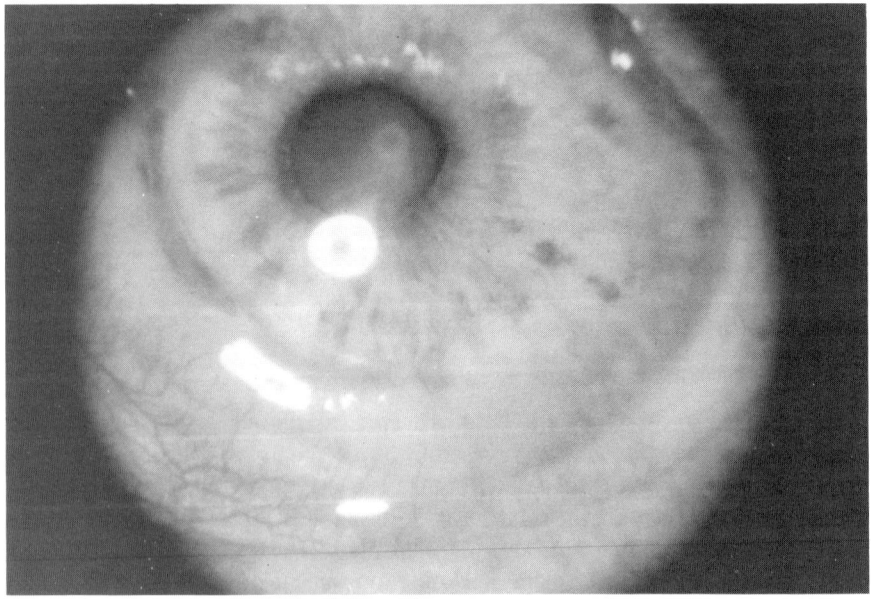

FIGURE 10-1. Noninfected peripheral corneal melt in a patient with long-standing rheumatoid arthritis.

Treatment modalities vary depending on the etiology of the inflammatory ulcer, but several guidelines are useful:

Rule out infection. Before treating an "inflammatory, noninfected" corneal ulcer, active infection must be ruled out. So-called nonvirulent bacteria or partially treated infections may have atypical presentations. If doubt exists, corneal scraping and culture are recommended.

Discontinue toxic medications. Many noninfected corneal ulcers develop secondary to drug toxicity from long-term "shotgun therapy." Discontinuing all potentially toxic topical agents is often efficacious. Close observation during the wash-out period, however, is required.

Ensure adequate lubrication. Nonpreserved artificial tears (e.g., Refresh) and ointments (e.g., Refresh PM) should be used frequently (every 1 hour to 2 hours while awake and several times during the night). In severely tear-deficient eyes, punctal occlusion (either permanent or temporary) prolongs tear retention (see Chapter 9).

Restore the lid anatomy. A well-positioned lid margin is a prerequisite for proper corneal wetting. If a lid abnormality exists (e.g., ectropion, entropion, trichiasis), it should be repaired. At times, a temporary tarsorrhaphy promotes epithelial healing.

Use bandage contact lenses. A therapeutic soft lens or a dissolvable collagen lens may offer adequate protection to the ingrowing epithelium and promote closure of an epithelial defect. Relatively nontoxic antibiotics can be added prophylactically (e.g., Polytrim or Chloroptic, four times per day).

Control of inflammation. Inflammatory mediators are a major source of collagenolytic activity. Control of the inflammatory response is necessary to suppress ulceration and can be achieved with topical steroids. When steroids are used, frequent observation is mandatory because they can potentiate an unrecognized infectious process. If the ulcer is peripheral in location, conjunctival resection is strongly recommended because it eliminates the source of many of the inflammatory cells (e.g., polymorphonucleocytes). This technically easy procedure can often be performed under topical anesthesia. Conjunctival resection also avoids the potential problems associated with topical steroids.

Specific therapy is based on the underlying pathogenesis of the "noninfected" ulcer. Examples of specific adjunctive therapy include the following:

Collagen vascular disease: Systemic steroids and immunosuppression.
Thyroid orbitopathy: Evaluation and treatment for thyroid disease (see Chapter 12).
Keratomalacia: Nutritional support.
Ocular cicatricial pemphigoid: Systemic immunosuppression.
Rosacea: Systemic tetracycline or erythromycin 250 mg 4 times per day or metronidiazole 0.75% topical gel every 12 hours for 3 weeks to 6 weeks, and lid hygiene.

Descemetocele

A number of noninfectious conditions lead to stromal thinning. If the process is progressive or the treatment delayed or ineffective, the ulcer may progress to loss of the entire corneal stroma. This condition, in which only the underlying Descemet's membrane and endothelium remain, is called a *descemetocele*. A descemetocele may be stable for a long period of time because the inflammatory process that led to the loss of stroma rarely involves Descemet's membrane. A descemetocele, however, is an ominous sign. Its presence should raise the suspicion that the initial treatment was inadequate or inappropriate. A careful review of the diagnosis and vigorous treatment of the underlying condition should be instituted.

Regardless of the cause, a cornea with a descemetocele requires structural support to facilitate stromal growth and prevent a corneal perforation. A number of steps can be taken.

The placement of a tight-fitting soft contact lens provides structural support and protects the ingrowing epithelium and stroma.

A conjunctival (Gundersen) flap provides a new nutrient vascular supply. It should not be performed, however, if the diagnosis is uncertain. Flaps are contraindicated if the descemetocele is filtering or if an infectious etiology is possible. The presence of a flap makes it difficult, if not impossible, to observe the disease process in the cornea. In addition, both the optical and cosmetic results of a conjunctival flap are poor (Figure 10–2).

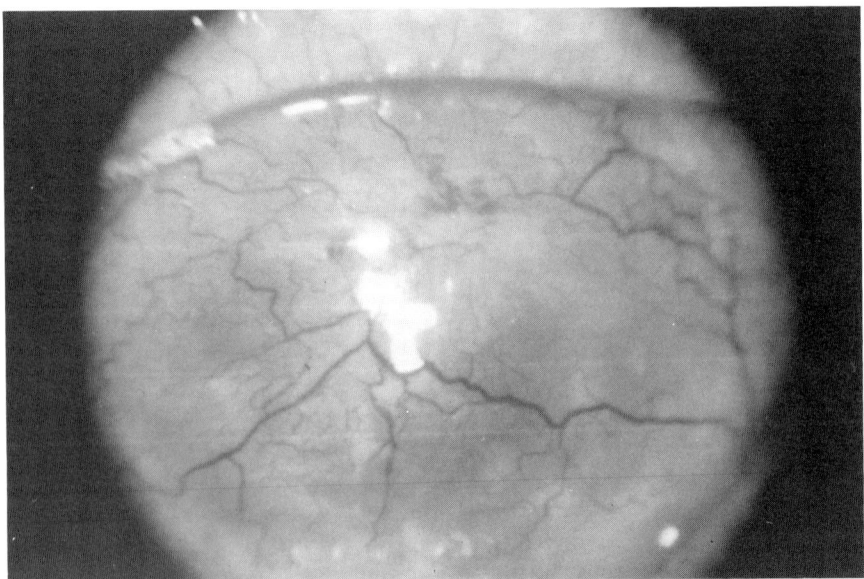

FIGURE 10–2. Conjunctival (Gundersen) flap.

The blowout patch technique consists of creating a small, usually lamellar bed around the thinned cornea, cleaning the necrotic tissue from the bed, and suturing a piece of donor stroma or sclera into the prepared bed. Fresh tissue is not needed, and glycerin-preserved corneal or scleral tissue can be used. In addition, lyophilized, cryolathed lamellar corneal tissue (Kerato-patch) is made for this procedure. If these materials are not available, autologous Tenon's capsule may be substituted.

There are many instances when surgical intervention (e.g., blowout patch graft) should be avoided. The surgical prognosis is especially poor when the descemetocele is associated with a stromal melting disorder (e.g., rheumatoid arthritis, progressive peripheral degeneration) or a disease that heals poorly (e.g., rosacea, collagen-vascular diseases). In these cases, the application of an adhesive may be more efficacious. The technique for applying an adhesive is relatively simple; it can be done in the office or clinic under slit lamp control.

The adhesives currently being used for ophthalmic purposes are members of the cyanoacrylate family, supplied as clear liquids. When they polymerize, or change into their adhesive state, they become opaque granular solids (Figure 10-3). The particles that make the adhesive polymerize are free anions, which are always available in tissue fluids. Polymerization is rapid (seconds to minutes), without a significant exothermic or endothermic reaction. Other advantages of these adhesives are that they require no catalyst, firmly bond to tissue, and break down very slowly.

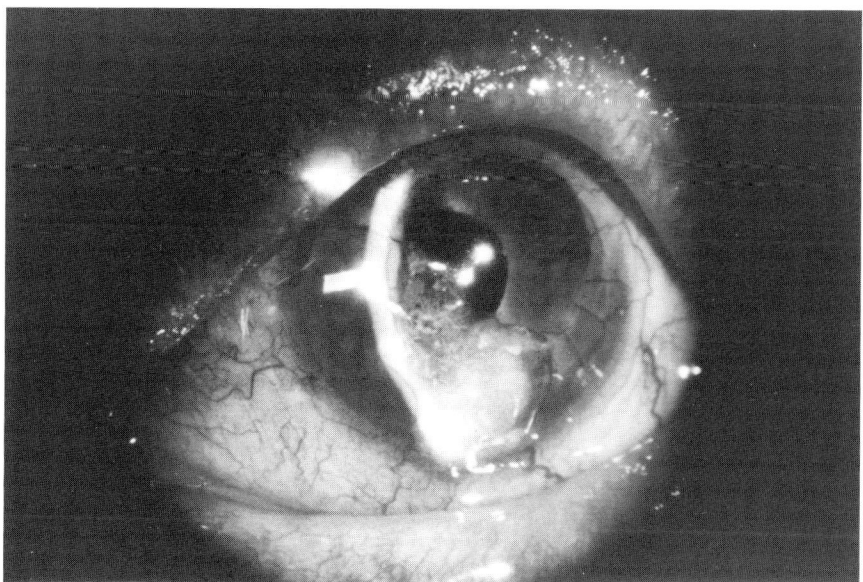

FIGURE 10-3. Midperipheral corneal perforation sealed with the application of cyanoacrylate adhesive.

The application technique is crucial to the success or failure of an adhesive. Prior to its application, all epithelium and necrotic tissue must be removed to provide a stable base for firm adhesion. The following specific situations lead to unsatisfactory results: the ulcer bed is too large (greater than 3.0 mm), or necrotic tissue or conjunctiva is adjacent to the perforation site (poor adhesion). The adhesive promotes vascularization but leaves an irregular surface that needs to be covered with a bandage contact lens. It will usually dislodge with time but may have to be removed if excessive corneal vascularization results.

Disorders Associated with the Use of Contact Lenses

Prior to the popularity of soft lenses and the advent of gas permeable lenses, the major disorder associated with contact lens wear was corneal hypoxia, due to the oxygen impermeability of hard lenses. With hard lenses, corneal oxygenation is dependent on an adequate exchange of tears beneath the lens. Lenses that were too tight (prohibiting movement) or too flat (prohibiting tear exchange) or were worn for too long a period resulted in corneal hypoxia. The hypoxia precipitated epithelial damage, leading to corneal epithelial erosions or abrasions, the so-called *contact lens overwear syndrome*. Treatment consisted of removing the lens, treating the abrasion, and refitting the contact or decreasing wearing time. Soft lenses and highly permeable rigid lenses have made this complication much less frequent, as evidenced by the number of patients who tolerate extended-wear contact lenses.

Soft contact lenses are more likely to cause allergic reactions, corneal vascularization, and serious corneal infections. These lenses are made of a hydrogel (water-containing) plastic and need to be cleaned and disinfected regularly. The materials used for these purposes can cause ocular sensitivity. When this occurs, the patient should be advised to use hydrogen peroxide disinfection and nonpreserved unit dose saline (e.g., Refresh). The use of disposable contact lenses can eliminate the need for these chemicals. Soft lenses can also cause a superior corneal pannus, an abnormal growth of blood vessels into previously clear cornea. While a small amount of growth (less than 2 mm) is well tolerated, larger amounts demand discontinuation of the lens (Figure 10–4). The vascular ingrowth is probably secondary to limbal hypoxia from the thicker peripheral part of the lens.

The most dangerous complication of soft contact lens use is the development of a corneal ulcer, which can be vision threatening. The incidence of corneal ulcers in contact lens wearers is significantly greater than the general population, and the incidence with extended-wear lenses is 7 to 10 times greater than with daily wear lenses. For this reason, a number of eye care practitioners no longer recommend extended-wear lenses for cosmetic purposes.

A corneal ulcer should be suspected in any soft lens wearer with a painful red

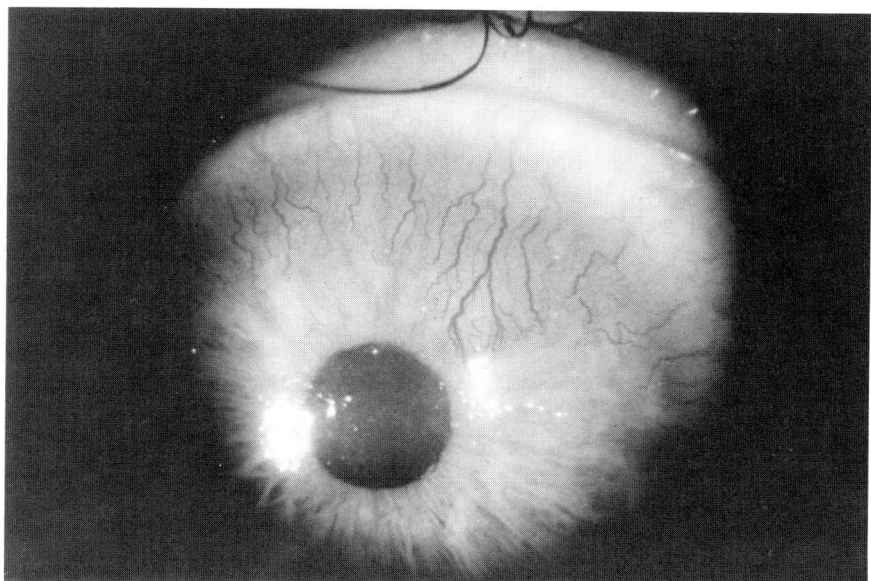

FIGURE 10–4. Extensive superior pannus (vascularization) in a soft contact lens wearer.

eye. On slit lamp examination, loss of corneal clarity, breakdown of the corneal epithelium, and surrounding cellular infiltrate can be appreciated (Figure 10–5). A rare and grave corneal infection associated with the use of nonsterile saline is caused by Acanthamoeba (see Chapter 16). While gas-permeable lenses are more time-consuming to fit, they can be as comfortable as soft lenses and appear to have fewer complications. In particular, they are less commonly associated with serious corneal infections.

Trauma to the cornea can occur with insertion or removal of any contact lens, and a foreign body can lodge under any lens. The abrasions these cause can be seen with the magnification of the slit lamp. They often become more apparent to the patient after removal of the lens because, while still in the eye, the lens bandages the corneal epithelium. Treatment consists of removing any foreign body and treating the corneal abrasion. The contact lens should be carefully examined to ensure that it has not been damaged before returning it to the patient, who should be instructed to clean and disinfect the lens prior to reinsertion.

Recurrent Corneal Erosions

A corneal abrasion is a painful loss of the corneal epithelium. The loss of the protective epithelium exposes the underlying basement membrane and sensitive nerve endings. The vast majority of corneal abrasions are traumatic in ori-

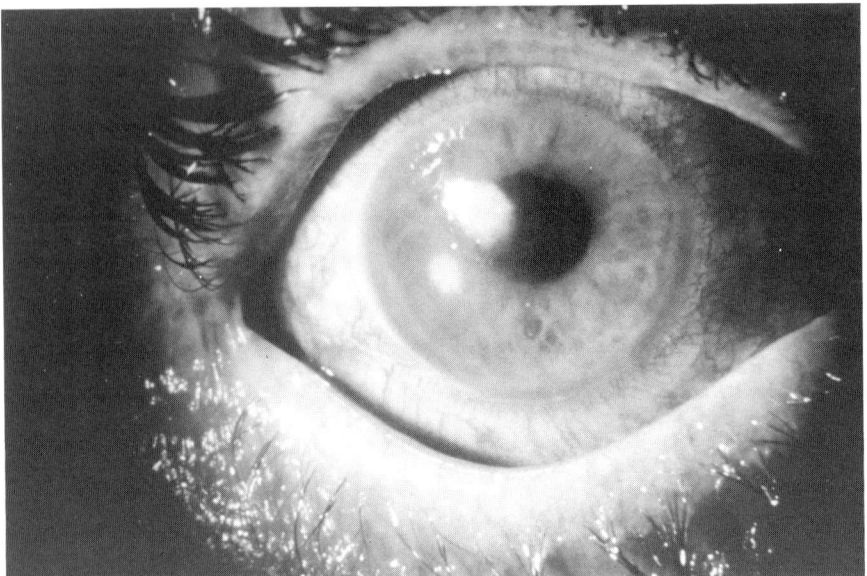

FIGURE 10-5. Pseudomonas corneal ulcer in a soft contact lens wearer.

gin. A group of patients exists, however, with either poor adhesion of the corneal epithelium to the underlying basement membrane or an inability to reform normal epithelial/basement membrane adhesions once these are disrupted. These patients are subject to painful recurring corneal abrasions that require a prolonged healing period. This condition is called *recurrent corneal erosions.*

Approximately 50% of patients with recurrent corneal erosions have evidence of map-dot-fingerprint corneal dystrophy (anterior membrane dystrophy), the result of an abnormality in epithelial turnover, maturation, and the production of basement membrane. Three types of lesions are seen within the epithelium and its immediately subjacent basement membrane: fingerprint lines, map lines, and dots or microcysts (Figure 10-6). These abnormalities occur in varying combinations and change in number and distribution from time to time. They are best seen at the slit lamp using sclerotic scatter, retroillumination, or a broad tangential beam (see Chapter 1). Fingerprint lines are thin, relucent, hairlike lines, often clumped in a concentric pattern resembling fingerprints. Map lines are thicker than fingerprint lines, more irregular, and surrounded by a faint haze. Dots are intraepithelial spaces containing the debris of epithelial cells that have collapsed and degenerated before reaching the epithelial surface. They are gray-white and have discrete edges. While 50% of patients with recurrent erosions have evidence of this dystrophy, only 10% of patients with map-dot-fingerprint dystrophy have symptoms of recurrent erosions.

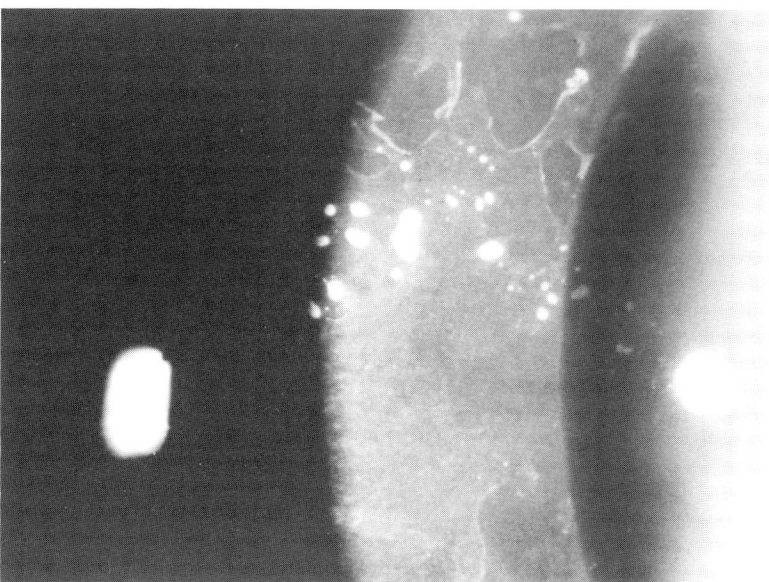

FIGURE 10-6. Map-dot-fingerprint corneal dystrophy. This patient's cornea exhibits dots, the light, small, sharply defined opacities, and maps, which are lighter, larger, and more diffuse.

The treatment of recurrent corneal erosions is directed at relieving pain, promoting epithelial healing, and preventing recurrences. The initial treatment is similar to that of any corneal abrasion, with semipressure patching and lid taping, or the frequent application of antibiotic ointment (e.g., erythromycin). Pain can often be relieved with cycloplegia (e.g., cyclopentolate 1% or scopolamine 0.25% three times per day) and/or systemic nonsteroidals. Patching may need to be continued for a number of days. If the abrasion heals quickly, daytime lubrication with artificial tears is recommended in addition to the application of 5% sodium chloride (hypertonic) ointment at bedtime. Hypertonic ointment acts to dehydrate the epithelium, allowing for better adhesion. If epithelial repopulation is slow or if the erosion has not healed in a few days, the loose epithelium should be debrided. Debridement can also be performed initially if the epithelium is extremely loose. If the eye does not subsequently heal with patching, a bandage contact lens (soft hydrogel contact lens) may be placed. This may not offer any healing advantage over patching, but it does allow the use of the eye and avoids long-term patching. Recently, dissolvable collagen lenses have become available. Their use is limited to short-term treatment in the acute period. Once a bandage lens has been used, it should be left in place for at least 3 months. The contact lens acts as a protective covering and allows the epithelium to heal and form adhesions to the underlying basement layer. After 3 months, the lens is usually discontinued, and artificial tears and bedtime ointment are used.

In recalcitrant cases, anterior stromal puncture of the epithelium may be employed using a 27-gauge or 30-gauge needle. Multiple small punctures disturb Bowman's layer, thereby promoting a tighter adhesion and stimulating the cornea to produce functional basement membrane complexes. Although recurrent corneal erosions may cause a great deal of pain and loss of work, they rarely lead to any loss of vision. If complications arise, they are usually from secondary infection. In the majority of patients, the frequency and severity of the recurrences appear to lessen with time.

Superficial Punctate Keratopathy

Superficial punctate keratopathy is a nonspecific sign, common to many disorders (Table 10–2). Patients present with mild pain, photophobia, and foreign body sensation. Examination reveals mild injection of the conjunctiva and pinpoint (punctate) staining of the cornea with fluorescein dye. The location of the staining can be helpful diagnostically. Involvement of the lower one-third of the cornea occurs with exposure keratopathy, ocular rosacea (Figure 10–7), chronic staphylococcal blepharitis, and toxic keratitis. Superior corneal involvement suggests superior limbic or vernal keratoconjunctivitis; central involvement suggests exposure keratopathy. A random distribution is consistent with Thygeson's keratitis, acute staphylococcal blepharitis, and adenovirus (epidemic keratoconjunctivitis).

The treatment of superficial punctate keratopathy is dependent on the etiology. The most common bacterial pathogen is staphylococcus. It is treated with topical antibiotics (erythromycin ointment 3 times per day or sulfacetamide drops 4 times per day). If corneal infiltrates are present, an antibiotic/steroid combination can be used (e.g., Blephamide, Vasocidin). Vernal keratoconjunctivitis without a "shield" ulcer is managed with cromolyn sodium 4% 4 times per day. Vernal patients with corneal ulcers also require a topical antibiotic (e.g., sulfacetamide 4 times per day, or erythromycin 3 times per day), a topical steroid (e.g., fluoromethalone [FML] or prednisolone acetate [Pred Forte] 1% 4 to 6 times per day), and a cycloplegic agent (e.g., cyclogel 1% 3 times per day). Contact lens wearers should temporarily discontinue use of their lens, and those with a great number of erosions should be placed on a prophylactic antibiotic (e.g., gentamicin or tobramycin, 4 times per day). The treatment for rosacea is detailed above, and the remaining disorders are treated supportively with nonpreserved artificial tears (e.g., Refresh) and lubricating ointments (Refresh PM, Lacrilube).

Filamentary Keratopathy

Filamentary keratopathy is characterized by moderate to severe ocular pain, foreign body sensation, conjunctival injection, photophobia, and the presence

TABLE 10-2. DIFFERENTIAL OF SUPERFICIAL PUNCTATE KERATOPATHY

CONDITION	COMMENT
Dry eye syndrome	Most common cause; decreased tear lake (< 1 mm), or tear film breakup time (< 10 seconds)
Exposure keratopathy	Inadequate or infrequent blinking, incomplete closure of the eyelids
Toxic keratopathy	Aminoglycoside antibiotics; topical beta-blockers; preservatives in many drops, including artificial tears
Radiation keratopathy	Arc weld (ultraviolet) and sunlamp burns
Chemical injury	Acid or alkali
Contact lens disorder	Overwear syndrome; giant papillary conjunctivitis; sensitivity from cleansers, disinfectants, or lubricants
Blepharitis	Squamous (eyelid crusting), staphylococcal (associated with punctate erosions and marginal infiltrates, which can ulcerate)
Viral infection	Adenovirus, herpes simplex, herpes zoster, molluscum contagiosum, varicella, measles
Chlamydial infection	Trachoma, adult inclusion conjunctivitis
Ocular rosacea	Chronic, acnelike disease of the nose, cheeks, and forehead; females > males; ages 30–50. Erythema telangectasia, papules, and pustules but no comedones; rhinophyma (thickening of the skin of the nose), recurrent chalazia, chronic blepharitis, conjunctivitis, and inferior corneal pannus
Superior limbic keratoconjunctivitis	Bilateral chronic keratinization of the superior bulbar conjunctiva, with papillae on the superior palpebral conjunctiva; females > males; 25% have hypothyroidism
Thygeson's keratitis	Bilateral and chronic; quiet-appearing eye without conjunctival injection
Vernal	Bilateral, chronic and recurrent, papillary reaction of superior tarsal conjunctiva; gelatinous elevations at the limbus; pseudomembrane and tenacious, sticky discharge; superior "shield" corneal ulcer with heaped-up margins; prominent itching
Trauma	Chronic eye rubbing

of short strands of epithelial and mucous cells attached to the anterior surface of the cornea (Figure 10-8). It is most commonly a complication of the dry eye syndrome but can also accompany superior limbic keratoconjunctivitis, recurrent corneal erosions, and prolonged ocular patching. Treatment consists of debridement of the filaments with a cotton-tipped applicator (after applying a topical anesthetic), and lubrication with a nonpreserved artificial tear (e.g., Refresh) every 1 hour to 2 hours during the day, and ointment (e.g., Refresh PM) at night. Hypertonic sodium chloride 5% drops and ointment and

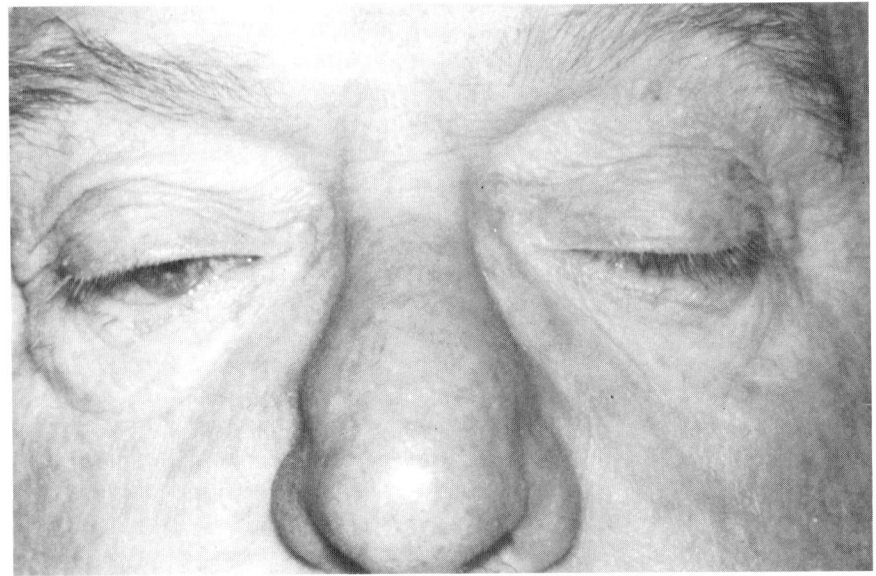

FIGURE 10-7. Rosacea.

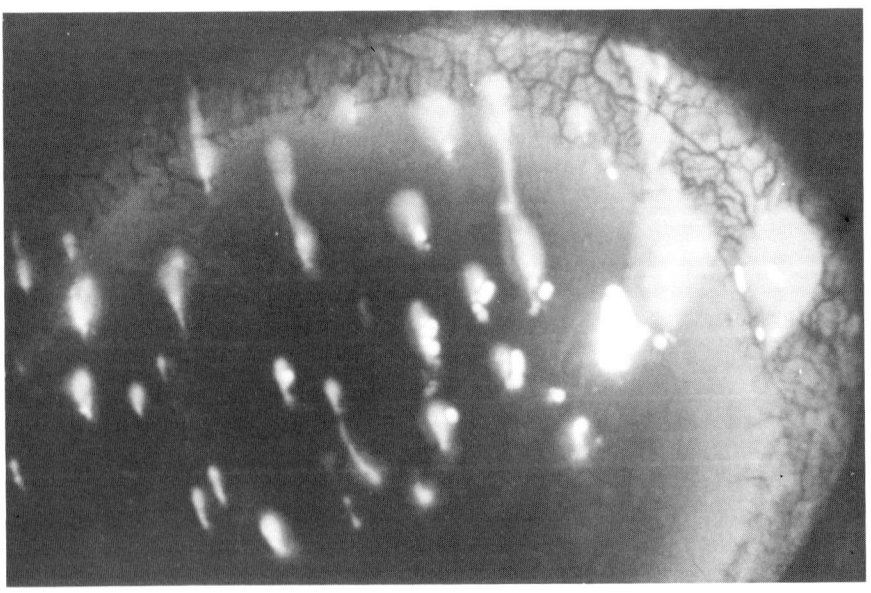

FIGURE 10-8. Filamentary keratopathy.

acetylcysteine 10% to 20% (Mucomyst), 4 times per day, can be added for severe cases. Except in patients with severe dry eyes, an extended-wear contact lens may also be efficacious.

Exposure Keratopathy

Exposure keratopathy results from inadequate or infrequent blinking or an inability to close the eyelids completely. Inadequate closure is a complication of thyroid ophthalmopathy, facial nerve palsy, blepharoptosis surgery, severe proptosis, and coma. Infrequent closure complicates Parkinson's disease and tardive dyskinesia.

Pain and ciliary injection accompany corneal drying and erosions. Corneal infection, perforation, and visual loss can follow. The treatment is directed at preventing corneal drying. This requires frequent instillation of nonpreserved artificial tears (e.g., Refresh), and lubricating ointments (Refresh PM, Lacrilube). In comatose patients, eyelid taping or a Saran wrap "moisture chamber" is advised (see Figure 4-15). In those with facial nerve paralysis, a temporary tarsorrhaphy, conjunctival flap, or soft contact lens may be indicated.

Neurotrophic Keratopathy

Dysfunction of the trigeminal nerve disrupts the sensory arc of protective ocular reflexes, rendering the cornea highly susceptible to trauma and dessication. The trigeminal nerve may also serve a metabolic role for the cornea.

Neurotrophic ulcers begin as oval epithelial erosions, with gray heaped-up margins, in the inferior cornea (Figure 10-9). Conjunctival injection and intraocular inflammation are common, but because of the trigeminal dysfunction, the patient is without pain. The disorder results subsequent to herpes zoster or simplex infection, or as a complication of trigeminal nerve surgery, irradiation to the eye, or brain stem tumor (particularly acoustic neuromas in individuals with neurofibromatosis). Treatment is similar to exposure keratopathy; infected ulcers require cultures and antibiotics (see Chapters 16 and 17).

Interstitial Keratitis

Interstitial keratitis is a disorder of the first or second decade characterized by pain, tearing, photophobia, conjunctival injection, corneal edema, and corneal stroma vascularization. Inflammatory cells in the anterior chamber and fine keratic precipitates may be present.

The most common cause of interstitial keratitis is congenital syphilis. Other causes include acquired syphilis, tuberculosis, Cogan's syndrome (associated

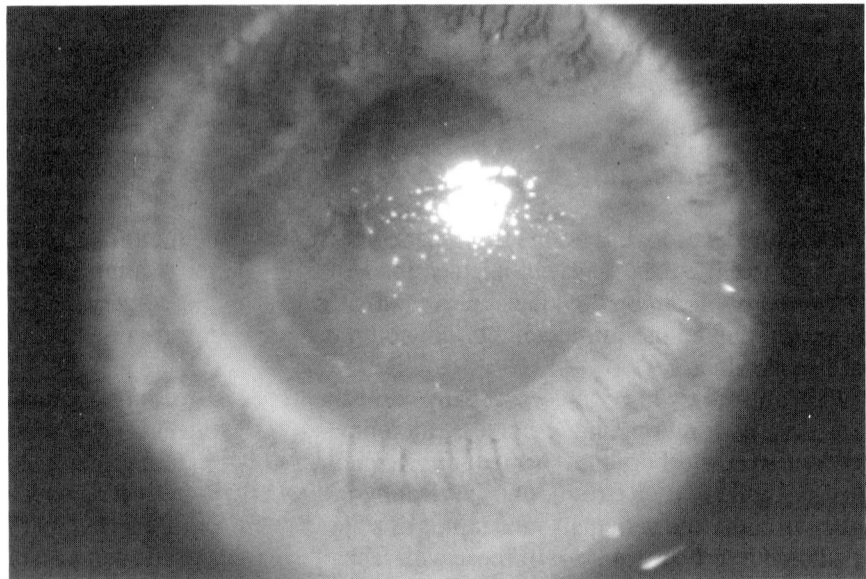

FIGURE 10-9. Neurotrophic keratopathy.

with hearing loss, vertigo, and tinnitus), leprosy, and herpes simplex virus. Syphilitic causes usually result in bilaterality within months to years, whereas tuberculosis is often unilateral and sectoral. Additional signs of congenital syphilis include a saddle nose, bossing of the frontal bones, poor development of the maxilla (Figure 10-10), anterior bowing of the tibias, and "Hutchinson's teeth" deformity of the permanent dentition (widely spaced, centrally notched, upper incisors, tapered like screwdrivers). Individuals with congenital syphilis can also have a "salt and pepper" chorioretinitis, optic atrophy, and a patchy hyperemia of the iris.

In addition to treating the underlying condition, topical steroids (e.g., fluoromethalone or prednisolone acetate 1%) every 1 hour to 6 hours, and cycloplegia (e.g., atropine 1%) 3 times per day are advocated. The workup for syphilis should include an FTA-ABS and VDRL of the cerebrospinal fluid. A chest X ray, and purified protein derivative (PPD) are necessary for undiagnosed tuberculosis.

NONTRAUMATIC EMERGENCIES OF THE OCULAR LENS

Nontraumatic emergencies of the ocular lens can be characterized as abnormalities of location (ectopia lentis), abnormalities in light transmission (pos-

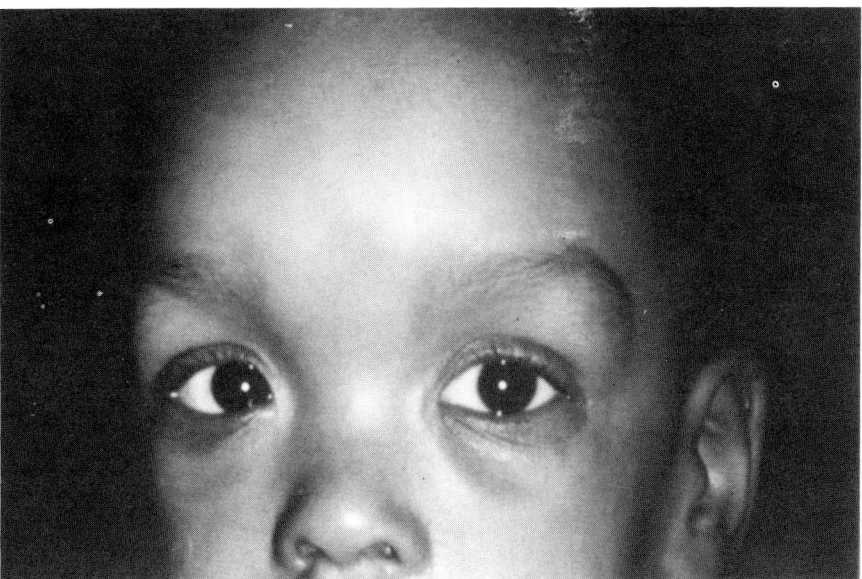

FIGURE 10-10. Facies of congenital syphilis. Note the frontal bossing, saddle nose, and maxillary hypoplasia.

terior subcapsular cataract) or lens-induced glaucoma (phacolytic and phakomorphic).

The normal crystalline lens is an aspherical, transparent, biconvex tissue devoid of blood vessels and nerves. It is supported by the zonular fibers, which originate from the pars plana of the ciliary body and insert on the peripheral anterior lens capsule. The normal lens is composed of approximately one-third lens protein and two-thirds water.

Ectopia Lentis

The normal lens is centered posterior to the iris and anterior to the vitreous face. Its central position enables it to function as a high-quality optical device without significant distortion. Changes in lens position (ectopia lentis) alter this relationship and are accompanied by complaints of decreased or distorted vision. Lenses may be partially dislocated from weakened or stretched zonules (the term *lens subluxation* is commonly used) (Figure 10-11) or totally dislocated due to complete zonular rupture (Figure 10-12). A subluxated lens remains in the pupillary area, while a dislocated lens may migrate anteriorly into the anterior chamber or posteriorly into the vitreous cavity. Signs of ectopia lentis include iridodonesis (a fine movement of the iris with ocular movement), phacodonesis (lens movement noted on ocular movement due to lens

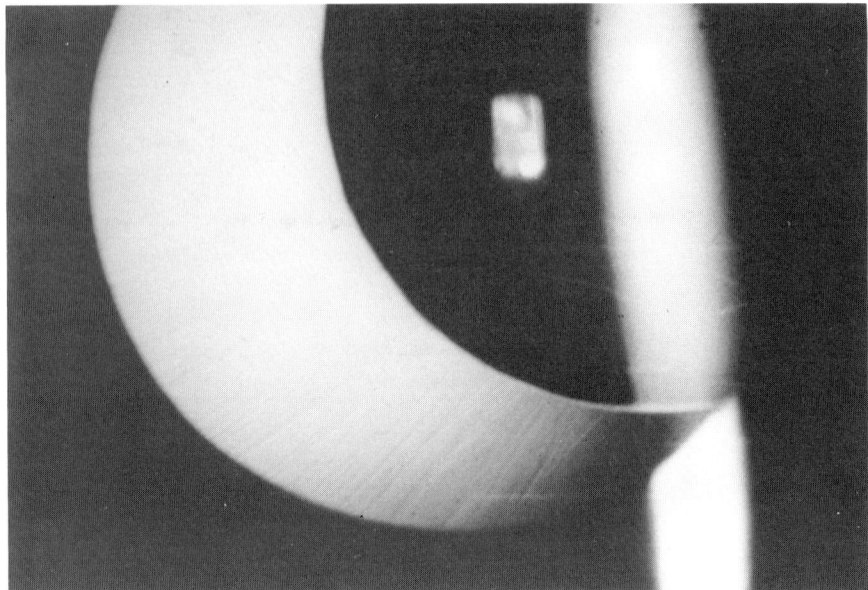

FIGURE 10-11. Partially dislocated (subluxed) ocular lens after ocular trauma.

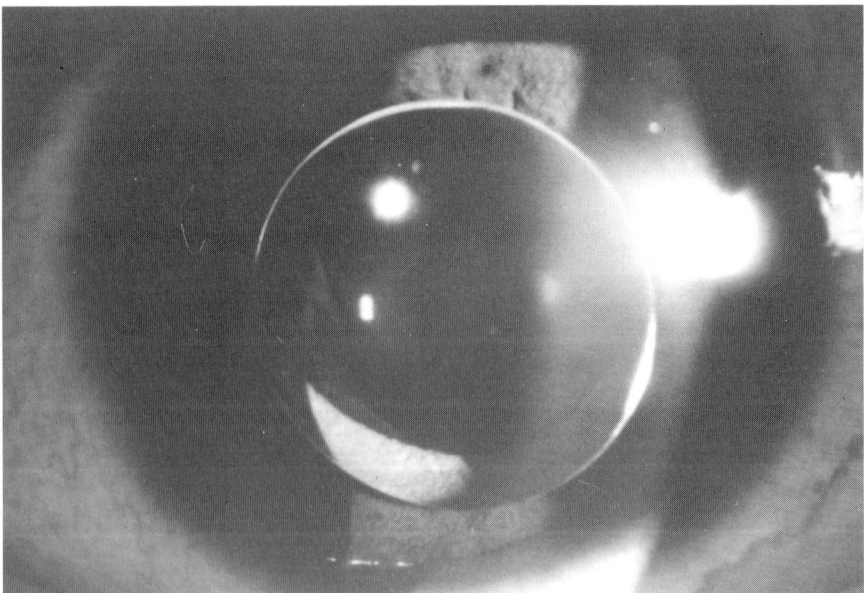

FIGURE 10-12. Complete dislocation of the ocular lens into the anterior chamber of the eye in a patient with Weill-Marchesani syndrome. Note the lens is smaller and more spherical than normal.

instability), noncorneal astigmatism, and the presence of vitreous in the anterior chamber.

Although trauma remains the most common cause of ectopia lentis (see Chapter 6), dislocation can also accompany other ocular abnormalities, particularly in association with a heredofamilial group of systemic syndromes, many of which share skeletal dysplasia as a common feature. Ectopia lentis may also be seen with severe ocular inflammation, aniridia (congenital absence of the visible portion of the iris, Figure 10–13), hypermature cataracts, and buphthalmos secondary to zonular stretching. Associated systemic syndromes include the following:

Marfan's syndrome, a dominantly inherited disorder in which more than 50% of affected individuals develop bilateral lens subluxations and/or dislocations. In these patients, the subluxated lens typically dislocates superiorly and temporally. Other associated abnormalities include joint hyperextensibility, arachnodactyly (slender, long fingers and limbs; Figure 10–14), pectus excavatus, and scoliosis. The most serious abnormalities involve aortic arch dilation and cardiac valve abnormalities, leading to premature death.

Homocystinuria, a group of recessively inherited inborn errors of amino acid metabolism resulting in deficiencies in the metabolism of homocysteine and methionine into cysteine. Other forms are a result of an impaired ability to convert homocysteine to methionine. These enzyme deficiencies lead to an accu-

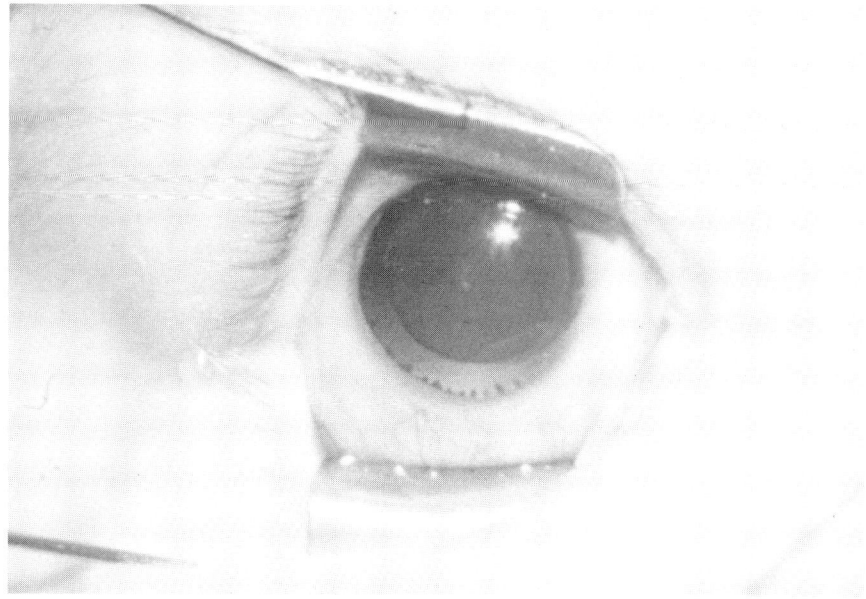

FIGURE 10–13. Aniridia with dislocated lens. (Photograph courtesy of John W. Simon, M.D.)

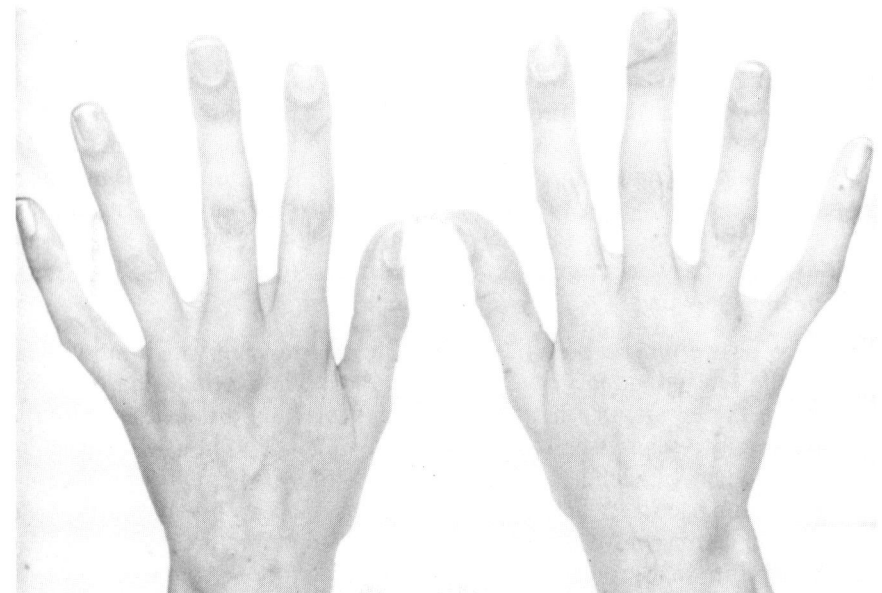

FIGURE 10–14. Long, slender fingers common to Marfan's syndrome.

mulation of methionine and/or homocysteine in both urine and blood. Patients appear tall and thin, similar to Marfan's syndrome. Unlike Marfan's, the lens dislocations tend to be inferior and medial and occur in over 90% of affected persons. There is generalized osteoporosis, and half of the patients have cognitive deficiencies. Death usually occurs secondary to thromboembolic events. Because clinical improvement occasionally follows vitamin supplements (pyridoxine, folate, or cobalamin), urine screening for homocystinuria should be performed in all cases of nontraumatic lens dislocations.

Weill-Marchesani, a syndrome comprised of brachymorphia (short, stocky build and short digits), limited joint mobility, and microspherophakia. In microspherophakia, the lens is increased in the anterior to posterior dimension and decreased in the horizontal dimension, resulting in a more spherical shape. Most patients exhibit high myopia due to the increased refractive power of the lens. The small lens size contributes to the frequency of lens dislocations into the anterior chamber (Figure 10–12).

Other. While much more rare, lens dislocations have also been reported in Ehlers-Danlos syndrome, hyperlysinemia, sulfite oxidase deficiency, and Refsum's syndrome.

Patients with subluxated lenses complain of distorted vision, monocular diplopia, and disabling glare. These symptoms relate to the poor optical quality of the peripheral lens and distortion when the edge of the lens is in the visual axis.

If the lens is tilted, significant lenticular astigmatism results. Occasionally a patient will have better vision with an aphakic correction, through a part of the pupil clear of the dislocated lens. When the subluxation is mild, visual complaints may be minimal. If the lens is totally dislocated into the vitreous cavity, the patient may notice a fluctuating decrease in vision depending on the position of the lens over the macula. A posteriorly dislocated lens may result in a posterior uveitis but more commonly is well tolerated. Anterior dislocations often result in pupillary block glaucoma, causing elevated intraocular pressure, pain, and decreased vision.

Treatment of a dislocated lens is required only if symptoms are visually disabling or if complications develop. If the lens is posteriorly dislocated and lens-induced inflammation develops, a pars plana lensectomy is indicated. An anterior dislocation with pupillary block requires emergent treatment to lower the intraocular pressure. The combined use of beta-blockers, osmotic agents, carbonic anhydrase inhibitors, and alpha agonists (apraclonidine) usually brings the acute pressure elevation under control. Laser iridotomy or surgical iridectomy is required to prevent further attacks. Lens extraction is the definitive treatment. If vitreous is already present in the anterior chamber, a pars plana approach is suggested. If the lens is partially dislocated and exhibits only minimal phacodonesis and there is no presenting vitreous, a careful extracapsular extraction can be entertained. The use of a posterior chamber intraocular lens implant, even in the presence of an intact posterior capsule, is contraindicated due to the inherent instability of zonular and capsular support.

Nontraumatic Acute Cataracts

Although cataracts are the leading cause of reversible visual loss, their progression is slow, and rarely do they present as an acute ocular emergency. There are instances, however, where the lens may acutely change in either optical clarity or refractive power. The diabetic eye is subject to a number of ocular abnormalities, including diabetic retinopathy, retinal vein occlusion, adult-onset cataract, and secondary glaucoma. Diabetics may also manifest sudden fluctuations in acuity secondary to changes in the crystalline lens. When there is a precipitous rise in blood sugar, there is a compensatory elevation in aqueous humor glucose and subsequently lens glucose. In the lens, glucose is converted to sorbitol by aldose reductase. Elevated levels of sorbitol cause an osmotic hydration of the lens. As water is drawn in, the lens swells, causing a myopic shift and a transient loss of clarity. At times, the change in vision can be dramatic. Both the myopic shift and the loss of clarity are reversible with adequate blood sugar control.

Occasionally a posterior subcapsular cataract can be the cause of rapidly progressive visual loss (Figure 10–15). Posterior subcapsular cataracts are associated with diabetes, prolonged steroid use, local irradiation, or inflammation.

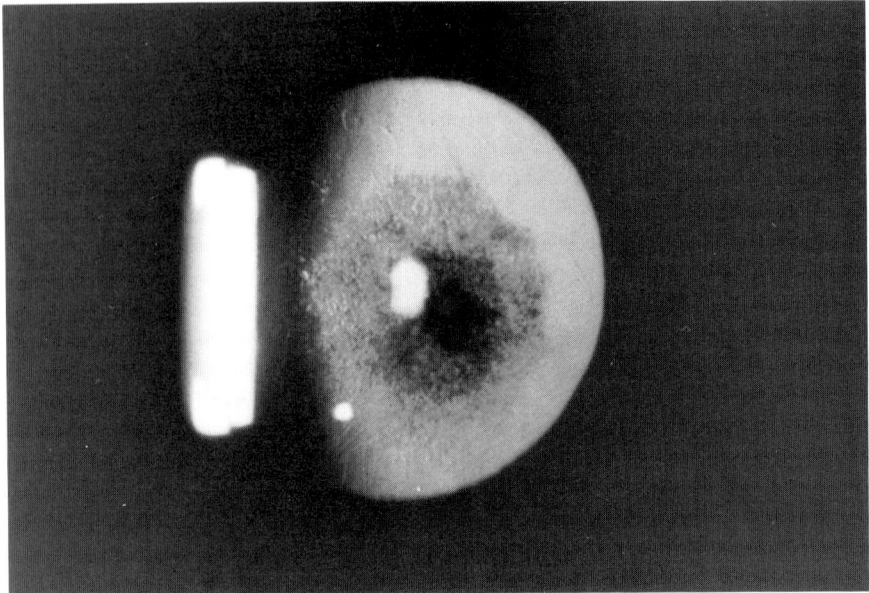

FIGURE 10–15. Posterior subcapsular cataract.

The lens opacity tends to progressively obscure the central visual axis. Once the pupillary zone is affected, vision may decrease precipitously. Early complaints are of glare, halos, and poor near vision. Near vision is particularly affected because the near response is linked to pupillary constriction. As the pupil constricts, the central posterior opacity completely obscures the pupillary aperture. Temporary visual improvement may be obtained with pupillary dilation or the use of tinted lenses to prevent pupillary constriction. Definitive therapy requires cataract extraction.

Phacolytic and Phakomorphic Glaucoma

A mature lens is one that transmits no light on routine examination and presents as a "white pupil" (Figure 10–16). As lenses mature, they swell in the anterior-posterior direction. A mature swollen lens is also called intumescent. With hypermaturity, the cataractous cortex undergoes liquefaction, allowing the opaque nucleus to float freely in the surrounding fluid; this is called a Morgagnian cataract (Figure 10–17). Eventually the lens capsule itself is altered, becoming hyperpermeable and allowing the passage of lens protein into the anterior chamber, leaving a dense, shrunken, cataractous lens. It is rare to encounter a patient in the United States with a hypermature cataract.

10—Emergencies of the Cornea and Ocular Lens 257

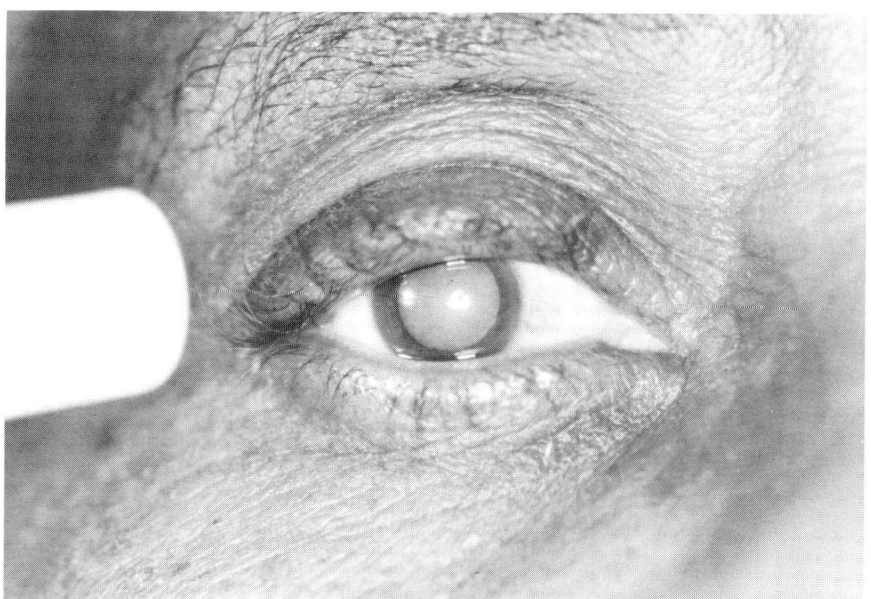

FIGURE 10-16. Mature cataract.

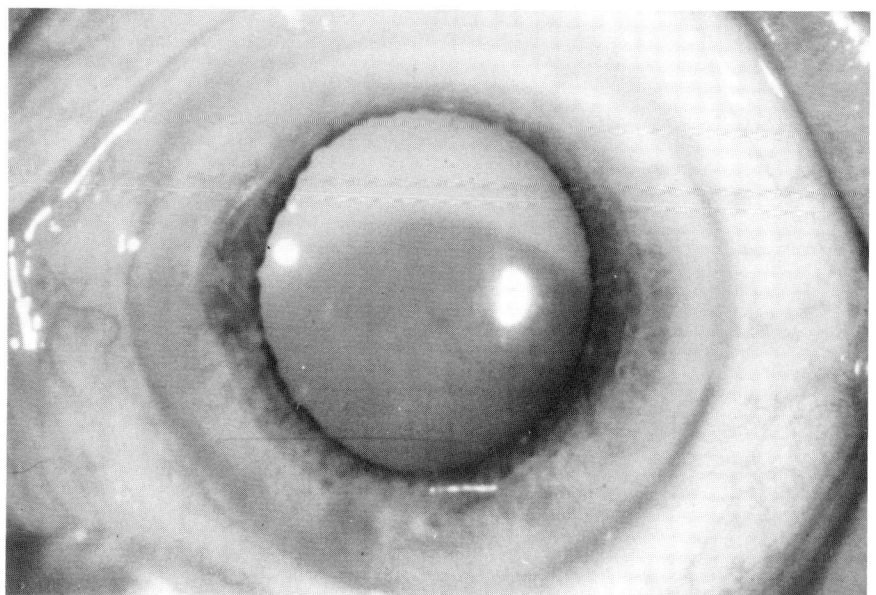

FIGURE 10-17. Hypermature Morgagnian cataract.

A swollen or intumescent lens can also shallow the anterior chamber, causing a secondary angle-closure glaucoma. The term for this is *phakomorphic glaucoma* (Figure 10–18). If angle closure develops suddenly, patients present with signs and symptoms of acute angle closure glaucoma (pain, nausea, elevated intraocular pressure, shallow anterior chamber). The acute management of phakomorphic angle-closure glaucoma differs from other causes of pupillary block glaucoma (see Chapter 11) only in that parasympathomimetics (pilocarpine) should be avoided. Pilocarpine causes an anterior movement of the lens, which could aggravate the secondary angle closure. Osmotic agents, carbonic anhydrase inhibitors, beta-blockers, and alpha agonists may be used. Secondary angle closure may also develop insidiously. One needs to consider phakomorphic glaucoma in any patient with angle closure associated with a shallow anterior chamber and a unilateral or asymmetric cataract. If medical management fails to lower the pressure to an acceptable level, a laser iridotomy or a surgical iridectomy should be performed. A peripheral iridotomy/iridectomy will relieve the angle closure unless extensive peripheral anterior synechiae (PAS) have formed. Once the pressure is controlled and the acute inflammation has subsided, cataract extraction should be performed. In cases of long-standing angle closure, cataract extraction may have to be combined with a filtering procedure to maintain adequate intraocular pressure control.

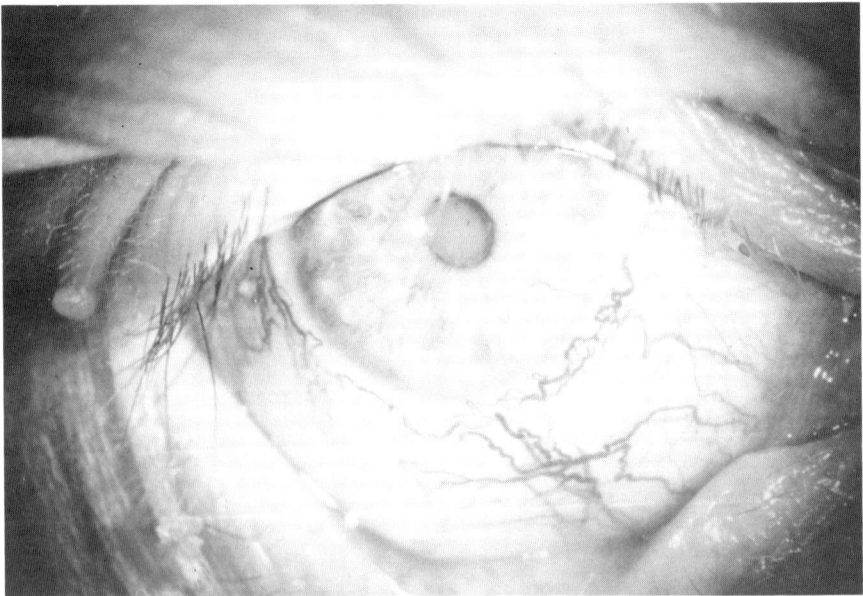

FIGURE 10–18. Phakomorphic glaucoma. The swollen, intumescent lens has caused a pupillary block glaucoma.

Lens-induced glaucoma can also occur in the absence of angle closure. Leakage of lens protein from a mature or hypermature cataract can block the trabecular meshwork and lead to outflow obstruction. This obstruction is secondary to direct blockage by the high molecular weight lens protein and/or protein-laden macrophages that have engulfed the lens material. Patients present with pain, redness, elevated intraocular pressure, and a mature or hypermature lens but with an open anterior chamber angle. Further examination reveals heavy flare and occasionally white flocculent material in the anterior chamber. The acute management involves lowering the intraocular pressure and controlling the inflammatory response. Definitive therapy requires cataract extraction, which is often complicated by the fact that the lens is mature or hypermature, the cortical material flocculent, and the lens capsule fragile. A complete cortical cleanup is mandatory, and an anterior chamber washout should be considered at the conclusion of the case.

REFERENCES

Corneal Disorders

Feder RS, Krachmer JH: Conjunctival resection for the treatment of the rheumatoid corneal ulceration. *Ophthalmology* 91:111, 1984.

Fujikawa LS, Nussenblatt RB: Recurrent and chronic corneal epithelial defects. In Abbott RL (ed): *Surgical Intervention in Corneal and External Diseases.* Orlando, Grune & Stratton, 1987, pp 59–67.

Kenyon KR: Recurrent corneal erosion: Pathogenesis and therapy. *Int Ophthalmol Clin* 19(2):169, 1979.

McLean EN, MacRae SM, Rich LF: Recurrent erosion: Treatment by anterior stromal puncture. *Ophthalmology* 93:784, 1986.

Mandelbaum S, Udell IJ: Noninfected Corneal Perforations. In Abbott RL (ed): *Surgical Intervention in Corneal and External Diseases.* Orlando, Grune & Stratton, 1987, pp 87–106.

Wagoner MD, Kenyon KR: Diagnosis and treatment of noninfected corneal ulcers. In *Focal Points: Clinical Modules for Ophthalmologists,* vol 8, no 7. San Francisco, American Academy of Ophthalmology, 1985.

Disorders of the Lens

Epstein DL, Jedzinak JA, Grant WM: Obstruction of aqueous outflow by lens particles and heavy molecular-weight soluble lens proteins. *Invest Ophthalmol Vis Sci* 17:272, 1978.

Glaucoma, Lens and Anterior Segment Trauma: Basic and Clinical Science Course, Section 8. American Academy of Ophthalmology, San Francisco, 1990.

Jarrett WH: Dislocation of the lens: A study of 166 hospitalized cases. *Arch Ophthalmol* 78:289, 1967.

Phelps CD: Examination and functional evaluation of crystalline lens. In Tasman W, Jaeger EA (eds): *Duane's Clinical Ophthalmology.* Philadelphia, JB Lippincott, 1990.

Sellyei LE Jr, Barraquer J: Surgery of the ectopic lens. *Ann Ophthalmol* 5:1127, 1973.

11

Glaucoma Emergencies

Robert A. Catalano

Glaucoma results from mechanical blockage of the flow of aqueous humor within the eye or limited egress of aqueous from the eye. Aqueous normally flows from the posterior chamber of the eye (behind the iris), where it is produced, to the anterior chamber of the eye (in front of the iris), where it is absorbed. It is then transmitted to vessels on the surface of the eye and eventually absorbed into the systemic circulation (Figure 11–1). Mechanical blockage anywhere along this pathway leads to increased intraocular pressure. Excessive distending force can result in excavation of the optic nerve (cupping) and loss of vision.

Glaucoma is divided into three categories: open angle, closed angle (angle closure), and infantile (congenital, developmental). In *open angle glaucoma,* aqueous has free access to the trabecular meshwork, the drainage apparatus in the anterior chamber. In *angle closure glaucoma,* access to trabecular meshwork is blocked by the iris. In *congenital glaucoma,* the outflow apparatus developed abnormally (trabeculodysgenesis). Glaucomas are further classified as being either *primary,* resulting from an unknown or developmental defect, or *secondary,* resulting from an associated or inciting abnormality (Table 11–1).

Although primary open angle glaucoma is much more common than the other forms of glaucoma, its onset is insidious and asymptomatic. It is encountered in the emergency setting only as an incidental finding. When it is discovered, sufficient time always exists for referral to an ophthalmologist; it will

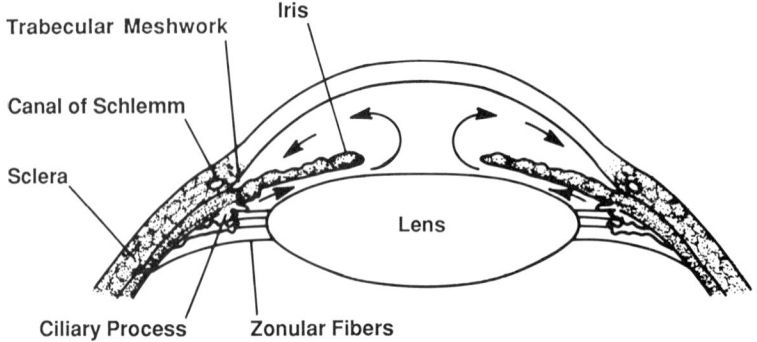

FIGURE 11-1. Flow of aqueous humor within the eye.

therefore not be considered in this book. Acute, symptomatic glaucomas include the primary and secondary angle closure glaucomas, infantile glaucoma, and, rarely, secondary open angle glaucoma.

Diagnosing Glaucoma in the Emergency Setting

Primary or secondary angle closure glaucoma is included in the differential diagnosis when adults present with ocular pain or inflammation. Angle closure is purported to occur in 1 of every 200 individuals. The incidence of occludable angles may be 10 times higher. Table 11-2 presents the differential diagnosis of a red eye (see also Chapter 16). Emphasis in this chapter is on angle closure glaucoma.

TABLE 11-1. CLASSIFICATION OF THE GLAUCOMAS

OPEN ANGLE	ANGLE CLOSURE	INFANTILE
Primary Cause unknown; the aqueous has free access to the trabecular meshwork. Usually insidious onset and asymptomatic.	**Primary** The iris root is anatomically displaced forward, and the entrance to the anterior chamber angle is narrow.	**Primary** The aqueous outflow apparatus develops abnormally or remains immature.
Secondary Increased episcleral venous pressure, trauma, inflammation, or steroids damage or block the flow of aqueous in the trabecular meshwork or episcleral vessels.	**Secondary** The lens-iris diaphragm is displaced forward due to a tumor, edema, or hemorrhage in the ciliary body; or adhesions between the iris and the lens or cornea develop.	**Secondary** Glaucoma associated with mesodermal dysgenesis, lens dislocation, aniridia, or other congenital malformation of the eye.

TABLE 11-2. DIFFERENTIAL DIAGNOSIS OF ANGLE CLOSURE GLAUCOMA

	ANGLE CLOSURE GLAUCOMA	ACUTE IRIDOCYCLITIS	VIRAL CONJUNCTIVITIS
History			
Onset	Sudden	Gradual	Gradual
Bilaterality	Unilateral	Unilateral	Bilateral
Pain	Severe, boring	Moderate	Burning, stinging
Photophobia	Moderate	Severe	Absent (except Adenovirus)
Examination			
Acuity reduction	Marked	Slight	None
Site of injection	Intense diffuse hue near limbus (ciliary flush)		Individual vessels dilated near the fornices
Injected vessels	Violaceous; do not move with conjunctiva; do not blanch with epinephrine 1:1000		Bright red; move with conjunctiva; blanch with epinephrine 1:1000
Discharge	Watery	Watery	Watery (purulent if bacterial infection)
Cornea	Cloudy if prolonged	Usually clear, +/− deposits on posterior surface	Clear
Pupil	Mid-dilated, unreactive	Miotic, reaction slow or absent	Normal size, normally reactive
Intraocular pressure	Increased	Normal or low	Normal
Gonioscopy	Angle closed	Angle open	Angle open

PRIMARY ACUTE ANGLE CLOSURE GLAUCOMA

History

Primary acute angle closure glaucoma usually affects individuals over age 50 years. Their history may suggest preceding attacks of angle closure during periods of pupillary dilatation. They may have experienced sudden ocular pain and blurred vision after viewing a movie or following emotional turmoil with sympathetic release. During these periods, colored, rainbowlike halos are seen surrounding lights, particularly streetlights and the headlights of oncoming cars.

After a series of attacks and occasionally at the initial occurrence, mechanical blockage of the trabecular meshwork does not remit (Figure 11-2). This usually occurs unilaterally and is associated with throbbing or boring pain. The pain mimics that of ocular migraine or an intracranial aneurysm and incites nausea and emesis. The gastrointestinal symptoms can become so severe that the patient may report these as the chief complaint.

Family history of a relative needing emergency treatment for acute glaucoma

ANGLE CLOSURE GLAUCOMA

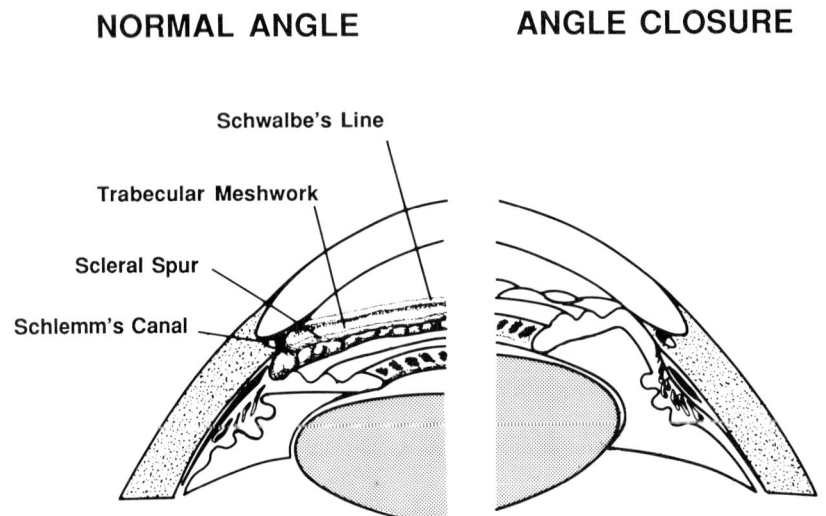

FIGURE 11-2. Mechanism of angle closure glaucoma: Pupillary block and mechanical obstruction of the trabecular meshwork by the iris.

is often elicited. Angle closure glaucoma is also more common among Eskimos and persons of northern European descent; it is rare in blacks. In whites, women are at a threefold to fourfold greater risk; in American blacks, the incidence between sexes is equal. Topical mydriatics and systemic anticholinergics (antihistamines and antipsychotics) can precipitate pupillary block in susceptible individuals. Farsightedness (hyperopia) is a predisposing condition; general anesthesia is an inciting state.

Ocular Findings

The affected eye develops a violaceous hue (ciliary flush) surrounding the limbus (the junction of the cornea and sclera) (Figure 11-3). Individual injected vessels are not distinguishable, and they do not constrict after application of topical epinephrine 1:1000. Additionally, the vessels do not move if the conjunctiva is moved with a cotton swab. Tearing may be profuse, and the cornea may appear cloudy or semiopaque secondary to edema that forms in the corneal stroma and epithelium. Microcystic bullae in the corneal epithelium give the surface an irregular appearance.

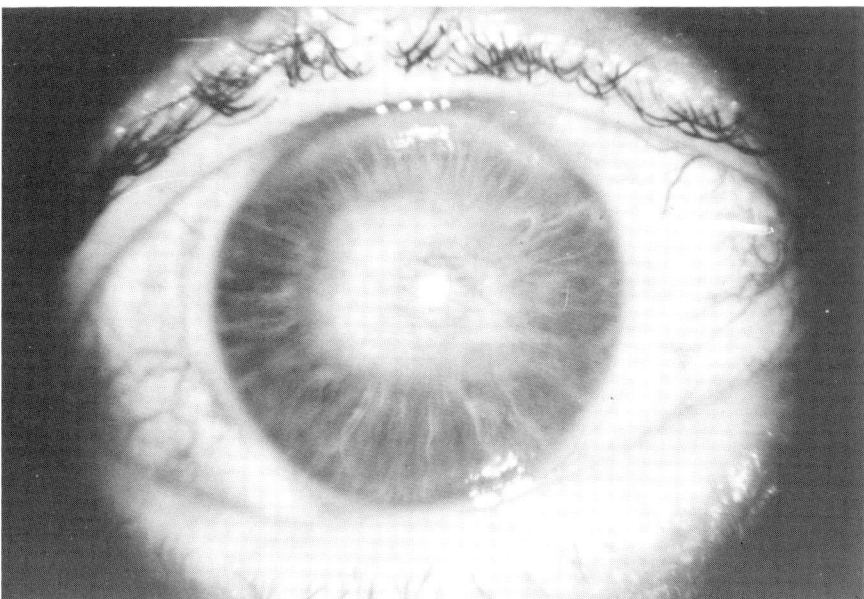

FIGURE 11-3. Acute angle closure characterized by corneal edema and conjunctival injection.

Corneal edema decreases the visual acuity, often to 20/200 or less. It also impedes the physician's view of the anterior chamber angle. In these instances, topical application of 50% glycerin usually temporarily detumesces the cornea. The pupil is usually mid-dilated and oval, with its long axis vertical. It usually bows forward (shallowing the anterior chamber) and does not react to light. Iris vessels are dilated, and the anterior chamber may be filled with pigment, inflammatory particles, and exudate. Small, irregular white opacities scattered under the anterior lens capsule *(glaucomaflecken)* may be present due to previous episodes of acutely increased intraocular pressure (Figure 11-4). The intraocular pressure is usually very high, often greater than 50 mm Hg.

The diagnosis of angle closure requires visualization by gonioscopy of a closed anterior chamber angle (Figures 11-5, 11-6). In some individuals, the peripheral iris is convex and inserted anteriorly on the ciliary body. This condition is called *plateau iris configuration.* In these patients, acute angle closure can occur with only a mild degree of pupillary block or due to blockage of the trabecular meshwork by the peripheral iris. The latter condition is called *plateau iris syndrome* and should be suspected when the iris plane is flat and the anterior chamber depth is normal in an eye with acute angle closure glaucoma. Furthermore, with this iris configuration, angle closure can occur despite a patent peripheral iridectomy.

If visualization of the anterior chamber angle is impossible because of

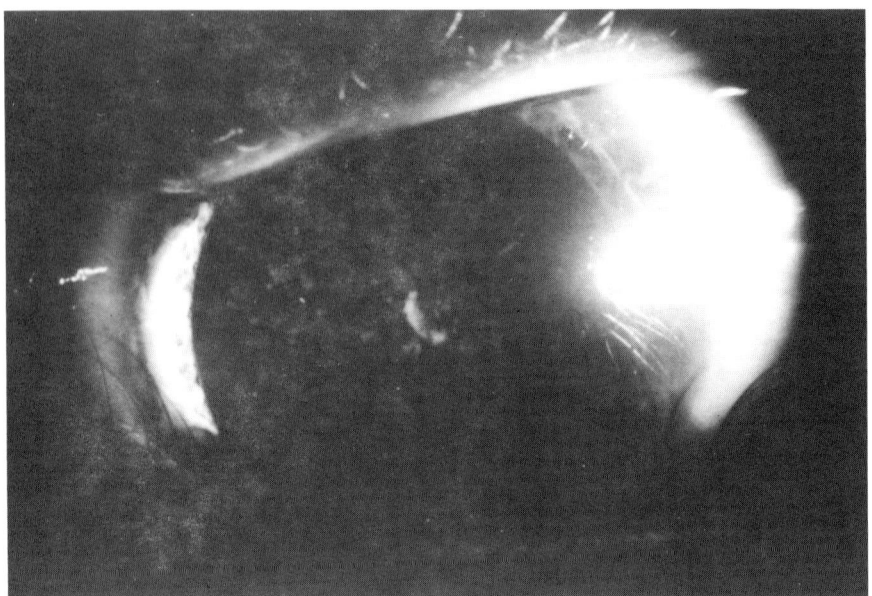

FIGURE 11-4. Glaucomaflecken due to previous episodes of angle closure glaucoma.

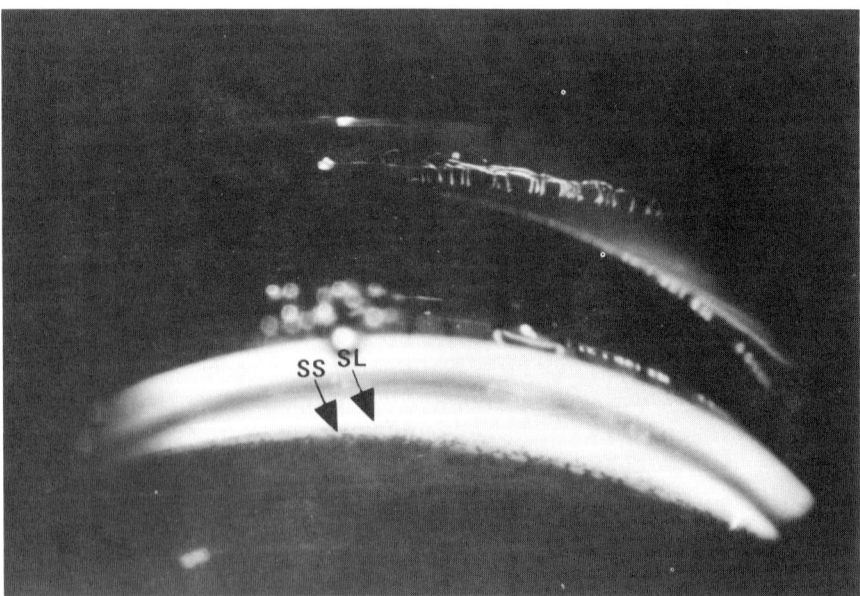

FIGURE 11-5. Gonioscopic view of an open angle (SS = scleral spur; SL = Schwabe's lines).

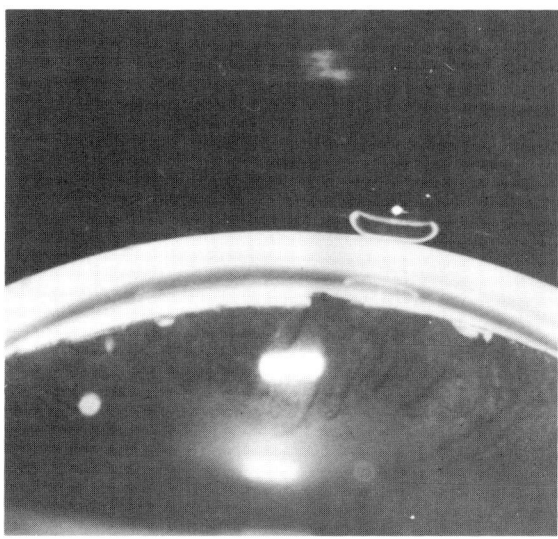

FIGURE 11-6. Gonioscopic view of a closed angle due to peripheral anterior synechia (abnormal peripheral adhesions of the iris to the cornea).

corneal edema, gonioscopy of the fellow eye will show a narrow angle. Approximately 50% of fellow eyes develop angle closure glaucoma, usually within 2 years of the attack in the presenting eye.

Treatment

A variety of agents, both topical and systemic, exist to treat an episode of acute angle closure. Alternately, if the episode is of recent onset and no corneal edema is present, an attack can occasionally be terminated by applying pressure to the center of the cornea with a small blunt object such as a muscle hook or a Zeiss goniolens (Figure 11-7). This bows the peripheral iris backward, opening the angle and forcing the aqueous behind the iris through the pupil. The cornea can be repeatedly indented for 10 seconds followed by release of pressure for 10 seconds. The patient should lie supine to allow gravity to move the lens posteriorly.

The initial medical treatment should include the following:

1. A topical beta-blocker (e.g., timolol ½% × 1).

2. A topical corticosteroid (e.g., prednisolone acetate 1% every 15 minutes to 30 minutes × 4 and then hourly).

3. A systemic carbonic anhydrase inhibitor (e.g., acetazolamide 250 mg to 500 mg slowly intravenously). Maximum effect noted at 2 hours; lasts 4 hours

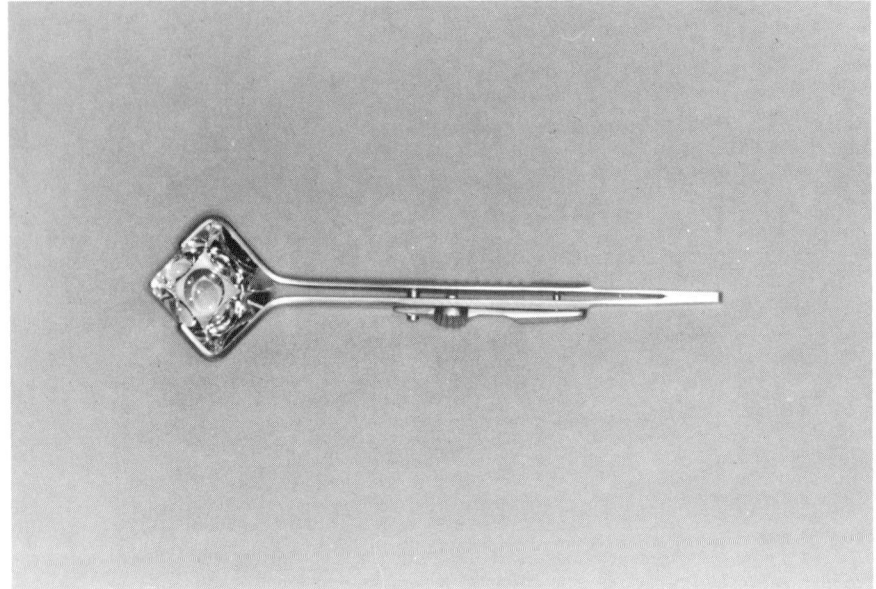

FIGURE 11-7. Zeiss goniolens.

to 6 hours. (Oral acetazolamide should be avoided due to nausea and vomiting until the acute attack is broken.) Or:

Systemic osmotic agent (e.g., oral isosorbide 50 mg to 100 mg [first choice]; hypertonic 20% mannitol 5 mL/kg to 10 mL/kg [equivalent to 1 g/kg to 2 g/kg] intravenously over 45 minutes, or a 50% solution of glycerol 1 g/kg to 1.5 gm/kg orally). Effect noted within 30 minutes to 60 minutes; lasts 5 hours to 6 hours.

4. A topical cholinergic (pilocarpine 1% to 2% every 15 minutes × 3. (Used only in phakic patients when the intraocular pressure is less than 50 mm Hg to 60 mm Hg.)

5. A topical mydriatic or cycloplegic (phenylephrine 2.5 or Mydriacyl 1% every 15 minutes × 4). (Used in pseudophakic or aphakic pupillary block.)

6. A systemic analgesic × 4 (acetaminophen 300 mg to 600 mg by mouth every 6 hours to 8 hours). Aspirin should be avoided because surgery may be needed.

Hyperosmotic agents induce headaches, dizziness, diuresis, and nausea (the latter occurs only with oral preparations). Oral glycerol also induces nausea and emesis and is very sweet. It should be sipped with ice. Mannitol increases blood volume and may precipitate congestive heart failure and pulmonary edema in patients with borderline cardiac function. Furosemide (Lasix) may be given in conjunction with this in patients with congestive heart failure. Mannitol can induce disorientation secondary to cerebral dehydration or a subarachnoid hemorrhage. Intracranial hemorrhage occurs due to rapid fluid overload of cerebral vessels, associated with shrinkage of the brain and traction on subarachnoid vessels. In diabetics, isosorbide is preferred to mannitol because it is metabolically inactive.

Once the intraocular pressure is less than 50 mm Hg to 60 mm Hg, the iris often becomes responsive to miotics, such as pilocarpine. Above this pressure, the iris is ischemic and the iris sphincter paralyzed. Multiple topical applications of pilocarpine can cause cholinergic toxicity, resulting in nausea, vomiting, diarrhea, abdominal cramps, diaphoresis, salivation, weakness, and bradycardia.

Miotics should be used only when pupillary block occurs in association with the eye's natural lens (phakic pupillary block). When angle closure occurs after cataract surgery, without (aphakic) or with an intraocular lens (pseudophakic) a mydriatric/cycloplegic agent such as Mydriacyl 1% or phenylephrine 2.5% should be used every 15 minutes, × 4. Cyclopentolate and atropine are too long lasting, increasing the difficulty of doing a peripheral iridectomy. Organophosphates such as phospholine iodide and di-isopropylfluorophosphate should never be used because they cause edema of the ciliary muscle, which can potentiate mechanical blockage of aqueous flow. Miotics are helpful if angle closure was induced by use of a mydriatic.

Definitive treatment such as a laser peripheral iridectomy is performed after the corneal edema has cleared. This often takes several days. In the interim, patients should have their intraocular pressure controlled using a combination of glaucoma medications, including the following:

Topical beta-blocker every 12 hours.
Acetazolamide 500 mg sequel every 12 hours.
Pilocarpine 1% to 2% every 6 hours (phakic cases only).
Prednisolone acetate 1% every 6 hours.

If examination of the other eye indicates that its angle is narrow and susceptible to closure, a peripheral iridectomy or laser iridotomy should be performed.

SECONDARY ACUTE ANGLE CLOSURE GLAUCOMA

History

A history of previous intraocular surgery, inflammation, or injury to an eye, in the setting of pain, redness, and blurred vision, suggests a secondary cause for an acute episode of angle closure. Additionally, if the angle in the fellow eye is open, one should suspect a secondary cause.

Causes

Obstruction at the Trabecular Meshwork

Obstruction of aqueous flow at the anterior chamber angle can occur from a variety of causes. Epithelium or fibrous tissue can grow on the posterior surface of the cornea and over the angle, from the site of a previous surgical incision *(epithelial downgrowth)* (Figure 11-8). Adhesions between the peripheral iris and the trabecular meshwork of the anterior chamber angle *(peripheral anterior synechia)* can occur following complicated cataract or glaucoma procedures (Figure 11-6). This especially occurs when the anterior chamber of the eye does not readily reform. Prolonged inflammation *(uveitis)* can lead to the development of similar adhesions.

An abnormal growth of vessels over the trabecular meshwork can also obstruct aqueous flow *(rubeosis iridis)* (Figure 11-9). In this condition, fibrous tissue, which accompanies the new vessels, contracts and pulls the peripheral iris against the cornea, blocking the anterior chamber angle. Rubeosis iridis occurs in some patients with advanced diabetic retinopathy, carotid occlusive disease, intraocular tumors, chronic uveitis or retinal detachment, or several months after a central retinal vein occlusion. *Ciliary body tumors* and *choroidal detachment* (Figure 11-10) provide another mechanism of anterior

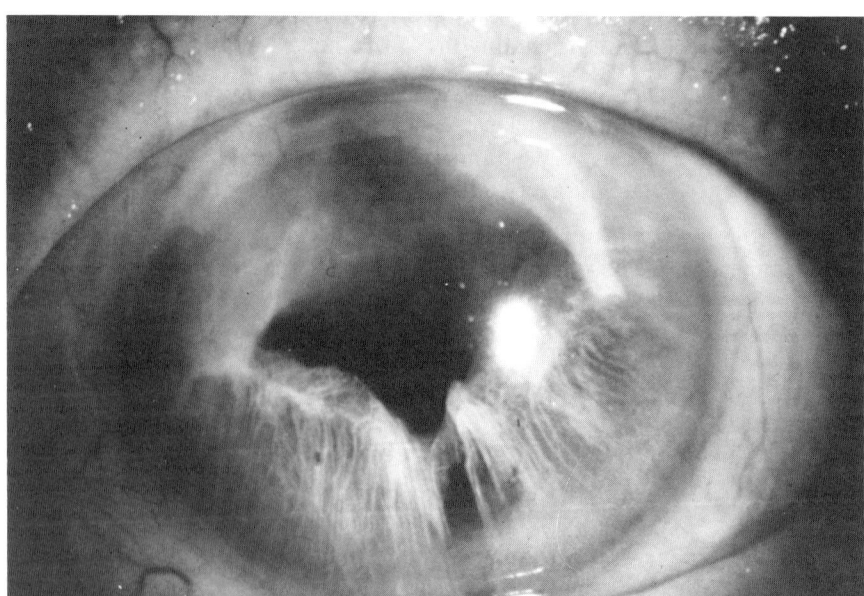

FIGURE 11-8. Epithelial downgrowth along the posterior surface of the cornea following cataract surgery.

11—Glaucoma Emergencies 271

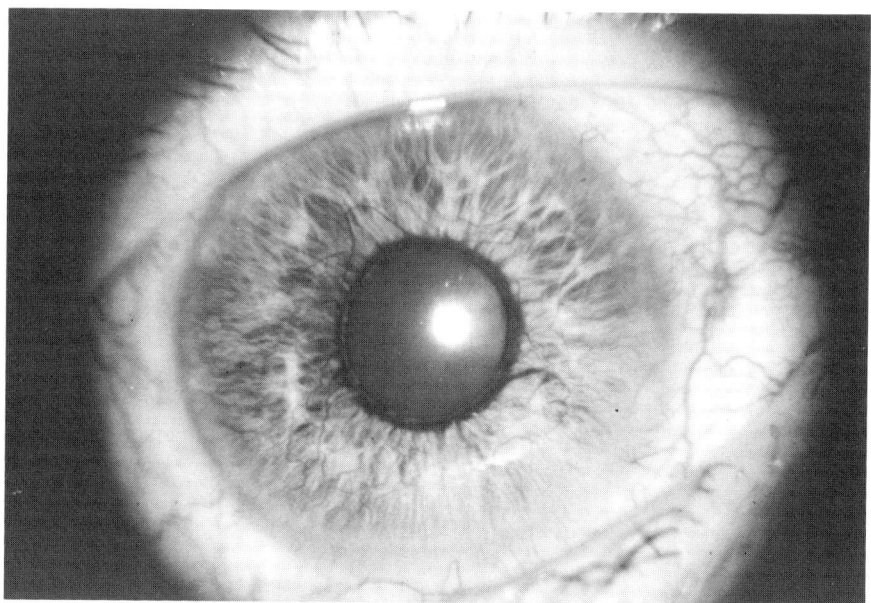

FIGURE 11-9. Rubeosis iridis.

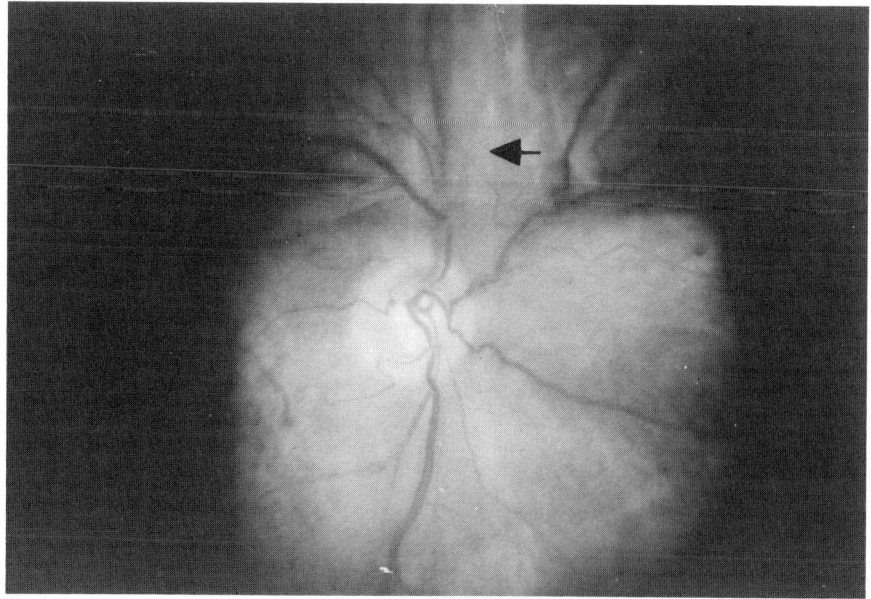

FIGURE 11-10. Choroidal detachment.

chamber angle obstruction by rotating the ciliary body/lens-iris diaphragm forward. A B-scan ultrasound may be helpful in diagnosing these causes.

Pupillary Block Glaucoma

Adhesions between the iris and lens *(posterior synechia)* can block the flow of aqueous from the posterior to anterior chamber, resulting in secondary angle closure glaucoma. Aqueous is blocked not only at the pupillary border *(pupillary block glaucoma),* but usually the peripheral iris bows forward *(iris bombé),* blocking the anterior chamber angle as well. Adhesions between the iris and lens can occur following surgery, inflammation (iritis), or ocular trauma (Figure 11-11). Similar blockage of aqueous at the pupillary margin can occur from a large intumescent cataract or a dislocated lens *(phacomorphic glaucoma)* (Figure 11-12) or from an anteriorly displaced vitreous face following removal of a cataractous lens. Pupillary block may also be precipitated by topical dilating agents (sympathomimetics and parasympathetic [muscarinic] antagonists) or systemic anticholinergics (antihistamines and antipsychotics).

Postoperative Angle Closure Glaucoma

Pupillary block can occur following cataract surgery when the pupil and any iridectomies are occluded by vitreous, lens remnants, or an intraocular lens.

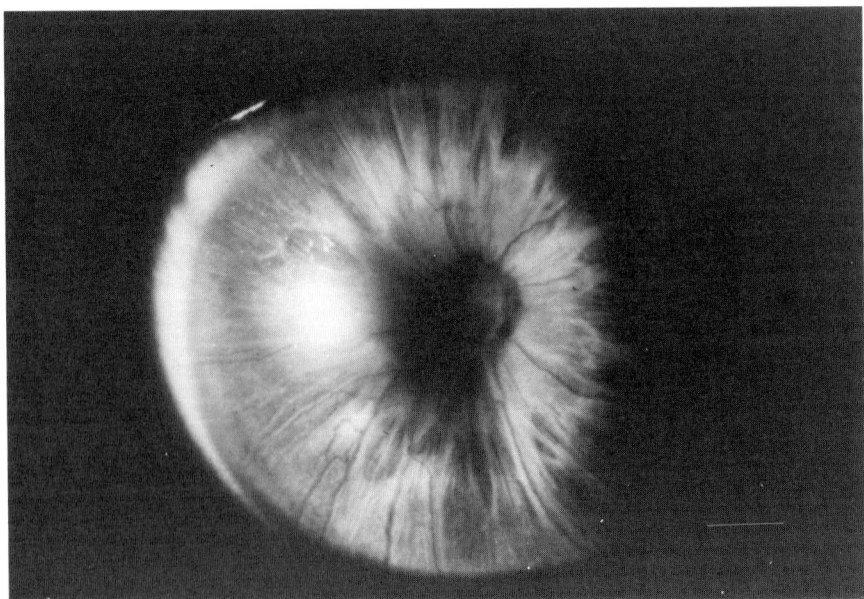

FIGURE 11-11. Iris bombé secondary to posterior synechia (abnormal adhesions of the iris to the lens) in chronic uveitis.

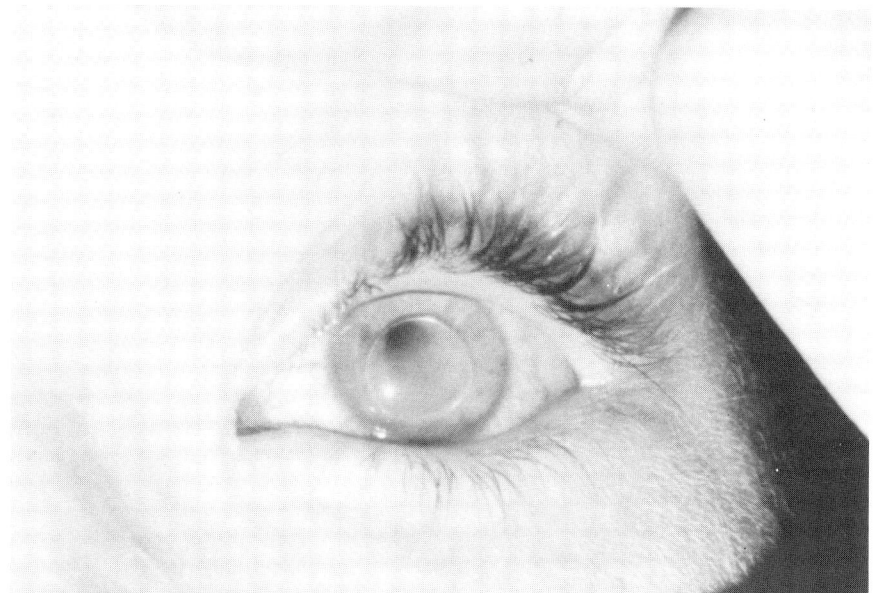

FIGURE 11-12. Angle closure glaucoma secondary to dislocation of the lens into the anterior chamber in Weill-Marchesani syndrome.

When an intraocular lens has been implanted, the condition is called *pseudophakic pupillary block* (Figure 11-13); without a lens, it is called *aphakic pupillary block*. Inflammatory adhesions between the iris and the vitreous or the intraocular lens often precipitate pupillary block. Aphakic pupillary block usually presents with a shallow anterior chamber, but in pseudophakia, the pupillary edge may be held posteriorly by the lens, keeping the central anterior chamber deep. Peripheral iris bombé still occurs. Cycloplegic and mydriatic agents (Mydriacyl 1% or cyclopentolate 1%) with a sympathomimetic (phenylephrine 2.5% or 10%) may be used. Atropine and scopolamine are usually avoided because they are too long acting and may result in poorer dilation. Topical steroids are used to decrease inflammation. Topical beta-blockers and systemic carbonic anhydrase inhibitors should also be used to reduce excessively elevated intraocular pressure. Even if medical therapy relieves the pupillary block, an iridectomy is required.

Malignant glaucoma is a condition in which the aqueous humor is misdirected posteriorly into or behind the vitreous. It usually follows surgical treatment of angle closure glaucoma or cataract extraction. Aqueous accumulates posteriorly and displaces the vitreous forward, shallowing the anterior chamber and occluding the trabecular meshwork. Atropine and phenylephrine along with agents to lower the intraocular pressure acutely should be used. Definitive treatment often includes laser or surgical therapy to disrupt the anterior vitreous face or a pars plana vitrectomy.

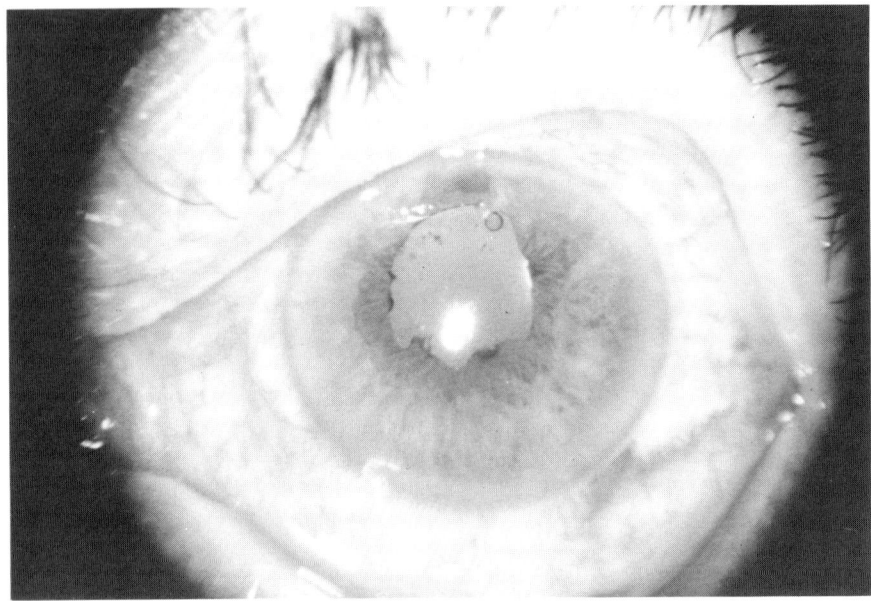

FIGURE 11-13. Pseudophakic pupillary block.

Generalized Treatment of Secondary Angle Closure Glaucoma

The initial treatment of secondary acute angle closure glaucoma is similar to that of primary acute angle closure, with one important exception. Unless the etiology of the attack is clear, miotics such as pilocarpine should not be administered. Miotics often cause vasocongestion, worsening some inflammatory secondary glaucomas. Carbonic anhydrase inhibitors, hyperosmotic agents, sympathomimetics, and topical beta-blockers are generally safe.

The long-term treatment of secondary glaucoma varies according to its etiology. It may include surgery, medications, photocoagulation, and/or cryotherapy after the acute episode is controlled. Glaucoma associated with inflammatory conditions may benefit from topical corticosteroids and cycloplegics. Pupillary block mechanisms usually necessitate laser or surgical iridectomies. Neovascular glaucomas often require laser or cryo-ablation of the retina, topical steroids, cycloplegic agents, and glaucoma medications. These managements are performed outside the acute setting and are beyond the scope of this book.

SECONDARY ACUTE OPEN ANGLE GLAUCOMA

Causes

Glaucoma Associated with Uveitis

Iridocyclitis (uveitis) is usually accompanied by a fall in intraocular pressure. An acute rise in intraocular pressure, however, can accompany herpes simplex and zoster infections, pars planitis, and sarcoidosis.

Posner-Schlossman syndrome, also known as *glaucomatocyclitic crisis,* is a syndrome in which a mild anterior chamber reaction occurs in association with a markedly elevated intraocular pressure of between 40 mm Hg and 60 mm Hg. It occurs predominantly in individuals between age 20 years and age 50 years. The anterior chamber angle is open, and occasionally a few fine precipitates on the posterior surface of the lower third of the cornea *(keratic precipitates)* are seen. The conjunctiva is minimally, if at all, injected, and symptoms are remarkably few relative to the markedly elevated pressure. Unilateral involvement is typical, and recurrent attacks may occur. Crises usually last a few weeks and are managed by systemic carbonic anhydrase inhibitors, topical epinephrine, and beta-blockers. Oral indomethacin, 75 mg/day to 150 mg/day, may also be effective. The mechanism responsible for the crises is unknown.

Increased intraocular pressure can occur in patients following cataract surgery with the implantation of an intraocular lens, associated with inflammatory cells, flare, and blood (hyphema) in the anterior chamber (Figure 11–14). Called *uveitis, glaucoma, and hyphema (UGH) syndrome,* treatment consists of atropine 1% three times a day and a topical steroid in addition to a carbonic anhydrase inhibitor and topical beta-blocker to lower the intraocular pressure acutely.

Pigmentary Dispersion Syndrome

Pigmentary dispersion syndrome is caused by the dislodging of iris pigment granules, which clog the trabecular meshwork. It occurs in nearsighted (myopic) young adults and may be exacerbated by exercise or pupillary dilatation. Although it is often asymptomatic, a rapid rise in intraocular pressure occasionally occurs, during which times ocular pain, blurred vision, and halos around lights occur. The diagnosis is made by observing spokelike transillumination of the iris (Figure 11–15) and heavy pigmentation of the trabecular meshwork. Additionally, a vertical spindle-shaped band of pigment, called *Krukenberg's spindle,* is often present on the posterior surface of the cornea. Miotics should be used because they eliminate the iris-zonule touch, which causes the pigmentary release.

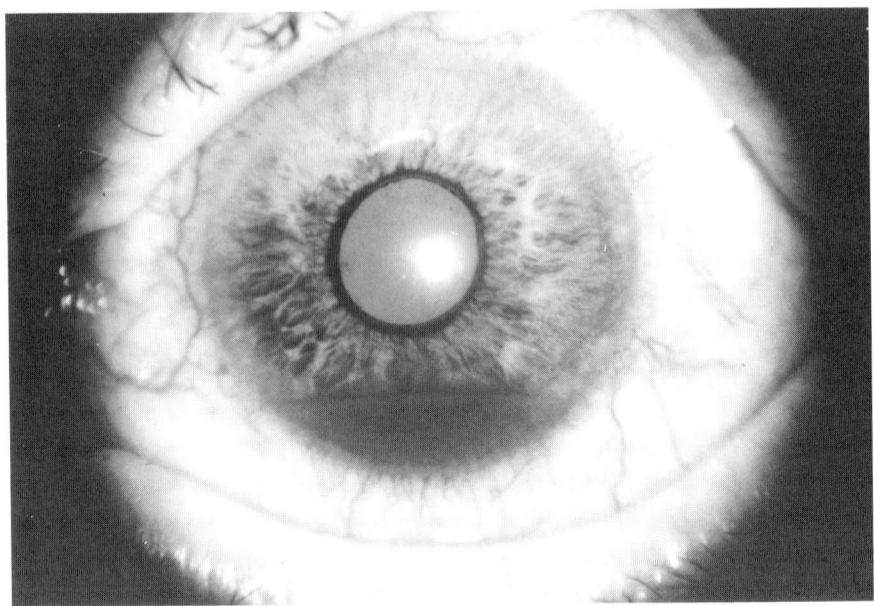

FIGURE 11-14. Uveitis, glaucoma, hyphema (UGH) syndrome following cataract surgery.

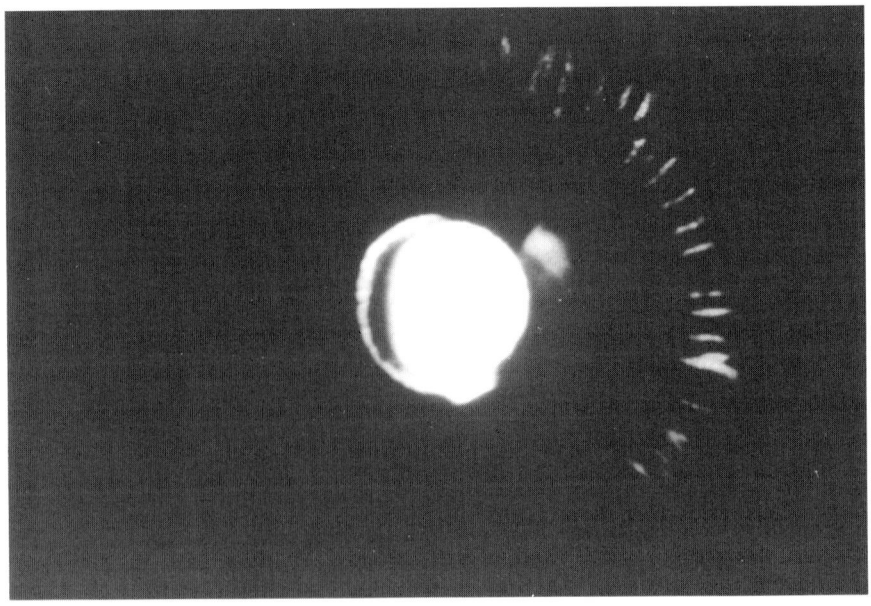

FIGURE 11-15. Iris transillumination in pigmentary dispersion syndrome.

Phacolytic Glaucoma

Lens protein can leak through the lens capsule of a hypermature cataract (Figure 11-16). This protein or macrophages laden with this protein can secondarily obstruct the trabecular meshwork. The intraocular pressure is usually markedly elevated, and the diagnosis is made by the presence of iridescent and white concretions within the anterior chamber (pseudohypopyon) or on the anterior lens capsule. Prominent white cells (macrophages) are seen in the anterior chamber, along with protein flare, and a hypermature cataract. The anterior chamber angle is open. Following abatement of the acute rise in intraocular pressure, definitive treatment requires cataract removal.

Lens Particle Glaucoma

The incomplete removal of lens particles during cataract surgery can result in elevated intraocular pressure due to obstruction of the trabecular meshwork. White fluffy remnants of lens cortex are visualized in the pupillary opening and over the trabecular meshwork, along with cells and flare in the anterior chamber (Figure 11-17). Trauma to the lens can result in a similar disorder; in this setting, a rent in the lens capsule is usually seen. Following cataract surgery, medical therapy is initially tried; if the intraocular pressure cannot be controlled, surgical removal of the residual lens material is necessary.

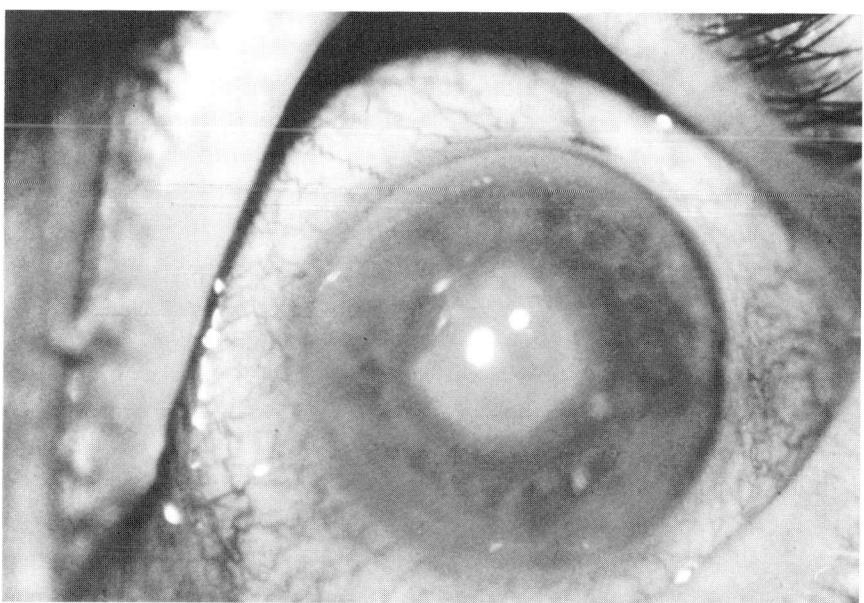

FIGURE 11-16. Phacolytic glaucoma.

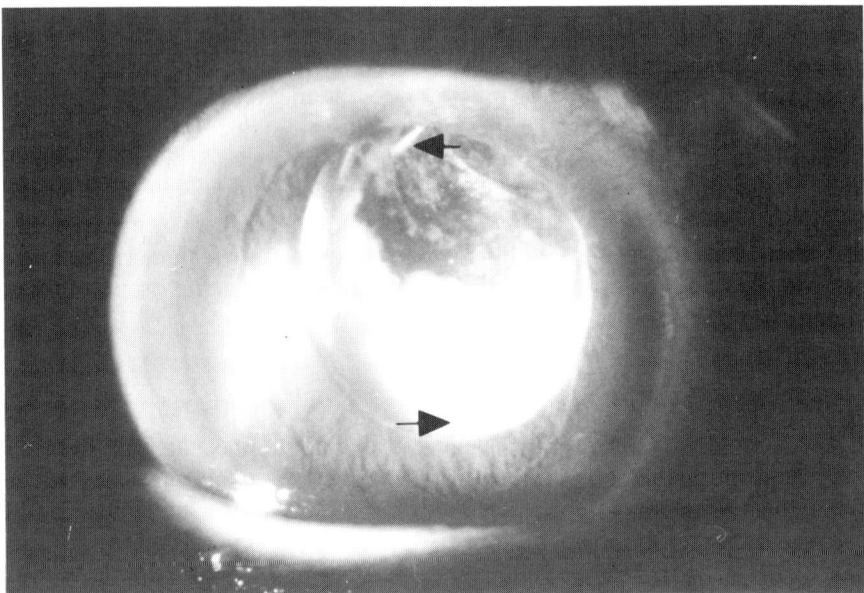

FIGURE 11-17. Incompletely removed lens particles following cataract surgery and implantation of an intraocular lens (arrows = haptics).

Phacoanaphylactic endophthalmitis is a rare condition seen 24 hours to 2 weeks following trauma or intraocular surgery in which a granulomatous inflammation occurs in response to liberated lens material. It rarely causes glaucoma and is usually associated with ocular hypotony. A hypopyon (accumulation of inflammatory cells inferiorly in the anterior chamber) is common, but fluffy white material is not seen.

Blood-induced Glaucoma

Mechanical obstruction of the trabecular meshwork can occur following trauma and hemorrhage into the anterior chamber (*hyphema*) or from denatured erythrocytes (*ghost cells*) passing anteriorly from the vitreous body.

A tear into the face of the ciliary body is the usual source of bleeding in traumatic hyphemas. Glaucoma is particularly common in patients with sickle cell anemia due to obstruction of the trabecular meshwork by sickled erythrocytes. Drugs that reduce aqueous formation and hyperosmotic agents frequently result in sufficient lowering of elevated pressure. If surgical intervention is necessary, total removal of the clot is unnecessary for resolution of the glaucoma.

Ghost cell glaucoma occurs subsequent to vitreous hemorrhage. It is often initiated by a precipitating event that ruptures the anterior hyaloid face, such as cataract surgery, vitrectomy, or trauma. The intraocular pressure rise is dependent on the number of ghost cells entering the anterior chamber; a large number can cause a rapid elevation to 60 mm Hg or 70 mm Hg, which can persist for several months. The conjunctiva is white because ghost cells do not incite an inflammatory response. Keratic precipitates do not form in ghost cell glaucoma and when seen suggest an inflammatory basis for the glaucoma. Tiny, khaki-colored cells, seen with 25× magnification, fill the anterior chamber and dot the posterior surface of the cornea. If a large number are present, they may form a pseudohypopyon. (A true hypopyon is composed of inflammatory white blood cells.) The emergency room treatment consists of standard medical therapy to lower the intraocular pressure; surgical intervention may be necessary.

Glaucoma Associated with Elevated Episcleral Pressure

A few rare systemic disorders cause glaucoma by raising the episcleral venous pressure and impeding the outflow of aqueous from the eye. The most common condition encountered in the emergency setting is a *carotid-cavernous fistula* (see also Chapter 13). Fistulas between the internal carotid artery and the surrounding cavernous sinus can develop spontaneously or with severe head trauma. Signs include ocular pulsation and a bruit over the eye. The episcleral veins are engorged, and ocular motility is restricted; ocular ischemia is usually present. Sturge-Weber syndrome, thyroid eye disease, retro-orbital tumors, and cavernous sinus thrombosis can also cause increased episcleral pressure but usually not acutely. Treatment in the emergency room is similar to that for other forms of glaucoma.

INFANTILE (CONGENITAL) GLAUCOMA

Similar to the glaucomas seen in adults, glaucoma in infants can be divided into primary and secondary types. Primary infantile glaucoma results from a developmental anomaly of the trabecular meshwork. Secondary infantile glaucoma occurs in association with a systemic or an ocular syndrome.

Primary Infantile Glaucoma

More than 80% of infants with *primary infantile glaucoma* present prior to age 12 months. Bilaterality occurs in 75% of the infants, and cardiac, auditory, and cerebral defects may be associated. Tearing (epiphora), sensitivity to light (photophobia), and eyelid squeezing (blepharospasm) are characteristic symptoms, but only half of affected infants present with all three. Signs of the disorder, corneal enlargement and clouding, may be more notable (Figure 11-18).

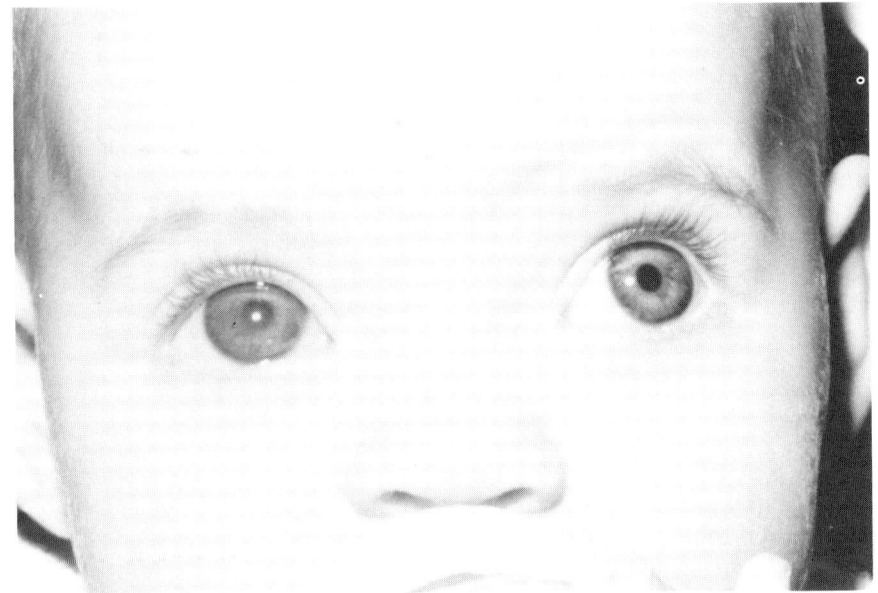

FIGURE 11-18. Unilateral infantile glaucoma in an infant with exotropia (divergent eyes).

Table 11-3 lists a differential diagnosis of signs and symptoms in infantile glaucoma.

Examination demonstrates a ground glass appearance of the cornea due to epithelial edema and enlargement of the corneal diameter from 10.5 mm to 12.0 mm or more. Horizontal breaks in the basement membrane of the corneal endothelium, called *Haab's striae,* may be visible on the posterior cornea. Other signs include a deeper than usual anterior chamber, enlargement of the cup-to-disc ratio of the optic nerve (Figure 11-19), nearsightedness (myopia), and marked enlargement of the entire globe (buphthalmos). The last is due to stretching of the globe and is seen when the glaucoma arises prior to age 3 years. Except in advanced cases, the pupils respond normally.

Intraocular pressure is best measured with a pneumotonographer or a hand-held Perkins applanation tonometer (Figure 11-20). Should examination under anesthesia be necessary, the surgeon should be prepared to treat the infant surgically, preventing the need for a second anesthetic. Most general anesthetic agents lower intraocular pressure; an intraocular pressure greater than 20 mm Hg under halothane anesthesia is suggestive of glaucoma. Primary infantile glaucoma is a surgical disorder, and several techniques, including goniotomy, trabeculotomy, or trabeculectomy, are used. Medical therapy is used as follows while awaiting definitive surgical treatment:

Topical beta-blocker (timolol ¼% to ½% every 12 hours).
Topical alpha agonist (dipiverin 0.1% every 12 hours).

TABLE 11–3. DIFFERENTIAL DIAGNOSIS OF SIGNS AND SYMPTOMS IN INFANTILE GLAUCOMA

Tearing
Nasolacrimal duct obstruction

Corneal irritation (conjunctival injection, blepharospasm, photophobia, epiphora, eye rubbing)
Abrasion or foreign body
Keratoconjunctivitis
Keratitis
Iridocyclitis

Corneal haziness
Interstitial keratitis (rubella or syphilis)
Mucopolysaccharidoses, lipidoses, or aminoacidosis
Cystinosis
Dystrophy (congenital hereditary endothelial dystrophy)

Corneal enlargement
Congenital megalocornea (usually without stria or edema)

Corneal stria
Forceps trauma (usually vertical or oblique with skin signs)

Scleral distension
Axial myopia

Optic nerve head cupping
Physiologic cupping
Heredofamilial optic atrophy
Optic pits or coloboma
Postneurotic atrophy
Toxic or vitamin-deficiency neuropathy
Compressive or infiltrative neuropathy
Hydrocephalus
Radiation optic neuropathy

(*From:* Stern JH, Catalano RA; Current status of diagnostic and therapeutic measures in infantile glaucoma. *Seminars of Ophthalmology* 5, no 4, 1990. Reprinted with permission.)

Systemic carbonic anhydrase inhibitor (acetazolamide 5 mg/kg to 10 mg/kg by mouth every 6 hours; use of the intravenous formulation orally may be easier than pulverizing tablets).

Secondary Infantile Glaucoma

Infantile glaucoma can be associated with several developmental abnormalities of the anterior eye. Peter's and Reiger's anomalies and aniridia can be recognized by grossly visible abnormalities of the iris and/or cornea (Figure 11–21). Glaucoma can also be seen in congenital rubella syndrome, usually associated with hearing and cardiac abnormalities. A rare systemic triad of glaucoma, cataracts, and renal disease, called Lowe's syndrome, is seen in males (X-linked) and is associated with frontal bossing, deep-set eyes, mental and motor retardation, muscular hypotonia, and hyperexcitability. The phako-

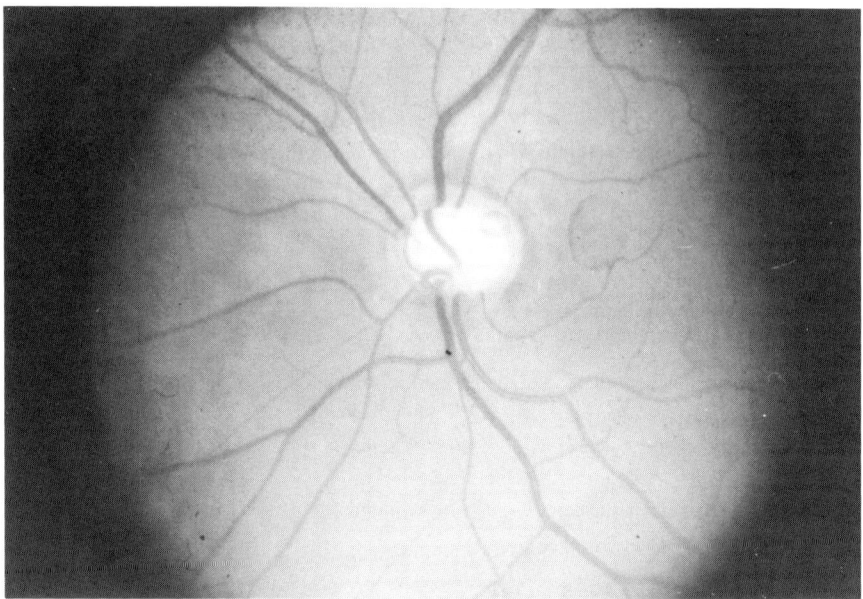

FIGURE 11-19. Increased cup-to-disc ratio in infantile glaucoma.

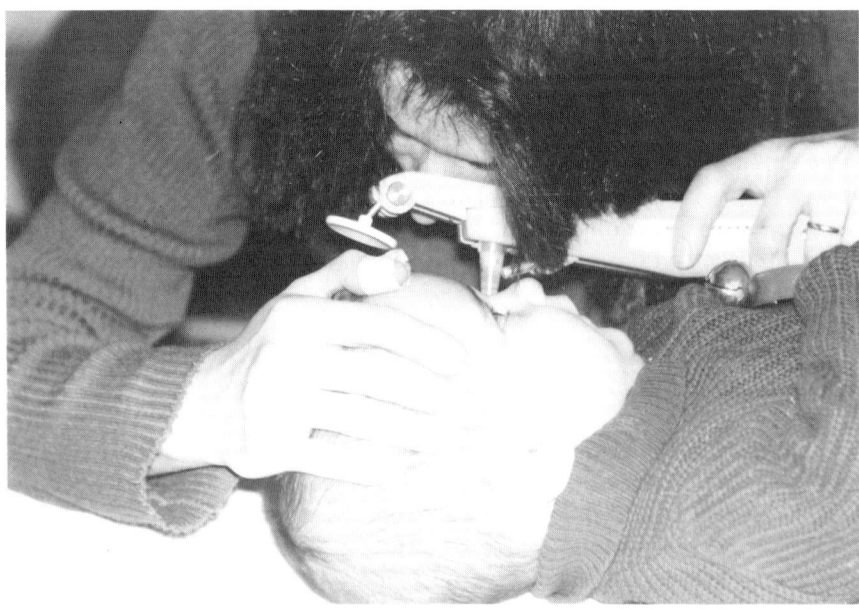

FIGURE 11-20. Measurement of intraocular pressure in an infant using a Perkins tonometer. (From Stern JH, Catalano RA: Current status of diagnostic and therapeutic measures in infantile glaucoma. *Seminars of Opthalmology* 5, no 4, 1990. Reprinted with permission.)

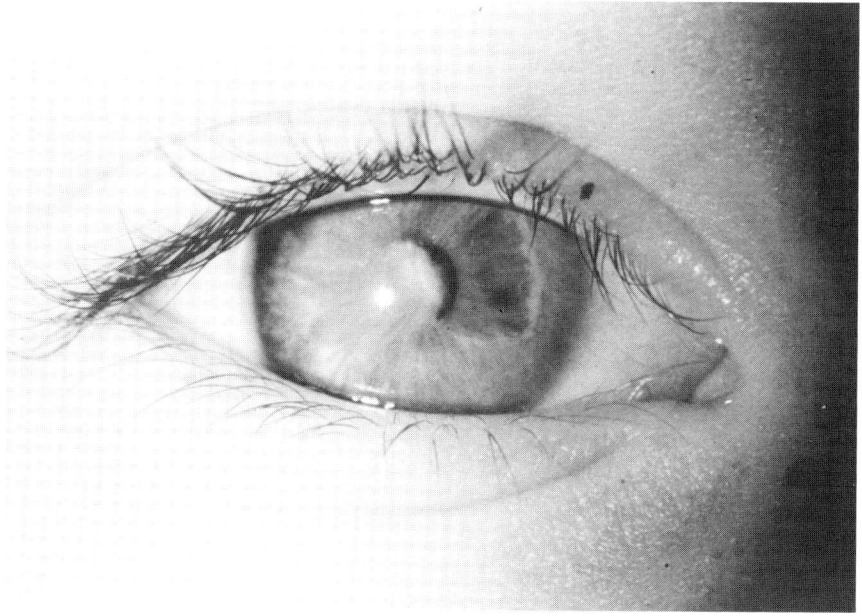

FIGURE 11-21. Peter's anomaly. Note central corneal opacity with iridocorneal adhesion.

matoses (particularly neurofibromatosis and Sturge-Weber) are also associated with infantile glaucoma, especially if the upper eyelid is involved (Figures 11-22 and 11-23). The glaucoma of Sturge-Weber syndrome is believed to be secondary to abnormalities in the anterior chamber angle or increased episcleral pressure. Other rare causes may have hand signs, including large thumbs (Rubenstein-Taybi syndrome) (Figure 11-24) or malformations of the digits (oculodental-digital syndrome). Table 11-4 lists secondary infantile glaucoma associations.

INDICATIONS FOR OPHTHALMOLOGIC REFERRAL

All patients with glaucoma need ophthalmologic care. The goal in the emergency department is to reduce the intraocular pressure to a level that will avoid ocular damage and allow the safe performance of a procedure specific to the inciting cause. An overriding principle in the treatment of secondary glaucoma in the acute setting is that no procedures or medications should be administered except for those that lower intraocular pressure. Procedures specific to a secondary cause of elevated intraocular pressure, and the use of antiinflammatory agents, should be deferred to an ophthalmologist once the diagnosis has been established.

284   III—Nontraumatic Ocular and Orbital Emergencies

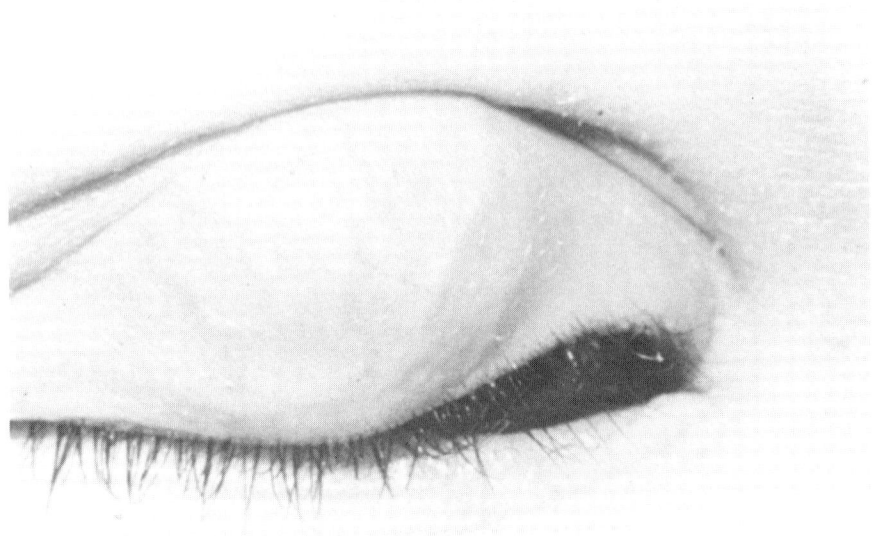

FIGURE 11-22.   Plexiform neurofibroma in the upper eyelid of a patient with neurofibromatosis.

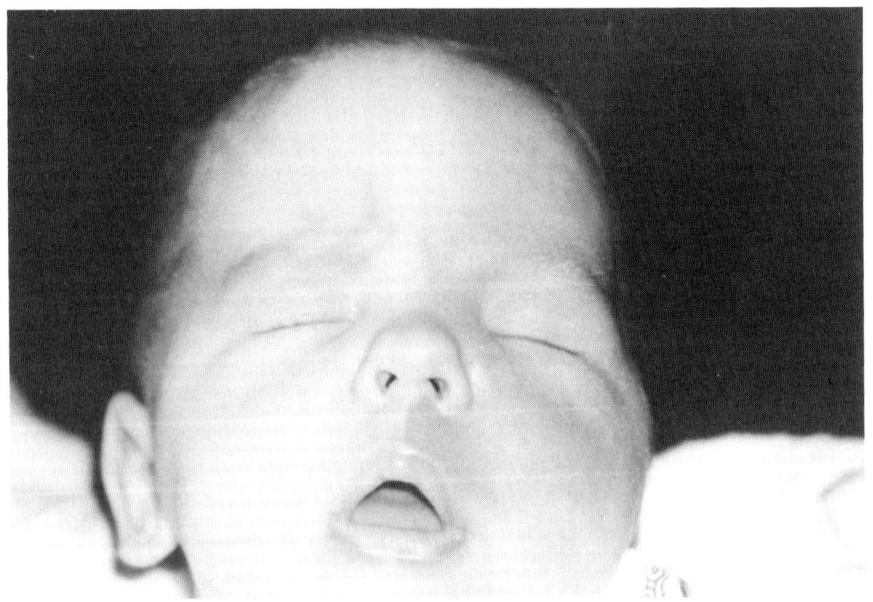

FIGURE 11-23.   Sturge-Weber syndrome.

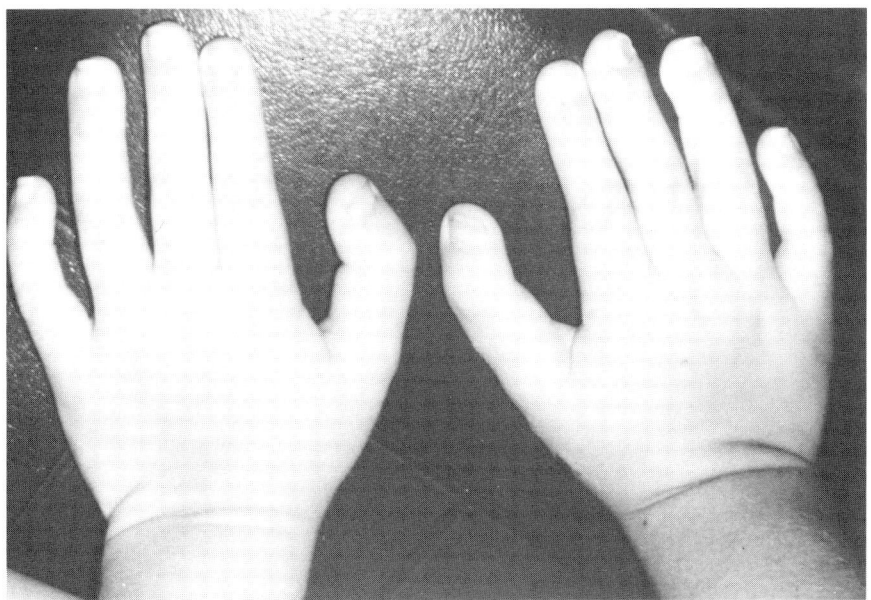

FIGURE 11-24. Rubenstein-Taybi syndrome.

TABLE 11-4. SECONDARY INFANTILE GLAUCOMA ASSOCIATIONS

Anterior cleavage or connective tissue abnormality
Axenfeld-Reiger's syndrome
Peter's anomaly
Posterior polymorphous dystrophy
Aniridia
Marfan's syndrome
Weill-Marchesani syndrome
Congenital microcornea

Phakomatoses and hamartomas
Neurofibromatosis
Sturge-Weber syndrome
Oculodermal melanocytosis
Cutis mamorata telangectasia congenita

Metabolic abnormality
Lowe's syndrome
Homocystinuria

Inflammation
Congenital rubella or syphilis
Herpes simplex
Uveitis

Mitotic abnormality
Juvenile xanthogranuloma
Retinoblastoma
Leukemia

Other congenital disorders
Rubenstein-Taybi syndrome
Oculo-dental-digital syndrome
Patau syndrome
Down syndrome
Persistent hyperplastic vitreous

Noncongenital disorders
Trauma
Aphakic or phacolytic glaucoma
Steroid induced glaucoma
Retinopathy of prematurity

(*From:* Stern JH, Catalano RA: Current status of diagnostic and therapeutic measures in infantile glaucoma. *Seminars of Ophthalmology* 5, no 4, 1990. Reprinted with permission.)

REFERENCES

Abbassi V, Lowe C, Calcagno PL: Oculo-cerebro-renal syndrome. A review. *Am J Dis Child* 115:145, 1968.
Anderson DR: Corneal indentation to relieve acute angle-closure glaucoma. *Am J Ophthalmol* 88:1091, 1979.
Brooks WE, Spalter HF: Haemolytic glaucoma occurring in phakic eyes. *Br J Ophthalmol* 70:603, 1986.
Campbell DG: Ghost cell glaucoma following trauma. *Ophthalmol* 88:1151, 1981.
Campbell DG, Shields MB, Liebman JM: Ghost cell glaucoma. In Ritch R, Shields MB, Krupin T: *The Glaucomas*. St. Louis, CV Mosby Co, 1989, pp 1239–1247.
DeLuise VP, Anderson DR: Primary infantile glaucoma (congenital glaucoma). *Surv Ophthalmol* 28:1, 1983.
Greenidge KC: Angle closure glaucoma. *Int Ophthalmol Clin* 30:177, 1990.
Hauviller V: Gonioscopic findings in trabeculotomies in young children. *J Pediatr Ophthalmol Strabismus* 26:133, 1989.
Herschler J, Cobo M: Trauma and elevated intraocular pressure. In Ritch R, Shields MB, Krupin T: *The Glaucomas*. St. Louis, CV Mosby Co, 1989, pp 1225–1237.
Hoskins HD Jr, Hetherington J Jr, Magee SD, et al: Clinical experience with timolol in childhood glaucoma. *Arch Ophthalmol* 103:1163, 1985.
Hoskins HD Jr, Shaffer RN, Hetherington J Jr: Anatomical classification of the developmental glaucomas. *Arch Ophthalmol* 102:1331, 1984.
Iwach AG, Hoskins HD, Hetherington J, Shaffer RN: Analysis of surgical and medical management of glaucoma in Sturge-Weber syndrome. *Ophthalmology* 92:904, 1990.
Kaufman JH, Tolpin DW: Glaucoma after traumatic angle recession: A ten year prospective study. *Am J Ophthalmol* 78:648, 1974.
Krupin T: *Manual of Glaucoma: Diagnosis and Management*. New York, Churchill Livingstone, 1988.
Lane SS, Kopietz LA, Lindquist TD, et al: Treatment of phacolytic glaucoma with extracapsular cataract extraction. *Ophthalmology* 95:749, 1988.
Lowe RF, Ritch R: Angle closure glaucoma: Mechanisms and epidemiology. In Ritch R, Shields MB, Krupin T: *The Glaucomas*. St. Louis, CV Mosby Co, 1989, pp 825–837.
Masuda K, Izawa Y, Mishima S: Prostaglandins and glaucomatocyclitic crisis. *Jpn J Ophthalmol* 19:368, 1975.
Mendelsohn AD, Jampol LM, Schoch D: Secondary angle-closure glaucoma after central retinal vein occlusion. *Am J Ophthalmol* 100:581, 1985.
Parks MM: Management of infantile glaucoma. *Trans New Orleans Acad Ophthalmol*. New York, Raven Press, 1986, pp 193–200.
Phelps CD, Thompson HS, Ossoinig KC: The diagnosis and prognosis of atypical carotid cavernous fistulas (red-eyed shunt syndrome). *Am J Ophthalmol* 93:423, 1982.
Reibaldi A, Avitabile T: Topical indomethacin in Posner and Schlossman's syndrome. *J Ocular Ther Surg* 4:28, 1985.
Samples JR, Bellows R, Rosenquist RC, et al: Pupillary block with posterior chamber intraocular lenses. *Arch Ophthalmol* 105:335, 1987.
Sears ML: Surgical management of black ball hyphema. *Trans Am Ophthalmol Otolaryngol* 74:820, 1970.
Seidman DJ, Nelson LB, Calhoun JH, et al: Signs and symptoms in the presentation of primary infantile glaucoma. *Pediatr* 77:399, 1986.
Stern JH, Catalano RA: Current status of diagnostic and therapeutic measures in infantile glaucoma. *Seminars of Ophthalmology* 5, no 2, 1991.
Van Buskirk EM: Pseudophakic glaucoma. In Weinstein GW: *Open Angle Glaucoma. Contemporary Issues in Ophthalmology*. New York, Churchill Livingstone, 1986, 3:133–154.
Wand M, Grant WM, Simmons RJ, et al: Plateau iris syndrome. *Trans Am Acad Ophthalmol Otolaryngol* 76:450, 1972.
Wappner R: Update: Lowe's syndrome. *Compr Ther* 13:3, 1987.
Warner LO, Bremer DL, Davidson PJ, et al: Effects of lidocaine, succinylcholine, and tracheal intu-

bation on intraocular pressure in children anesthetized with halothane-nitrous oxide. *Anesth Analg* 69:687, 1989.

Watcha MF, Chu FC, Stevens JL: Effects of halothane on intraocular pressure in anesthetized children. *Anesth Analg* 71:181, 1990.

Weiss JS, Ritch R: Glaucoma in the phakomatoses. In Ritch R, Shields MB, Krupin T: *The Glaucomas.* St. Louis, CV Mosby Co, 1989, pp 905–929.

12

Nontraumatic Orbital Disorders

Robert A. Catalano

The differential diagnosis for a patient with ocular pain or distorted, decreased, or double vision is extensive (Chapters 13 and 14). An orbital disorder is suggested when the patient also has proptosis (bulging eyes), globe displacement, eyelid swelling, or restriction of ocular motility. The first part of this chapter reviews historical, physical, radiologic, ultrasonographic, and laboratory findings in orbital disorders. The remainder of the chapter reviews specific entities. Because orbital disorders are often age dependent, discussion of childhood and adult entities are segregated.

HISTORY AND PHYSICAL FINDINGS

Krohel, Stewart, and Chavis (1981) first suggested that orbital disorders be evaluated using six Ps: pain, progression, proptosis, palpation, pulsation, and periorbital changes. The first two relate to the history and the latter four to findings on examination. We will follow this useful technique. The history should also review prior disease (Graves' disease, sinus infection, carcinoma), injury (head trauma), or treatments (radiation). The family history (orbital tumors) and old photographs may likewise be helpful.

The Six Ps in Evaluating Orbital Disease*

(Each of the six Ps will be presented with a different diagnosis.)

Pain

Tension headache: Bilateral, retrobulbar, worse in the evening.

Infection: Preseptal cellulitis (lid swelling and erythema), orbital cellulitis, (the addition of chemosis, proptosis, motility disturbance and visual loss), sinusitis (localized tenderness over sinus, upper respiratory infection), phycomycosis (diabetic, immunocompromised, acute visual loss, proptosis, ophthalmoplegia, and facial palsy).

Inflammation: Optic neuritis (aggravated by eye movement); vasculitis, foreign body reaction, pseudotumor (proptosis, motility disturbance, injection, lid swelling), posterior scleritis (deep orbital pain with radiation to the temple, mild proptosis, injection, localized choroidal effusions).

Aneurysm: Intermittent pain and associated neurologic signs.

Hemorrhage (sudden pain, proptosis, nausea and vomiting, with ecchymosis, motility disturbance, choroidal folds, disc edema, or visual loss): Orbital varix, cavernous sinus thrombosis, lymphangioma, hypertension, blood dyscrasia.

Ischemia: Sickle cell disease, carotid-cavernous fistula (ocular ischemia and glaucoma, subjective bruit, motility disturbance, episcleral injection, visual loss).

Carcinoma: ADULTS: Malignant lacrimal gland (deep, gnawing, sometimes episodic pain, loss of sensation in distribution of lacrimal nerve, palpable mass in superior temporal quadrant of orbit), nasopharyngeal carcinoma (facial and orbital pain with cranial nerve palsy and Horner's syndrome), metastatic tumor (acute pain, ptosis, visual loss, proptosis, diplopia).

CHILDREN: Orbital hemorrhage with lid ecchymosis: metastatic neuroblastoma (before age 4 years), granulocytic sarcoma (mean age 7 years), Ewing's sarcoma (ages 10–25); rhabdomyosarcoma (rapid progression of proptosis, pain less common), Burkitt's lymphoma (pain uncommon).

Progression

Days to weeks: Tender, palpable masses; diplopia [in adults] usually present:
Infection: Cellulitis, orbital or subperiosteal abscess.
Inflammation: Vasculitis, pseudotumor.
Hemorrhage: Lymphangioma.

---

*Modified with permission from: Krohel GB, Stewart WB, Chavis RM: *Orbital disease: A Practical Approach.* New York, Grune and Stratton, 1981.

Carcinoma: Rhabdomyosarcoma, neuroblastoma, granulocytic sarcoma, Burkitt's lymphoma.

Months to years: Diplopia and pain often absent

Tumors: Dermoid, benign mixed lacrimal tumor, neurofibroma (S-shaped upper eyelid deformity), cavernous hemangioma (second to fifth decade, slow progression of proptosis, motility disturbance, and subsequent visual loss), fibrous histiocytoma (diplopia secondary to extraocular muscle infiltration), fibrous dysplasia (facial asymmetry), lymphoma (if anterior, palpable mass; if posterior, proptosis), sinus mucocele (may become infected—mucopyocele—suggested by the acute onset of pain, proptosis, and globe displacement), metastatic carcinoma (breast and lung), malignant lacrimal tumor (symptoms less than 1 year in duration and pain), capillary hemangioma (enlarges over the first year of life).

Thyroid ophthalmopathy: Lid swelling, erythema, tearing, diplopia, vague discomfort, especially on upward gaze.

Orbital varix: Recurrent lid swelling and proptosis over months to years, especially with Valsalva maneuver. Sudden pain, nausea, and proptosis suggest secondary orbital hemorrhage.

Proptosis

Pseudoproptosis: Enlarged globe, asymmetry of bony orbit or lid fissures, extraocular muscle palsy, contralateral enophthalmos.

Unilateral proptosis (greater than 2 mm asymmetry): ADULTS: Thyroid ophthalmopathy, pseudotumor, carotid-cavernous fistula, cavernous sinus thrombosis. CHILDREN: Cellulitis.

Bilateral proptosis: ADULTS: Thyroid ophthalmopathy, cavernous sinus thrombosis, carotid-cavernous fistula, vasculitis (Wegener's granulomatosis), lymphoma, metastases. CHILDREN: Neuroblastoma, pseudotumor, leukemia.

Recurrent proptosis: Orbital varix (exacerbation with Valsalva maneuver, phleboliths on skull X ray, positive venography), lymphangioma (exacerbation with upper respiratory infection), pseudotumor, infected sinus mucocele, ruptured dermoid cyst with granulomatous reaction.

Proptosis with globe displacement:

Axial: Cavernous hemangioma, optic nerve glioma or meningioma, carotid cavernous fistula (axial proptosis, conjunctival chemosis, and injection), neurilemoma, most rhabdomyosarcomas, metastatic tumors.

Superior: Maxillary sinus tumor (pain and inferior chemosis), fibromatosis (firm, painless, tumor in childhood).

Inferior: Capillary hemangioma (with or without involvement of upper eyelid), metastatic tumor, fibrous dysplasia.

Inferior and medial: Dermoid, lacrimal gland mass.

Inferior and lateral: Frontal mucocele or osteoma, some rhabdomyosarcomas.

Medial: Neuroblastoma with metastases to zygomatic bone.

Palpation

Should be performed with eyelids open and gaze in primary position.

Resistance to retropulsion: thyroid ophthalmopathy, retrobulbar tumor, inflammation.

Rise in blood pressure with palpation: metastatic carcinoid tumor or pheochromocytoma.

Mass in the superior nasal quadrant: Encephalocele (midline, fluctuant, transilluminating, pulsatile, in infancy), plexiform neurofibroma ("bag of worms"), sinus mucocele (boggy), dermoid (smooth, firm, oval, and freely movable), metastatic (fixed to bone, rock-hard, tender), capillary hemangioma (compressible), lymphoma (firm and not fixed to bone), fibrous histiocytoma (cystic).

Mass in the superior temporal quadrant: Dermoid, prolapsed lacrimal gland, lacrimal gland tumor (fixed to bone, radiographic changes), lymphoma, pseudotumor (tender and associated with inflammatory signs), metastases.

Pulsation

Observe pulsation from patient's side, at the slit lamp, or in mirror of exophthalmometer. Listen for bruits with bell stethoscope over closed eyelid, with opposite eye open.

Without bruits: Encephalocele, neurofibromatosis and absence of sphenoid wing, surgical removal of orbital roof, vascular orbital metastases, cranial or sinus trauma with bony defects.

With or without bruits: Arteriovenous malformations, carotid-cavernous fistulas, sinus mucocele.

Periorbital Changes

Injection over horizontal rectus muscle insertions: Thyroid ophthalmopathy (purple in color).

Corkscrew epibulbar vessels: Arteriovenous malformation, carotid-cavernous fistula (dark red in color with white sclera); pseudotumor, orbital abscess (sclera is injected).

Strawberry birthmark: Capillary hemangioma.

Other discoloration of lid skin: Lymphangioma, varix (dilated, bluish, may involve conjunctiva).

Salmon-colored mass under superior conjunctiva: Lymphoma.

Yellow, fleshy mass under lateral conjunctiva: Dermolipoma.

S-shaped lid, "bag of worms" texture: Plexiform neurofibroma.
Bilateral ecchymoses: Neuroblastoma, granulocytic sarcoma.
Lid retraction and lid lag on downward gaze: Thyroid ophthalmopathy.
Prominent mass in temple: Sphenoid wing meningioma.
Swelling of lateral lower eyelid: Orbital apex meningioma.
Partial immobility of eye: Thyroid disease, metastatic tumor, pseudotumor, myositis, orbital cellulitis, large orbital tumor.
Complete immobility of eye: Metastatic tumor, mucormycosis, orbital cellulitis, pseudotumor, venous thrombosis.
Black, crusted infarcted tissue on palate, nasal mucosa, or skin: Phycomycosis (Mucor and Rhizopus).
Facial asymmetry: Neurofibromatosis, fibrous dysplasia.

Associated Ocular Findings

Abduction blindness: Optic nerve sheath meningioma (pupil may also briskly dilate).
Anterior uveitis: Scleritis, sarcoidosis, pseudotumor in children.
Posterior uveitis: Sarcoidosis, reticulum cell sarcoma.
Optic nerve dysplasia: Encephalocele.
Optociliary shunt vessels at disc: Optic nerve sheath or sphenoid wing meningioma. These also occur following central retinal vein occlusion, chronic papilledema, or bony compression of the optic nerve.
Choroidal folds: Thyroid ophthalmopathy, papilledema, ocular hypotony, orbital tumor.
Smooth indentation of globe: Orbital tumor.

Radiographic Signs

Ocular calcification: Retinoblastoma, phthisis bulbi, cicatricial retinopathy of prematurity, choroidal osteoma.
Orbital calcification: Meningioma (with hyperostosis and bone destruction), hemangioma, varix, malignant lacrimal gland tumor, dermoid cyst.
Blurring of oblique (innominate line): Sphenoid ridge meningioma (usually with hyperostosis of the lesser wing).
Absence of sphenoid wing: Neurofibromatosis.
Local compression lacrimal gland fossa: Dermoid, benign lacrimal tumor, lymphangioma.
Bone destruction, sclerosis, calcification of lacrimal fossa: Malignant epithelial tumors, histiocytic or metastatic tumor.
Osteoblastic lesions: Metastatic prostate and breast tumors.
Enlargement of optic canal: Optic nerve glioma or meningioma, invasive retinoblastoma, optic nerve granuloma, ophthalmic artery aneurysm.

Sinus opacification: Sinusitis.
Sinus expansion: Mucocele (bony margins may be round, thickened, or destroyed; sinus may be opaque).
Optic nerve enlargement: Optic nerve glioma or meningioma, metastatic tumor, granulomatous disease, pseudoenlargement (contralateral optic atrophy).
Thickened extraocular muscles: Thyroid ophthalmopathy, myositis (pseudotumor involving extraocular muscles), arteriovenous fistulas, metastatic disease. Tendons uninvolved in thyroid ophthalmopathy.
Enlarged superior ophthalmic vein: Arteriovenous malformation or fistula.
Scleral enhancement: Scleritis, pseudotumor.

Ultrasonographic Signs

Good transmission: Cystic and angiomatous tumors (dermoid, cavernous hemangioma, mucocele, lymphangioma).
Poor transmission: Solid and infiltrative tumors (meningioma, glioma, neurofibroma, metastatic tumor, pseudotumor).
Few internal echoes: Cystic lesions, tumors containing compact cells with little intercellular substance (lymphoma).
Strong internal echoes: Angiomatous tumors.
Rounded borders: Cystic and solid tumors.
Irregular borders: Infiltrative and angiomatous tumors.
Thickened optic nerve: Optic nerve tumors.
Thickened extraocular muscles: Thyroid ophthalmopathy, myositis, arteriovenous fistulas, metastatic disease. Tendons uninvolved in thyroid ophthalmopathy.

Laboratory Studies

Carcinoembryonic antigen (CEA): > 5.0 ng/mL suggests metastatic disease, especially breast, colon, lung, prostate, pancreas.
Thyroid function (see also Table 12–2): T_3 and T_4; if normal, a thyrotropin-releasing hormone (TRH) test should be performed in those suspected of thyroid disease.
Urine vanillylmandelic acid: Elevated in children with metastatic neuroblastoma.

NONTRAUMATIC ORBITAL DISORDERS IN CHILDREN

Because the orbit is a bony cavity, closed on every side except anteriorly, pathologic processes that involve the orbit present with proptosis (forward displacement of the eye) or as a mass, hemorrhage, or inflammation in or behind the eyelids. Orbital disorders in children should be evaluated with regard to the rate of progression and the presence of pain, proptosis, hemorrhage, fever, or inflammation. Figure 12-1 is a flowchart that can be used to narrow the differential diagnosis for the child who presents with signs and symptoms of orbital swelling or inflammation. Pathologic entities to be considered under each of these categories are listed below.

A. Infectious disorders
   1. Preseptal cellulitis
   2. Orbital cellulitis
      a. With orbital or subperiosteal orbital abscess
   3. Mucormycosis (see adult disorders)
B. Inflammatory disorders
   1. Orbital pseudotumor
   2. Tolosa-Hunt syndrome
C. Ischemic disorder
   1. Sickle cell disease
D. Hamartomas
   1. Capillary hemangioma
   2. Lymphangioma
   3. Neurofibroma
   4. Neurilemoma (see adult disorders)
E. Choristomas
   1. Dermoid cyst
   2. Epidermoid cyst
   3. Lipodermoid
   4. Teratoma
F. Malignant neoplasms
   1. Rhabdomyosarcoma
   2. Metastatic neuroblastoma
   3. Acute leukemia
      a. Lymphoblastic leukemia
      b. Granulocytic sarcoma (chloroma)
   4. Burkitt's lymphoma
   5. Eosinophilic granuloma
   6. Optic nerve glioma
   7. Optic nerve sheath meningioma
   8. Other primary sarcoma

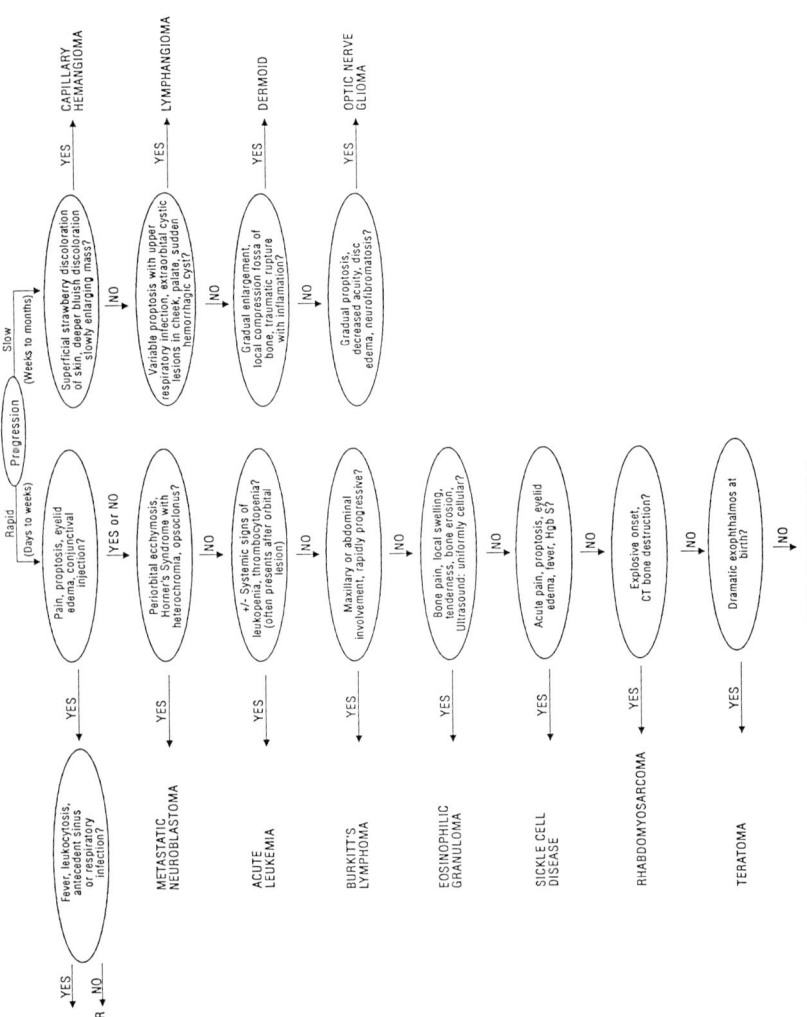

FIGURE 12–1. Flowchart for nontraumatic orbital disorders in children.

G. Encephaloceles
   1. Nasal
   2. Sphenoid wing
H. Pseudoproptosis
   1. Enlarged globe (myopia, congenital glaucoma)
   2. Cranial nerve palsy
   3. Asymmetric palpebral fissures
   4. Asymmetric orbital size
   5. Orbital floor fracture of other eye (see Chapter 5)
   6. Horner's syndrome of other eye (see Chapter 13)

Infectious Disorders

An infectious process that has not penetrated deeper than the orbital septum is called *preseptal cellulitis.* The modifier *preseptal* indicates that the process involves only the subcutaneous tissue of the eyelid, brow, or forehead. Involvement deeper than the orbital septum is called *orbital cellulitis.* The latter is the most common cause of sudden proptosis in a child. Cellulitis is heralded by conjunctival chemosis, decreased ocular motility, reduced visual acuity, pain on ocular movement, and proptosis (Figure 12–2). Fever, leukocytosis, lid

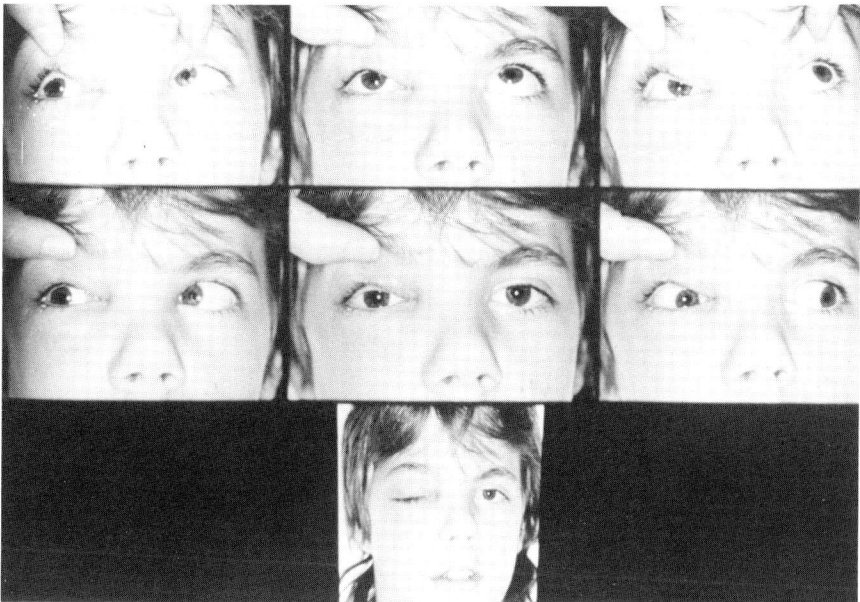

FIGURE 12-2. Orbital cellulitis right eye. Erythema and edema with decreased ocular motility, especially in upward gaze. (From: Nelson LB, Catalano RA: *Atlas of Ocular Motility.* Philadelphia, WB Saunders Co, p 201, with permission.)

edema, and rhinorrhea are also usually present. Table 12–1 differentiates the clinical findings in preseptal and orbital cellulitis.

The pathogen in *preseptal cellulitis* is usually *Staphylococcus aureus* (especially in traumatic cases) or *Streptococcus pyogenes* or *pneumoniae*. Anaerobic infections, particularly clostridia and bacillus, can occur with dirty wounds. If purulent material is present, it should be cultured and fluctuant abscesses drained. A 48-hour to 72-hour course of a penicillinase-resistant oral penicillin or cephalosporin (Augmentin, cefuroxime) is generally acceptable in older children and adults with preseptal cellulitis. If signs of orbital cellulitis develop or if the infection does not respond to oral antibiotics, hospitalization and intravenous therapy are usually indicated. Most clinicians suggest hospitalization for all children under age 5 years because of the possibility of *Hemophilus influenza* infection.

Children with *H. influenza* infection present with markedly swollen, violaceous eyelids, irritability, and coryza. They may have high fever, leukocytosis, or positive blood cultures. The presence of any of these is not useful in differentiating *H. influenza* preseptal from orbital cellulitis. Rapid treatment is necessary because bacteremia, meningitis, epiglottitis, and pneumonia can develop quickly. *H. influenza* coverage is obtained with cefuroxime. Strains resistant to ampicillin are common, and chloramphenicol is generally avoided in children because it can suppress the bone marrow.

Orbital cellulitis usually results from the spread of infection in the paranasal sinuses; in children, the ethmoid is the most commonly involved sinus. Additional precipitants include puncture wounds deep to the orbital septum, surgical trauma, acute dacryocystitis (infection of the lacrimal sac), extension from intracranial or dental infections, and endogenous bacteremias. *H. influenza* type B is the most common bacteremic cause of cellulitis in children. Uncontrolled orbital cellulitis can lead to damage to the ocular blood supply

TABLE 12–1. DIFFERENTIAL CLINICAL FINDINGS IN PRESEPTAL AND ORBITAL CELLULITIS

SIGN OR SYMPTOM	PRESEPTAL CELLULITIS	ORBITAL CELLULITIS*
Proptosis	Absent	Marked
Motility	Normal	Restricted
Ocular pain	Absent	Present
Visual acuity	Normal	May be reduced
Fever	Absent or minimal	High
Leukocytosis	Absent to moderate	Marked
Lid swelling	Mild to marked	Marked
Chemosis	Absent to moderate	Marked
Sensation over V1, V2	Normal	May be reduced
Mean age	2 years	7–9 years

*With the progressive and combined involvement of multiple cranial nerves, the pupil, disc edema, congestion of retinal veins, infarction of the retina or choroid, and bilaterality, consider cavernous sinus thrombosis.

and infarction of the retina and choroid, cavernous sinus extension and thrombosis, orbital apex syndrome, and intracranial abscess. Orbital or subperiosteal orbital abscesses can result; the former are suggested by the lack of response to adequate antibiotic therapy.

Material for Gram's stain and culture is difficult to obtain in deep orbital cellulitis. Occasionally culturable purulent material is present on the nasal or nasopharyngeal mucosa. Urine antigen studies, which identify fractions of the infecting organism's cell wall polysaccharides, excreted in the patient's urine, may be helpful if available. Chest and paranasal sinus X rays may reveal the source of infection, but the sinuses are not well developed in young children, and in this population sinus X rays are not generally helpful. Computed tomography (CT) images the extent of orbital involvement and the presence of orbital abscesses. CT is also useful in distinguishing tumor-simulating cellulitis, particularly rhabdomyosarcoma and neuroblastoma in children. Bone destruction would suggest the latter. The CT criteria to distinguish subperiosteal abscesses from reactive inflammatory edema, however, are not well established.

The pathogens in orbital cellulitis are the same as in preseptal cellulitis, with the addition of *Pseudomonas auerginosa, Escherichia coli, Bacteroides,* and *Peptococcus.* The latter two are more commonly seen after human or animal bites. Intravenous nafcillin and chloramphenicol are the drugs of choice pending culture results; in children under age 5 years, cefuroxime 100 mg/kg to 150 mg/kg per day intravenously (IV) in three doses, for up to 2 weeks, is used to cover *Hemophilus.* Nafcillin, cephalosporin, or vancomycin is the treatment of choice if gram-positive cocci are found. For human or animal bites or other possible anaerobic infections, penicillin G, cefuroxime, or chloramphenicol (100 mg/kg per day in four divided doses) is recommended. Ceftazidine (150 mg/kg per day in four divided doses) is useful against gram-negative bacteria. Sinus decongestants, either topically or systemically, should also be considered. Oral antibiotics should not be used as the initial treatment of orbital cellulitis. After an appropriate course of intravenous therapy, dictated by clinical findings, outpatient treatment with oral cloxacillin or cefaclor (for minor staphylococcal or streptococcal infections) or Augmentin 40 mg/kg per day in three doses (for nonresistant strains of *H. influenza*) can be instituted. Generally, antibiotic treatment should continue for 5 days to 7 days or until there is complete clinical resolution; streptococcal infections require a minimum of 10 days of treatment.

The presence of an orbital abscess, suspected by lack of improvement and corroborated by CT, is an indication for surgical drainage. Surgical treatment of a subperiosteal orbital abscess (SOA) in children, however, remains controversial. Several recent reports have documented CT evidence of an SOA that was not found at surgery and have suggested that SOA in children may be successfully managed with medical treatment alone. We suggest that the management of a suspected SOA in children be based principally on clinical signs.

Clinical findings should govern whether surgical intervention in children with radiographically detected subperiosteal masses is indicated. CT scanning can be useful in preventing surgical intervention in patients who clearly show no radiographic signs of SOA, and scanning should be performed when there is evidence of clinical deterioration to delineate the extent of disease. Ultrasound may be of value in differentiating an abscess if it demonstrates a low reflective space between the high spikes of the dense periorbital and the bony wall. Ultrasound is of less value, however, when the SOA is located posteriorly.

Inflammatory Disorders

Children as young as age 3 years and adults can be afflicted with an idiopathic inflammation of the orbit called *orbital pseudotumor*. Patients with this disorder present with lid erythema and swelling, ptosis, and an S-shaped deformity of the upper eyelid, restricted eye movements, orbital pain, proptosis, conjunctival chemosis and vascular congestion, and reduced corneal sensitivity (Figure 12-3). One-third of children with pseudotumor present with bilateral involvement, and only rarely in children is there an associated systemic disorder. In contrast, bilateral involvement in adults suggests a systemic vasculitis or lymphoproliferative disorder.

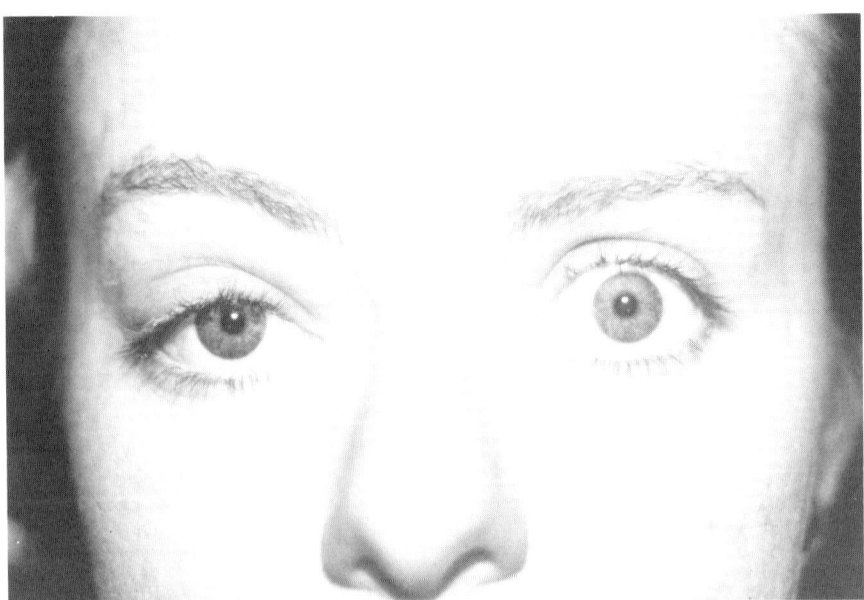

FIGURE 12-3. Orbital pseudotumor, right orbit. Note S-shaped curve to upper eyelid.

Nearly half of the children with pseudotumor have headache, abdominal discomfort, fever, and lethargy. Eosinophilia, an elevated erythrocyte sedimentation rate, antinuclear antibodies, and mild spinal fluid pleocytosis are occasionally found. The absence of marked leukocytosis and a left shift helps differentiate this condition from bacterial orbital cellulitis. Children with pseudotumor may also have papillitis or iridocyclitis. The latter are not usually seen in adults.

In both children and adults, pseudotumor variants include myositis (principal involvement of extraocular muscle[s]), sclerotenonitis (sclera and Tenon's capsule), dacryoadenitis (lacrimal gland), or papillitis (dural sheath of the optic nerve). Of these, myositis and dacryoadenitis are the most common forms encountered in children. The *Tolosa-Hunt syndrome* is another variant, in which inflammation primarily occurs around the superior orbital fissure and optic canal. Involvement of this area results in restriction of ocular movements and reduction of visual acuity.

Clinical, CT, and ultrasound findings are often sufficiently characteristic to exclude the need for biopsy prior to treatment. CT may demonstrate infiltration within the retrobulbar fat and thickening of the extraocular muscles if a myositic component is present and/or contrast enhancement of the sclera (ring sign) if sclerotenonitis is present (Figure 12-4). In contrast to thyroid ophthalmopathy (see Figure 12-16) both the extraocular muscle and tendon are thickened in pseudotumor, whereas the muscle insertions are spared in thyroid disease. Neoplastic involvement of an extraocular muscle usually produces more focal, globular enlargement. B-scan ultrasonography can demonstrate an acoustically hollow, edematous Tenon's capsule in sclerotenonitis and thickened extraocular muscles if myositis is present. Biopsy findings include patchy infiltrates of lymphocytes, plasma cells, and eosinophils (especially in children) and lymphoid hyperplasia embedded in a loose, fibrous stroma. Scarring (sclerosing pseudotumor) is a late finding.

The treatment of pseudotumor consists of systemic corticosteroids. The initial dose is 1.0 mg/kg to 1.5 mg/kg; in adults, the dose does not usually exceed 60 mg to 80 mg of Prednisone per day. The use of intravenous corticosteroids is generally not needed, but topical steroids will alleviate iridocyclitis if it is present. Acute cases should respond rapidly, but recurrences can occur if steroids are tapered too rapidly. If systemic steroids do not result in a rapid improvement, a biopsy is indicated. If the biopsy confirms pseudotumor, treatment can continue with corticosteroids, orbital irradiation, and/or cyclophosphamide.

Ischemic Disorder

Acute orbital pain, proptosis, eyelid edema and fever can occur in *sickle cell disease* with sickling crises. Orbital bones become infarcted with secondary

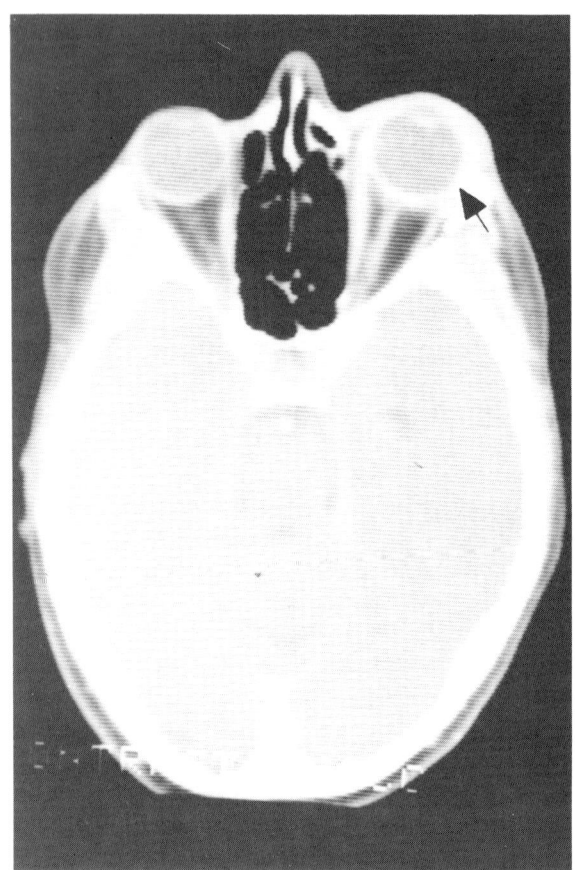

FIGURE 12-4. Scleral enhancement (ring sign = arrow) in pseudotumor of right eye.

inflammation. The disorder is differentiated from osteomyelitis with subperiosteal abscess by the decreased uptake of radionucleotides in sickle cell infarction but increased uptake in infection. Furthermore, subperiosteal abscesses are more likely to occur adjacent to an opacified sinus.

Hamartomas

A *hamartoma* is a tumor arising from tissue components normally present at the involved site. *Choristomas* contain tissue elements not normally found at the site. Capillary hemangiomas and neurofibromas are classic examples of hamartomas; choristomas include dermoid cysts and teratomas. Debate continues as to whether lymphangiomas are hamartomas or choristomas.

Capillary hemangiomas are usually first noted between birth and age 6 weeks. They grow rapidly during the first 6 months of life and may double in size in days to weeks. The surfaces of superficial lesions are elevated, red, and irregularly dimpled, hence the name *strawberry nevus* (Figure 12-5). Unlike port wine stains, hemangiomas blanch with pressure. Deeper tumors are more bluish. Hemangiomas can occur in the eyelid, the orbit, or in both locations. Eyelid lesions are more common, and isolated orbital tumors may be difficult to diagnose with certainty. The most common respective sites of involvement are the medial upper eyelid and superior nasal quadrant of the orbit. Additional hemangiomas are present in one-fourth of affected children, especially on the scalp, neck, face, or shoulders. CT may be useful if the diagnosis is uncertain. Because of the propensity of encephaloceles and rhabdomyosarcomas to involve the superior nasal quadrant, CT scanning is advised prior to treating an orbital hemangioma in this area. A homogeneous mass, with possible orbital expansion but without bony clefts or destruction, is characteristic of an orbital hemangioma. Contrast enhancement is not useful because malignant tumors also enhance. A-scan ultrasonography demonstrates high-amplitude spikes from vessel lumen/cellular interfaces, in contrast to low-amplitude spikes seen in densely cellular rhabdomyosarcomas.

Hemangiomas gradually involute during childhood. Small eyelid tumors can, however, induce astigmatism and anisometropic amblyopia, and large

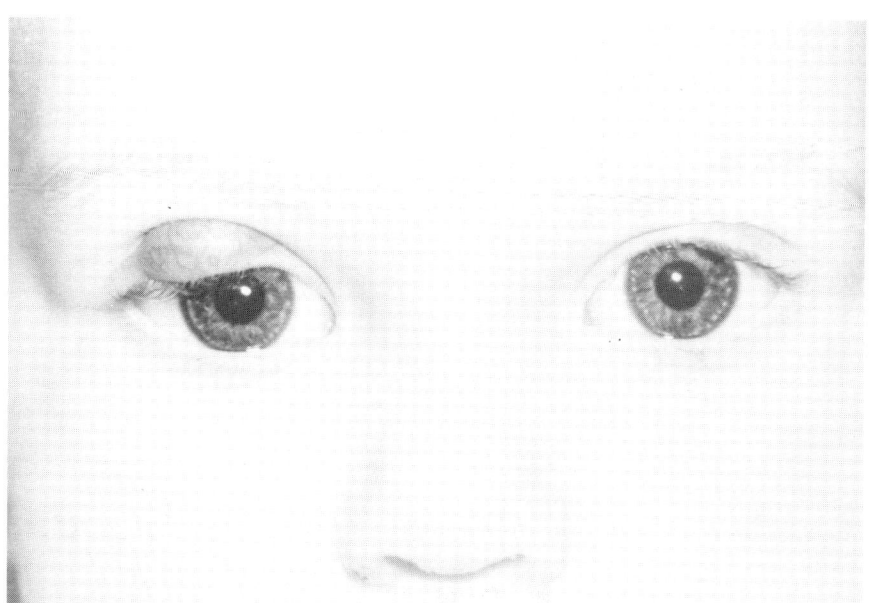

FIGURE 12-5. Capillary hemangioma, right upper eyelid.

tumors can cause occlusion amblyopia. Patching therapy and glasses to correct an induced astigmatism may be necessary. Intralesional steroids may also be necessary. The tumor mass is injected at several different sites with up to 40 mg of triamcinolone (prolonged acting) and 6 mg of an equal mixture of betamethasone sodium phosphate and betamethasone acetate (rapidly acting), using a 27-gauge needle. Because epinephrine can potentially enhance the action of the steroid, lidocaine hydrochloride 1% with 1:1,000,000 epinephrine is often used as the dilutant for the steroid. Orbital hemangiomas that cause proptosis or globe displacement may also have to be treated. Deep orbital injections carry increased risks of hemorrhage and retinal artery embolus of steroid. Other options include systemic steroids (2 mg/kg per day or 4 mg/kg on alternate days), ortho-voltage radiotherapy (single treatment of 200 rads), and surgical resection. Pediatric consultation is advised.

The lymphatic (or vascular) channels that comprise *lymphangiomas* are likely present at birth, but the tumor usually becomes apparent only after an acute hemorrhagic episode, during the first decade of life (see Figure 12–19). Interstitial capillaries hemorrhage, leading to acute proptosis and the formation of loculated "chocolate cysts," containing old, dark blood. There may be a history of variable proptosis related to upper respiratory infections and reactive hyperplasia of lymphoid tissue present in the tumor. Lesions can be found in the conjunctiva, eyelids, orbit, facial sinuses, or palate. CT may demonstrate expansion of the orbit without bone destruction and a multilobed mass. Ultrasound will show very low internal reflectivity, except when clots are present.

Lymphangiomas usually stabilize in size by the third decade. Spontaneous regression can occur but not as characteristically as capillary hemangiomas. Unless massive proptosis and optic nerve compression occur, hemorrhagic cysts are treated conservatively. Uninvolved portions of a hemorrhagic lymphangioma should not be evacuated because of the risk of greater hemorrhage. Bovie electrocautery or carbon dioxide laser surgery may prevent this complication. Occasionally orbital decompression is necessary for cosmetic or functional treatment.

Neurofibromas are tumors composed of proliferating Schwann cells, axons, endoneural fibroblasts, and mucin. They are encountered in the von Recklinghausen form of neurofibromatosis (NF1). They may be discreet and nodular or diffuse and plexiform. Plexiform neurofibromas of the upper eyelid can cause an S-shaped deformity to the lid (Figure 12–6). They have a texture similar to a bag of worms and are associated with a higher incidence of congenital glaucoma.

Plexiform orbital neurofibromas are enclosed within a perineural sheath. Similar to plexiform neurofibromas of the eyelid, they are more likely to be associated with neurofibromatosis and present during the first decade of life. Because the lesions are diffuse, enveloping the optic nerve, extraocular muscles, and lacrimal gland, their surgical removal is difficult. These tumors frequently coexist with bony orbital defects, particularly of the sphenoid bone. When associated with neurofibromatosis, malignant transformation can occur

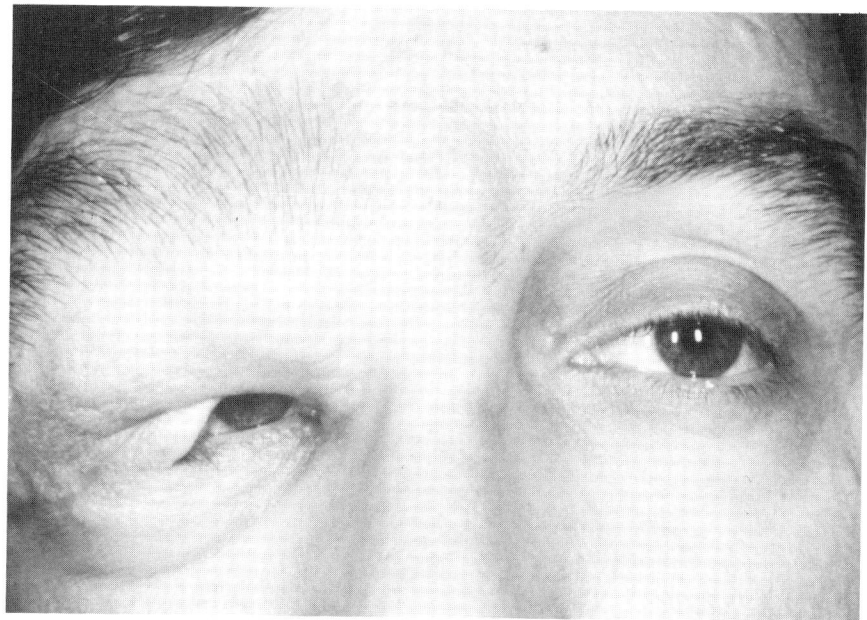

FIGURE 12-6. Plexiform neurofibroma, right upper eyelid, in a patient with neurofibromatosis. (Courtesy Dale R. Meyer, M.D.)

in up to 10% of cases. *Neurilemomas (schwannomas)* are composed only of Schwann cells. Like neurofibromas, they can be associated with neurofibromatosis (presenting at a younger age) or unassociated (presenting in middle age). Unlike neurofibromas, neurilemomas rarely, if ever, undergo malignant transformation. When not associated with neurofibromatosis, *orbital neurofibromas* and *neurilemomas* are easier to excise surgically and less likely to recur. Because these variants usually develop in early to middle adulthood, they are discussed under adult disorders.

Choristomas

Dermoid cysts arise from dermal elements and *epidermoid cysts* from epidermal elements that get pinched off at suture lines during embryonic development. Dermoid cysts are lined by keratinizing epithelium and contain components of dermal appendages, such as hair, teeth, and sebaceous and sweat glands, in the cyst wall. Epidermoid cysts are lined by epidermis only. They are usually filled with keratin and do not contain dermal elements. Half of the cysts that present in childhood are located anterior to the orbital septum, in the lateral brow and upper eyelid, adjacent to the zygomaticofrontal suture (Figure 12-7). Twenty-five percent of cysts occur at the nasofrontal suture. These need

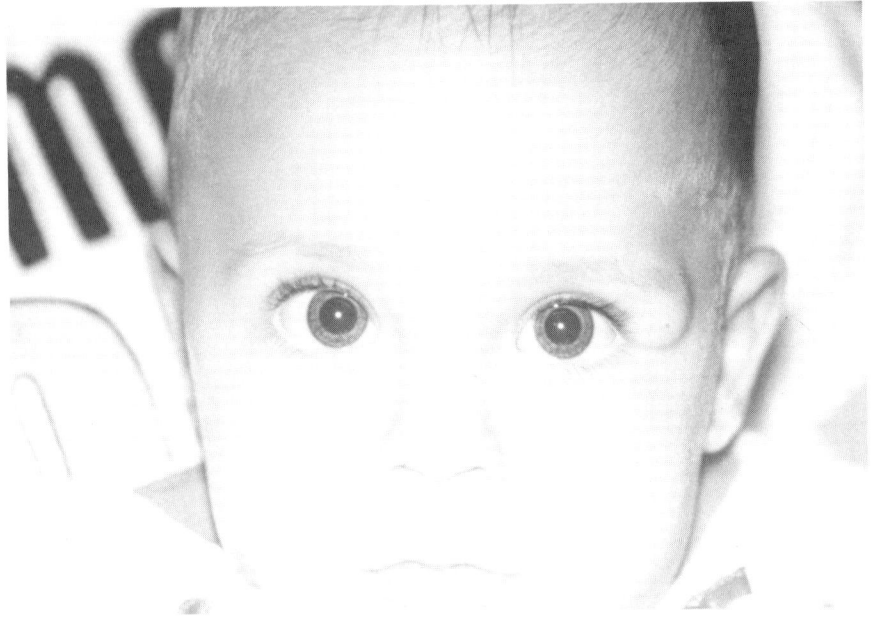

FIGURE 12-7.   Dermoid cyst, left orbit.

to be distinguished from capillary hemangiomas and orbital encephaloceles. A bony defect and herniation of brain tissue on radiologic studies is characteristic of the latter. Cysts that present in adulthood are usually located posterior to the orbital septum.

Dermoid and epidermoid cysts are smooth, oval, and painless to palpation. They slowly enlarge and are freely movable. Because bony structures are under pressure from the cyst, well-corticated osseous depressions can occur. Usually no palpable bony defect is felt, but bony dehiscences can occur and can enlarge with time. This is particularly true of posteriorly located dermoids. If the entire extent of the cyst cannot be palpated, radiologic studies are indicated to rule out a dumbbell-shaped cyst with possible dural exposure at surgery or an encephalocele. Traumatic rupture of the cyst can lead to an acute inflammatory process, resembling orbital cellulitis or pseudotumor; surgical excision through the upper eyelid crease is therefore generally suggested. Rarely, patients with orbital dermoids may present with spontaneous draining fistulas. Fistulas usually result after incomplete removal.

Lipodermoids are solid fat-containing tumors, usually located over the lateral surface of the globe beneath the conjunctiva (Figure 12-8). They may extend deep toward the muscle cone, lacrimal gland, or levator muscle. Restrictive strabismus can result from incomplete removal and the development of an extraocular muscle adhesion syndrome. Resection can also damage lacrimal gland ducts. Lipodermoids are therefore best left alone unless cosmetically dis-

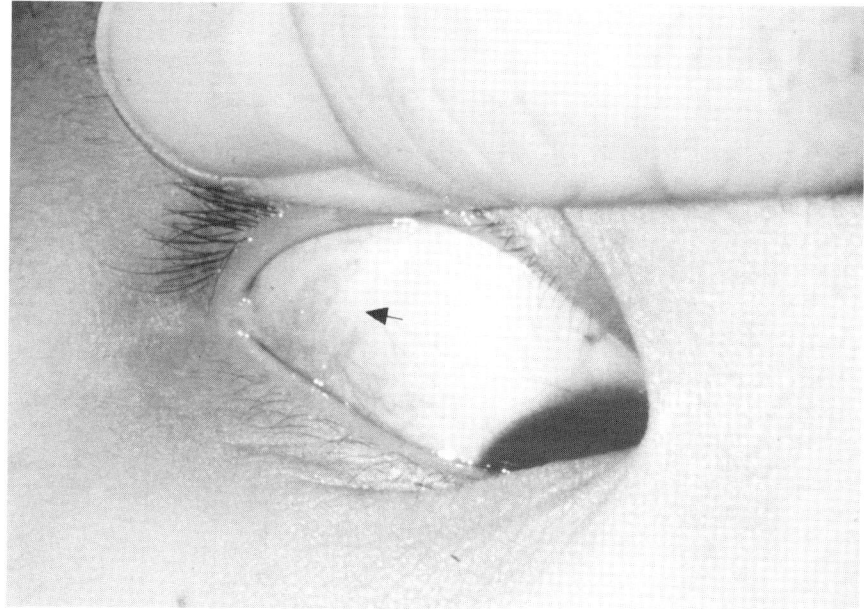

FIGURE 12-8. Lipodermoid, right eye (arrow).

figuring. Lipodermoids are present from a young age; simulating lesions presenting in adulthood include prolapsed orbital fat, prolapsed palpebral lobe of the lacrimal gland, and lymphomas.

Teratomas are rare tumors that often present at birth with marked proptosis and disfigurement. Histologically, they are composed of tissue elements from two or more germinal layers. They are usually cystic and often contain intracranial contents. An enlarged orbit and zygomaticofrontal suture separation are seen on X ray. Some teratomas can be removed without exenteration, preserving ocular function.

Malignant Neoplasms

Rhabdomyosarcoma is the most common primary orbital malignancy in childhood. It most commonly originates in the superior nasal orbit and causes a rapid (days to weeks) downward and outward displacement of the globe (Figure 12-9). It may be present at birth but more commonly develops during the latter part of the first decade. A marked adnexal response with lid edema and discoloration is usually concomitant. Sinus extension can result in nasal stuffiness and nosebleeds. A history of antecedent trauma is not unusual, often causing a delay in diagnosis.

If the mass is in the superior nasal quadrant, it may be palpable. CT scanning

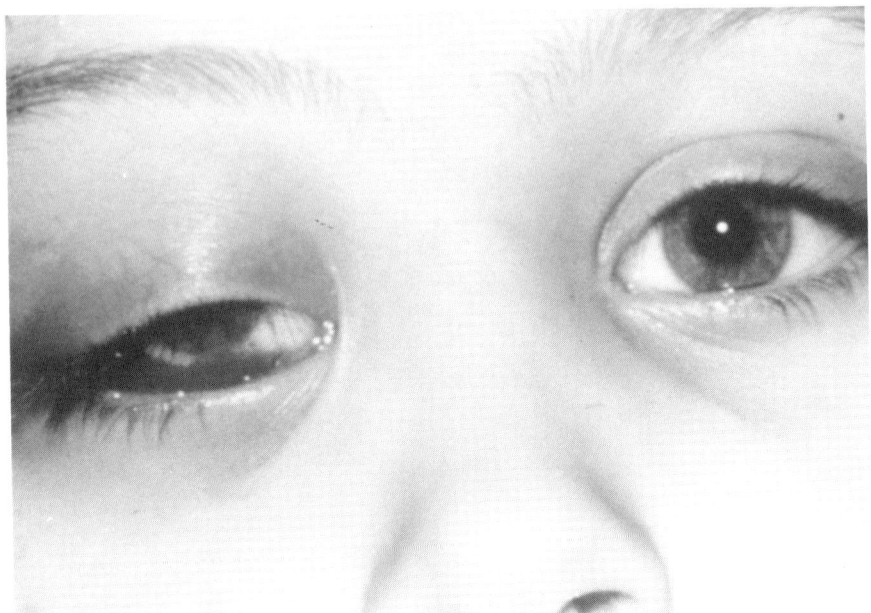

FIGURE 12-9. Rhabdomyosarcoma, superior right orbit, displacing globe inferiorly. (Courtesy Dale R. Meyer, M.D.)

will demonstrate bone destruction in advanced cases; ultrasonography (echography) findings include a relatively well-circumscribed mass with low to moderate internal reflections. Biopsy is needed for diagnosis. A transconjunctival or eyelid incision is recommended to prevent tumor seeding along the biopsy tract. The periosteum also presents a relative barrier and should not be violated. Spindle-shaped cells with prominent cross-striations and "tadpole" cells with tapered cytoplasmic processes are hallmarks of the tumor in tissue biopsies. Because these findings may be present only in more differentiated tumors, electron microscopy may be necessary. This requires glutaraldehyde fixation of fresh biopsy specimens.

Upon diagnosis, complete evaluation requires bone marrow biopsy, complete blood count, liver function tests, bone scanning chest X ray, and lumbar puncture to search for distant metastases. Therapy is based on guidelines established by the Intergroup Rhabdomyosarcoma Study. Local radiation of 4500 to 6000 rads is given over 6 weeks, combined with systemic chemotherapy (Vincristine, Adriamycin, and Cyclophosphamide). Extraorbital extension decreases 3-year survival from 90% to 30%.

Neuroblastoma is the most common metastatic orbital tumor in children. It usually originates in the adrenal medulla or an adjacent retroperitoneal site but can arise in the neck or mediastinum. It generally presents in children between age 18 and 36 months but can present at birth or as late as the mid-teens.

Ophthalmologic findings occur in 20% of cases, and in nearly half of these patients, orbital findings were the presenting complaint. The classic finding is periorbital ecchymosis. It occurs when the rapidly growing tumor outgrows its blood supply, causing hemorrhagic necrosis (Figure 12-10). Proptosis can also occur. Orbital presentations generally signify disseminated disease and herald a poor prognosis. Additional ocular findings include Horner's syndrome (with heterochromia), from involvement of the cervical sympathetic ganglia, and opsoclonus (chaotic, bilateral, back to back, rapid movements of the eyes in various directions). The latter is a paraneoplastic sign.

Diagnostic studies include urinalysis for catecholamine metabolites and CT of the orbit to determine metastatic extent and of the abdomen or thorax to demonstrate the primary tumor. Biopsy is required for definitive diagnosis, and specimens should be fixed in formalin for light microscopy and glutaraldehyde for electron microscopy. The latter may demonstrate neurosecretory granules

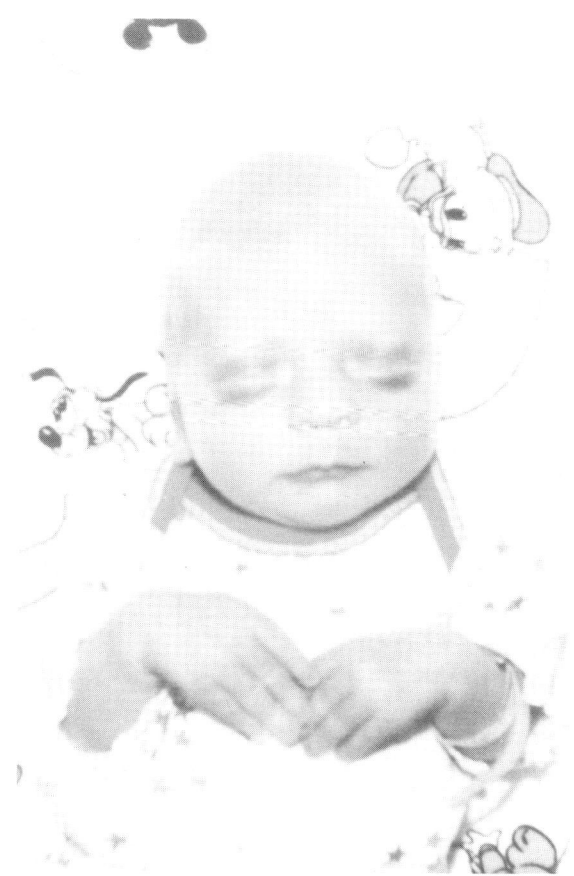

FIGURE 12-10. Periorbital ecchymosis in metastatic neuroblastoma.

containing catecholamines. Homer-Wright pseudorosettes are rarely found in orbital metastases. Management includes surgical excision, radiation and chemotherapy, and autologous bone marrow transplantation.

The most common malignancy in childhood is *acute leukemia,* especially lymphoblastic leukemia. Almost all intraocular involvement and most orbital involvement is secondary to this type. Although less common, myelogenous leukemia disproportionately involves the orbit. A rare form called *granulocytic sarcoma* or *chloroma* may present months in advance of blood or bone marrow signs of leukemia. It may present bilaterally in up to 50% of cases. Diagnosis is made using the Leder stain, which demonstrates cytoplasmic esterase in cells obtained at biopsy. Electron microscopy may also reveal early granule formation. In this disorder, chemotherapy is more effective if it can be instituted prior to the development of the leukemic phase.

Orbital involvement in acute leukemia results in proptosis secondary to acute hemorrhage or leukemic infiltration. Imaging studies are usually nonspecific, and biopsy is necessary for diagnosis. Treatment may involve radiation, systemic, and intrathecal chemotherapy.

Burkitt's lymphoma is endemic in East Africa, where it accounts for the majority of pediatric orbital tumors. It is rare but not unheard of in North America. It presents between ages 3 and 15 years (mean 7 years) with unilateral or bilateral proptosis or extranodal masses in the maxilla, mandible, or abdominal viscera. Its progression may be explosive, with a doubling time of only 24 hours. Histologically, the tumor demonstrates a "starry-sky" pattern due to the presence of large histiocytes interspersed among homogeneous neoplastic lymphocytes.

Eosinophilic granuloma (Langerhans cell granulomatosis) is a relatively benign and probably reactive lesion composed of histiocytes and mature eosinophils. It is the subset of histiocytosis X, which most commonly involves the orbit. It usually involves the superior temporal quadrant and occurs as a solitary lesion within bone rather than a systemic disorder. Symptoms include localized bone pain, tenderness, and swelling. Radiologic studies demonstrate bone erosion similar to that which can occur with lacrimal tumors. Ultrasonography, however, demonstrates its uniformly cellular nature, and electron microscopy reveals Langerhans or Birbeck granules in biopsy specimens. Treatment of an eosinophilic granuloma includes intralesion steroids, low-dose radiation, and surgical excision.

Other histiocytic tumors (Letterer-Siwe and Hand-Schuller-Christian disease) can also produce proptosis. In addition, they usually also cause lytic skull lesions, visceral abnormalities, and/or diabetes insipidus from encroachment of hypothalamus and pituitary gland. They should be excluded by bone scans, liver function tests, and a 24-hour urine collection after water deprivation.

Optic nerve gliomas occur predominantly in children during the first decade of life. The associated incidence of neurofibromatosis varies between 12% to 40%. Clinically, they present as gradual, painless proptosis with loss of vision and an afferent pupillary defect (Figure 12-10). Depending on the stage when diagnosed, disk edema or optic atrophy may be seen; strabismus due to ocular displacement can also occur. If the chiasm is involved (50% of cases), pituitary dysfunction and signs of increased intracranial pressure may be present. Intracranial involvement is suggested by nystagmus, headache, vomiting, or seizures.

In children the tumor is almost always a benign juvenile pilocytic (hairlike) astrocytoma, but some tumors progress. Tumors in patients with neurofibromatosis proliferate within the subarachnoid space, whereas tumors in patients without neurofibromatosis do not usually invade the dura. Plain X rays and tomography will demonstrate enlargement of the optic foramen (Figure 12-11); CT scan shows a fusiform enlargement of the nerve. MRI scanning, however, best demonstrates the extent of intracranial involvement. Treatment of optic nerve gliomas is controversial. Some clinicians suggest surgical excision if the tumor is growing rapidly, if the affected eye is blind and there is corneal exposure and disfigurement, or if a mass effect by the tumor causes increased intracranial pressure. Radiation therapy can be used for nonresectable tumors involving the chiasm and optic radiations.

Orbital *meningiomas* occur more frequently in the second through fifth decades and are discussed under adult disorders. Those that occur in childhood are more aggressive than those occurring in adulthood. Similar to optic nerve gliomas, there is a higher than expected incidence in patients with neurofibromatosis.

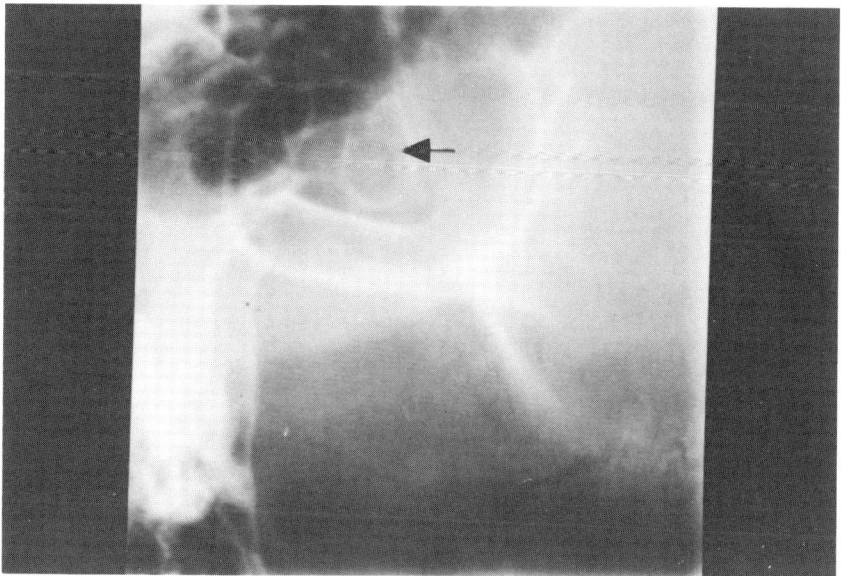

FIGURE 12-11. Enlargement of the optic foramen (arrow) in optic nerve glioma.

Sarcomas other than rhabdomyosarcoma can also present with a relatively abrupt onset of proptosis. Included are alveolar soft-part sarcomas and liposarcomas. Prompt biopsy and treatment is imperative.

Encephaloceles

Congenital facial clefts usually involve the orbit and/or maxilla. Clefts involving orbital bones can result in the herniation of meninges (meningocele), brain tissue (encephalocele), or both (meningoencephalocele). Most commonly, these present as a subcutaneous mass near the medial canthus, over the bridge of the nose (Figure 12-12). Straining or crying may increase the size of the mass, and the globe may be displaced. The differential includes an orbital capillary hemangioma.

Dysplasia of orbital bones can occur in neurofibromatosis. Hypoplasia of both the greater and lesser wing of the sphenoid, with elevation of the lesser wing, widening of the superior orbital fissure, and herniation of the temporal lobe into the orbit, can occur (Figure 12-13). Transmission of the cerebrospinal fluid pulsation can result in a pulsatile exophthalmos, in concert with the radial pulse. Orbital neurofibromas are often associated with these bony defects.

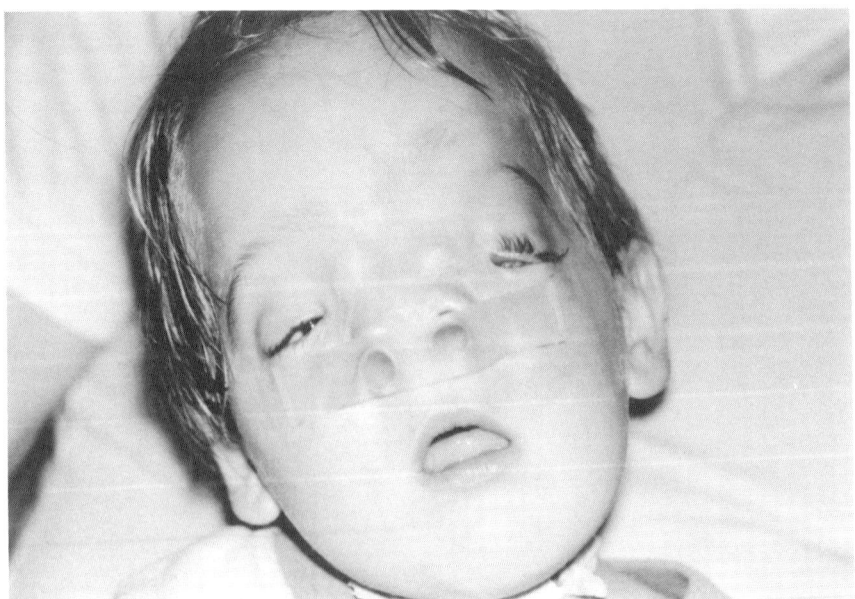

FIGURE 12-12. Nasal encephalocele in child undergoing facial reconstruction.

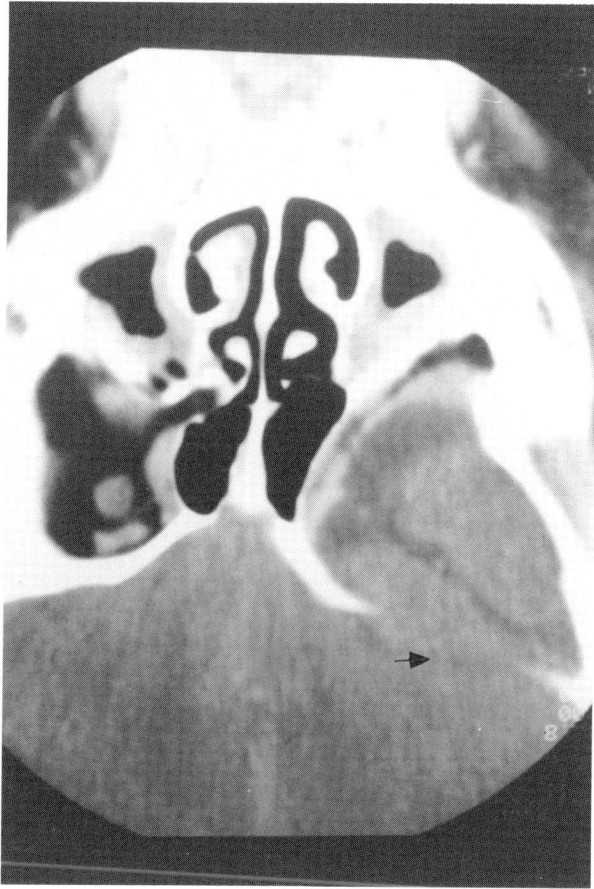

FIGURE 12-13. Sphenoid wing dysplasia and herniation of brain tissue into the orbit in a child with neurofibromatosis.

NONTRAUMATIC ORBITAL DISORDERS IN ADULTS

Similar to disorders in children, orbital disorders in adults should be evaluated with regard to their rate of progression, and the presence of pain, proptosis, or hemorrhage (Figure 12-14) can be used to narrow the differential diagnosis for the adult who presents with signs and symptoms of orbital swelling or inflammation. Entities to be discussed under each of these categories are listed below.

A. Thyroid ophthalmopathy
B. Infectious disorders
   1. Preseptal cellulitis (see childhood disorders)

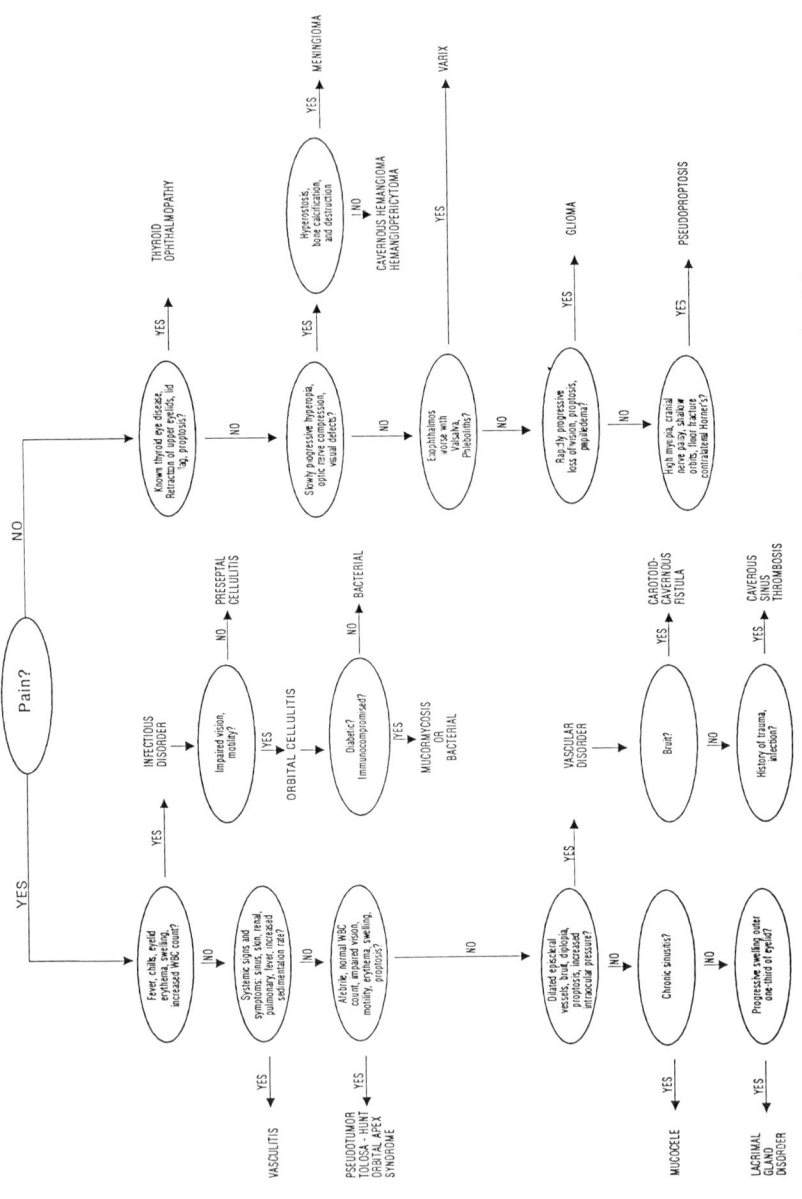

FIGURE 12–14. Flowchart for nontraumatic orbital disorders in adults.

    2. Orbital cellulitis (see childhood disorders)
    3. Mucormycosis
    4. Aspergillosis
    5. Mucopyocele (an infected mucocele; see below)
C. Inflammatory disorders (see childhood disorders)
    1. Orbital pseudotumor
    2. Tolosa-Hunt syndrome
D. Orbital vasculitis
    1. Polyarteritis nodosa
    2. Wegener's granulomatosis
    3. Lethal midline granuloma
E. Vascular disorders other than vasculitis
    1. Spontaneous orbital hemorrhage
    2. Orbital varix
    3. Carotid-cavernous fistula (see also Chapter 13)
    4. Cavernous sinus thrombosis (see also Chapter 13)
F. Orbital tumors
    1. Dermoid (see childhood disorders)
    2. Cavernous hemangioma
    3. Hemangiopericytoma
    4. Lymphoid tumors
    5. Neurofibroma
    6. Neurilemoma
    7. Optic nerve glioma
    8. Meningioma
    9. Fibrous histiocytoma and mesenchymal sarcomas
   10. Metastatic tumors
   11. Tumors of the lacrimal gland (see below)
G. Lacrimal gland disorders
    1. Benign mixed epithelial tumor
    2. Malignant mixed epithelial tumor
    3. Adenoid cystic carcinoma
    4. Lymphoid tumor
    5. Sarcoidosis
    6. Acute dacryoadenitis
    7. Chronic dacryoadenitis
H. Fibrous dysplasia
I. Mucoceles
J. Pseudoproptosis (see childhood disorders)

Thyroid Ophthalmopathy

Thyroid ophthalmopathy (orbitopathy) is the most common cause of both unilateral and bilateral exophthalmos in adults. It usually presents between age

20 years and age 45 years; women are affected eight times more often than men. Thyroid eye disease may precede, follow, or occur concomitant with hyperthyroidism. A history of weight loss, palpitations, tremor, sweating, heat intolerance, and hair or skin changes suggests hyperthyroidism. Some patients, however, may never develop clinical or laboratory evidence of thyroid dysfunction. Furthermore, thyroid function studies do not correlate with the level of activity of thyroid orbitopathy.

Eyelid signs include upper or lower eyelid retraction (Dalrymple sign), upper eyelid lag on downward gaze (von Graefe sign), lower eyelid lag on upward gaze, tremor of the lids on gentle closure, infrequent and incomplete blinking, and eyelid edema. Additional signs include restriction of ocular motility (the inferior rectus muscle is usually the first affected muscle, followed by the medial rectus) and vascular congestion of the conjunctiva (especially over the insertion of the lateral rectus muscle; Figure 12–15). All of the extraocular muscles may become involved, resulting in bizarre ocular motility patterns, simulating myasthenia gravis, multiple cranial nerve palsies, or chronic progressive external ophthalmoplegia. An additional diagnostic sign is elevation of intraocular pressure on upward gaze, secondary to inferior rectus restriction. Forced duction testing will also be positive for mechanical restriction.

In contrast to many acute orbital syndromes, pain is not an early sign. Vision can be threatened by corneal exposure and drying (secondary to eyelid retrac-

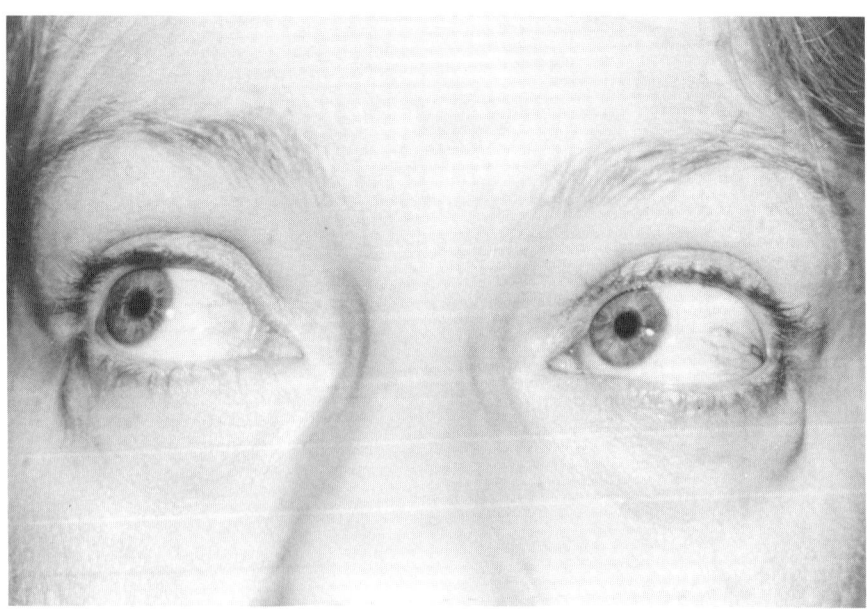

FIGURE 12–15. Vascular congestion of conjunctiva over horizontal rectus muscles in thyroid ophthalmopathy.

tion and exophthalmos) or optic nerve compression (due to thickened muscles in the orbital apex). These are also usually late findings. Corneal decompensation can lead to corneal ulceration and perforation. The active stage of thyroid orbitopathy lasts only months to years; soft tissue changes, however, do not readily regress.

The diagnosis of thyroid orbitopathy is usually made clinically. Laboratory testing is usually performed to determine if the patient is also hyperthyroid (Table 12-2). CT can demonstrate enlarged extraocular muscles with sparing of the extraocular tendons (Figures 12-16 and 12-17). This can also be demonstrated with ultrasonography. Coronal sections are especially useful in diagnosing optic nerve compression in the orbital apex. Because there is an association between thyroid eye disease and myasthenia gravis, testing for acetylcholine receptor antibodies, or Tensilon testing, may be indicated.

The management of different findings in thyroid eye disease is summarized in Figure 12-18. Topical guanethidine 5% to 10% can be used for lid retraction, but its duration of action is short. Radiation therapy for optic neuropathy is usually 1500 rads to 3000 rads directed to the posterior orbit. It is used only in the treatment of dysthyroid optic neuropathy and has no effect on proptosis or ocular motility disturbances. Steroid therapy is usually 80 mg to 150 mg per day of Prednisone. A response to steroids should be apparent within 24 hours; maximal response occurs in 2 weeks to 8 weeks. Cyclophosphamide or azathioprine may also be useful in acute cases if the patient has a positive leukocyte migration test. Plasmapheresis may offer temporary benefit. Occasionally orbital decompression is necessary. The percentage increase in orbital volume and degree of reduction of orbital "stiffness" correlate well with the reduction of proptosis in orbital decompression. Strabismus surgery should be performed only after the orbitopathy has been quiescent for at least 6 months. Eyelid surgery should be performed after extraocular muscle surgery or orbital decompression because either can alter the resting position of the eyelids.

TABLE 12-2. LABORATORY TESTING IN THYROID AND OTHER DISORDERS

TEST	HYPERTHYROIDISM	HYPOTHYROIDISM	MALNUTRITION	↑ ESTROGEN
Serum total T_4	Increased	Decreased	Decreased	Increased
Serum total T_3	Increased	Decreased	Decreased	Increased
T_3 resin uptake	Increased	Decreased	Increased	Increased
Serum TSH	Decreased	Elevated	Normal	Normal
TRH stimulation	No TSH response	↑TSH in thyroid failure ↓ TSH in pituitary failure		

T_4 = thyroxine; T_3 = triiodothyronine; TSH = thyroid stimulating hormone; TRH = thyrotropin-releasing hormone; ↑ = increased; ↓ = decreased; ↑ Estrogen = increased estrogen level (either exogenous or endogenous). T_3 toxicosis = increased T_3 and decreased TSH with normal T_4.

318 III—Nontraumatic Ocular and Orbital Emergencies

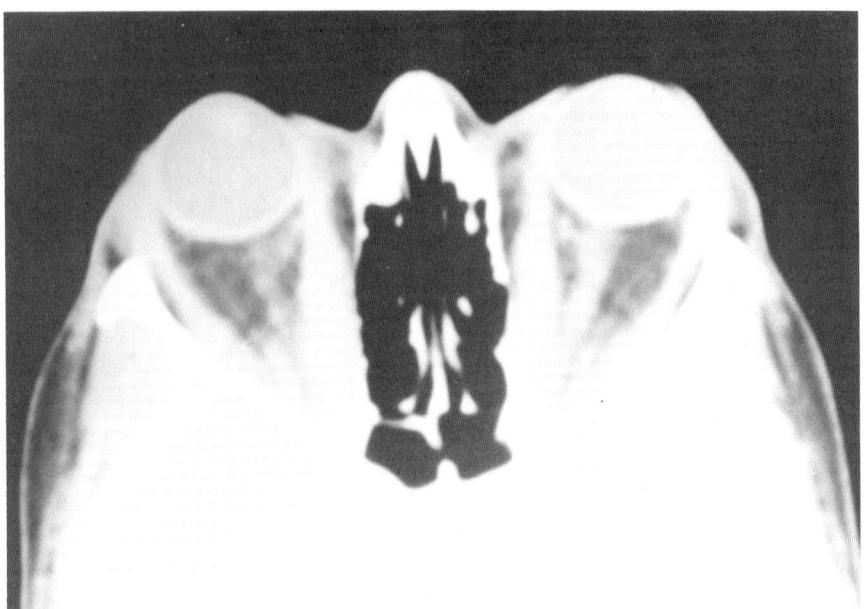

FIGURE 12–16. CT demonstrating thickened extraocular muscles with sparing of the extraocular muscle tendons.

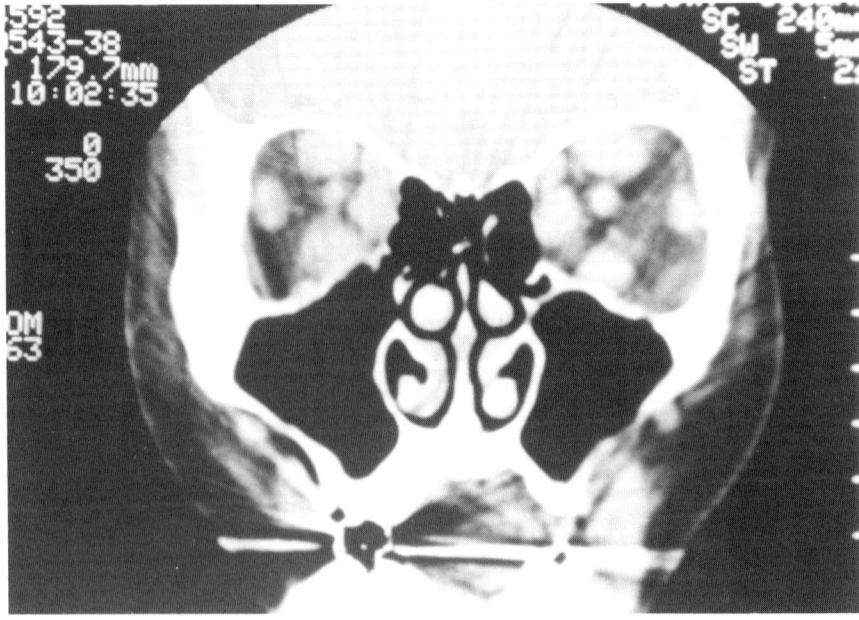

FIGURE 12–17. Coronal CT demonstrating thickened extraocular muscles in orbital apex.

MANAGEMENT OF THYROID EYE DISEASE

	Findings					
Treatments	Ocular Irritation	Diplopia with EOM Restriction	LID Retraction and Exophthalmos	Exposure Keratopathy Mild to Moderate	Severe	Optic Neuropathy
	Topical lubricants	Prisms	Levator and/or Müller's muscle recession; lateral tarsorrhaphy, and/or medial canthoplasty, sclera or fascia spacer grafts	Topical lubricants, moisture chamber	Systemic corticosteroids	Systemic corticosteroids
	Moisture chamber	Extraocular muscle surgery		Levator and/or Müller's muscle recession, lateral and/or medial tarsorrhaphy, canthoplasty, sclera or fascia spacer grafts	Orbital decompression, eyelid surgery	Oribal decompression
					Irradiation	Irradiation

EOM: extraocular muscle.
Modified from Krohel GB, Stewart WB, Chavis RM: Orbital Disease: A Practical Approach. New York, Grune & Stratton, 1981, p. 120.

FIGURE 12-18. Management of thyroid eye disease.

Infectious Disorders

Preseptal and orbital cellulitis can occur in adults as well as children. In addition to the infections discussed under childhood disorders, fungal infections can be encountered in ketoacidotic, debilitated, or immunocompromised adults and rarely in dehydrated children in metabolic acidosis. *Rhizopus* and *Mucor* are the most commonly encountered fungi; *Aspergillosis* is infrequently seen. Fungi extend to the orbit from infected paranasal sinuses. Successful treatment is contingent on early recognition and treatment; mortality is high.

Phycomycosis should be considered in the immunocompromised patient with orbital cellulitis who rapidly develops proptosis, orbital apex syndrome (internal and external ophthalmoplegia, ptosis, decreased corneal sensation), seventh nerve palsy, decreased vision, fever, rhinorrhea, headache, and deep orbital pain. *Mucor* can invade blood vessels and cause their thrombosis. Black, crusted, infarcted tissue on the palate, nasal mucosa, or skin is suggestive of mucormycosis. Necrotic material should be submitted for Gram's, Giemsa, and calcofluor white stains and cultured in blood, Sabouraud's, and brain-heart infusion agar, and an anaerobic medium. CT will demonstrate sinus involvement and bone destruction; biopsy will reveal nonseptate, large, branching hyphae. Management involves wide surgical excision and the administration of topical and systemic amphotericin B. Hyperbaric oxygen treatment may also be helpful (see Chapter 16).

Aspergillosis usually occurs in otherwise healthy adults and is more commonly encountered in hot or humid climates. The maxillary sinus is the most frequently involved sinus. Similar to mucormycosis, thrombotic arteritis occurs but with a much more granulomatous, rather than necrotic, reaction. Infection is generally very slowly progressive; proptosis, persistent severe pain, and visual loss are the most common symptoms. Biopsy specimens should be stained with Gomori methenamine silver (GMS) stain to demonstrate septate, branching hyphae of uniform width. Treatment includes surgical debridement and intravenous amphotericin B, flucytosine, and/or rifampin; mortality is high when the central nervous system is involved.

Orbital Vasculitis

Polyarteritis nodosa is a multisystem inflammatory disorder characterized by polymorphic inflammation (neutrophils and eosinophils) and necrosis of the full thickness of the walls of large and medium-sized arteries. The disorder is more common in males and usually occurs between age 20 years and 40 years. Signs of orbital involvement include acute pain and proptosis, lid erythema, chemosis, and a motility disturbance, simulating pseudotumor. Episcleritis, corneoscleral ulcers, and retinal, choroidal, and cranial or peripheral nerve lesions may be associated. Cardiovascular, renal, gastrointestinal, and cutaneous signs may be present. Management consists of high-dose systemic corticosteroids.

Wegener's granulomatosis is characterized by fibrinoid degeneration of vessels and necrotizing granulomas in the walls of vessels in the vicinity of the vasculitis. The tissues affected are the sinus mucosa, lungs, and kidneys. It can occur at any age but most commonly presents in the fourth and fifth decades. Clinical features include mucosal ulcerations and bony erosions of the nasopharynx, tracheobronchial necrosis, cavitary lesions at the base of the lungs, glomerulonephritis, and hemorrhagic and gangrenous skin lesions. Orbital involvement simulates pseudotumor with proptosis, eyelid edema, dacryocystitis, and diffuse granulomatous involvement. Symptoms include diplopia, decreased vision, and headaches. Scleritis, scleral necrosis, central retinal vein congestion, disc edema, and retinal vasculitis can occur. Cyclophosphamide, methotrexate, chlorambucil, and azathioprine have been used with variable results, and lobectomy of lung lesions may be helpful. Corticosteroids have no effect.

Lethal midline granuloma is the clinical term used to describe a relentless, progressive destruction of the nose, paranasal sinuses, and palate. It can be caused by phycomycosis, parasites, neoplasms, and idiopathic inflammation. Biopsy is necessary to distinguish this disorder from Wegener's granulomatosis. The former is treated with radiation therapy and the latter with cytotoxic agents.

Vascular Disorders Other Than Vasculitis

Spontaneous orbital hemorrhage is unusual but may occur with an unsuspected lymphangioma or orbital varix (Figure 12–19). Systemic conditions associated with spontaneous hemorrhage include hypertension, scurvy, leu-

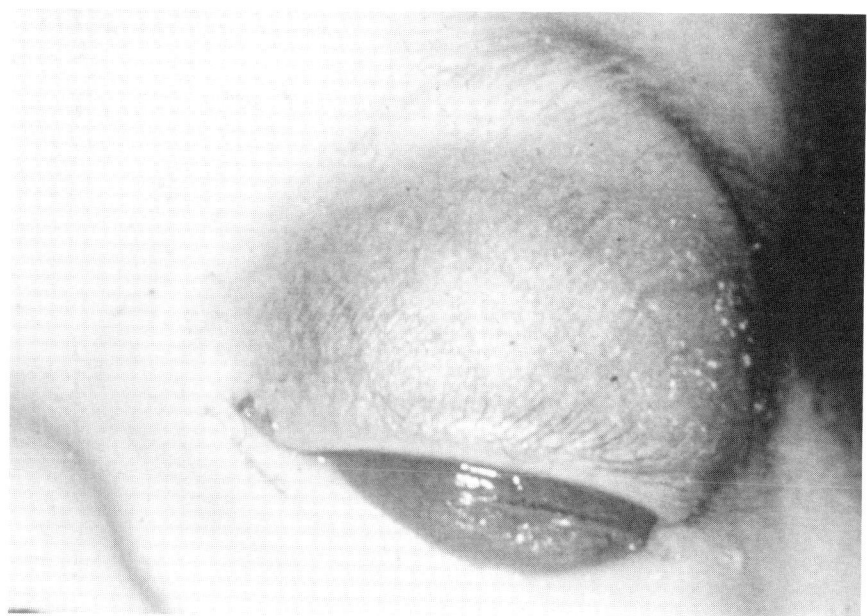

FIGURE 12-19. Spontaneous orbital hemorrhage in infant with lymphangioma.

kemia, hemophilia, and rupture of an ophthalmic artery aneurysm. Acute proptosis, with restriction of ocular motility and chemosis and dissection by hemorrhage under the eyelids and conjunctiva, may occur. To prevent visual loss from excessively elevated intraocular or intraorbital pressure, orbital decompression by way of a lateral canthotomy and cantholysis may be necessary (see Chapter 4). Anterior chamber paracentesis and intravenous acetazolamide can be used to reduce intraocular pressure. If visual loss is not threatened, the patient is treated conservatively; the hemorrhage resorbs over several months.

Orbital varices are congenital venous malformations. They are usually unilateral and may involve conjunctival vessels, the eyelids, and the retinal vasculature. Spontaneous hemorrhage within a varix can result in acute proptosis, pain, vomiting, eyelid ecchymosis, chemosis, motility disturbance, and/or visual loss. A history of intermittent proptosis associated with a Valsalva maneuver or positional change is nearly always pathognomonic. Contrast-enhanced CT or venography can demonstrate the abnormal vasculature. Plain film X rays may demonstrate phleboliths. Orbital varices are managed conservatively; surgery is attempted only if vision is threatened.

Arteriovenous fistulas arise from either spontaneous or traumatic communication between the arterial and venous systems in the region of the cavernous sinus. Spontaneous communications tend to be low-flow shunts between dural vessels and the cavernous sinus *(dural sinus fistula)*. They occur most frequently in postmenopausal females and can result from a congenital malformation, such as an aneurysm or an arteriovenous malformation. They are also associated with atherosclerosis, collagen vascular disease, or childbirth. Signs include dilated conjunctival veins, mild proptosis, and bruit. Traumatic communications are usually high-flow shunts between the internal carotid artery and cavernous sinus *(carotid-cavernous fistula)*. Signs include pulsating exophthalmos, arteriolization of episcleral and conjunctival vessels (corkscrew configuration), bruit, limited ocular motility, increased intraocular pressure, venous stasis retinopathy, and hemorrhagic central retinal vein occlusion (Figure 12-20). CT and orbital ultrasound can demonstrate enlargement of the superior ophthalmic vein and congested extraocular muscles. High-flow fistulas may require balloon embolization. Indications include visual deterioration, diplopia due to vascular engorgement of the extraocular muscles, intolerable bruit or headache, or corneal exposure due to proptosis. Low-flow shunts are less symptomatic and resolve spontaneously in up to 60% of cases.

Cavernous sinus thrombosis results from infection and phlebitis of the veins draining the face, sinuses, ear, or pharynx; embolic involvement in mucormycosis; or traumatic phlebothrombosis. Signs and symptoms include exophthalmos, eyelid and orbital edema and discoloration, retinal vein congestion, and variable involvement of the third, fourth, fifth, or sixth cranial nerves. Severe aching pain around the eye is secondary to involvement of the fifth (ophthalmic) nerve. Acute hypopituitarism can occur due to the proximity of

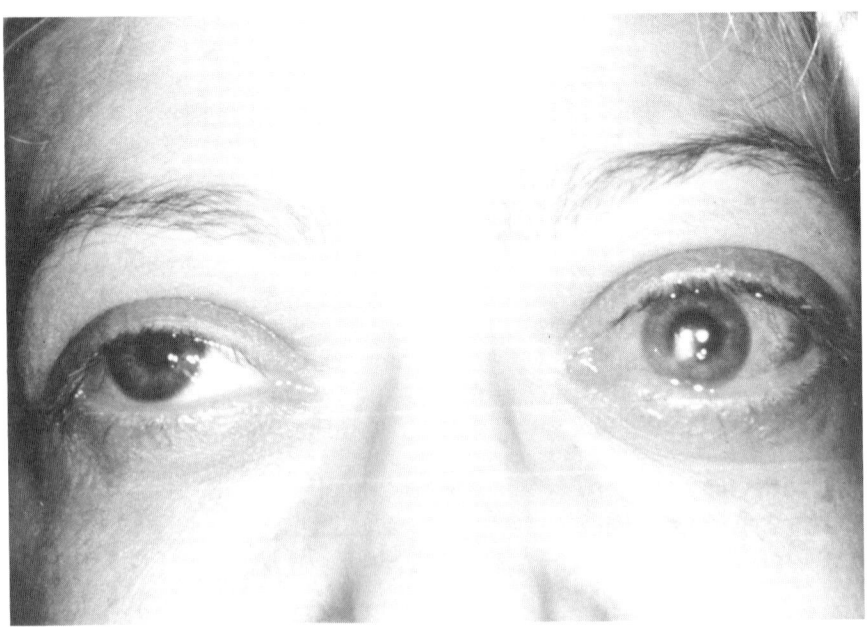

FIGURE 12-20. Left carotid cavernous fistula, with glaucoma.

the pituitary gland. Progression to bilaterality often occurs within hours to days and is heralded by the development of a contralateral sixth nerve palsy. Cavernous sinus thrombosis can be a sequela of orbital cellulitis, and it may be difficult to differentiate whether increasing proptosis, chemosis, or ocular motility deficits signifies progression to thrombosis. Systemic signs of infection, including headache, fever, tachycardia, sweating, vomiting, and mental status changes, are more severe with cavernous sinus thrombosis. Additionally, with thrombosis, the eyelids and orbit are bluish due to vascular congestion, and the pain is severe and aching. In cellulitis, the eyelids are red and tender and the pain associated more with eye movement. Cranial nerve deficits (e.g., internal ophthalmoplegia), retinal vein congestion, and bilaterality signify cavernous sinus involvement.

With infectious etiologies, treatment consists of high-dose, broad-spectrum antibiotics. Steroids are useful for hypopituitarism and also reduce orbital inflammation. The use of anticoagulants and antifibrinolytic agents is controversial.

Orbital Tumors

Cavernous hemangioma is the most frequently encountered, benign, primary orbital tumor of adults. A vascular hamartoma, it is more frequent in women and usually presents in the third to fifth decade of life as a slowly progressive proptosis. The globe is usually displaced axially and occasionally also vertically or horizontally. The tumor can occur anywhere in the orbit, but usually it is within the muscle cone (Figure 12–21). If it is large enough, pressure on the globe can cause hyperopia, choroidal folds, optic nerve compression, and increased intraocular pressure. Restriction of ocular motility with diplopia in extreme gazes can also occur. CT demonstrates the rounded or oval contour of the tumor, with internal heterogeneity, loculation, and usually contrast enhancement. Ultrasonography reveals the presence of a circumscribed mass with good transmission and high internal reflectivity. Because the tumors are well circumscribed and encapsulated, they are very amenable to surgical excision and do not recur even after incomplete removal. Radiation and corticosteroids are ineffective.

Hemangiopericytomas are uncommon tumors that arise from the pericytes surrounding the endothelial cells of capillaries. They may occur primarily in the orbit, extend into the orbit from an adjacent sinus, or metastasize to the orbit. Primary tumors present similar to cavernous hemangiomas but may also cause engorgement of conjunctival vessels and conjunctival prolapse. CT and ultrasound findings are similar to those of cavernous hemangiomas, but at surgery the tumor is bluish; hemangiomas are purplish-red. Treatment is surgical excision. Unlike cavernous hemangiomas, incompletely removed tumors can recur, often malignantly.

Lymphoid hyperplasia and *lymphoma* are lymphoid tumors that can occur

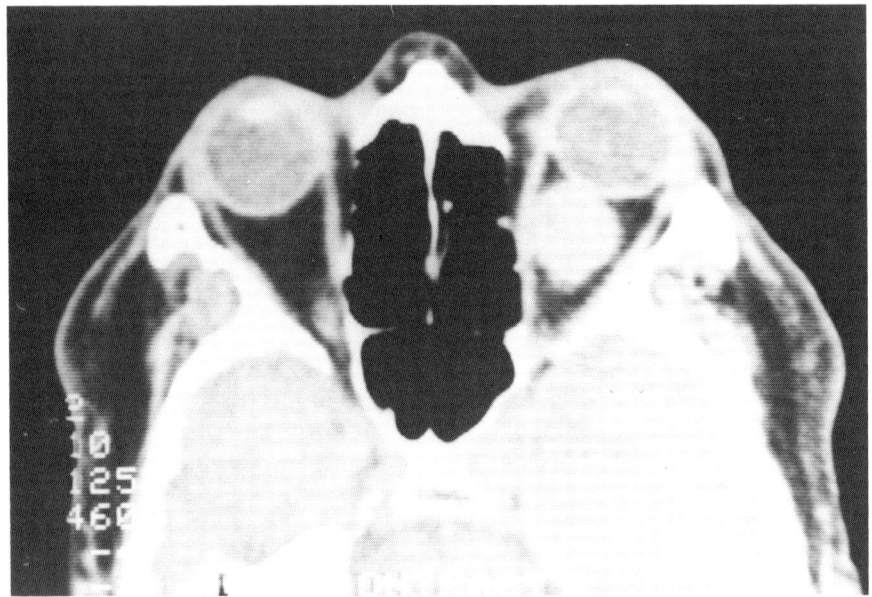

FIGURE 12-21. Cavernous hemangioma in muscle cone of right eye.

in the adult orbit. The first is a localized benign and reactive disease of uncertain origin. The second is a malignant tumor that may occur primarily in the orbit or be one of several foci of disseminated disease. Either tumor can occur in the lacrimal gland, anterior orbit, or conjunctiva; the last are visible as fleshy, salmon-colored masses in the conjunctival fornix. They have a predilection for superior locations (Figure 12-22). If located in the posterior orbit, they can cause painless progressive proptosis with visual and ocular motility disturbances. CT scanning demonstrates a putty-like molding of the infiltrating tumor to preexisting orbital structures (Figure 12-23). Bone erosion does not occur. Systemic evaluation includes bone marrow biopsy, complete blood count, liver, spleen, and bone scans, chest X ray, retroperitoneal studies, and serum electrophoresis. Biopsy is necessary to distinguish benign hyperplasia from malignant lymphoma. Biopsy specimens should be prepared for light and electron microscopy, and fresh tissue should be sent for cell surface marker studies. Benign hyperplasia can be treated with 1000 rads to 2500 rads; malignant lymphomas require 1500 rads to 3000 rads and chemotherapy if disseminated.

Simple neurofibromas are comprised of proliferating Schwann cells, endoneural cells, and axons. They may be circumscribed, but they are not encapsulated. They can occur in the upper eyelid, the superior orbit, or posterior to the globe. When not associated with neurofibromatosis, orbital neurofibromas

12—Nontraumatic Orbital Disorders 325

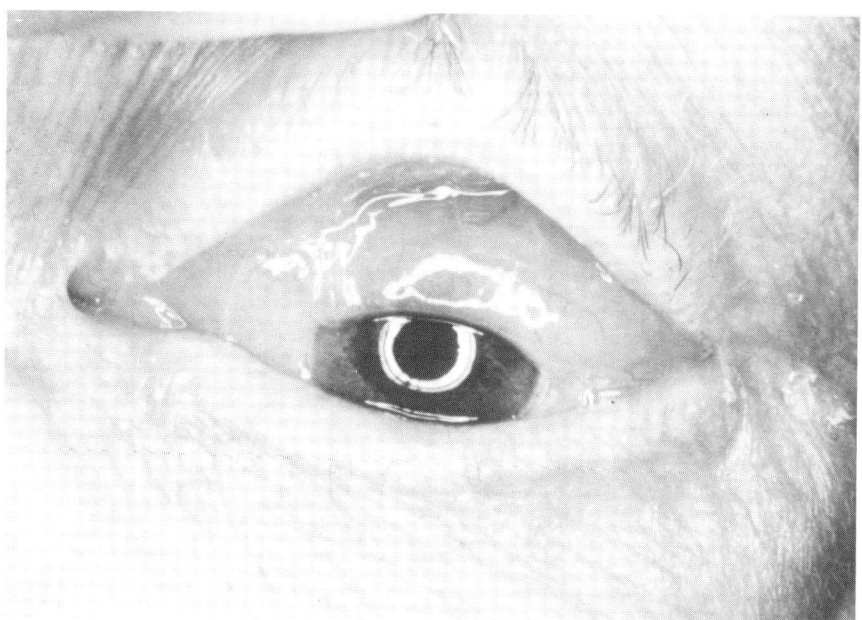

FIGURE 12-22. Lymphoma presenting as a salmon-colored mass in superior conjunctiva.

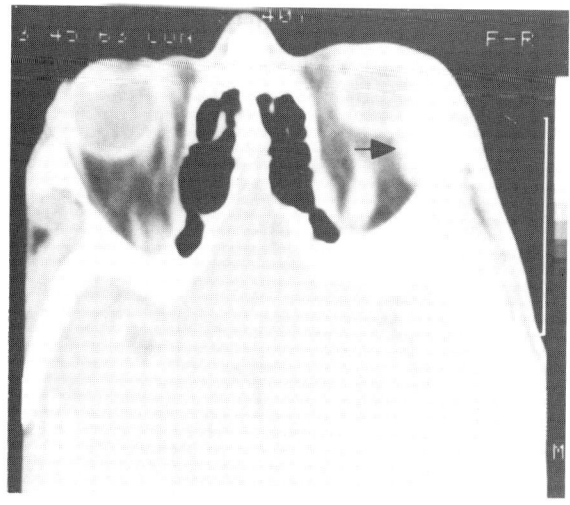

FIGURE 12-23. "Putty-like" molding of lymphoma to preexisting structures (arrow).

generally develop in early to middle adulthood. Neurofibromas in association with neurofibromatosis are more extensive than those seen in the absence of this disorder. They tend to be enclosed within perineural sheaths and are called *plexiform neurofibromas*. The plexiform type is generally present during the first decade of life. They are less solitary, more difficult to excise surgically, and more likely to recur than simple neurofibromas.

Neurilemomas (schwannomas) are slow-growing tumors comprised only of Schwann cells. They arise in middle age and can produce proptosis of up to 10 mm. Neurilemomas compress the nerve of origin, resulting in pain on retropulsion of the orbit. This can be useful in distinguishing these tumors from unencapsulated and painless neurofibromas. Neurilemomas can occur anywhere in the orbit. If located in the muscle cone, optic nerve compression can result in disk edema and visual loss. Unlike neurofibromas, schwannomas rarely, if ever, undergo malignant transformation. Because they are encapsulated, surgical removal, without recurrence, is possible.

Nearly 80% of *optic nerve gliomas* are diagnosed by age 15 years; these tumors are discussed under childhood disorders. Childhood gliomas generally behave benignly. Gliomas that occur in adults, especially in the absence of neurofibromatosis, are usually aggressively malignant, resulting in death within 1 year of the onset of symptoms. Signs and symptoms include headaches, proptosis, loss of vision, and papilledema.

Orbital meningiomas can arise within the cranium and invade the orbit secondarily or (less commonly) can arise directly from the meninges of the optic nerve (Figure 12-24). They are much more common in females, and the mean age of diagnosis is the late thirties. Pregnancy may be an exacerbating factor, for unknown reasons. Meningiomas usually present as progressive loss of vision or progressive exophthalmos. Visual field loss, optic atrophy, retinal striae, and/or optociliary shunt vessels are commonly found on examination. Meningiomas arising from the lateral portion of the sphenoid bone produce a temporal fossa mass and proptosis (Figure 12-25). Orbital apex meningiomas can cause swelling of lateral lower eyelid.

Radiographic findings in sphenoid ridge meningiomas include hyperostosis (bone thickening), bone resorption and destruction, and blurring of oblique (innominate) line. CT scanning demonstrates a lucid center in optic nerve sheath meningiomas. In contrast, optic nerve gliomas have a denser center and a more fusiform shape. Surgical manipulation of optic nerve sheath meningiomas can result in blindness. Intervention is usually reserved for tumors that have already caused blindness or threaten intracranial structures. Irradiation is not of value.

Fibrous histiocytomas and *mesenchymal sarcomas* (liposarcoma, fibrosarcoma, and osteogenic sarcoma) occur rarely in the orbit. Fibrous histiocytomas are very firm tumors that displace normal tissues and may resemble hemangiopericytomas histologically. Osteogenic sarcoma can develop within orbital bones and soft tissues in patients with inherited retinoblastoma. It is more com-

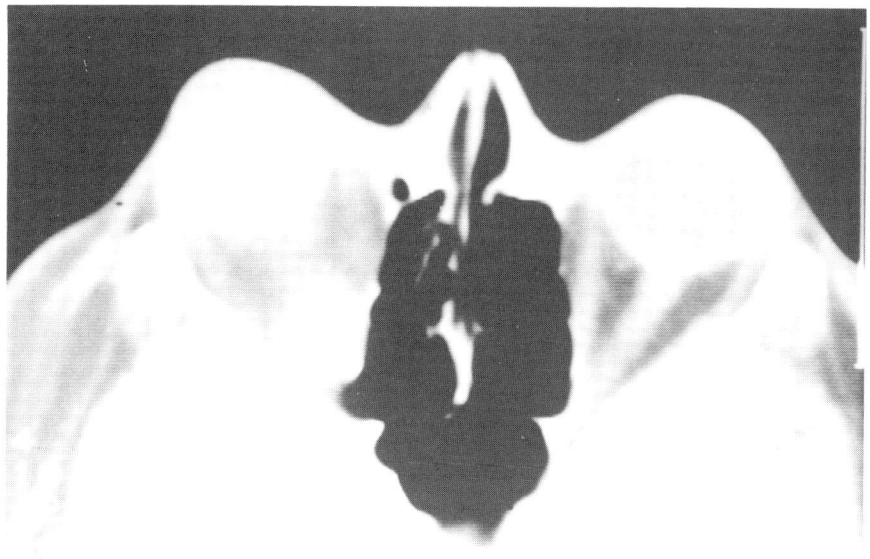

FIGURE 12-24. Optic nerve sheath meningioma.

mon in those who received radiation therapy but can occur even in its absence. The prognosis is poor when it occurs in previously irradiated bones or when it is not amenable to surgical resection.

The two most common primary sites for *metastatic orbital tumors* are the breast in females and the lung in males. Renal, gastrointestinal, and prostatic tumors and malignant melanoma can also metastasize to the orbit. Orbital metastases may be the presenting sign of a tumor or may occur many years after discovery of the primary tumor. Syndromes of presentation, in order of frequency, include: mass effect (palpable mass with displacement of the globe), infiltrative effect (resulting in diplopia, enophthalmos, limitation of eye movement, and a firm orbit), functional effect (cranial nerve disorder and/or loss of vision), and inflammatory effect (acute or subacute inflammatory symptoms). Pain, conjunctival chemosis and injection, and rapidly developing proptosis, ophthalmoplegia, and inflammation characterize the usual presentation. Rarely, metastatic breast carcinoma causes a fibrous response and enophthalmos. Metastatic prostate carcinoma can simulate acute pseudotumor.

Metastatic tumors infiltrate and entrap structures, resulting in restriction of ocular movement, visual loss, and bone destruction. When anterior, they are palpable as rock-hard masses fixed to bone. Incisional biopsies are performed to provide tissue for immunohistochemical (e.g., estrogen receptor) studies and to facilitate the diagnosis when the primary site is unknown. Fine needle biopsy may be considered for anteriorly located masses. Treatment is palliative local

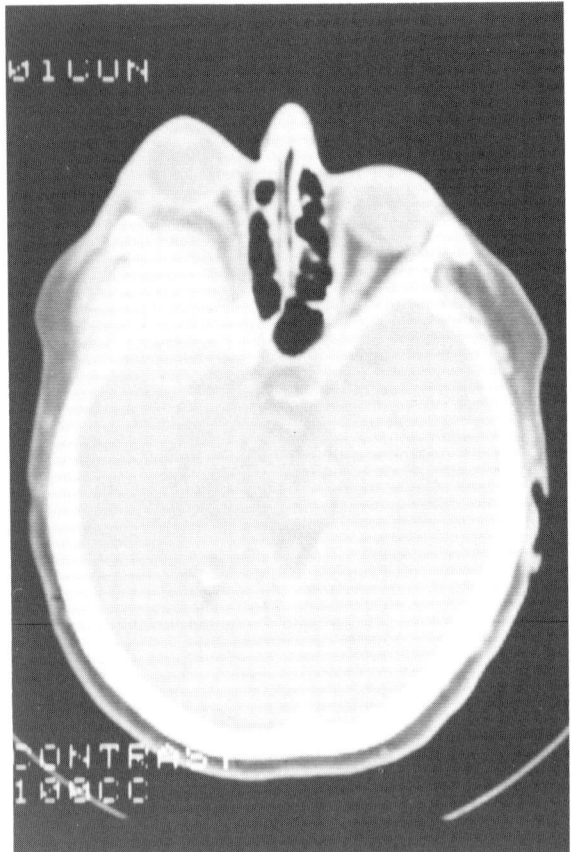

FIGURE 12-25. Sphenoid wing meningioma.

radiation therapy. Carcinoid tumors, however, should be widely excised as patients may survive for many years if only the primary lung or gastrointestinal tumor remains.

Lacrimal Gland Disorders

Lacrimal tumors include benign and mixed epithelial tumors, adenoid cystic carcinoma, and lymphoid tumors. Epithelial parenchymal tumors comprise half of all lacrimal tumors. The most common is *benign mixed tumor* (pleomorphic adenoma). It presents in adults during the fourth and fifth decades as a firm lobular mass in the lacrimal fossa that slowly but progressively displaces the globe inferiorly and medially. The presence of pain is unusual due to the slow growth and encapsulation of this tumor. Pressure enlargement of the lacrimal gland fossa is found on radiographic studies. Treatment consists of complete excision of the tumor and its pseudocapsule. Incisional biopsies can spread tumor cells in the orbit, resulting in infiltrative, difficult-to-resect recurrences, and occasionally malignant degeneration. *Malignant mixed tumors* arise either from benign mixed tumors or de novo. Malignant transformation of a benign mixed tumor results in rapid tumor growth and invasion of adjacent structures.

Adenoid cystic carcinoma (cylindroma) is the second most common epithelial tumor of the lacrimal gland. It is highly malignant, with a rapid course heralded by pain and cavernous sinus involvement (with corresponding neurologic deficits). Pain occurs from perineural invasion and bone destruction.

Nonepithelial lesions of the lacrimal gland comprise the remaining 50% of lacrimal tumors and include pseudotumor, sarcoidosis, lymphoid hyperplasia and lymphoma, and the lymphoepithelial infiltration of Mikulicz syndrome.

CT helps define the size and shape of lacrimal masses and demonstrates bony changes. Lymphoid tumors mold around preexisting structures (Figure 12–23), whereas epithelial tumors are globular and displace or distort associated structures. Inflammatory and lymphomatous lesions also cause more diffuse lacrimal gland enlargement than epithelial tumors. Benign tumors may cause well-corticated concavities in the lacrimal fossa, but bone destruction is a hallmark of malignancy.

The duration of symptoms and the presence of systemic abnormalities, inflammatory signs, pain, or X ray findings help guide management decisions (Figure 12–26). If a malignant tumor is diagnosed, a metastatic workup is necessary. If distant metastases are not found, exenteration and/or orbitectomy are required. Radiation may be necessary, but chemotherapy has not been proved to be of value.

Acute dacryoadenitis may occur as a secondary or primary infection. Secondary infections most frequently arise from generalized gonorrhea, mumps, infectious mononucleosis, or histoplasmosis. Secondary infections can also arise from contiguous conjunctivitis, hordeola, or orbital cellulitis. Secondary infections are also more likely to be bilateral than primary infections. Either the palpebral or the orbital lobe, or both, may be involved. Involvement of the orbital lobe results in more severe symptoms, simulating cellulitis. Proptosis and globe displacement are also more likely to occur with orbital lobe involvement. Signs include an S-shaped curve to the upper eyelid, preauricular adenopathy, and tender swelling of the lacrimal gland (see Figure 16–7). Localized chemosis, conjunctival injection, and bulging of the palpebral lobe are often visible. Systemic signs include fever, leukocytosis, malaise, and headache. Primary acute dacryoadenitis is self-limiting and resolves within 1 week to 2 weeks with warm compresses and aspirin. Antibiotics should be used if systemic signs of infection are present. Failure to respond rapidly to antibiotics suggests the possibility of pseudotumor, in which case corticosteroids are indicated.

Chronic dacryoadenitis is characterized by a hard, nonfixed, lobulated mass

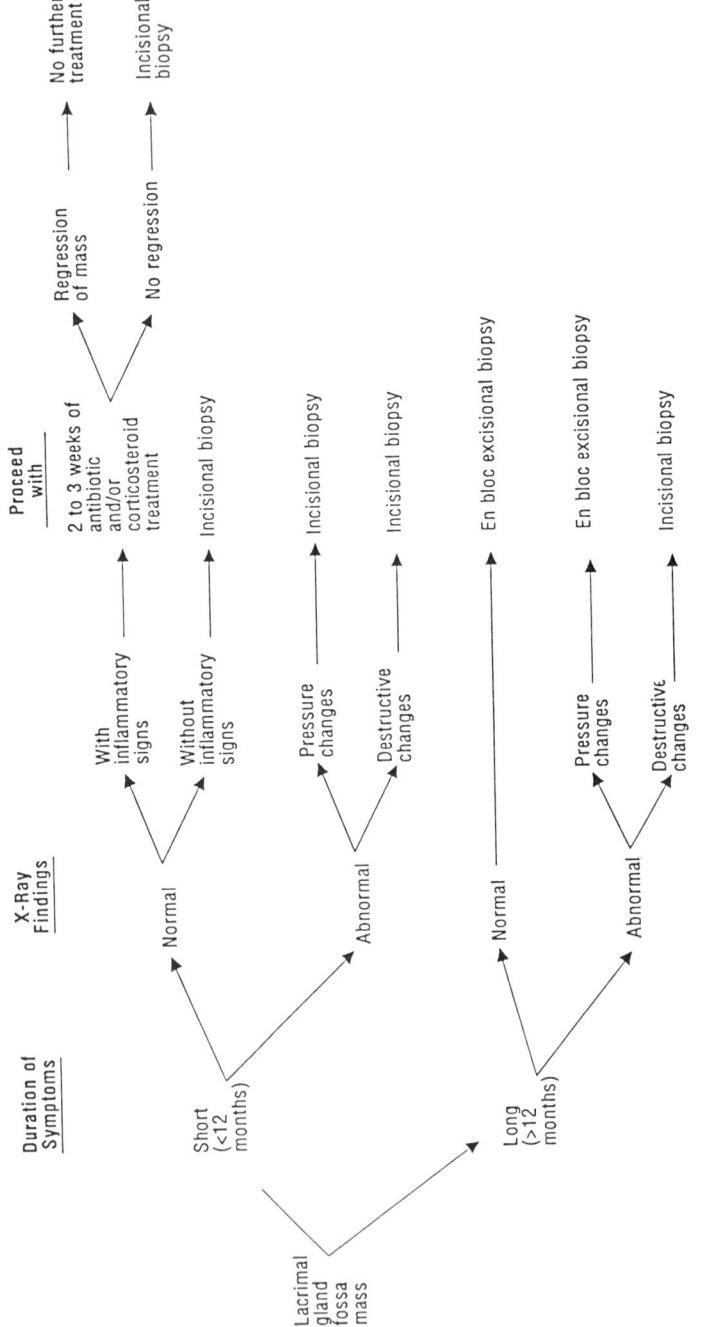

FIGURE 12-26. Management of lacrimal gland/fossa masses.

in the region of the lacrimal gland. The mass may be tender to palpation, but pain is not a cardinal feature. The disorder is usually bilateral. Upper eyelid inflammation and swelling can cause ptosis, and the globe is usually displaced inferiorly and medially. An incisional biopsy is advised for diagnosis. When benign mixed tumor is in the differential, en bloc excisional biopsy should be performed. Common etiologies include sarcoidosis, benign lymphoepithelial lesion, pseudotumor, and thyroid orbitopathy. Less common etiologies include syphilis, tuberculosis, leprosy, and trachoma.

Fibrous Dysplasia

Fibrous dysplasia is a nonneoplastic bone disorder characterized by the replacement of osteogenesis by proliferating fibro-osseous tissue. Depending on which bone is involved, proptosis, displacement of the globe, nasal lacrimal duct obstruction, and sinus obstruction (resulting in infections and mucoceles) can occur. Rarely, optic nerve compression and atrophy can occur. Surgery may be attempted if visual acuity is threatened, but it is usually undertaken with a guarded prognosis. Dysplasia may occur in a single bone or be polyostotic. Albright's syndrome is the association of polyostotic fibrous dysplasia, cutaneous hyperpigmentation, and precocious puberty in females.

Mucoceles

A *mucocele* is a benign, encapsulated, mucoid-filled mass within a paranasal sinus (Figure 12-27). The pathogenesis of mucoceles is uncertain, but they may arise following obstruction of one or more ducts of mucus glands in the submucosa of the sinus. They can occur secondary to trauma, osteoma formation, or chronic sinusitis and most commonly occur in the frontal or ethmoidal sinus. Proptosis, displacement of the globe, and obstruction of the lacrimal drainage system can give rise to symptoms of diplopia, nasal obstruction, epiphora, and headache. Sphenoid mucoceles may also produce decreased vision, optic atrophy, and a pulsating exophthalmos. Extension of a sphenoid mucocele into the cranium, by bony erosion, may result in meningitis, abscess, or increased intracranial pressure. A *mucopyocele* is an infected mucocele. When infection occurs, signs and symptoms of acute sinusitis are superimposed on the findings.

CT scanning is most useful in demonstrating mucoceles. Most have a homogeneous appearance; infection (mucopyocele) results in enhancement of the rim. CT also demonstrates any bony erosion by the mucocele. The treatment of mucoceles is surgical removal. Because coexisting malignant neoplasms are occasionally associated with paranasal mucoceles, biopsy specimens should be obtained if surgery is required.

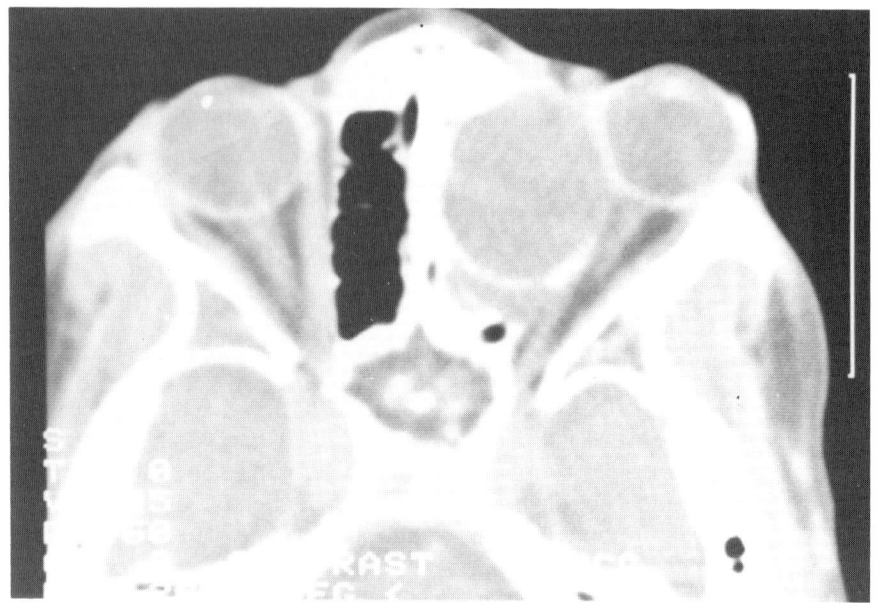

FIGURE 12-27. Ethmoidal sinus mucocele.

REFERENCES

Abdul-Rahim AS, Savino PJ: Orbital apex syndrome. In Lindberg JV (ed): *Oculoplastic and Orbital Emergencies.* Norwalk, CT, Appleton & Lange, 1990, pp 125-143.
Alper MG: Mucoceles of the sphenoid sinus: Neuro-ophthalmologic manifestations. *Trans Am Ophthalmol Soc* 74:53, 1976.
Barthold HJ, Harvey A, Markoe AM, et al: Treatment of orbital pseudotumors and lymphoma. *Am J Clin Oncol* 9:527, 1986.
Bennett CL, Putterman A, Bitran JD, et al: Staging and therapy of orbital lymphomas. *Cancer* 57:1204, 1986.
Boldt HC, Nerad JA: Orbital metastases from prostate cancer. *Arch Ophthalmol* 106:1403, 1988.
Bray WH, Giangiacoma J, Ide CH: Orbital apex syndrome. *Surv Ophthalmol* 32:136, 1987.
Bullen CL, Liesegang TJ, McDonald TJ, et al: Ocular complications of Wegener's granulomatosis. *Ophthalmology* 90:279, 1983.
Bullock JD, Goldberg SH, Rakes SM, et al: Primary orbital neuroblastoma. *Arch Ophthalmol* 107:1031, 1989.
Burde RM: Double vision, visual loss, and an enhancing orbital apex. *Surv Ophthalmol* 33:55, 1988.
Catalano RA, Smoot CN: Subperiosteal orbital masses in children with orbital cellulitis: Time for a reevaluation? *J Ped Ophthalmol Strabismus* 27:141, 1990.
Char DH: *Thyroid Eye Disease.* 2d ed. New York, Churchill Livingstone, 1991.
Char DH, Ablin A, Beckstead J: Histiocytic disorders of the orbit. *Ann Ophthalmol* 16:867, 1984.
Char DH, Norman D: Orbital tumor diagnosis: Imaging techniques. *Ophthalmic Forum* 3:16, 1985.
Chavis RM, Everson MH: Acute proptosis in adults. In Lindberg JV (ed): *Oculoplastic and Orbital Emergencies.* Norwalk, CT, Appleton & Lange, 1990, pp 105-123.
Curtin HD: Pseudotumor. In *Imaging in Ophthalmology, Part I.* Radiol Clin North Am. Philadelphia, WB Saunders Co, 1987, pp 583-589.
Feldman M, Lowry LD, Rao VM, et al: Mucoceles of the paranasal sinus. *Trans PA Acad Ophthalmol* 39:614, 1987.

Ferry AP, Abedi S: Diagnosis and management of rhino-orbitocerebral mucormycosis (phycomycosis). *Ophthalmology* 90:1096, 1983.
Freedman MI, Folk JC: Metastatic tumors to the eye and orbit. *Arch Ophthalmol* 105:1215, 1987.
Glover AT, Grove AS: Eosinophilic granuloma of the orbit with spontaneous healing. *Ophthalmology* 94:1008, 1987.
Goldberg RA, Rootman J, Cline RA: Tumors metastatic to the orbit: A changing picture. *Surv Ophthalmol* 35:1, 1990.
Gorman CA, Waller RR, Dyer JA (eds): *The Eye and Orbit in Thyroid Disease.* New York, Raven Press, 1984.
Grove AS: Orbital disease: Examination and diagnostic evaluation. *Ophthalmology* 86:854, 1979.
Harris GJ: Subperiosteal abscess of the orbit. *Arch Ophthalmol* 101:751, 1983.
Harris GJ, Beatty RL: Acute proptosis in childhood. In Lindberg JV (ed): *Oculoplastic and Orbital Emergencies.* Norwalk, CT, Appleton & Lange, 1990, pp 87–103.
Hornblass A: Lacrimal evaluation. In Hornblass A: *Oculoplastic, Orbital, and Reconstructive Surgery.* Baltimore, Williams and Wilkins, 1990, 1348–1355.
Hornblass A, Herschorn BJ, Stern K, et al: Orbital abscess. *Surv Ophthalmol* 29:169, 1984.
Israele V, Nelson JD: Periorbital and orbital cellulitis. *Pediatr Infect Dis* 6:404, 1987.
Jakobeic FA, Font RL: Orbit. In Spencer WH, Font RL, Green WR, et al (eds): *Ophthalmic Pathology: An Atlas and Textbook.* Philadelphia, WB Saunders Co, 1986, pp 2765–2811.
Jordan DR, Nerad J, Hansen SO: Case report: Orbital lymphangioma. *Ophthalmic Practice* 8:242, 1990.
Katowitz JA, Kropp TM: Congenital abnormalities of the lacrimal drainage system. In Hornblass A: *Oculoplastic, Orbital, and Reconstructive Surgery.* Baltimore, Williams and Wilkins, 1990, 2:1397–1416.
Keltner JL, Satterfield D, Dublin AB, Lee BCP: Dural and carotid cavernous sinus fistulas: Diagnosis, management, and complications. *Ophthalmology* 94:1585, 1987.
Kennerdell JS, Dresner SC: The nonspecific orbital inflammatory syndromes. *Surv Ophthalmol* 29:93, 1984.
Kline LB: The Tolosa-Hunt syndrome. *Surv Ophthalmol* 27:79, 1982.
Kohn R, Hepler R: Management of limited rhino-orbital mucor-mycosis without exenteration. *Ophthalmology* 92:1440, 1985.
Krohel GB, Stewart WB, Chavis RM: *Orbital Disease: A Practical Approach.* New York, Grune and Stratton, 1981.
Krohel GB, Wright JE: Orbital hemorrhage. *Am J Ophthalmol* 88:254, 1979.
Kushner BJ: Treatment of periorbital infantile hemangioma with intralesional corticosteroid. *Plast Reconstr Surg* 76:517, 1985.
Kushner BJ: Infantile orbital hemangiomas. *Int Pediatr* 5:249, 1990.
Kwan ESK, Wolpert SM, Hedges TR, et al: The Tolosa-Hunt syndrome revisited: Not necessarily a diagnosis of exclusion. *AJR* 150:413, 1988.
Lawless M, Martin F: Orbital cellulitis and preseptal cellulitis in children. *Aust N Z J Ophthalmol* 14:211, 1986.
Leone CR Jr, Lloyd WC III: Treatment protocol for orbital inflammatory disease. *Ophthalmology* 92:1325, 1985.
McDonald HR, Char DH: Adenoid cystic carcinoma presenting as an orbital apex syndrome. *Ann Ophthalmol* 17:757, 1985.
Maurer HM, Donaldson M, Gehan EA, et al: The intergroup rhabdomyosarcoma study: Update— November 1978. *J Natl Cancer Inst Monogr* 56:61, 1981.
Mauriello JA, Flanagan JC: Management of orbital inflammatory disease. *Surv Ophthalmol* 29:104, 1984.
Mottow LS, Jakobiec FA, Smith M: Idiopathic inflammatory orbital pseudotumor in childhood. II. Results of diagnostic tests and biopsies. *Ophthalmology* 88:565, 1981.
Musarella MA, Chan HSL, DeBoer G, et al: Ocular involvement in neuroblastoma: Prognostic implications. *Ophthalmology* 91:936, 1984.
Nelson LB, Melnick JE, Harley RD: Intralesional corticosteroid injections for infantile hemangioma of the eyelid. *Pediatrics* 74:241, 1984.
Nicholson DH, Green WR: Ocular tumors in children. In: Nelson LB, Calhoun JH, Harley RD: *Pediatric Ophthalmology.* 3d ed. Philadelphia, WB Saunders Co, 1991, pp 382–426.
Orbit, eyelids, and lacrimal system, section 9. In *Basic and Clinical Science Course.* San Francisco, American Academy of Ophthalmology, 1988.

Orcutt JC, Garner A, Henk JM, et al: Treatment of idiopathic inflammatory pseudotumor by radiotherapy. *Br J Ophthalmol* 67:570, 1983.

Robin JB, Schanzlin DJ, Meisler DM, et al: Ocular involvement in the respiratory vasculitides. *Surv Ophthalmol* 30:127, 1985.

Rootman J, Hay E, Graeb D, et al: Orbital-adnexal lymphangiomas. *Ophthalmology* 93:1558, 1986.

Rootman J, Nugent R: The classification and management of acute orbital pseudotumors. *Ophthalmology* 89:1040, 1982.

Rootman J, Robertson W, Lapointe JS, et al: Lymphoproliferative and leukemic lesions. In Rootman J (ed): *Diseases of the Orbit.* Philadelphia, Lippincott 1988, p 227.

Rosenthal AR: Ocular manifestations of leukemia: A review. *Ophthalmology* 90:899, 1983.

Rubin SE, Rubin LG, Zito J, et al: Medical management of subperiosteal orbital abscess in children. *J Pediatr Ophthalmol Strabismus* 26:21, 1989.

Schwartz JN, Donnelly EH, Klintworth GK: Ocular and orbital phycomycosis. *Surv Ophthalmol* 22:3, 1977.

Seibert RW, Seibert JJ, Frazier EA: Infarction of the orbit and paranasal sinuses in sickle cell anemia. *South Med J* 80:1569, 1987.

Sherman RP, Rootman J, Lapointe JS: Orbital dermoids: Clinical presentation and management. *Br J Ophthalmol* 68:642, 1984.

Shetlar DJ, Font RL, Ordonez N, et al: A clinicopathologic study of three carcinoid tumors metastatic to the orbit. *Ophthalmology* 97:257, 1990.

Shields CL, Shields JA, Peggs M: Metastatic tumors to the orbit. *Ophthalmol Plast Reconstr Surg* 4:73, 1988.

Shields JA: *Diagnosis and Management of Orbital Tumors.* Philadelphia, WB Saunders Co, 1989.

Shields JA, Bakewell B, Augsburger JJ, et al: Classification and incidence of space-occupying lesions of the orbit: A review of 645 biopsies. *Arch Ophthalmol* 102:1606, 1984.

Shields JA, Bakewell B, Augsburger JJ, et al: Space-occupying orbital masses in children. *Ophthalmology* 93:379, 1986.

Shorr N, Lessner AM, Goldberg RA: Proptosis: A systematic approach to its diagnosis and management. *Ophthalmic Pract* 8:95, 1990.

Spires JR, Smith RJH: Bacterial infections of the orbital and periorbital soft tissues in children. *Laryngoscope* 96:763, 1986.

Stefanyszyn MA, Harley RD, Penne RB: Disorders of the orbit. In Nelson LB, Calhoun JH, Harley RD: *Pediatric Ophthalmology.* 3d ed. Philadelphia, WB Saunders Co, 1991, pp 355–381.

Steinberger AA: Cavernous sinus thrombosis. In Hornblass A (ed): *Oculoplastic, Orbital, and Reconstructive Surgery.* Baltimore, Williams & Wilkins, 1990, pp 933–935.

Steinkuller PG, Jones DB: Preseptal and orbital cellulitis and orbital abscess. In Linberg JV: *Oculoplastic and Orbital Emergencies.* Norwalk, CT, Appleton & Lange 1990, pp 51–66.

Weaver DT, Bartley GB: Malignant neoplasia of the paranasal sinus associated with mucocele. *Ophthalmology* 98:342, 1991.

Weber AL, Mikulis DK: Inflammatory disorders of the paraorbital sinuses and their complications. *Radiol Clin North Am* 25:615, 1987.

Weichselbaum RR, Cassady JR, Albert DM, et al: Multimodality management of orbital rhabdomyosarcoma. *Int Ophthalmol Clin* 20:247, 1980.

Wharam M, Beltangady M, Hayes D, et al: Localized orbital rhabdomyosarcoma. An interim report of the intergroup rhabdomyosarcoma study committee. *Ophthalmology* 94:251, 1987.

Wilson ME, Parker PL, Chavis RM: Conservative management of childhood lymphangioma. *Ophthalmology* 96:484, 1989.

Wilson WB: Meningiomas of the anterior visual system. *Surv Ophthalmol* 26:109, 1981.

Wilson WB, Manke WF: Orbital decompression in Graves' disease: The predictability of reduction of proptosis. *Arch Ophthalmol* 109:343, 1991.

Wolff MH, Sty JR: Orbital infarction in sickle cell disease. *Pediatr Radiol* 15:50, 1985.

Wright JE, Stewart WB, Krohel GB: Clinical presentation and management of lacrimal gland tumors. *Br J Ophthalmol* 63:600, 1979.

Ziegler JL: Burkitt's lymphoma. *Cancer* 32:144, 1982.

Zimmerman LE, Font RL: Ophthalmologic manifestations of granulocytic sarcoma (myeloid sarcoma or chloroma). *Am J Ophthalmol* 80:975, 1975.

Zinreich SJ, Kennedy DW, Malat J, et al: Fungal sinusitis: Diagnosis with CT and MR imaging. *Radiology* 169:439, 1988.

13

Neuro-Ophthalmologic and Nontraumatic Retinal Emergencies

Robert A. Catalano

A patient who splashed bleach in his eye can clearly articulate why he came to the Emergency Department, and his treatment can be readily instituted. Patients with neuro-ophthalmologic and nontraumatic retinal emergencies, however, do not present with their diagnosis. They present with symptoms, which are usually not exclusive to a specific region of the eye or cause.

This chapter and the next discuss 12 such symptoms and one sign that commonly present as ophthalmic emergencies (Table 13–1). Each constitutes a separate section, which begins with a differential diagnosis. Understandably, there is some overlap among the sections. Specific conditions may be listed under more than one differential but are discussed only under their most common or most incapacitating symptom. In addition, some symptoms may be due to conditions that mimic neuro-ophthalmologic or retinal disorders but in fact are due to problems occurring in some other ocular structure. The differential will include these disorders and direct readers to the appropriate chapter in this book.

The symptom of sudden loss of vision encompasses a great many disorders. For clarity, the workup of a patient who presents with this symptom is discussed separately (Chapter 14). Most of the nontraumatic retinal emergencies and many of the neuro-ophthalmologic emergencies that an ophthalmologist may encounter are included under the discussion of this symptom.

TABLE 13-1. PRESENTING SYMPTOMS OF A POSSIBLE NEURO-OPHTHALMOLOGIC OR RETINAL DISORDER

Sudden onset of diplopia (double vision)

Sudden development of a pupillary abnormality

Headaches

Painful ophthalmoplegia (pain and restricted eye movements)

Visual hallucinations

Oscillopsia (perception that the environment is moving)

Metamorphopsia (distortion of vision)

Photophobia (sensitivity to light)

Photopsia (flashes of light or colored spots)

Floaters

Blinking and blepharospasm (spasm of the facial muscles)

Leukocoria (white reflex in the pupil; a *sign*)

Sudden visual field loss or abnormality

Sudden loss of vision (see Chapter 14)

SUDDEN ONSET OF BINOCULAR DIPLOPIA (DOUBLE VISION)

A. History
B. Physical findings and evaluation techniques
C. Due to cranial nerve palsies
   1. Associated with neoplasia
   2. Associated with trauma
   3. Associated with vascular disorders
      a. Aneurysm
      b. Diabetes
      c. Arteriosclerosis and hypertension
      d. Temporal arteritis (see also Chapter 14)
   4. Associated with cavernous sinus or superior orbital syndromes
      a. Carotid-cavernous fistula
      b. Cavernous sinus thrombosis
      c. Metastatic tumors (lymphoma, leukemia)
      d. Mucormycosis (see below and Chapter 12)
      e. Tolosa-Hunt syndrome (see Chapter 12)
      f. Mucocele (see Chapter 12)
      g. Herpes zoster (see below and Chapter 16)

5. Associated with infectious diseases
   a. Bacterial
      i. Meningitis
      ii. Lyme disease
   b. Viral
   c. Fungal (mucormycosis)
6. Associated with neurogenic disorders
   a. Multiple sclerosis
   b. Internuclear ophthalmoplegia
   c. Guillain-Barré syndrome
   d. Wernicke's encephalopathy
7. Associated with increased intracranial pressure
   a. Neoplasia
   b. Pseudotumor cerebri
   c. Hydrocephalus
8. Associated with ophthalmoplegic migraine (see below)

D. Special considerations for isolated cranial nerve palsies

1. Sixth nerve palsies
2. Fourth nerve palsies
3. Third nerve palsies

E. Muscular disorders and the sudden onset of diplopia

1. Myasthenia gravis
2. Thyroid ophthalmopathy
3. Pseudotumor/myositis

F. Orbital disorders and diplopia (see Chapter 12)

1. Orbital fracture/hematoma
2. Orbital pseudotumor/tumor
3. Orbital cellulitis/mucormycosis

G. Subluxation of the ocular lens and diplopia (see Chapter 7)

H. Macular edema and diplopia (see Chapter 14)

History

A few simple questions and examination techniques can narrow the differential diagnosis when a patient presents with diplopia.

Is the patient a child or adult? In children, neoplastic, traumatic, and inflammatory causes are more common. In adults, aneurysmal, neoplastic, vascular (especially diabetes), and traumatic causes predominate.

Is the diplopia monocular or binocular? If the diplopia persists with one eye occluded, the disorder is almost assuredly not neuro-ophthalmologic. Monocular diplopia can be caused by an uncorrected refractive error, corneal irregularity, dislocated lens, cataract, vitreous or retinal disorder, or a nonorganic disorder.

Is there associated pain? Painful ophthalmoplegias (pain associated with paralysis of the extraocular muscles) are due to tumors, pseudotumor, infections, bleeding aneurysms, diabetes, or temporal arteritis. Pain that remits with the onset of third nerve palsy in children suggests ophthalmoplegic migraine. Persistent pain suggests a cavernous sinus or superior orbital syndrome. Pain in association with obtundation or stupor suggests a ruptured aneurysm. Myasthenia gravis and thyroid ophthalmopathy are painless.

Is the pupil dilated? The presence of a fixed dilated pupil and diminished ability to focus near objects (accommodation) suggests a compressive disorder or aneurysm affecting the third nerve. Myasthenia and dysthyroidism spare the pupil and accommodation; this is also generally true with diabetic infarcts.

Is the diplopia intermittent or persistent? An intermittent or remitting palsy in an adult suggests diabetes, a vascular accident, or myasthenia; in children, intermittent palsies are seen following viral-like illnesses, inflammation, migraine, and trauma.

Is more than one cranial nerve involved? It is very useful to distinguish solitary oculomotor paresis from conditions that simultaneously involve multiple cranial nerves or extraocular muscles. Generally, the simultaneous onset of multiple palsies suggests an orbital or cavernous sinus syndrome, brain stem lesion, pituitary apoplexy, acute polyneuropathy *(Guillain-Barré syndrome),* carcinomatous meningitis, basal sarcoidosis, ocular myasthenia, or thyroid ophthalmopathy. The last two are usually painless, involve the eyes bilaterally, and spare the pupils. Unilateral involvement and pain are more typical of orbital and cavernous sinus syndromes. The latter may also be associated with proptosis, facial hypesthesia, and periocular pulsation.

Physical Findings and Evaluation Techniques

Localization to Involved Muscle or Nerve

Localization to vertical or horizontal acting extraocular muscles can be achieved by asking the patient with binocular diplopia whether the images are separated vertically or horizontally. If the diplopia is horizontal, further localization to the medial or lateral recti muscles can be achieved. Diplopia worse at distance fixation directs attention to the lateral recti and sixth cranial nerves; diplopia greater at near fixation directs attention to the medial recti. If, in addition, the patient notes that the displacement of images is greater on right or left gaze, the physician can specifically isolate the abnormally acting muscle or nerve. For instance, if the patient notes horizontal diplopia, worse at distance fixation, and in left gaze, attention should be directed to the left lateral rectus muscle and left abducens nerve.

Ductions and Versions

Formal examination techniques include testing ocular ductions and versions. There are six cardinal positions of gaze, and a single extraocular muscle is the prime mover of each eye into each position (Table 13-2; see also Figure 5-3). To diagnose a subtle extraocular muscle palsy, a dissimilar image test can be performed. A red lens or red Maddox rod is placed in front of one of the patient's eyes as they fixate a penlight. The patient's fixation is then directed into each of the cardinal positions of gaze. The image seen with one eye is the light of the penlight. In the other eye, a red light (if a red lens is used) or a red line (red Maddox rod test) is seen. With the acute onset of diplopia, the separation of images increases as the eyes move into the field of action of the paretic muscle. Furthermore, the separation of images will be greater when the patient fixates the penlight with the eye with the paretic muscle (the secondary deviation) than when he or she fixates the penlight with the sound eye (the primary deviation). Cover testing, using prisms to neutralize the misalignment of an eye with a paretic muscle, is a more objective method for isolating a single paretic muscle.

Ocular Saccades, Pursuit, and Vestibulo-Ocular Reflex Testing

Additional diagnostic techniques include directing the patient to quickly move the eyes in a certain direction (testing ocular saccades) or to follow a slowly moving object (testing ocular pursuit). Note is made of any lag in the movement of one eye. When directing the patient to look to the side, a lag in the adducting (turning in) eye is one sign of an *internuclear ophthalmoplegia*. Inability to look upward can signify a periaqueductal *(Parinaud's)* syndrome. Doll's head (oculocephalic) maneuvers and caloric testing make use of the ves-

TABLE 13-2. POSSIBLE PARETIC MUSCLE WHEN DIPLOPIA IS WORSE IN A SPECIFIC CARDINAL POSITION OF GAZE

POSITION OF GAZE	POSSIBLE PARETIC MUSCLE	
	Right Eye	*Left Eye*
Up and to the right	Right superior rectus	Left inferior oblique
Straight to the right	Right lateral rectus	Left medial rectus
Down and to the right	Right inferior rectus	Left superior oblique
Down and to the left	Right superior oblique	Left inferior rectus
Straight to the left	Right medial rectus	Left lateral rectus
Up and to the left	Right inferior oblique	Left superior rectus

tibular system to move the eyes into a paretic field of gaze. Deviation of the eyes into the paretic field establishes the etiology as being supranuclear or above the cranial nerve nucleus and extraocular muscle pathway.

Forced Duction and Tensilon Testing

Mechanical movement of the eye into various fields of gaze (forced duction testing) is used to detect restriction to ocular movements. Tensilon testing involves the intravenous use of up to 10 mg (1 cc) of edrophonium chloride to test for immunologic blockade of the acetylcholine receptor sites on the extraocular muscles; a positive response is diagnostic of *myasthenia gravis* (see below).

Laboratory Examinations

Adults who present with the sudden onset of diplopia should be tested for diabetes with a glucose tolerance test. Adults older than age 55 years should also be tested for temporal arteritis, diagnosed by an elevated Westergren erythrocyte sedimentation rate (W-ESR) and, if positive, a temporal artery biopsy. A normal W-ESR is approximately the age of the individual divided by two in males with the addition of 5 mm per hour to this calculation in females (see Chapter 14). Diplopia can be the first indication of either of these disorders. Children should have a peripheral blood count for lymphocytosis. In the absence of other signs, an elevated white blood cell count could suggest a benign postviral illness.

Neuroimaging Studies

In traumatized patients, a computed axial tomography (CT) scan provides good visualization of soft tissues, bony structures, acute hematomas, and foreign bodies. Coronal or sagittal scans may be particularly useful to visualize entrapped extraocular muscles in patients with facial fractures and diplopia but may be unobtainable in acutely injured patients. For orbital floor fractures, a combination of oblique sagittal and coronal projections will best display all fracture margins (see Chapter 2).

In nontraumatized patients, CT scan or magnetic resonance imaging (MRI) is immediately indicated in patients with third nerve palsies involving the pupil and should be strongly considered even if the pupil is spared. This is especially the case in patients without long-standing diabetes or with incomplete or nonresolving third nerve palsies, multiple cranial nerve abnormalities, or aberrant regeneration of the third nerve. If these studies are normal and the patient is older than age 20 years, cerebral angiography is usually indicated. MRI is superior to CT scan in evaluating posterior fossa disease (see Chapter 2). MRI is preferable for children with diplopia to rule out a posterior fossa tumor.

Table 13-3 lists several diagnostic studies to be considered in the patient who presents with acute diplopia.

TABLE 13–3. DIAGNOSTIC STUDIES TO CONSIDER FOR PATIENTS WITH DIPLOPIA

Forced duction test	Peripheral blood count for lymphocytosis (children)
Tensilon test	
Glucose tolerance test	Neuroradiographic studies
Erythrocyte sedimentation test (older adults)	Cerebral angiography

Cranial Nerve Palsies and the Sudden Onset of Diplopia

Discussion of the orbital disorders that cause diplopia is found in Chapter 12. Diplopia in these disorders is caused by displacement of the globe and misalignment of the common visual direction of the two eyes. In addition to diplopia, proptosis, restricted eye movement, pain, periorbital masses, and pulsation suggest an orbital disorder.

Cranial Nerve Palsies Associated with Neoplasia

Children with papilledema, decreased corneal sensitivity, nystagmus, and the acute onset of diplopia almost always have a brain tumor. Bilaterality of the paresis is a further indication of tumor. A history of trauma is often given in cases where tumors are eventually diagnosed. This is likely because uncoordination, ataxia, and falling are early manifestations of posterior fossa tumors. The majority of associated tumors in children with sixth nerve palsies are brainstem gliomas, followed by posterior fossa astrocytomas and medulloblastomas. Approximately 40% of tumors responsible for sixth nerve palsies in adults are metastatic.

Tumor involvement of the cavernous sinus is also usually metastatic; lymphomas and leukemias are the most common. Metastatic involvement of the cavernous sinus is heralded by a combination of unilateral third, fourth, and sixth nerve palsies with facial pain or numbness in the distribution of the first or second branch of the fifth cranial nerve. *Carcinomatous meningitis* can also rapidly produce bilateral sequential cranial nerve palsies. This diagnosis requires positive cytology in three lumbar punctures. *Nasopharyngeal carcinoma* is another neoplastic syndrome that results in sequential cranial nerve palsies. The sixth cranial nerve is typically involved first; the patient may also have ear pain and nasal and eustachian tube obstruction. The last results in serous otitis media, cervical lymphadenopathy, and exophthalmos.

Pituitary apoplexy is the syndrome of sudden infarction of a pituitary tumor that has extrasellar extension. It is characterized by severe headache, oculomotor disturbances, and variable visual field defects. The last may include bitemporal hemianopsia or abrupt bilateral blindness. Signs and symptoms usually progress rapidly. Slow-growing pituitary tumors, which produce visual symptoms due to insidious chiasmal compression, usually do not produce ophthalmoplegia. Neuroradiographic studies demonstrate the enlarged sella turcica (see Chapter 2).

Cranial Nerve Palsies Associated with Trauma

Head trauma is a common cause of cranial nerve palsies. The sixth, third, and fourth nerves are affected, in this order. The position of the fourth nerves with respect to the tentorial edge increases their susceptibility to injury in closed-head, sudden-deceleration injuries. Bilateral palsies are not uncommon in these situations. A few cases of minor head trauma precipitating a third nerve palsy have been reported. In each case, a large basicranial tumor, which encased and stretched the third nerve, was present.

Severe crushing injuries, manifest by loss of consciousness and skull fractures, are usually necessary to cause traumatic sixth nerve palsies. Seventh nerve palsies are often associated. Blood or cerebral spinal fluid draining from the external ear or ecchymosis of the mastoid bone *(Battle's sign)* may be evidence of a basal skull fracture.

The presence of certain signs in traumatic third nerve palsies may help localize the site of injury. Bilateral ptosis with unilateral motility disturbances localizes the injury to the third nerve nucleus. Damage in the brain stem may be associated with contralateral weakness *(Weber syndrome)* or hemidyskinesia *(Benedikt syndrome)*. Isolated mydriasis suggests damage in the middle cranial fossa, where the pupillary fibers run peripherally in the nerve, in the ciliary ganglion, or to the iris itself *(traumatic mydriasis)*.

The association of trauma with rapid onset of redness, conjunctival swelling (chemosis), proptosis, diplopia, and a bruit suggests the development of a *carotid-cavernous fistula. Cavernous sinus thrombosis* (Figure 13-1) may also occur. In both, the first division of the fifth nerve is usually affected, and the second division is affected if the entire sinus is involved. The *orbital apex syndrome* includes all of these features, with the addition of optic neuropathy.

Cranial Nerve Palsies Associated with Vascular Disorders

Several vascular disorders are included in the differential diagnosis of all oculomotor pareses. Precipitous dilatation of a posterior communicating artery aneurysm is the most common cause of an acute, spontaneous third nerve palsy with pupillary involvement. Hypertension and diabetes are frequent causes of cranial nerve palsy in elderly patients and should be suspected if the paresis is remitting. Temporal arteritis is a rare but treatable cause of isolated cranial nerve palsy and may be seen in association with polymyalgia rheumatica or arteritic optic neuropathy.

Although the incidence of ophthalmoplegia in diabetes is relatively rare, a

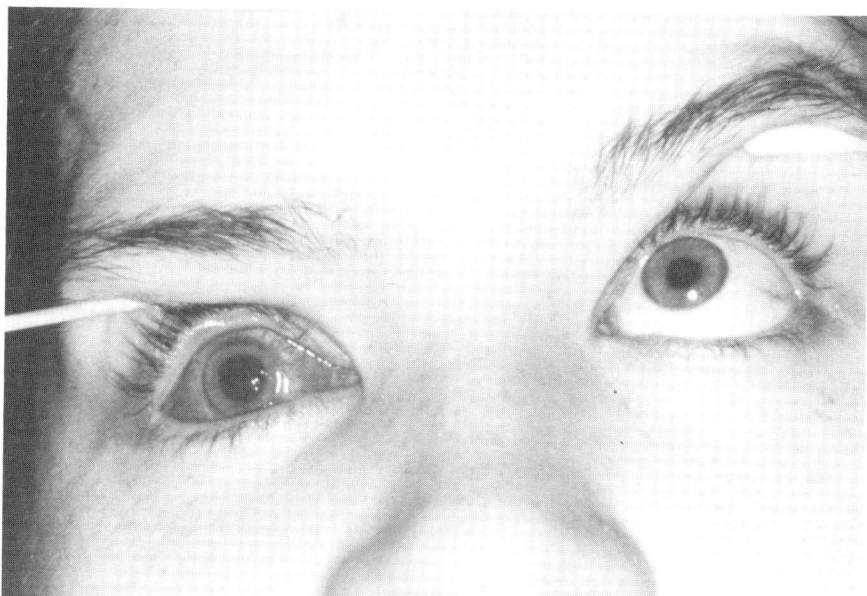

FIGURE 13-1. Traumatic cavernous sinus thrombosis.

cranial nerve palsy may be the first sign of diabetes. Recurrences in the same or other nerves may also occur. The simultaneous occurrence of multiple cranial nerve palsies, however, is exceedingly rare with diabetes, and an alternate diagnosis should be considered. The absence of pupillary involvement in third nerve palsy is helpful in differentiating a diabetic third nerve palsy from a palsy due to a compressive disorder or ruptured aneurysm. Pupillary fibers course the periphery of the third nerve; ischemic infarcts due to diabetes usually spare these peripheral fibers and pupillary function. In addition, pain, headache, or mild ocular discomfort may occur with diabetic palsies. The pain may precede the palsy and may be severe. Persistent pain, however, is more characteristic of cavernous sinus and superior orbital fissure syndromes and nasopharyngeal carcinoma involving the clivus. Recovery from diabetic palsies usually occurs from several weeks to 3 months.

Cranial Nerve Palsies Associated with Cavernous Sinus or Superior Orbital Fissure Syndromes

Cavernous sinus and superior orbital fissure syndromes are distinguished by multiple cranial nerve palsies and pain and numbness around the eye in the distribution of the first (trigeminal) or second (maxillary) branch of the fifth cranial nerve. Concomitant sympathetic paresis may diminish pupillary dilatation even in the presence of a total third nerve palsy. The occasional appearance of a normal-sized pupil and asymmetric involvement of the different fibers of the third nerve may cause confusion of cavernous sinus syndromes with myasthenia. The majority of cavernous sinus syndromes are vascular in etiology. Tumors, infection, and inflammation in this or the superior orbital fissure *(Tolosa-Hunt syndrome),* however, can cause similar signs.

When diplopia is accompanied by severe pain, dilated tortuous conjunctival and episcleral vessels, exophthalmos, ocular bruit, and increased intraocular pressure, a *carotid-cavernous fistula* should be suspected. These abnormal communications between a branch of the carotid artery and the cavernous sinus can result from head trauma (75% of cases) or occur spontaneously. The latter is usually seen in postmenopausal women. Traumatic fistulas usually result in a direct connection between the internal carotid and cavernous sinus and have a high flow rate. These are more likely to manifest as a rapid onset of redness, proptosis, bruits, severe pain, conjunctival swelling (chemosis), and ophthalmoplegia. Spontaneous fistulas usually result in the connection between a meningeal (dural) branch of the internal or external carotid artery and the sinus. Dural fistulas are usually of lower flow, and the signs may mimic thyroid disease; the latter, however, is usually bilateral. A distinguishing sign of low flow shunts is the arteriolization of episcleral and conjunctival vessels, which become dilated and tortuous. The major organ at risk is the eye, with visual loss occurring secondary to elevated intraocular pressure. Diplopia results most commonly from paresis of the sixth nerve or mechanical limitation of movement of the eye caused by enlarged, engorged extraocular muscles. Abnormal pulsation of the globe may be present but difficult to observe. Neuroradiographic studies are useful to demonstrate an enlarged superior ophthalmic vein (see Chapter 2). Balloon embolization of the fistula may be ameliorative.

Infection (particularly *Staphylococcus aureus*) carried by the bloodstream from the face, sinuses, nasal cavity, orbit, or mouth is the most common cause of *cavernous sinus thrombosis.* This can also result following a fracture through the cavernous sinus or a neurosurgical procedure in the area of the sinus (Figure 13-1). When it occurs in association with orbital cellulitis, the earliest signs are headache, fever, nausea, vomiting, and altered consciousness. In contrast to the bright red appearance of the eyelids with cellulitis, the lids in this disorder appear bluish-purple due to venous congestion. Proptosis and swelling of the conjunctiva are also seen. Ocular motor palsies and decreased sensation in the maxillary distribution of the facial nerve appear early, seemingly out of proportion to the amount of proptosis and edema. Eventually engorgement of the retinal veins, disc edema, and elevated intraocular pressure develop. The occurrence of a contralateral sixth nerve palsy is the earliest indication of contralateral spread of the cavernous sinus thrombosis. Infectious causes require intravenous antibiotics; aseptic cavernous sinus thrombosis can be treated with systemic anticoagulation.

Cranial Nerve Palsies Associated with Infectious Diseases

Fifty years ago, basilar meningitis due to syphilis and tuberculosis was not an unusual cause of cranial nerve palsy. The third nerve was usually involved bilaterally, and other cranial nerve and brain stem findings were associated. Meningococcic meningitis is a rare cause of third nerve palsy today.

Lyme disease is a tick-borne illness caused by the spirochete *Borrelia burgdorferi*. It is most common in the eastern United States, Pacific Northwest, and Midwest. Neuro-ophthalmologic manifestations include meningitis with papilledema, optic neuritis, neuroretinitis, and sixth nerve paresis. Additional findings include multiple cranial nerve neuropathies, radiculopathy, conjunctivitis, episcleritis, keratitis, and iridocyclitis. The illness usually begins in the summer, following a tick bite. The first stage includes a localized blotchy red skin rash, known as erythema chronicum migrans, stiff neck, fever, headache, fatigue, malaise, myalgias, and/or arthralgias. Not all patients, however, develop a fever or rash. The second stage, occurring in up to 15% of patients, includes meningitis with or without facial nerve palsy and carditis. The third stage, occurring months to years later in up to 60% of untreated patients, is characterized by an oligoarticular arthritis. Central nervous system manifestations can occur during either the second or third stage; cranial neuropathies occur most commonly during the second stage, approximately 4 weeks after the onset of the rash. Most patients with neurologic manifestations also have headache, spinal fluid lymphocytic pleocytosis, and occasionally elevated cerebrospinal fluid (CSF) protein, but normal CSF glucose and opening pressure; half have a facial palsy.

An enzyme-linked immunosorbent assay (ELISA) is available for diagnosis through Microbiology Reference Laboratory (MRL), 10703 Progress Way, Cypress, California. A panel of tests, including a quantitative ELISA test and Lyme immunofluorescent IgG and IgM titers, are provided. Additional tests, also available through MRL, include a Lyme Western blot, a Lyme lymphocyte stimulation test, and a Lyme polymerase chain reaction test. The recommended treatment is tetracycline (250 mg by mouth 4 times per day) or doxycycline (100 mg 2 times per day) for 10 days to 20 days. For children, penicillin 50 mg/kg per day in four divided doses (not < 1 g or > 2 g per day), or erythromycin 30 mg/kg per day in three to four divided doses, for 15 days to 20 days, can be used. If the central nervous system is involved, intravenous ceftriaxone (2 g every 12 hours for 14 days), cefotaxime, or intravenous penicillin G (2 million to 4 million units every 4 hours for 10 days) is recommended.

Benign recurrent sixth nerve palsies also occur as postviral illnesses in children. Rarely, they follow an immunization for rubella, rubeola, mumps, diphtheria, or pertussis. The onset is typically 1 week to 4 weeks after illness or immunization, and resolution occurs in 1 month to 3 months. For unknown reasons, the left sixth nerve is more commonly involved. With the onset of acquired immune deficiency syndrome, diplopia secondary to cranial nerve involvement by infectious agents (e.g., herpes zoster) is again becoming more prevalent. Complete or partial third nerve palsy occurs more commonly than fourth or sixth nerve palsy in *herpes zoster ophthalmicus.* Occasionally only the pupil is involved. Full recovery of motor function usually occurs, but the pupil may remain mid-dilated and poorly responsive to light.

In diabetics, especially those in ketoacidosis or debilitated patients, an acute orbital inflammatory syndrome may arise due to the fungus *mucormycosis.* The organism causes thrombosis of orbital arteries, leading to ischemic necrosis of orbital structures. This often progresses to cavernous sinus thrombosis and death. Nasal examination may reveal blood and a black crusty material. Surgical debridement and amphotericin B is the treatment of choice (see Chapters 12 and 16).

Cranial Nerve Palsies Associated with Neurogenic Disorders

Diplopia and strabismus are the most common features of brain stem and cranial nerve involvement in *multiple sclerosis.* The abducens is the most frequently involved nerve. Another sign of multiple sclerosis is *internuclear ophthalmoplegia* (INO), a disorder characterized by weakness or the inability of an eye to look inward (nasally) when the opposite eye looks outward (temporally). The outward-looking eye also manifests nystagmus. The misalignment of the eyes on side gaze results in diplopia. Myasthenia gravis, vascular infarcts of the brain stem (elderly patients), and brain stem lesions (tumors, aneurysms) are other causes of INO.

Rapidly progressive and painless, bilateral cranial nerve palsies may occur in the *Miller-Fisher bulbar variant of Guillain-Barré syndrome.* Facial paralysis and pupillary involvement usually accompany the inability to move the extraocular muscles. Ataxia, areflexia, and sensory signs are also usually present. This condition often follows a viral illness, fever, or infectious mononucleosis.

Cranial Nerve Palsies Associated with Increased Intracranial Pressure

An early sign of increased intracranial pressure may be a decrease in the ability to turn the eyes outward (an abduction deficit). Clinically, symptoms mimic divergence paralysis; patients complain of horizontal diplopia when viewing distant objects. Headache, vomiting, circulatory (slow pulse), and respiratory (increased rate, Cheyne-Stokes breathing) disturbances and psychic changes are other nonlocalizing signs of increased intracranial pressure.

In the setting of increased intracranial pressure, a localizing sign is the *clivus-ridge syndrome,* which is clinically manifest as a unilateral mydriatic pupil, which is usually still reactive to light and convergence. Increased intracranial pressure compresses the superficial dorsal pupillomotor fibers of the third nerve against the clivus ridge of the tentorial notch. When present, it suggests an ipsilateral space occupying supratentorial mass. In the early stages, it may be present in the absence of paresis of any of the extraocular muscles.

Ophthalmoplegic Migraine

Ophthalmoplegic migraine is a disorder usually seen in children in their first decade who have a family history of migraine. The third nerve, including the pupil, is most commonly involved. Ophthalmoplegia is often preceded by pain in and about the involved eye, nausea, and vomiting. These symptoms remit with the onset of the third nerve palsy. The paresis typically resolves within 1 month, but may last for years. The disorder may be more common in blacks with hemoglobin AS, for unknown reasons.

Special Considerations for Isolated Cranial Nerve Palsies

Isolated Sixth Nerve Palsies

The sixth nerve innervates only the lateral rectus muscle, which pulls the eye outward. Eyes with sixth nerve palsies deviate inward; their ability to turn outward is diminished (Figure 13-2).

The intracranial course of the sixth nerve is long; lesions from the brain stem to the orbit can cause a sixth nerve palsy. Associated findings are often helpful in locating the lesion. Disorders in the area of the sixth nerve (abducens) nucleus cause an ipsilateral gaze paresis rather than an isolated sixth nerve palsy. Lesions in the dorsal pons *(Foville's syndrome)* result in ipsilateral facial weakness, facial analgesia, deafness, and Horner's syndrome (small pupil, lid droop, and decreased sweating). If the lesion is in the ventral pons *(Millard-Gubler's syndrome),* contralateral hemiplegia will accompany the abduction weakness. These lesions are usually due to vascular disease in the elderly, but occasionally they can be caused by demyelinating disease or tumor. Meningiomas and acoustic neuromas in the cerebellopontine angle result in sixth nerve palsies in association with seventh and eighth nerve disorders, corneal hypesthesia, nystagmus, and cerebellar signs.

After leaving the brain stem, the sixth nerve travels in the basal cistern, where it is susceptible to basilar tumors such as nasopharyngeal carcinoma, more common in patients of Chinese ancestry. Increased intracranial pressure from tumors, hydrocephalus, or pseudotumor cerebri can also stretch the sixth nerve between its exit from the brain stem and its attachment to the clivus. Elevated intracranial pressure manifests as sixth nerve paresis accompanied by nausea, vomiting, papilledema, and headache. Farther anteriorly, the sixth nerve passes beneath the petroclinoid ligament. Mastoiditis, arising from middle ear infections, can cause a petrositis with involvement of the facial nerve (facial

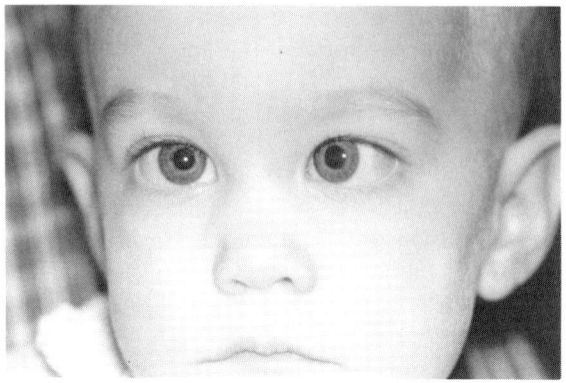

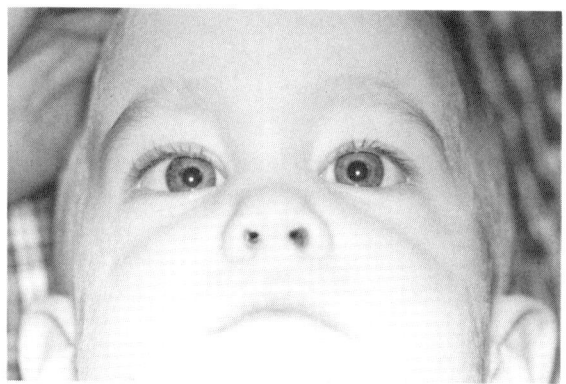

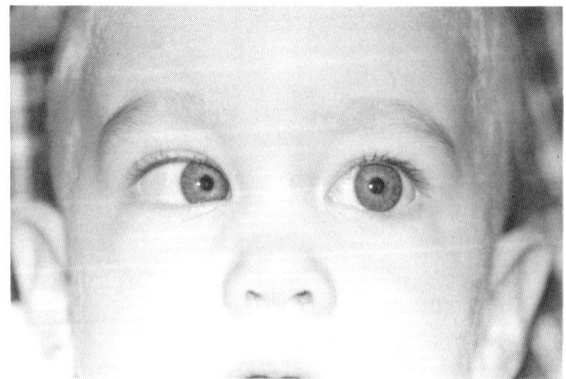

FIGURE 13–2. Bilateral sixth nerve palsy.

palsy), trigeminal ganglion (facial pain), and sixth nerve *(Gradenigo's syndrome)*. The sixth nerve then traverses through the middle of the cavernous sinus, where, in association with the third and fourth nerves, it is susceptible to traumatic, vascular, and inflammatory disorders. Lesions in the superior orbital fissure or orbital apex typically involve multiple cranial nerves and/or produce proptosis.

It is important to recognize that the cause of sixth nerve paresis differs in pediatric and adult populations (Table 13-4). Tumors and trauma are encountered more frequently in the pediatric age range. Inflammatory disease as a cause of sixth nerve palsy, including meningoencephalitis, Gradenigo's syndrome, and brain abscess, also occurs almost exclusively in children. With the exception of congenital anomalies, however, vascular disease is essentially a nonexistent cause in children. Rare causes in either group include lumbar puncture or spinal anesthesia.

A transient sixth nerve palsy after an otherwise benign viral illness in children has also been described. The palsy develops 7 days to 21 days following a fever or upper respiratory infection and usually resolves within 10 weeks. The age range of reported patients has been 18 months to the early teenage years. Hydrocephalus, pseudotumor cerebri, leukemia, and subdural hematomas comprise some of the more common miscellaneous causes of this paresis in children and young adults.

Although the prognosis is poor when the cause is neoplastic, complete spontaneous resolution usually occurs in over 50% of patients with traumatic sixth nerve palsies. The prognosis is even better when the cause is inflammatory; greater than 90% of inflammatory pareses resolve completely and spontaneously.

Isolated Fourth Nerve Palsies

The fourth cranial nerve innervates only the superior oblique muscle. This muscle serves to rotate the eye inward, depress, and slightly turn the eye out-

TABLE 13-4. ETIOLOGY OF SIXTH NERVE PARESIS

ETIOLOGY	CHILDREN < 15 YEARS OF AGE	PATIENTS OF ALL AGE GROUPS
Neoplasm	39%	31%
Head trauma	20	11
Inflammatory	17	—
Vascular disease	3	9
Aneurysm	—	3
Undetermined	9	22
Other	12	24

(Modified from Harley RD: Paralytic strabismus in children. *Ophthalmology* 87:24, 1980.)

ward. The eye with a fourth nerve palsy is higher than the contralateral eye, and this difference becomes greater upon tilting the head to the affected side (Figures 13-3 and 13-4).

Isolated fourth nerve palsies occur less frequently than sixth or third nerve palsies. Superior oblique palsies that present spontaneously in late childhood or early adulthood often represent "decompensated" congenital palsies that can no longer be controlled by fusional mechanisms. Increased vertical fusion amplitudes are indicative of congenital palsies that decompensated. Head tilts in old photographs also suggest a long-standing condition.

Because of its long intracranial course within the subarachnoid space, the peripheral fourth nerve is especially vulnerable to contrecoup shearing forces in closed-head trauma. Microvascular injuries, particularly diabetes, are second only to trauma as a cause of isolated fourth nerve palsy. Compression from hydrocephalus, tumors, and vascular loops also occurs, but compression from aneurysmal dilatation rarely occurs as an isolated finding.

Herpes zoster ophthalmicus, inflammation, and injury to the trochlea that suspends the superior oblique tendon are rare causes of isolated fourth nerve palsy.

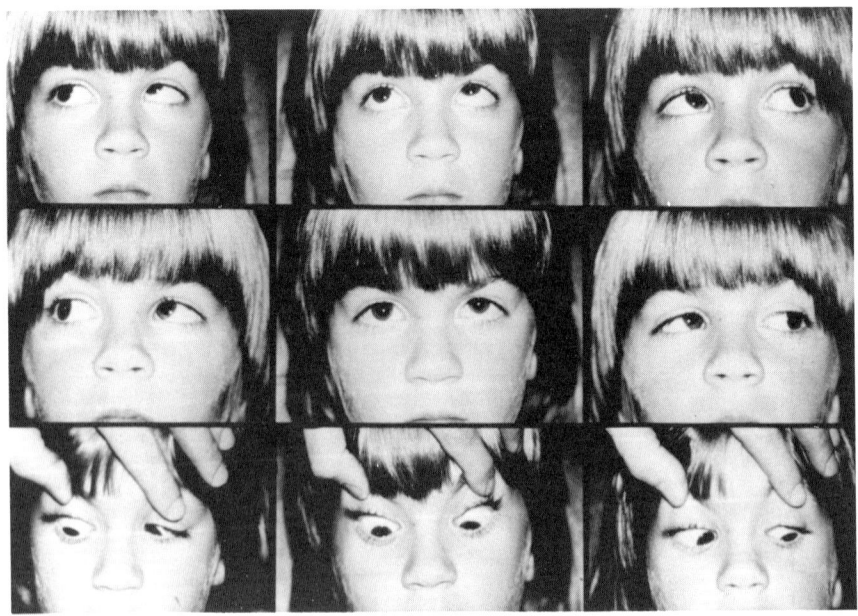

FIGURE 13-3. Left fourth cranial nerve palsy. Note underaction of left superior oblique (lower left) and overaction of its antagonist, the left inferior oblique (upper left).

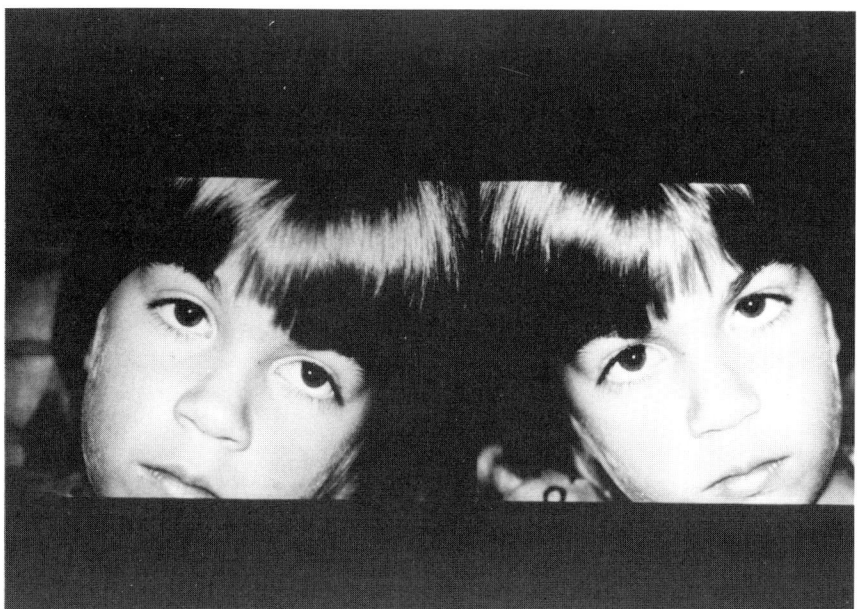

FIGURE 13-4. Head tilt to the left increases hyperdeviation in left fourth cranial nerve palsy.

Isolated Third Nerve Palsies

The third nerve functions to elevate, depress, and turn the eye in. In addition, the upper eyelid, pupil, and ciliary body are innervated by the third nerve. Signs of third nerve palsy include an outward and downward deviation of the eye and ptosis (lid droop) of the eyelid. If the pupillary fibers are involved, the pupil is enlarged and responds poorly to light (Figure 13-5).

Similar to the sixth nerve, the association of findings is helpful in localizing an isolated third nerve palsy. A lesion of the third nerve nucleus should be suspected with bilateral total third nerve palsy, bilateral ptosis, or bilateral pupillary involvement. Unilateral ptosis, pupillary involvement, and unilateral involvement of the extraocular muscles with sparing of the contralateral superior rectus muscle cannot represent a nuclear lesion. Oculomotor palsy in association with contralateral hemiplegia *(Weber's syndrome)* indicates involvement of the corticospinal tracts. If the red nucleus is involved, the patient will also have contralateral ataxia and intention tremor *(Benedikt's syndrome)*. These brain stem syndromes usually signify vascular infarction, demyelination, or tumor.

The most common lesion causing an acute spontaneous third nerve palsy is rupture of a posterior communicating artery aneurysm. Patients present with intense pain and other signs of subarachnoid hemorrhage. They are usually

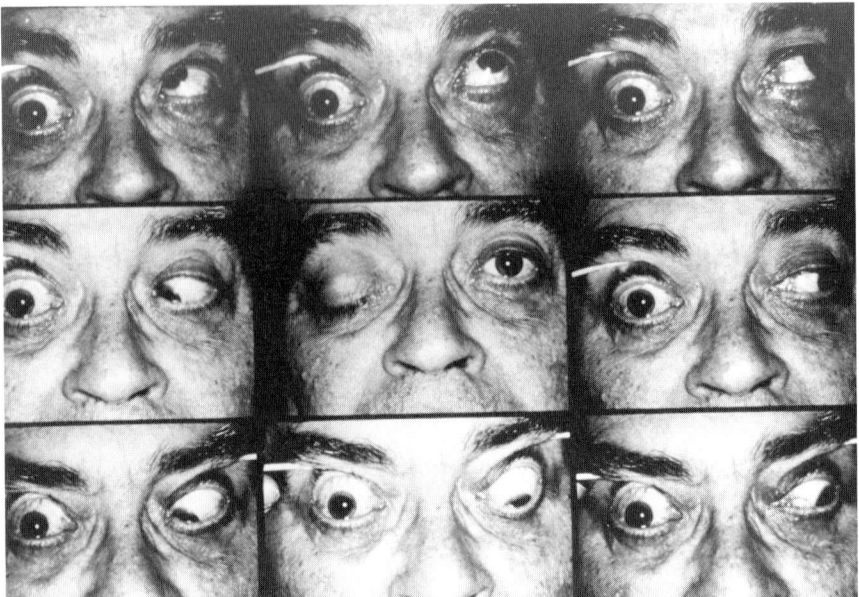

FIGURE 13-5. Right third nerve palsy: Complete ptosis and limited motility of the right eye.

obtunded or comatose at presentation. Because the pupillary fibers course the periphery of the third nerve, the pupil is nearly always involved in bleeding aneurysms. Even in known diabetics, patients with third nerve palsies and fixed dilated pupils should undergo cerebral angiography.

Muscular Disorders and the Sudden Onset of Diplopia

Myasthenia gravis, thyroid ophthalmopathy, and pseudotumor involving an extraocular muscle are the most common myopathic causes of diplopia. (The last two are discussed in Chapter 12.) It is important to remember that pseudotumor is associated with acute pain, but dysthyroidism and myasthenia are not. Proptosis and resistance to retropulsion are usually present with pseudotumor and dysthyroidism but not with myasthenia.

Myasthenia gravis is an autoimmune disease caused by antibodies directed against acetylcholine receptors in muscles. It is associated with other immune-related illnesses, particularly thyroid disease and systemic lupus erythematosis. Muscular weakness, without signs of muscle atrophy, sensory loss, or neurologic deficit, characterizes the disorder. Fatigability and fluctuation (remissions, exacerbations, and variability) are hallmarks. Myasthenia preferentially involves the extraocular, facial, and oropharyngeal muscles. Approximately

75% of patients present with ocular complaints, and 20% never develop other manifestations. Ptosis (lid droop) is almost invariable, but involvement of the other extraocular muscles is quite variable. Myasthenia occasionally mimics an internuclear ophthalmoplegia or a central gaze palsy. Any or all extraocular muscles may be involved, but the pupil is clinically spared (not to pupillography). The disorder may be unilateral.

Myasthenia can occur at any age, and *Tensilon testing* is diagnostic. Several methods of administering this test exist. A common way is to administer 0.2 mL (2 mg) of edrophonium chloride intravenously as a test dose. If the lid or extraocular muscle function is not improved within 1 minute, an additional 0.8 mL (8 mg) is administered over 30 seconds. The absence of response within 3 minutes to 4 minutes is considered a negative test. The presence of acetylcholine receptor antibodies is also diagnostic but does not correlate with the clinical state. The electromyogram may also be abnormal. Clinically, one can test for orbicularis or levator weakness. The former is confirmed by noting forceful eyelid closure weakness and the latter by ptosis on prolonged upward gaze or lid twitch after prolonged downward gaze.

Treatment involves systemic anticholinesterase (mestinon or prostigmin), immunosuppression (corticosteroids, cyclophosphamide, azathioprine), plasmaphoresis, and, rarely, whole body or splenic radiation. When myasthenia is associated with a thymoma, a thymectomy may be therapeutic. Certain medications aggravate myasthenia, including topical timolol, respiratory depressants, aminoglycoside antibiotics, and certain antiarryhthmics (quinidine, procainamide). Certain toxins and drugs may also cause symptoms that mimic myasthenia. These include insecticides, spider venom, snake venom, tick paralysis, botulinum, and D-penicillamine.

SUDDEN DEVELOPMENT OF PUPILLARY ABNORMALITIES

A. History
B. Anatomy of the pupillary pathways
C. Acute onset of anisocoria (asymmetric pupil size)
   1. Physiologic anisocoria
   2. Due to one pupil's being too small (miosis)
      a. Horner's syndrome
      b. Tadpole pupil
      c. Aortic or carotid artery aneurysm
      d. Pharmacologic (miotics)
      e. Trauma
      f. Cerebrovascular accident
      g. Raeder's paratrigeminal syndrome (see below)
      h. Cluster headache (see below)
      i. Orbital infection (see Chapter 12)

j. Inflammation of the anterior eye (keratitis/iridocyclitis) (see Chapter 16)
3. Due to one pupil's being too large (mydriasis)
   a. Amaurotic pupil
   b. Trauma
   c. Pharmacologic (mydriatics)
   d. Iris infarct/atrophy
   e. Irritative sympathetic lesions
   f. Ciliary ganglion lesions
   g. Adie's syndrome
   h. Migraine
   i. Third nerve palsy (see above)
   j. Acute glaucoma (see Chapter 11)
D. Bilaterally small pupils
   1. Drug abuse
   2. Toxins (insecticide poisoning)
   3. Parinaud's syndrome
   4. Midbrain and pontine cerebrovascular accident
   5. Epidemic encephalitis
   6. Purulent meningitis
   7. Tetanus
   8. Severe hypoxia
   9. Spasm of the near reflex
   10. Argyll-Robertson pupil
E. Bilaterally large pupils
   1. Drug abuse
   2. Toxins
   3. Medullary cerebrovascular accident
   4. Epidural or subdural hemorrhage
   5. Midbrain injury
   6. Irritative sympathetic lesion
   7. Coma

History

Several intrinsic ocular or optic nerve disorders and a variety of toxic, traumatic, infectious, and vascular insults are accompanied by pupillary signs. The common involvement of the pupil is related to the dual innervation of the iris by both sympathetic and parasympathetic nerves. Often pupillary findings are incidental to the chief complaint, but they can be very useful diagnostically.

The most common presenting abnormality specific to the pupil is anisocoria, or asymmetric pupil size. Occasionally individuals with an enlarged pupil may note slightly blurred vision in the affected eye. More often patients with anisocoria are otherwise asymptomatic. The history should elicit whether the smaller pupil is always on the same side or whether it reverses sides within hours or days (physiologic anisocoria). The latter is commonly familial. If it never reverses, the patient is questioned regarding previous unilateral trauma, suggesting damage to the pupillary sphincter (in the eye with the larger pupil) or dilator muscle (eye with the smaller pupil). A history of unilateral glaucoma requiring eyedrops in an eye with a small pupil suggests the use of miotics. Finally, the patient is asked whether the asymmetry is greater in dim illumination (sympathetic system) or bright illumination (parasympathetic).

A small pupil that dilates poorly is consistent with *Horner's syndrome.* This syndrome occurs due to any interruption along the sympathetic pathway from the hypothalamus to the iris. The duration of findings and any history of recent surgery that may have damaged the sympathetic chain should be asked. A long duration of miosis, without other signs or symptoms, suggests a benign etiology; a lighter color of the affected iris suggests a congenital origin. Further questioning should elicit hypothalamic symptoms such as diabetes insipidus or disturbed temperature regulation, evidence of a pulmonary tumor (smoking, hemoptysis), cervical trauma, brachial plexus abnormalities, enlarged gland or mass in the neck, associated sensory or motor deficits, or headache.

A large pupil that constricts poorly is suggestive of inadvertent instillation of a mydriatic (dilating) agent, a third nerve palsy, or *Adie's syndrome,* which usually affects young women and occasionally occurs bilaterally. Individuals with an enlarged pupil may note slightly blurred vision in the affected eye due to chromatic and spherical aberrations and decreased depth of focus.

Patients who present with bilaterally large or small pupils usually have other localizing signs or symptoms. It is important to recognize, however, that many drugs and toxins can cause mydriatic (large) or miotic (small) pupils. It is also important to remember that the pupils are smaller in infancy, old age, and sleep. Hypermetropic (farsighted) individuals tend to have smaller pupils than myopes (nearsighted). Additionally, the pupil is generally smaller with brown irides than blue, in men, and when fatigued.

The physician who incidentally notes an irregularly shaped pupil will usually find a history of ocular trauma, surgery, inflammation (iridocyclitis), or a congenital abnormality (e.g., a coloboma—key-shaped defect in the inferior nasal iris; Figure 13–6).

Anatomy of the Pupillary Pathways

Light Reflex Pathway and Parasympathetic Fibers

Light impulses are transmitted by the optic nerve to the optic chiasm, where decussation occurs. Temporal optic nerve fibers from each eye travel to the ipsilateral optic tract and brain, while nasal fibers cross to the opposite side of the brain at the chiasm. The first synapse for fibers carrying light impulses occurs in the midbrain in an area called the pretectum, near the superior col-

356 III—Nontraumatic Ocular and Orbital Emergencies

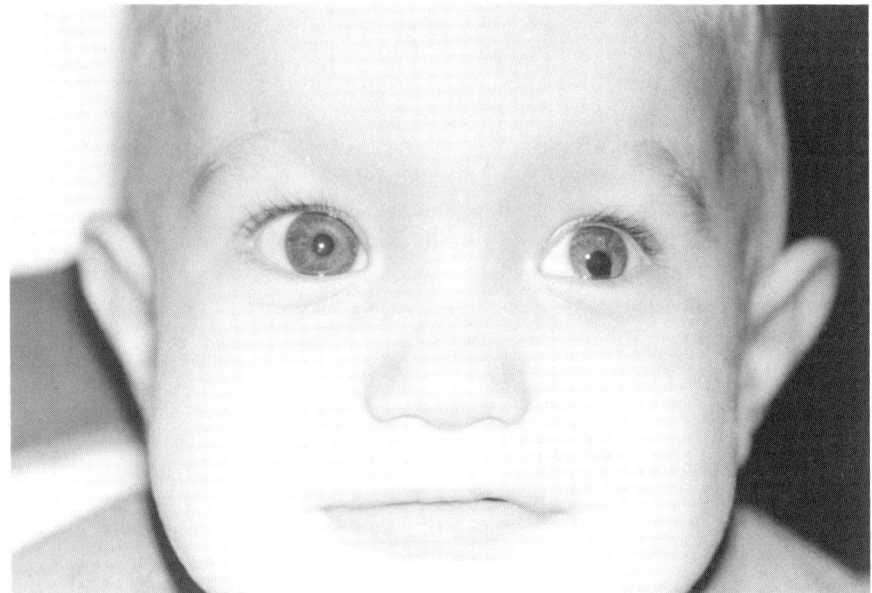

FIGURE 13-6. Unilateral coloboma of the left eye.

liculus. Further splitting occurs in the pretectum, and fibers are sent from here to both the ipsilateral and contralateral Edinger-Westphal nuclei, which form the parasympathetic centers of the third cranial nerve. From here, efferent fibers travel with the extraocular motor fibers of the third cranial nerve, departing their company in the orbit to synapse in the ciliary ganglion. Postganglionic fibers from the ciliary ganglion enter the eye and innervate the iris sphincter (controlling pupillary constriction) and ciliary body (controlling accommodation of the lens).

Sympathetic Fibers

Impulses from the hypothalamus travel via first-order neurons to the cervical spinal cord, where they synapse in the ciliospinal center of Budge in the lower cervical and upper thoracic spinal cord. Second-order (preganglionic) neurons then travel cephalad to synapse in the superior cervical ganglion. Third-order (postganglionic) neurons course various pathways without synapsing, to enter the eye and innervate the dilator muscle of the iris (Figure 13-7).

Acute Onset of Anisocoria

Figure 13-8 presents a flowchart that is useful in the evaluation of anisocoria (asymmetric pupil size). Disorders where the abnormal pupil is the smaller one

OCULOSYMPATHETIC PATHWAY

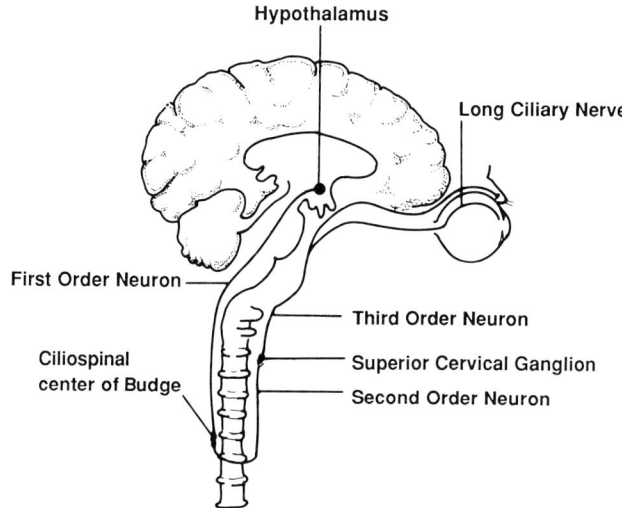

FIGURE 13-7. The oculosympathetic pathway.

(a problem with dilation—sympathetic system) are separated from disorders with an enlarged pupil (a problem with constriction—parasympathetic nervous system). The first step determines whether the anisocoria changes depending on the degree of illumination. If there is no accentuation of the anisocoria based on illumination and if both eyes constrict briskly to light without dilation lag in darkness, the patient likely has *physiologic* or *simple anisocoria*. If the anisocoria is accentuated in darkness and the smaller pupil fails to dilate with cocaine, the patient has *Horner's syndrome*. Greater anisocoria in light than darkness suggests a parasympathetic defect due to a third nerve palsy, anticholinergic agent, or iris damage.

The presence of ptosis (lid droop) associated with a large pupil further suggests a third nerve disorder, but ptosis associated with a small pupil suggests a sympathetic disorder *(Horner's syndrome)*. In this disorder, the lower lid on the involved side is also 1 mm higher than the opposite side (upside-down ptosis).

Physiologic Anisocoria

Physiologic anisocoria is also called simple or central anisocoria and in the past was called springing or alternating anisocoria or seesaw mydriasis. Distinguishing characteristics include the absence of other visual or neuro-ophthalmologic deficits. Both pupils constrict briskly to light and accommodation, and both pupils dilate normally to cocaine. If one were to plot the anisocoria against time, the pupillary inequality would be found to be irregular and would likely

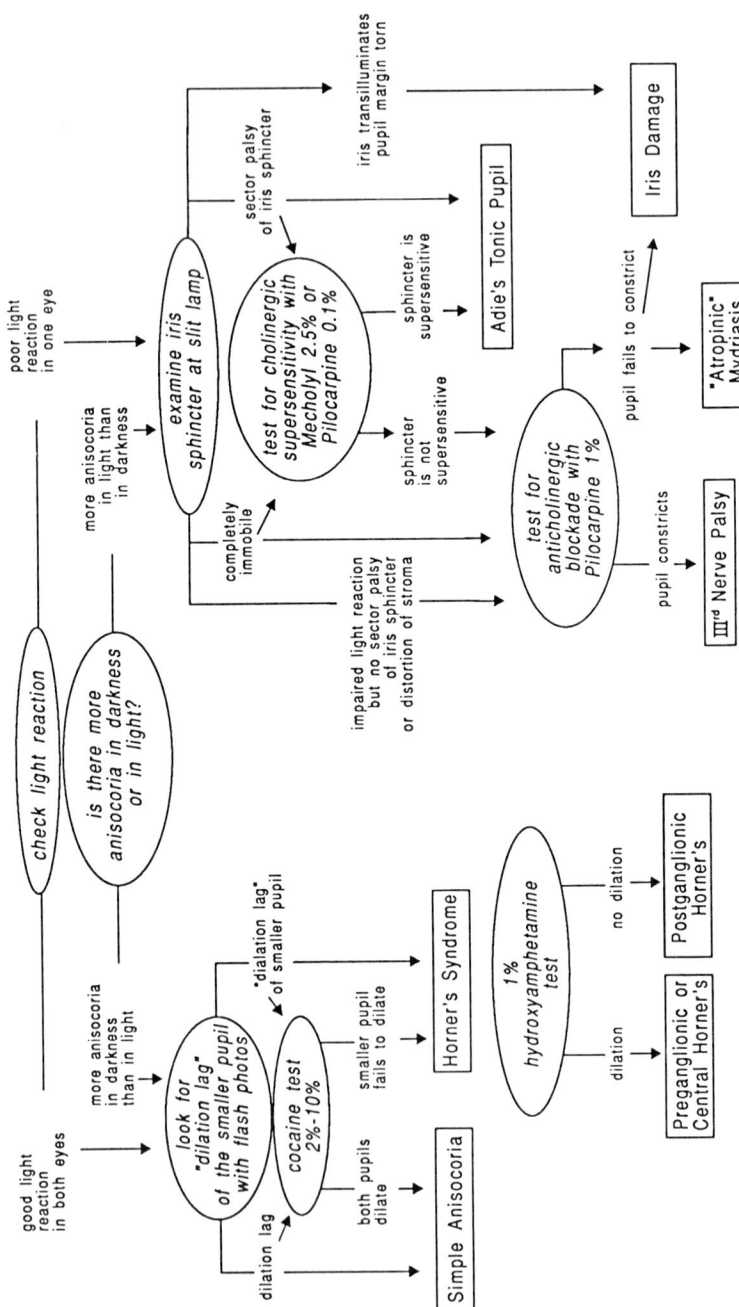

FIGURE 13–8. Flowchart used for patients with anisocoria. Reproduced by permission from: Thompson, HS, Pilley SFJ: Unequal pupils. Survey of Ophthalmology 21:45, 1976.

reverse over a few hours or days. Because it is difficult to see pupillary inequalities of less than 0.3 mm, many investigators use this difference as a threshold for diagnosing anisocoria. There is evidence that it may be caused by asymmetries of the supranuclear inhibitory control of the Edinger-Westphal nucleus. It is more common in older individuals and tends to run in families.

Anisocoria Due to One Pupil's Being Too Small

Horner's syndrome (Figure 13-9) results from disruption of the ipsilateral sympathetic outflow to the eye and face. It is characterized by miosis, ptosis (droopy eyelid), anhydrosis (decreased sweating on the homolateral side), and enophthalmos (less protrusion of the affected eye). The last is seldom clinically striking; usually the difference in protrusion between the eyes is less than 2 mm. The anisocoria is greater in dim illumination because the affected smaller pupil dilates poorly.

Horner's syndrome can be congenital or acquired. When congenital, it is usually secondary to birth trauma. Trauma to the spine can be associated with injury to the lower brachial plexus (Klumpke's paralysis). Although less than 5% to 10% of infants with "congenital Horner's syndrome" have neuroblastoma, screening for this curable malignancy is appropriate in infants. All cases of true congenital Horner's syndrome will have heterochromia, with the affected iris being lighter.

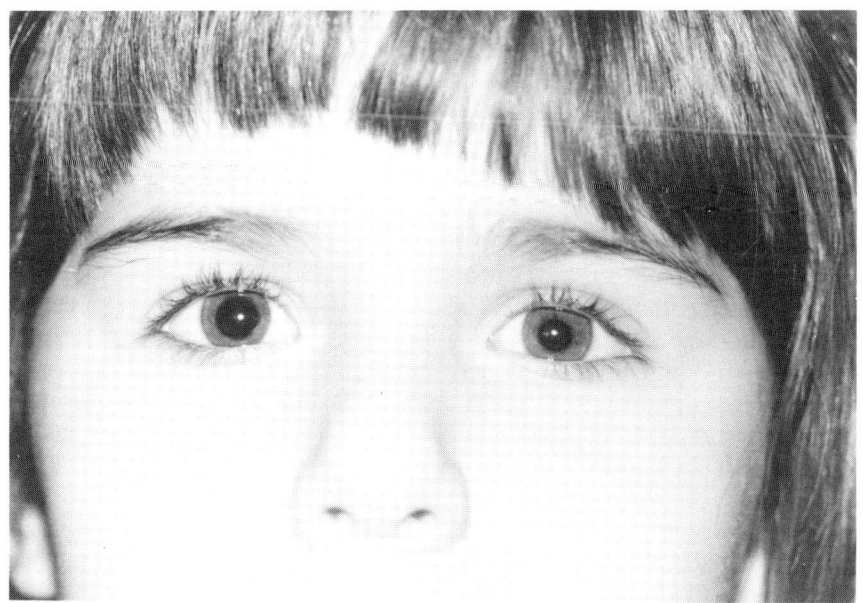

FIGURE 13-9. Horner's syndrome of the left eye: Ptosis and miosis.

Pharmacologic testing is employed to diagnose and localize the lesion in acute acquired Horner's syndrome (Figure 13-8). The syndrome occurs due to an interruption of the sympathetic pathway. The end result of this interruption is a decrease in the amount of norepinephrine released from the third order (postganglionic) nerve ending. Cocaine prevents the reuptake of norepinephrine from sympathetic nerve endings. With the topical administration of cocaine, the normal pupil dilates because more norepinephrine is available to act on the dilator muscle. The absence of iris dilation with cocaine diagnoses Horner's syndrome. The cocaine test is performed by placing 1 drop of cocaine 2% to 10% in each eye, followed by a second drop in 10 minutes, and checking for asymmetric dilatation in 15 minutes to 30 minutes.

The cocaine test does not help localize the lesion because any interruption along the sympathetic pathway will decrease the amount of norepinephrine at the postganglionic nerve ending. There is no reliable test to differentiate a first- from a second-order neuron disorder. Hydroxyamphetamine 1% (Paredrine), however, will differentiate first- and second- from third-order neuron disorders. This is important because third-order (postganglionic) lesions are most often benign; they are often related to vascular headaches. In contrast, almost 50% of first- and second-order neuron defects result from neoplastic processes (Table 13-5). Paredrine causes the release of norepinephrine from the postganglionic nerve ending, stimulating the iris dilator muscle. Lesions involving the postganglionic neuron result in an absence of norepinephrine at the nerve ending and absence of iris dilation with paredrine. Lesions of the first- and second-order neurons do not interfere with the integritiy of the third-order neuron; iris dilation still occurs. Two drops of Paredrine 1% are used, 1 minute apart. The test is positive for a third-order neuron defect if the affected pupil remains miotic after 30 minutes. The cocaine and Paredrine tests should be done on separate days because they interfere with each other's actions. They should also not be done on the same day as other tests that disrupt the corneal epithelium, such as intraocular pressure testing. Following corneal manipulation, the absorption of drugs may be unequal between the two eyes, giving false-positive or false-negative results.

A *tadpole pupil* is a rare, benign, and transitory finding. It is usually reported by the affected patient, who notes episodic slightly blurred vision and a peaked pupil. Episodes occur several times a day for several weeks and can be interspersed by months. Strenuous exercise can elicit the disorder. A history of migraine may be given, but these episodes do not usually occur during a migraine attack. In one study (Thompson et al., 1983) many of the patients had a partial postganglionic Horner's syndrome.

A *dissecting aortic artery aneurysm* should be considered in atherosclerotic individuals with unilateral periorbital pain, a droopy eyelid, and miosis. The pain often arises over days to weeks and is localized to the orbit, forehead, ear, throat, or neck; it may shift in location.

Unilaterally applied *topical miotics,* such as pilocarpine, can also be the cause of anisocoria. A history of unilateral glaucoma requiring the instillation

TABLE 13-5. HORNER'S SYNDROME

LOCALIZATION	DIFFERENTIAL DIAGNOSIS
First-order neuron	Hypothalamic syndrome Basal meningitis (syphilitic) Brain stem infarction/hemorrhage Cerebral infarction/hemorrhage Pituitary or brain stem tumor Cervical spine: transection, tumor, meningitis, poliomyelitis, syringomyelia, syphilis, amyotrophic lateral sclerosis, vascular malformation Multiple sclerosis Trauma (including surgery)
Second-order neuron	Spinal birth injury (Klumpke's paralysis) Cervical rib Tumor in thoracic apex (Pancoast) Tumors of: mediastinum, esophagus, sympathetic chain (neuroma) retropharynx, intraoral Aortic aneurysm Lymphadenopathy (Hodgkin's disease) Thyroid adenoma, multinodular goiter, surgery Trauma (including surgery—tonsillectomy)
Third-order neuron	Raeder's paratrigeminal syndrome Migraine/cluster headaches Cavernous sinus/Tolosa-Hunt syndrome Herpes zoster ophthalmicus Orbital tumor/cyst Otitis media Aneurysm of internal carotid Trauma (including surgery)

of eyedrops is suggestive. Children who experiment with an older family member's medications can present this way. The affected pupil dilates poorly, if at all, in dim illumination. A history of *unilateral trauma,* with damage to the pupillary dilator muscle, is also easily ascertained. Finally, the pupil is also small in association with vascular headaches. In addition to pain and miosis, the eye may be red and watery with vascular headaches (see below).

Anisocoria Due to One Pupil's Being Too Large

A blind eye often has a larger pupil than a seeing eye *(amaurotic pupil).* In addition, the pupil in a contused eye may be transiently or permanently dilated. The use of *topical mydriatics* also causes pupillary enlargement. The latter is seen in health personnel who inadvertently or functionally place atropine, or adrenergic agents such as nasal sprays, in an eye. Pharmacologically dilated pupils react poorly to both light and the near reflex and constrict minimally, if at all, with the instillation of pilocarpine 1% (Figure 13-8).

Iris infarcts or atrophy, which occur in the elderly, and *irritative sympathetic lesions,* which occur secondary to cranial or cervical cord lesions, or aortic dilatation, can also cause unilateral mydriasis. *Lesions of the ciliary ganglion,* either destructive (herpes zoster, tumor) or traumatic (postretrobulbar block), should be included in the differential. Fixed, dilated pupils result either from pharmacologic blockade of the iris sphincter or a more generalized midbrain or third nerve lesion. The presence of other third nerve signs distinguishes the latter.

The pupil is often mid-dilated and fails to constrict in acute glaucoma and may be enlarged during glaucomatocyclitic crisis *(Posner-Schlossman syndrome),* characterized by a high intraocular pressure, mild pain, decreased vision, a white eye, and a very mild anterior chamber reaction.

Adie's tonic pupil is characterized by an irregularly dilated pupil that reacts minimally, if at all, to light, slowly constricts to convergence or accommodation, and slowly redilates upon going from near to far gaze (reducing accommodation). The condition is unilateral in 80% of cases, and deep tendon reflexes (knees, ankles) are reduced in up to 90% of cases.

Patients with Adie's pupil are often asymptomatic but occasionally may have photophobia or presbyopic-like symptoms related to a reduced accommodative ability. Slit lamp examination of the iris may show segmental constriction of the iris sphincter. The affected pupil is also suprasensitive to topical parasympathomimetics. Two solutions, mecholyl 2.5% and pilocarpine 0.1%, are often recommended diagnostically (Figure 13-8). Neither is readily available, but the latter can be concocted by diluting commercially available pilocarpine 1% with normal saline. It is important to note that suprasensitivity may not be noticed until several weeks after the acute onset of the disorder. The associated photophobia can be treated with pilocarpine 0.05%; accommodative symptoms usually resolve spontaneously within a few months. Over several months to years, the pupil usually becomes smaller and may even become smaller than the normal pupil.

Adie's syndrome occurs predominantly in females; the etiology is unknown, but the condition is benign. Herpes zoster, varicella, temporal arteritis, syphilis, diabetes, and Guillain-Barré syndrome can produce similar findings and should be ruled out. The presence of Adie's pupil, with or without suprasensitivity, in an infant less than 1 year of age is suggestive of familial dysautonomia *(Riley-Day syndrome).* This syndrome of Ashkenazi Jews includes feeding difficulties, hypotonia, delayed development, labile body temperature and blood pressure, corneal hypesthesia, decreased tearing, and the absence of fungiform papillae on the tongue. Breath-holding episodes, recurrent pneumonias, and intractable vomiting crises also occur.

Bilaterally Small Pupils

Many insecticides function by inhibiting acetylcholinesterase and cause marked bilateral miosis. Several antipsychotics, barbiturates, injection and inhalation anesthetics, morphine, codeine, levodopa, and propranolol also induce miosis. An acute *pontine angle lesion,* due to a hemorrhage or tumor, causes bilateral miosis, partial to total loss of the pupillary light reaction, but an intact near (accommodative) reaction. Conjugate gaze is usually disturbed. Other irritative central nervous system conditions such as encephalitis and meningitis can cause bilateral miosis. *Spasm of the near reflex* is a functional disorder marked by induced accommodation, myopia, and convergence (see Chapter 15). It cannot be sustained for more than a few seconds to minutes.

Bilateral miotic (less than 2 mm in size) and irregular pupils that constrict poorly to light but better to accommodation (fixation on a near object) are suggestive of tertiary syphilis involving the central nervous system *(Argyll-Robertson pupils).* Frequently iris atrophy also occurs, with portions of the iris transilluminating. In this condition, the FTA-ABS will be positive. Several disorders can mimic this, including diabetes, chronic alcoholism, multiple sclerosis, encephalitis, midbrain tumors, malaria, and senile and degenerative diseases of the central nervous system.

Bilaterally Large Pupils

Amphetamine, digoxin, LSD, marijuana, mescaline, prednisone, quinine, reserpine, and thioridazine induce mydriasis. Clostridium, tetanus, lead, and carbon monoxide are toxic causes of mydriasis. In comas due to alcohol ingestion, diabetes, uremia, meningitis, eclampsia, and epilepsy, the pupils are dilated and unresponsive to stimulation.

Cerebrovascular accidents involving the medulla and epidural or subdural hemorrhages are often associated with bilaterally dilated pupils. Midbrain lesions may cause *Parinaud's syndrome,* which is characterized by bilaterally dilated pupils that respond poorly to light but constrict normally with convergence. The presence of eyelid retraction and retraction nystagmus on attempted upward gaze suggest this diagnosis. A pinealoma or craniopharyngioma should be sought. Other causes include stroke, multiple sclerosis, and hydrocephalus.

HEADACHES

A. Traction and inflammatory headaches
 1. Intracranial tumors
 2. Subdural hematoma
 3. Subarachnoid hemorrhage
 4. Intraparenchymal hemorrhage
 5. Ischemic cerebrovascular disease
 6. Meningitis/encephalitis
 7. Temporal arteritis (see also Chapter 14)
 8. Pseudotumor cerebri (see also Chapter 14)

9. Orbital pseudotumor (see also Chapter 12)
10. Trigeminal neuralgia
11. Malignant hypertension
12. Hydrocephalus
13. Diabetic neuropathy
14. Herpes zoster ophthalmicus (see also Chapter 16)
15. Retrobulbar neuritis (see Chapter 14)

B. Vascular headaches
   1. Migraine headaches
   2. Cluster headaches (Raeder's paratrigeminal syndrome)
   3. Postconvulsive
   4. Postconcussional

C. Tension or muscle contraction headaches

D. Asthenopia

E. Toxic headaches

F. Metabolic headaches

G. Acute angle closure glaucoma (see Chapter 11)

H. Uveitis (see Chapter 16)

Traction and Inflammatory Headaches

Most patients with the chief complaint of headaches have tension or muscle contraction headaches rather than a life- or vision-threatening problem. Patients with headaches associated with major illnesses usually seek medical attention due to some other manifestation of their illness. Additionally, individuals with inflammatory headaches usually cite an onset of hours to weeks; individuals with tension headaches cite an onset of months to years.

To differentiate some of the more serious causes of headache, the patient should be asked about the quality, location, duration, frequency, and rapidity of onset of the headache, as well as any accompanying or preceding symptoms. Age, gender, concurrent illness, and medication histories are also important. Patients who complain of suffering the "worst headache I have ever experienced" should be examined for signs of subarachnoid or intraparenchymal hemorrhage, meningitis, or ischemic cerebrovascular disease. Subacute, persistent, or recurrent headaches can signify tumors, abscesses, subdural hematomas, pseudotumor cerebri, temporal arteritis, cluster headaches, or orbital pseudotumor. Chronic episodic headaches include migraine, exertional, and tension headaches. Accompanying neurologic signs, decreased vision, stiff neck, fever, scalp tenderness, or jaw claudication usually signify a major illness.

Similarly, a serious illness may be heralded by headaches that are atypical for the individual, unresponsive to mild analgesics, awaken the person from sleep, had an "explosive" onset, change with head position, or are always located in the same area.

Table 13-6 lists some inflammatory disorders associated with headaches. Findings and suggested diagnostic tests are included.

TABLE 13-6. TRACTION AND INFLAMMATORY HEADACHES

DISORDER	DESCRIPTION	DIAGNOSTIC TESTS
Intracranial tumor	Slowly progressive focal neurologic deficit, with dizziness, lethargy, gait disturbance, cognitive dysfunction, progressive unilateral or bilateral visual loss, and diffuse or localized headache. Headache can be worse in morning, dull or throbbing, and often is not severe. It can be intermittent or recurrent, start suddenly and last minutes to hours. Syncope, transient blindness, or vomiting can accompany headaches.	CT or MRI scan Ophthalmoscopy looking for papilledema Visual fields
Subdural hematoma	Slowly progressive neurologic deficits, worse in morning, without fever or stiff neck. Individual may have personality changes, focal signs, and changes in cognitive ability.	CT scan
Subarachnoid hemorrhage	Rapidly evolving, diffuse pain, stiff neck, photophobia, confusion, lethargy, and brief loss of consciousness at onset. Headache becomes worse with head movement or cough. No fever or leukocytosis. Headaches act as a sentinel for berry aneurysms, when occur in the middle-aged; females > males.	CT scan Lumbar puncture Ophthalmoscopy looking for subhyaloid hemorrhages
Intraparenchymal hemorrhage	Headaches are associated with focal neurologic signs, obtundation, or coma. Headache, gait ataxia, and vomiting suggest cerebellar lesion. Occurs more frequently in hypertensive and elderly or after sudden extreme elevation of blood pressure (cocaine, medications, trauma).	MRI or CT scan
Ischemic cerebrovascular disease	Precedes or begins at the onset of a stroke and can be ipsilateral and nonthrobbing. Carotid artery dissection is manifest by sudden severe pain, bruit, Horner's syndrome, visual scintillations.	CT scan Ophthalmoscopy looking for retinal emboli
Meningitis or encephalitis	Rapidly evolving headache, stiff neck, fever, leukocytosis, confusion, lethargy, retro-orbital pain, and cranial nerve palsies. Pain worsened by eye movements.	Lumbar puncture

Table continued on following page

TABLE 13-6. TRACTION AND INFLAMMATORY HEADACHES (continued)

DISORDER	DESCRIPTION	DIAGNOSTIC TESTS
Temporal arteritis	Gradual onset of unilateral, sharp, severe pain, with jaw claudication, scalp tenderness, nocturnal worsening, weight loss, malaise, and fever. Polymyalgia rheumatica, transient monocular visual loss, diplopia, and central or altitudinal field defects may be present. Occurs in females > males, whites > blacks, and elderly ($\geq$ 55 years).	Westergren sedimentation rate (elevated) Temporal artery biopsy
Pseudotumor cerebri	Diffuse chronic headache and obscurations of vision, in obese females, in their teens to thirties, with menstrual irregularities, nausea and vomiting, and diplopia. Associated with the use of nalidixic acid, corticosteroids, vitamin A, tetracycline, and pregnancy.	Ophthalmoscopy looking for papilledema and absent venous pulsations Lumbar puncture
Orbital pseudotumor	Severe, steady, boring pain with a subacute onset, localized behind the affected eye, with decreased ocular motility, diplopia, proptosis, and numbness of the forehead.	CT or MRI scan Orbital biopsy Blood tests
Trigeminal neuralgia	Jabbing, electric sensations of brief duration in a division of the trigeminal nerve. Occasionally, interepisodic dull, burning pain, ipsilateral tearing, rhinorrhea, conjunctival injection, and facial swelling may be present. Pain can often be evoked by moving the mouth or tactile stimulation of trigger point. Occurs in females > males, with an increased incidence over age 60.	History Exclusionary brain MRI
Malignant hypertension	Occipital headaches, heart failure, renal failure, various degrees of obtundation, decreased mentation, and blurred vision.	Ophthalmoscopy looking for disc edema, cotton wool spots, hemorrhages
Herpes zoster ophthalmicus	Severe retrobulbar pain and vesicular eruption in the distribution of the ipsilateral ophthalmic (V) nerve. Skin eruption can occur several days after the headache begins. Malaise, blurred vision, eye pain, and injection are common. Can involve the cornea, optic nerve, and retina and cause uveitis.	Cutaneous findings Immunocompromised or AIDS patients
Diabetic neuropathy	Severe retrobulbar pain preceding an oculomotor defect. Diabetic retinopathy is frequently present.	History of diabetes Glucose tolerance test

Vascular Headaches

Migraine Headaches

Migraines are thought to be a reaction pattern related to a number of endogenous and exogenous factors. Endogenously, neurovascular instability, disturbances in the autonomic system, and alterations in monoamine oxidase and platelets have been shown. Exogenously, a number of factors that trigger the release of serotonin from platelets have been implicated: stress (particularly just after the stress is resolved); depression; rapid hormonal changes; certain foods with a high content of tyramine (cheeses, sour cream, alcohol), phenylethylamine (chocolate), or vasodilator substances (monosodium glutamate); medications (estrogen, reserpine, nitroglycerin); and physical stimuli (bright sunlight, stuffy rooms, oversleeping).

These endogenous and exogenous factors trigger the release of serotonin from platelets. This produces capillary dilatation and constriction of the extra- and intracranial arteries. The latter is the cause of the aura that precedes the headache in about 20% of migraineurs. Serotonin is subsequently absorbed and metabolized, causing a rebound effect of vasodilation of arteries and constriction of capillaries. Headache occurs due to the arterial distension and inflammation.

Migraine usually begins after puberty and affects women three times as often as men, with a prevalence as high as 20% to 25% of the population. A family history is often elicited, as is a childhood history of motion sickness or cyclic vomiting. The frequency of attacks is as often as one to three times per week to as few as one every 2 years. The duration ranges from several hours to days. Unilateral, holocephalic, bifrontal, and occipital headaches are all encountered. The pain may be limited to half the head at the onset and subsequently involve the entire cranium. Half the patients describe the headache as pulsatile or throbbing with occasional superimposed brief jabs of sharp pain. During an episode, the patient appears sick; her skin is pale and sweaty, and she may be tense and irritable, speaking in a low voice through tight lips with a clamped jaw. She usually seeks a quiet, dark room to rest. Additional associated findings are listed in Table 13-7.

Migraine is often classified as classic or common. Three components are necessary for the less common (10% of cases) diagnosis of *classic migraine:* aura, headache, and autonomic symptoms. The aura is most commonly a scintillating scotoma. It is described as a shadowy gray darkness, beginning near fixation, with a slowly expanding border of brilliant, intense, zigzag lines, flickering at 5 cycles to 10 cycles per second. The blind (scotomatous) area expands slowly, over 10 minutes to 20 minutes, into the periphery. Parasthesias or other focal neurologic symptoms may also occur. The aura typically lasts about 20 minutes and may precede or occur concurrent with headache. The headache usually lasts 2 hours to 4 hours and rarely longer than 12 hours. Patients with

TABLE 13-7. ASSOCIATED FINDINGS IN MIGRAINE

Nausea	90%
Photophobia	80
Blurred vision	67
Scalp tenderness	67
Light-headedness	67
Vomiting	50
Diarrhea	15
Aura	10
Other (vertigo, tremor, pallor, chills)	10

(From: Drexler ED: Severe headaches. *Postgrad Med* 87:164, 1990.)

unusual patterns, such as the aura occurring during or after the headache or with strict unilaterality of all attacks, should be suspected of having a mass lesion or vascular malformation. Occasionally the aura may occur without headache *(acephalgic headache)*. This is more common beyond the third and fourth decade, when many patients lose the headache component and develop only isolated auras thereafter.

Common migraine is characterized simply by headaches and a variety of associated findings (Table 13-7). Unlike classic migraine, the headache may last days. In further contradistinction to classic migraine, which often occurs precipitously, common migraine has a more typical periodicity, with more predictable symptom-free intervals and precipitating factors.

The term *complicated migraine* is used when vasoconstriction results in a persistent neurologic deficit. When ischemia or infarction occurs, it most often involves the occipital lobes, but it can involve the retinal arteries (retinal migraine) or other arteries supplying the brain, brain stem, or cranial nerves (ophthalmoplegic migraine). Rarely, patients may experience only the vasoconstriction phase of migraine, without vasodilation and headache *(migraine equivalents)*. These patients are usually over age 40 years with a history of classic migraine at a younger age.

Retinal migraines, due to central retinal artery vasospasm, are characterized by monocular visual loss, either full or altitudinal, preceded by a scintillating scotoma. Retinal migraines frequently occur without headache and, rarely, may result in central retinal artery occlusion. They occur more frequently in young females, with a history of classic or common migraine and recurrent episodes of monocular visual loss. Rarely, ischemic papillitis, retinal hemorrhage, vitreous hemorrhage, or central serous retinopathy may occur. There may be a relationship to oral contraceptive use (see Chapter 14).

Ophthalmoplegic migraine occurs due to paralysis of the third, fourth, or sixth cranial nerve. Typically this form of migraine occurs in children under age 10 years. The oculomotor nerve, with pupillary involvement, is affected during or as the headache is resolving. The ophthalmoplegia usually resolves over several days to weeks. The necessity of neuroradiologic testing in a child with a typical history is controversial. This diagnosis should be suspect, however, in patients over age 20 years, especially if there is no history of migraine or with persistent headache and ophthalmoplegia. These patients should be considered to have an aneurysm until proved otherwise.

Treatment of Acute Migraine Attack. During acute migraine attacks, the drugs of choice are acetaminophen or aspirin when effective; moderate to severe migraines, however, rarely respond to these mild medications. Other medications include the following:

Ergotamine tartrate: 2 mg orally or sublingually at the onset and 1 mg every half-hour subsequently as needed. Dosage should not exceed 6 mg per day or 12 mg per week; also available as inhalor, suppository, intramuscular, or subcutaneous preparations. Side effects include abdominal cramps, nausea, diarrhea, uterine contractions, and intermittent claudication. Pregnancy, coronary heart disease, hepatic or renal dysfunction, thyrotoxicosis, Raynaud's phenomenon, anemia, and thrombophlebitis are contraindications.

Dihydroergotamine: 1 mg intramuscularly at the onset of migraine and repeated hourly for a maximum dose of 3 mg per day. Similar actions, side effects, indications, and contraindications as ergotamine.

Steroids: Dexamethasone 16 mg intramuscularly. May be of benefit to patients with prolonged migraine attacks lasting 2 days to 7 days. Steroids are believed to relieve sterile intravascular inflammation.

Metoclopramide: 10 mg intravenously, followed in 10 minutes by dihydroergotamine mesylate 0.5 mg intravenously.

Prochloroperazine: 10 mg intravenously over 2 minutes.

Preventative Treatment of Migraines. A number of medications are tried preventively when migraine occurs three or more times per month:

Propranolol: Prevents vasodilation; 20 mg, 4 times per day, with the nighttime dose increased to 40 mg in 2 weeks. The dose can be gradually increased to a maximum of 240 mg per day.

Cyproheptadine: Blocks histamine and serotonin receptors; it works better in children; 4 mg to 12 mg per day.

Methysergide: Blocks vasoconstriction and inflammatory effects of serotonin; 4 mg to 8 mg per day. Because it can cause fibrotic and vasoconstrictor effects, it is not a first-line medication and should be discontinued for 1 month every 6 months. It also causes nausea, gastrointestinal pain, diarrhea, weight gain, muscle cramps, anxiety, and hallucinations.

Amitriptyline: Prevents uptake of serotonin; 25 mg at bedtime increased every 1 week to 2 weeks by 25 mg until the dosage reaches 100 mg to 200 mg.

Platelet inhibitors: Aspirin, one tablet, 3 times per day; sulfinpyrazone, 200 mg, 2 to 4 times per day; dipyridamole, 50 mg, 4 times per day.

Clonidine: A central sympatholytic, especially effective in preventing dietary migraine; 0.1 mg, 2 to 3 times per day.

Verapamil: A calcium channel blocker; 240 mg per day.

Patients with migraines should be instructed to avoid foods containing tyramine, phenylethylamine, nitrate, and monosodium glutamate; to wake up and eat breakfast at the same time every day (avoid relative hypoglycemia in morning); and to get sufficient rest and sleep.

Cluster Headaches

Cluster headaches begin abruptly and are characterized by unilateral, excruciating, deep pain around or behind one eye. The pain may radiate to the ipsilateral temple, jaw, nose, or upper neck. Ipsilateral lacrimation, conjunctival injection, nasal congestion, and rhinorrhea occur during the attack. A transient partial Horner's syndrome may also occur and become permanent with repeated attacks.

This headache type occurs six times more commonly in men, especially between the ages of 20 and 50 years. The headaches last 10 minutes to several hours and occur once or twice a day, often at the same time each day. They may occur as often as six times each day to as infrequently as once per week and can awake the individual from sleep (usually 1 hour to 2 hours after falling asleep, during the first period of rapid eye movement sleep). Two patterns of cluster headache have been described. The episodic type occurs in 1-month to 2-month cycles, often at the same time each year. Headaches may occur once or twice daily for several weeks followed by symptom-free intervals of months to years. Chronic cluster headaches occur without remission.

Daily cluster headaches with postganglionic oculosympathetic defects comprise the *benign form of Raeder's paratrigeminal syndrome.* These also occur more commonly in men, with a slightly older age of onset. Attacks often last 1 month or 2 months and rarely recur. An atypical history, or neurological involvement other than third-order sympathetics, suggests a parasellar mass lesion; neuroradiologic testing is indicated.

Treatment of Acute Cluster Headache

1. Aspirin or acetaminophen.
2. Ergotamine tartrate: Inhalant: 9 mg/mL, with 1 inhalation every 5 minutes (maximum of 3 inhalations per 24-hour period); sublingual: 2 mg (maximum 3 tablets taken 30 minutes apart).
3. Inhalation of 100% oxygen at 8 L/min to 10 L/min for 10 minutes.
4. Application of 4% topical lidocaine to the nasal mucosa.
5. Prednisone: 40 mg to 60 mg per day, tapered after 1 week to 2 weeks.

6. Methysergide maleate: 4 mg to 10 mg per day. The dose needs to be built up, and the effect may be delayed.
7. Verapamil: 240 mg to 480 mg per day.

Prophylactic Treatment of Cluster Headaches

1. Lithium carbonate: 600 mg to 900 mg per day (response within 1 week).
2. Ergotamine: 1 mg to 2 mg orally 30 minutes to 60 minutes prior to the expected episode. It is used when headache occurs regularly.
3. Surgical trigeminal gangliorhizolysis (radiofrequency-produced lesions of the trigeminal ganglion).
4. Abstinence of alcohol and cigarette smoking during the cluster period.

Tension or Muscle Contraction Headaches

Tension headaches are the most commonly encountered headache syndrome. They occur in the absence of suspicious signs of traction or inflammation. Often there is a family history and a situational history of an inescapable unpleasant situation. Chronic myositis, cervical osteoarthritis, dental malocclusion, and posttraumatic reactions should be ruled out as causes of this type of headache. Additionally, depressive, delusional, hypochondrical, and conversional headaches overlap tension headaches.

Asthenopia

Asthenopia is ill defined ocular discomfort associated with use of the eyes. Common causes of asthenopia include very specific uncorrected errors of refraction, wearing the wrong glasses, or a refractive imbalance between the two eyes. Individuals with headaches often obtain eye examinations, believing they may need glasses. Generally refractive errors do not cause "headaches." When they do, the problem is usually secondary to an excessive need for the eye to accommodate (increase its refractive power through contraction of the ciliary muscle in the eye, increasing the thickness and curvature of the ocular lens). This occurs when nearsighted glasses are too strong or farsighted glasses are too weak or when accommodative ability decreases in middle age (presbyopia). Similar discomfort occurs with refractive imbalances or a need for one eye to accommodate more than the other secondary to errors in the spectacle prescription or localized ocular disease (Adie's syndrome, herpes zoster ophthalmicus).

Uncorrected or miscorrected refractive errors do not cause severe, incapacitating headaches. Furthermore, headaches due to refractive errors are relieved when the eyes are not used. "Excessive use of the eyes" does not cause headaches, although the tension accompanying the associated activity may. Furthermore, headaches upon awakening and migraines are not caused by "eye strain."

Less common causes of asthenopia include convergence insufficiency, subclinical open angle glaucoma (see Chapter 11), Parinaud's syndrome, and accommodative spasm (the last discussed in Chapter 15). *Convergence insufficiency* is characterized by eye discomfort, blurred vision, and headaches with reading or other close work, usually presenting in the late teenage years. It is often idiopathic but may be associated with Adie's syndrome, uveitis, illness, or drug use. The demonstration of a reduced amplitude of fusional convergence is diagnostic. This can be tested by asking the patient to report when diplopia or blurred vision occurs as a small, interesting target is brought closer to the eyes. Normally, diplopia occurs at less than 6 cm to 8 cm from the eyes; a displaced near point of accommodation is suggestive of convergence insufficiency. Another useful test is the base-out prism test. Base-out prisms, placed before an eye, cause the eye to turn in. The average individual can not maintain fusion when a base-out prism greater than 25 to 30 prism diopters is placed in front of one eye; they report diplopia. The patient with convergence insufficiency will note diplopia with 10 to 15 diopters or less of base-out prism. This disorder is treated with exercises that increase convergence (pencil push-ups) or prisms in the bifocal segment in older individuals.

Other Headache Types

Headaches can also be caused by toxic agents or metabolic disorders or can follow concussions, convulsions, pneumoencephalograms, myelograms, or lumbar punctures. Toxic headaches include alcohol hangovers, carbon monoxide poisoning, caffeine withdrawal, foreign protein reactions, and systemic infections (particularly viral influenza). Metabolic headaches include hypoxia, hypercapnia, and hypoglycemia. Certain vasodilator agents (histamine, nitrates, and monosodium glutamate) and pressor agents (as occurs with a catecholamine-releasing pheochromocytoma, and ingested tyramine in patients taking monoamine oxidase inhibitors) can also elicit headaches.

PAINFUL OPHTHALMOPLEGIA

A. Orbital disorders (see above and Chapter 12)
   1. Pseudotumor and Tolosa-Hunt syndrome
   2. Trochleitis
   3. Carotid-cavernous fistula
   4. Cavernous sinus thrombosis
   5. Mucormycosis
   6. Sphenoid sinus mucocele
   7. Lymphoma

8. Metastatic tumor
9. Nasopharyngeal carcinoma
10. Orbital cellulitis/sinusitis
11. Herpes zoster ophthalmicus

B. Cranial syndromes (see above)
1. Pituitary apoplexy
2. Meningioma/chordoma
3. Metastatic tumor
4. Carcinomatous meningitis
5. Aneurysm
6. Petrositis (Gradenigo's syndrome)

C. Other (see above and Chapter 14)
1. Temporal arteritis
2. Ophthalmoplegic migraine
3. Diabetic ophthalmoplegia

Painful ophthalmoplegia is the term used to describe pain associated with single or multiple ocular motor nerve palsies. The majority of affected individual's also note diplopia, and most of these conditions are described under this heading. Orbital disorders are discussed in Chapter 12. It is worth repeating that pain may precede ophthalmoplegia in several conditions: temporal arteritis, herpes zoster ophthalmicus, ophthalmoplegic migraine, diabetic ophthalmoplegia, and carcinomatous meningitis. The first two occur in the elderly, and the third occurs principally in children. Rapid, sequential cranial nerve abnormalities with headache is usually a late manifestation of carcinomatous meningitis, and, rarely, it may be the presentation of occult carcinoma.

Ophthalmoplegia due to myasthenia and ocular myopathy (chronic progressive external ophthalmoplegia) is not associated with pain. Similarly, ophthalmoplegia due to thyroid ophthalmopathy is, at most, associated with a vague foreign body sensation.

VISUAL HALLUCINATIONS

A. Release hallucinations
B. Temporal lobe disease—formed
C. Occipital lobe disease—unformed
D. Palianopia (visual preservation)
E. Complicated migraine (Alice in Wonderland syndrome)
F. Epilepsy
G. Psychoses
H. Insulin hypoglycemia
I. Delirium of fever

J. Advanced syphilis
K. Sensory deprivation
   1. Sundown syndrome
   2. Secondary to dense bilateral cataracts
L. Poisoning
M. Drug intoxication and withdrawal
N. Functional hallucinations (see Chapter 15)

A lesion anywhere in the visual pathway can result in *release hallucinations.* These can be formed (e.g., faces) or unformed (e.g., flashes) and typically occur in an area where the visual field is blind. They often occur secondary to posterior cerebral artery occlusion, tend to be continuous over long periods of time (minutes to hours), and vary in their pattern from one time to the next. They are not usually associated with other sensory or motor phenomema.

More commonly, visual hallucinations are due to irritative phenomena. These tend to be brief and intermittent, stereotypically repetitive, and associated with other sensory or motor discharges. Highly organized hallucinations (people, objects) usually signify temporal lobe disease. In temporal lobe disease, they may also be associated with perceiving foul odors. Unformed hallucinations (flashes of white or colored light, zigzag lines) occur with occipital lobe disease. *Palianopia* (paliopsia), or visual preservation, is a specific type of visual hallucination in which the sensation of visual perception remains or recurs after the stimulus is removed. It may represent an enhancement of normal afterimage phenomena and occurs with tumors, vascular disease, and seizure activity and after cranial trauma.

Alice in Wonderland syndrome is a rare form of complicated migraine, believed to be secondary to parietal lobe ischemia. Affected patients usually report distortion of body parts, but visual and other sensory hallucinations are occasionally described. Visual hallucinations can also be a sign of psychosis or disorientation, or accompany insulin hypoglycemia, high fever (especially in children), or advanced syphilis.

Sensory deprivation is a well-known cause of hallucinations. Deprivation can occur in elderly patients following bilateral eye patching for trauma or surgery or following hospitalization and separation from familiar surroundings. Symptoms typically start at night when external stimuli are at a minimum. The episodes are best classified as transient psychotic events. Individuals suffer paranoid delusions and become noisy, abusive, confused, and hyperactive. Sedatives and tranquilizers worsen the condition. A rare and fascinating sensory deprivation hallucination can occur in patients with bilateral dense cataracts. These occur without associated behavioral disturbances, and affected individuals are aware they are only mirages. They tend to occur with the individual resting in a quiet, dimly illuminated room, just prior to reclining. Affected patients "see" vividly colored images. These images are short in duration but may occur daily; some patients may derive pleasure from experiencing these hallucinations.

Poisoning with certain mushrooms, gasoline, mullet (a Hawaiian fish), oloiuqui (morning glory seeds), and nutmeg may elicit hallucinations. Marijuana, hashish, mescaline, lysergic acid, psilocin, cocaine, and alcohol are common recreational drugs that induce visual hallucinations. They can also be induced as a side effect of many pharmaceuticals, including digitalis, cortisol, and scopolamine. Finally, visual hallucinations occur in some drug withdrawal states, most notable alcohol withdrawal.

OSCILLOPSIA

A. Vestibular dysfunction
B. Cerebellar/posterior fossa dysfunction
C. Paraneoplastic syndrome
D. Internuclear ophthalmoplegia
E. Fixation and voluntary nystagmus
F. Superior oblique myokymia
G. Drug induced

Oscillopsia is the illusionary perception that the world is moving or fluttering. It usually accompanies an acute loss of vestibular function and can follow sectioning of the vestibular nerve (VIII) for vertigo or streptomycin toxicity; it can also occur spontaneously. In vestibular dysfunction, oscillopsia is associated with horizontal nystagmus, which is accentuated by head or body movement due to the absence of vestibular modulation of eye movements. Nystagmus and oscillopsia are at their maximum initially and decrease during the course of the disease.

Oscillopsia also commonly accompanies acquired nystagmus associated with vascular or demyelinating disease affecting the brain stem or cerebellum, suggested by the presence of opsoclonus and ocular flutter. *Opsoclonus* is characterized by involuntary, erratic, rapid eye movements in all directions. *Ocular flutter* is spontaneous to-and-fro oscillations that interrupt fixation; they may occur in the recovery phase of opsoclonus. Occasionally, an occult neoplasm, particularly neuroblastoma, induces opsoclonus and oscillopsia. This effect has been termed *paraneoplastic.*

A lesion of the medial longitudinal fasiculus, *internuclear ophthalmoplegia,* whether due to multiple sclerosis, tumor or vascular accident, results in monocular nystagmus in the contralateral abducting (outward-looking) eye and may be accompanied by oscillopsia. Oscillopsia can also occur with fixation or voluntary nystagmus and has been rarely reported with myokymia (fluttering) of the superior oblique muscle. Multiple drugs, particularly barbiturates, may induce this symptom. *Superior oblique myokymia* is a brief, recurrent microoscillation of the superior oblique muscle that is difficult to see with the unaided eye. Occasionally patients complain of vertical diplopia or fluttering of an eye with blurring of vision, but usually on questioning they also note torsional oscillopsia. The ocular movement can be verified using the magnification of the slit lamp or ophthalmoscope. In some patients, the myokymia can be induced by having the patient look in the direction of action of the suspected superior oblique muscle (downward and inward); in other cases, it can be induced by convergence. The prognosis for this condition is excellent; resolution usually occurs within several years. If the condition is debilitating, carbamazepine 200 mg, 3 times per day, may be helpful.

METAMORPHOPSIA

A. Macular disease (see Chapter 14)
   1. Central serous retinopathy
   2. Age-related macular degeneration
   3. Cellophane maculopathy

B. Retinal detachment (see Chapter 14)

C. Choroidal tumor (see Chapter 14)

D. Orbital tumor (see Chapter 12)

E. Scleral buckle

F. Aura of classic migraine (see above)

G. Complicated migraine (Alice in Wonderland syndrome)

H. Disorders of the temporal cortex

I. Topical miotic eyedrops

J. Recently changed glasses prescription

K. Venous stasis retinopathy (See Chapter 14)

Metamorphopsia is the condition in which objects appear distorted. Most commonly, straight lines, patterns, or edges appear irregularly curved. Occasionally objects appear too small *(micropsia)* or too large *(macropsia)*. Metamorphopsia almost always suggests a macular abnormality, with abnormal compression or separation of photoreceptor elements in the fovea. Micropsia results if the photoreceptors are abnormally separated but maintain their axial alignment to the optical system. Metamorphopsia results when the photoreceptors are partially misaligned and a scotoma (absence of vision) occurs when the misalignment is so great that the photoreceptors are no longer axial to the impinging light. Macular edema, a retinal detachment or hemorrhage, or a choroidal tumor should be sought. The last causes metamorphopsia due to an accompanying serous retinal detachment or compressive distortion of the macula. Compressive orbital tumors (Figure 13-10) or scleral buckles for retinal detachment may have a similar affect.

The aura of classic migraine is typically a shimmering, scintillating scotoma.

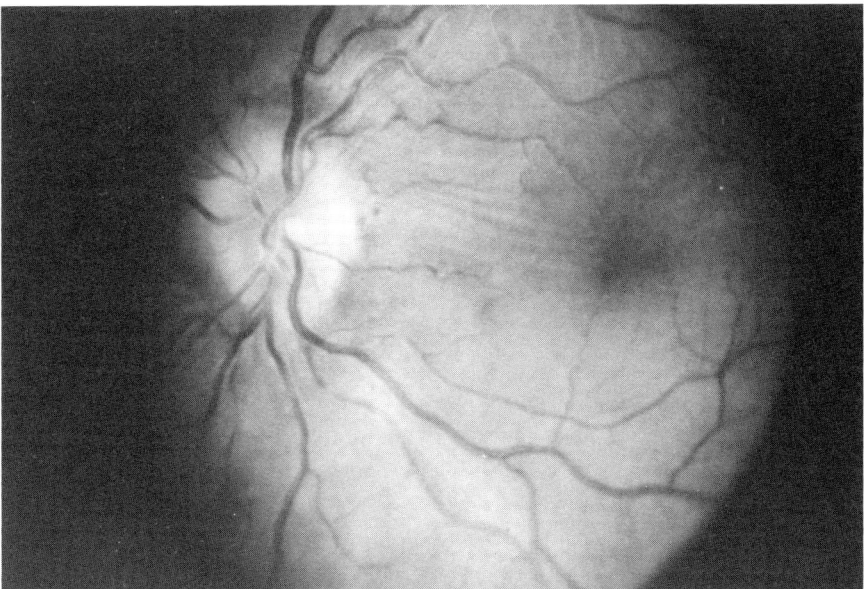

FIGURE 13-10. Optic disk edema and secondary macular edema (note choroidal folds) in a patient with an orbital tumor. The presenting complaint was metamorphopsia.

Some patients report this as a distortion of vision rather than the more typical description of an expanding gray area of scotoma with peripheral bright, zigzag lines or arcs. A rare form of complicated migraine, also called the *Alice in Wonderland syndrome,* is characterized by perceived distortions of the size and shape of body parts. Olfactory, auditory, and gustatory hallucinations are also common. This migraine variant is thought to be related to parietal lobe ischemia, and the name of the syndrome is given for Lewis Carroll's description of such hallucinations. It occurs most frequently in young adults, and headache is variable. The differential diagnosis includes drug intoxication, temporal lobe epilepsy, and schizophrenia. Temporal lobe disorders usually cause micropsia. Topical miotics may cause relative micropsia through induced myopia. Recently changed glasses, especially astigmatic corrections, may also induce metamorphopsia, especially in adults.

SUDDEN ONSET OF PHOTOPHOBIA

A. Ocular causes
1. Optic neuritis
2. Cone degenerations or abnormalities
3. Strabismus
4. Noninfectious corneal abnormality (see Chapter 9)

5. Keratoconjunctivitis (see Chapter 16)
   a. Secondary to Lyme disease (see above)
6. Angle closure glaucoma (see Chapter 11)
7. Anterior uveitis (see Chapter 16)
8. Cataract (gradual onset)

B. Central nervous system abnormality
   1. Migraine
   2. Meningitis
   3. Subarachnoid or subdural hemorrhage
   4. Posterior fossa tumor
   5. Trigeminal neuralgia

C. Certain systemic diseases

D. Certain inborn errors of metabolism

E. Toxic and drug induced

F. Functional (see Chapter 15)

Photophobia means "intolerance or fear of light." It is physiologic when it occurs due to excessive light (sun gazing) or excessive contrast (bright areas juxtaposed with dark areas). Glare describes the discomfort that results from viewing reflected (and usually polarized) light. Photophobia is a common complaint in those with ocular neuroses (see Chapter 15).

When photophobia occurs secondary to a pathologic central nervous system abnormality, it is usually superseded as a presenting complaint by other symptoms, including headache, obtundation, and disorientation. Photophobia often accompanies several ocular disorders, including keratoconjunctivitis, acute glaucoma, uveitis, or optic neuritis. Other symptoms generally outweigh the complaint of photophobia in these conditions as well. Several notable exceptions, however, occur in children. A cone degeneration may be first discovered upon ophthalmoscopic examination in a photophobic child with reduced vision. A history of preferred dim illumination (hemeralopia) and a reduction in visual acuity as illumination increases further suggest this disorder. Monocular eyelid closure in bright sunlight is common in children with intermittent exotropia and not unusual in children with other forms of strabismus and in nonstrabismic children. One theory, although it is controversial, is that this occurs to reduce photophobia and is not related to the avoidance of diplopia. A few children have been reported who presented with a triad of photophobia, torticollis (head tilt), and epiphora (tearing) and were found to have posterior fossa tumors.

Individuals with certain inborn abnormalities, such as erythropoietic porphyria, cystinosis, or hypoparathyroidism, may have a gradual onset of photophobia, as may those with systemic diseases such as botulism, rabies, schistosomiasis, or psittacosis. Individuals with albinism or achromatopsia (total absence of cones) are photophobic from birth; they do not present with an acute onset of photophobia. Photophobia can also be induced by mercury poisoning and multiple drugs, including atropine, chloroquine, digitoxin, tetracycline, tolbutamide, and antipsychotics. Some topical medications, including timolol and aminoglycoside antibiotics, may cause toxic epithelial defects of the cornea and photophobia.

PHOTOPSIA

A. Digital pressure on the eye
B. Rapid eye movements
C. Retinal traction or break (see Chapter 14)
D. Posterior vitreous detachment (see Chapter 14)
E. Retinal microembolization (see Chapter 14)
F. Central retinal vein thrombosis (see Chapter 14)
G. Optic neuritis (see Chapter 14)
H. Optic nerve compression (see Chapter 14)
I. Auditory induced phosphenes
J. Focal occipital lobe disorders
K. Migraine headaches (see above)
L. Ionizing radiation striking the eye

Photopsia, or the sensation of phosphenes (flashes of light), can occur normally with digital pressure on the eye or with rapid eye movements *(Flick phosphene).* The latter occur more commonly in axial myopes. Phosphenes in the temporal periphery associated with retinal traction at the vitreous base are called *Moore's lightning streaks.* More severe vitreous traction may cause a retinal break or *posterior vitreous detachment* The presence of hemorrhage in the vitreous suggests one of the latter two disorders. Occasionally, patients with retinal microembolization or central retinal vein thrombosis note light flashes occurring as a result of retinal ischemia. Optic nerve compression from tumors or masses may also elicit phosphenes. An interesting phenomenon in some patients with optic nerve or chiasmal disease is the induction of phosphenes by sound. In these disorders, phosphenes usually occur as part of a startle reaction during a state of relaxation. The photisms occur in the defective portion of the visual field when sound is perceived in the ipsilateral ear. This phenomenon has also been called *auditory-induced phosphenes.*

Eye movement and sound-induced phosphenes occur in optic neuritis and occasionally are seen in ischemic optic neuropathy. Phosphenes may also occur with focal occipital lobe disorders, especially neoplastic or arteriovenous malformations involving the calcarine fissure. Occipital and temporal lobe seizures may induce phosphenes.

FLOATERS

A. Vitreous abnormality
   1. Vitreous degeneration
   2. Vitreous hemorrhage (see Chapter 14)
   3. Posterior vitreous detachment (see Chapter 14)
   4. Metastatic endophthalmitis
   5. Parasitic cysts (echinococcus)
B. Retinal abnormality
   1. Retinal break (see Chapter 14)
   2. Venous stasis retinopathy (see Chapter 14)
C. Uveitis (see Chapter 16)
   1. Tuberculosis
   2. Sarcoidosis
   3. Toxoplasmosis
   4. Pars planitis
   5. Amyloidosis
D. Tumor
   1. Malignant melanoma with hemorrhage or pigment
   2. Reticulum cell sarcoma
   3. Retinoblastoma
   4. Medulloepithelioma

The most common etiology of floaters is benign liquification of the vitreous body. Vitreous liquefaction occurs with age in nearly all individuals. It occurs as early as the second decade in myopes and accompanies peripheral uveitis, retinitis pigmentosa, Wagner and Stickler syndromes, and trauma. Benign floaters are seen as curved lines or dots that drift by themselves or with eye movement. They are especially noticeable when staring at a brightly illuminated paper or when gazing at the sky on a bright day. Long periods of time may elapse between times when the patient notices or is attentive to them. In distinction, the vitreous opacity that occurs with a posterior vitreous detachment is generally seen at all times and in the same location.

Pathologic floaters should be suspected when the patient reports that they began as a sudden "shower of floaters," were associated with flashes of light, and/or were followed by decreased vision. The association of the acute onset of new floaters with flashes of light almost always indicates a retinal tear or posterior vitreous detachment. Because most of these disorders are associated with sudden loss of vision, they are discussed in Chapter 14. Uveitic entities are discussed in Chapter 16.

Although ocular tumors require urgent treatment, many are asymptomatic until they grow large or are discovered incidentally on ophthalmologic exam. This is especially true in infants or with slow-growing tumors. Exceptions include malignant melanomas that hemorrhage, some metastatic tumors (usually from the breast or lung), and reticulum cell sarcoma, a bilateral malignant lymphoma that occurs in individuals beyond age 50 years. It is not unusual for ocular findings to be the first manifestation of the latter tumor. Examination reveals yellow-white chorioretinal infiltrates and vitreous opacities. Central nervous system involvement should be suspected when generalized, nonlocalizing neurologic symptoms and/or dementia occur. Corticosteroids may exacerbate the condition.

BLINKING, BLEPHAROSPASM, AND EYELID TWITCHING

A. Physiologic reflex
   1. Associated with conditions that cause photophobia
   2. Associated with conditions that cause ocular pain
B. Associated with systemic conditions
   1. Frontal seizures
   2. Hypoparathyroidism
   3. Giles de la Tourette syndrome
   4. Tic douloureux
   5. Tardive dyskinesia
   6. Medication induced
C. Associated with muscular conditions
   1. Essential blepharospasm
   2. Hemifacial spasm
   3. Facial myokymia
D. Functional blinking (see Chapter 15)

Blinking is a physiologic reflex that maintains the tear film and protects the eye from noxious stimuli, dryness, confrontational threat, bright light, and tactile stimulation. In infancy, blinking occurs approximately at two times per minute; by age 15 years, physiologic blinking increases to 14 times to 17 times per minute. Physiologic blinking increases with ocular conditions that cause intraocular scattering of light and photophobia—for example, uveitis and acute glaucoma with corneal edema. Painful ocular conditions, such as conjunctivitis, corneal abrasions, foreign bodies, and trichiasis (misdirected eyelashes), also cause blepharospasm or blinking.

Excessive blinking can also be caused by certain systemic conditions. These include focal *frontal seizures,* with ipsilateral facial twitching, and *hypoparathyroidism,* with hypocalcemia and signs of hyperreflexia and tetany. Blinking can also occur as a component of *Giles de la Tourette syndrome,* which is principally characterized by convulsive motor spasms and uncontrolled vocalizations of bizzare sounds or vulgar words. It can occur with *tic douloureux,* characterized by episodic pain in the distribution of the fifth cranial nerve, which is usually associated with wincing. Finally, antipsychotic and analeptic medications can result in *tardive dyskinesia,* or oculogyrate crises, with excessive blinking, and antiemetics and nasal decongestants have occasionally been reported to cause facial dyskinesias and excessive blinking.

Blinking can suggest essential blepharospasm, hemifacial spasm, or facial myokymia. *Essential blepharospasm* is characterized by bilateral uncontrolled twitching or closure of the eyelids and other facial muscles. It occurs episodically and disappears during sleep. Its etiology is unknown, but it is treated with botulinum toxin or doxorubicin injections into the orbicularis muscles or with surgical stripping of the orbicularis muscle from the upper eyelids and brow. *Hemifacial spasm* (Figure 13-11) is the simultaneous contracture of all of the facial muscles on one side of the face. Twitches may start around the eye and subsequently generalize to all the facial muscles innervated by the ipsilateral facial nerve. It does not disappear during sleep and occurs secondary to lesions compressing the facial nerve extra-axially. An aneurysm of the posterior communicating artery, arteriovenous malformation, or tumor involving the cerebellar pontine angle area should be suspected. Botulinum toxin injection of the facial muscles and surgical decompression of the facial nerve may be helpful. About one-third of patients also report benefit from carbamezepine. Injected doxorubicin has been used to treat blepharospasm and hemifacial spasm. Upon injection of doxorubicin, the eyelids usually become swollen and

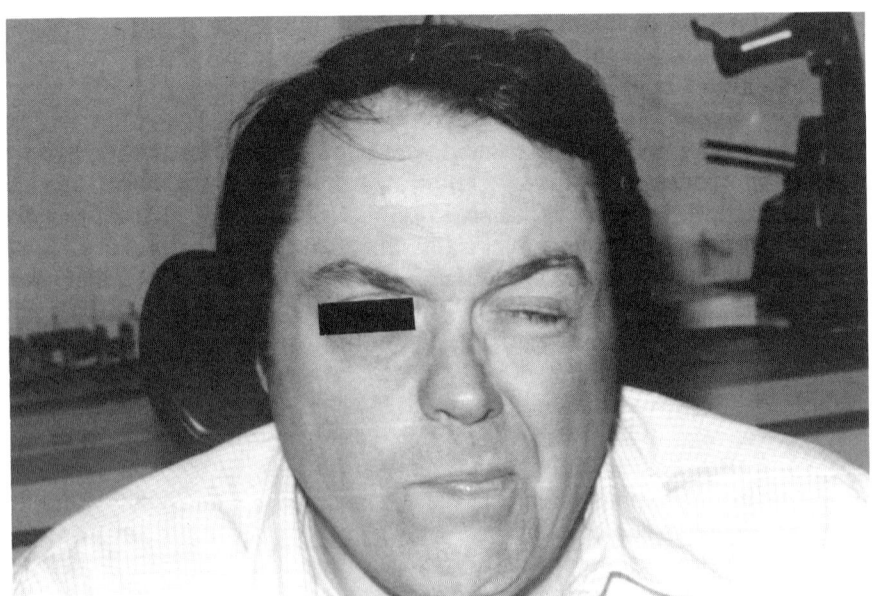

FIGURE 13-11. Hemifacial spasm.

inflamed for up to 3 months; no long-term, irreversible complications have been reported, however. The maximum safe single injection dose is 1 mg in the upper eyelid and 1.5 mg in the lower eyelid. Multiple injections, separated by at least 2 months, may be needed before an effect is noted. Botulinum injections do not result in permanent cures, and there remains no assurance that a permanent cure will result with doxorubicin.

Facial myokymia is an episodic twitching of the orbicularis oculi muscle. In some individuals, it is characterized by fine, undulating contractions; in others, episodic twitches are reported. When it involves only a single muscle, facial myokymia is almost always a benign condition. A history of periods of episodic twitching, lasting a few hours each day for several days to weeks and occurring during times of fatigue or stress, is often elicited in otherwise healthy individuals. Facial myokymia may, however, be a presenting feature of multiple sclerosis, a brain stem neoplasm, a brain stem vascular lesion, or the Guillain-Barré syndrome. In children, it can occur in association with a brain stem glioma. In these instances, it persists indefinitely. The treatment of facial myokymia in adults is initially conservative. Ocular irritation is treated with antihistamines or artificial tears. If the myokymia persists more than 3 weeks to 4 weeks or other neurologic abnormalities arise, MRI is indicated to rule out a tumor or vascular anomaly of the posterior fossa. If no abnormality is detected, a muscle relaxant, such as orphenadrine citrate (Norgesic) (one to two tablets every 4 hours to 6 hours) should be tried. If this is not effective with 1 week to 2 weeks, botulinum or surgical myectomy should be considered.

Conditions that cause ocular pain and photophobia usually have associated signs or symptoms, including tearing, decreased visual acuity, or conjunctival injection. The underlying pathology is usually readily diagnosed and the increased blink rate understood as a secondary phenomenon. Similarly, systemic abnormalities are suggested by associated findings or known use of particular medications. Muscular abnormalities are also generally easily recognized by the history and findings. Another condition, seen predominantly in children, is *functional blinking* (see Chapter 15). In fewer than half of these children, a temporally related stressful event is identified, and the disorder is believed to be self-limited. The main secondary gain is usually increased attention from the caretaker.

LEUKOCORIA

A. Corneal abnormality
   1. Peter's anomaly
   2. Congenital corneal opacity

B. Congenital cataract

C. Persistent hyperplastic primary vitreous

D. Ocular tumor
   1. Retinoblastoma
   2. Medulloepithelioma
E. Congenital developmental defect
   1. Coloboma of the choroid and retina
   2. Medullated nerve fibers
   3. High myopia with retinal degeneration
   4. Retinal dysplasia
   5. Juvenile retinoschisis
   6. Falciform fold of retina/congenital retinal detachment
F. Progressive retinal disorder
   1. Cicatricial retinopathy of prematurity
   2. Coats's disease
   3. Organized vitreous hemorrhage
   4. Incontinentia pigmenti
   5. Norrie disease
   6. Familial exudative vitreoretinopathy
   7. Retinal astrocytoma (tuberous sclerosis or neurofibromatosis)
G. Infectious
   1. Nematode endophthalmitis (toxocariasis)
   2. Metastatic endophthalmitis

Leukocoria means "white pupil" (Figure 13-12). Although it is a sign rather than a symptom, it is discussed as a separate entity, because it is often the way children with serious ocular disorders present. A complete discourse on these topics is beyond the scope of this book. A few salient points, however, will be made.

A family history of retinal tumor, blind eye in childhood, congenital cataracts, or other developmental or progressive retinal disorder should be determined. The personal history should indicate prematurity, contact with puppies (toxocariasis in older children), or the presence of skin blisters and verrucous lesions within the first few months of life (incontinentia pigmenti).

In all cases, a complete ocular examination must be performed. Corneal opacities can be readily recognized, as can congenital cataracts (Figure 13-13), either directly or with the hand-held slit lamp. A small eye suggests persistent hyperplastic primary vitreous or incontinentia pigmenti. Cells in the anterior chamber of the eye (pseudohypopyon) or iris neovascularization suggest retinoblastoma (an intraocular tumor of retinal elements; Figure 13-14). Vitreous haze in a 6 to 10 year old suggests toxocariasis (infection with the larval stage of an intestinal parasite of dogs; Figure 13-15). A dilated fundus examination is essential, and infants may have to be examined under anesthesia. This is particularly true if the parents note leukocoria when the child looks in certain directions, but the entire retina cannot be visualized with the child awake

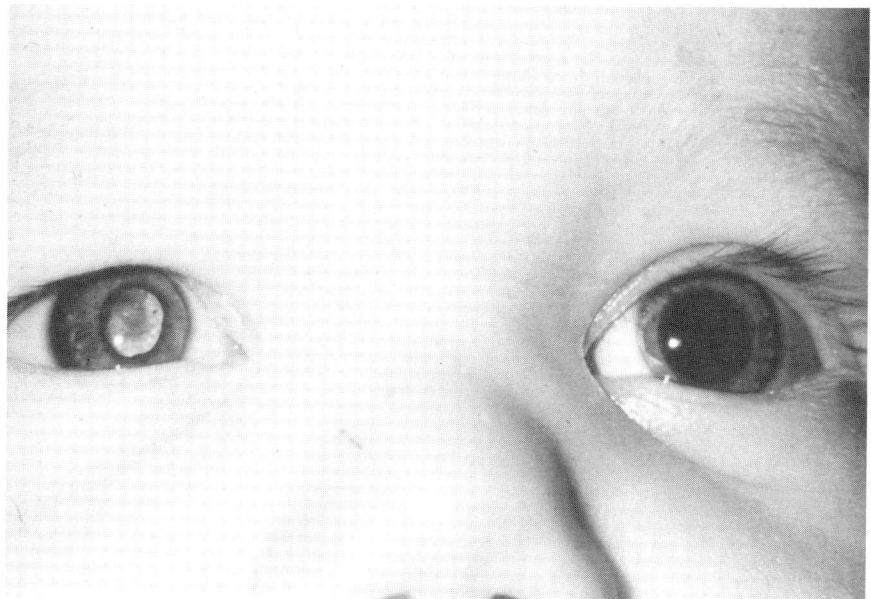

FIGURE 13-12. Leukocoria secondary to persistent hyperplastic primary vitreous.

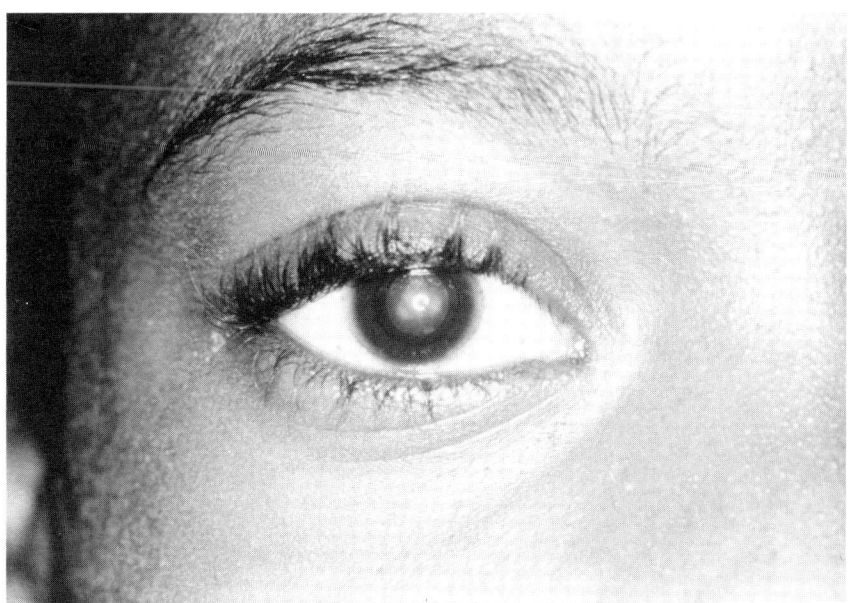

FIGURE 13-13. Congenital cataract.

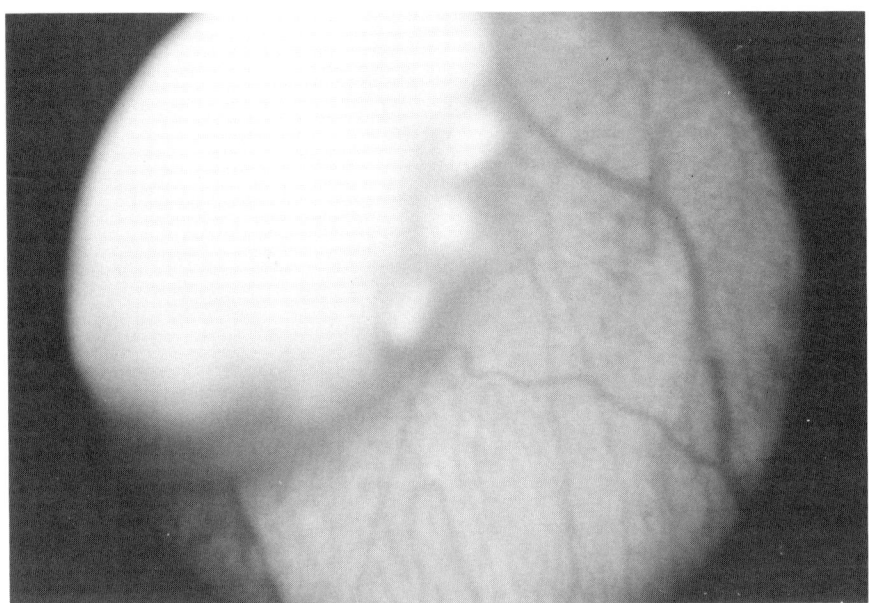

FIGURE 13–14. Retinoblastoma.

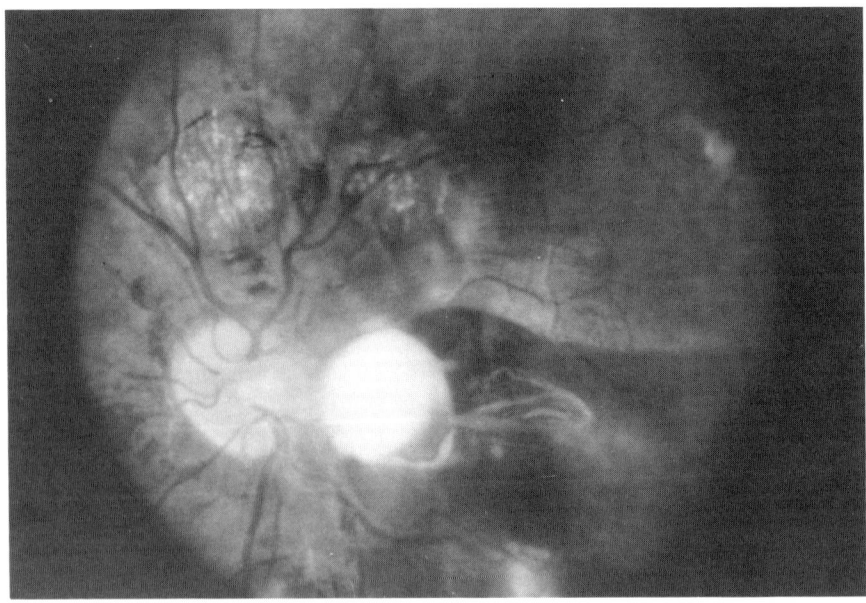

FIGURE 13–15. Toxocariasis.

because of limited cooperation. Treatable conditions such retinoblastoma, toxocariasis, Coats's disease (a vascular abnormality manifest by subretinal exudation (that may involve the macula), serous retinal detachment, and retinal ischemia; Figure 13-16), and retinopathy of prematurity need to be ruled out.

SUDDEN VISUAL FIELD LOSS OR ABNORMALITY

The following outline details lesions corresponding to specific visual field abnormalities:

1. Monocular field defects that do not respect the vertical midline
   a. Lesions in the ipsilateral retina
   b. Lesions in the ipsilateral optic nerve
2. Altitudinal (superior or inferior visual field) loss (see Chapter 14)
   a. Ischemic optic neuropathy
   b. Optic nerve or chiasmal lesion
   c. Segmental retinal artery or vein occlusion
3. Nerve fiber bundle (arcuate) scotoma (see Chapters 11 and 14)
   a. Glaucoma

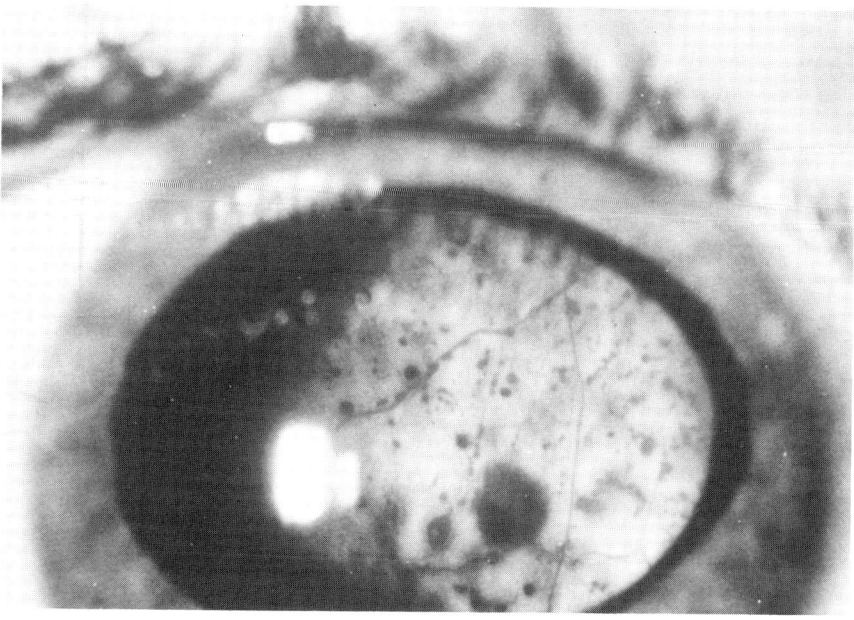

FIGURE 13-16. Coats's disease.

b. Ischemic optic neuropathy
   c. Optic pit
   d. Optic drusen
   e. Chronic papilledema
4. Central loss of vision (see Chapter 14)
   a. Optic neuritis
   b. Ischemic optic neuropathy
   c. Compressive lesion of the optic nerve
   d. Nutritional/toxic/hereditary disorders
   e. Macular disease
5. Central loss of vision that includes the blind spot (cecocentral field loss) (see Chapter 14)
   a. Toxic optic neuropathy
   b. Any condition above that can also cause a central loss of vision
   c. Optic pit with serous retinal detachment
6. Bitemporal visual field loss
   a. Pituitary adenoma
   b. Meningioma
   c. Craniopharyngioma
   d. Aneurysm
   e. Glioma
7. Binasal visual field loss
   a. Tumor compressing both optic nerves or chiasm
   b. Aneurysm compressing both optic nerves or chiasm
   c. Bilateral occipital disease
   d. Bitemporal retinal disease
   e. Glaucoma
8. Homonymous hemianopsia
   a. Lesion of the optic tract, lateral geniculate body, temporal, parietal, or occipital lobes; due to stroke, tumor, aneurysm, or trauma
   b. Migraine
9. Constriction of peripheral fields
   a. Migraine (transient)
   b. Chronic papilledema
   c. Bilateral occipital lobe infarction with macular sparing
   d. Central retinal artery occlusion with cilioretinal artery sparing (see Chapter 14)
   e. Peripheral retinal disorder
   f. Glaucoma
   g. Nonorganic visual loss (see Chapter 15)

A complete discourse on visual field defects is beyond the scope of this book. In addition to the differential noted, a few caveats are listed in Table 13–8.

TABLE 13-8. CAVEATS REGARDING VISUAL FIELD DEFECTS

SITE OF LESION	FINDING
Retina and optic nerve	A monocular defect that may not respect the vertical midline
Anterior optic chiasm	Visual loss in one eye with a superior temporal defect in the opposite eye (junctional scotoma)
Body of optic chiasm	Bitemporal hemianopsia without visual acuity loss
Posterior optic chiasm	Central bitemporal hemianopic scotomas due to damage of crossing macular fibers
Posterior to the chiasm	Homonymous field defect that respects the vertical midline
Optic tract	Associated with memory loss, +/− contralateral hemiparesis, and incongruous when not complete
Temporal lobe	Denser above and less congruous, +/− seizures, and formed hallucinations
Parietal lobe	Denser below and more congruous +/− optokinetic nystagmus asymmetry (greater nystagmus with drum rotated away from the side of the lesion), hemiparesis, agnosias, and acalculia
Occipital lobe	Sparing of an ipsilateral peripheral temporal crescent of vision, very congruous, with +/− macular sparing, brain stem dysfunction (dysarthria), and +/− unformed visual hallucinations

Special notations
Binasal defects are usually caused by lesions of both optic nerves or retinas.
Visual acuity is usually not reduced by lesions posterior to the optic tract.
True bitemporal defects arise only from lesions involving the optic chiasm.
Nerve fiber layer and optic nerve atrophy are caused by lesions anterior to the optic radiations.
Bilateral homonymous altitudinal defects (usually inferior) suggest infarction or trauma to both superior occipital lobes.
90% of isolated homonymous hemianopsias are due to strokes.
A complete homonymous hemianopsia is nonlocalizing.

REFERENCES

Blinking, Blepharospasm, and Eyelid Closure

Elston JS: Botulinum toxin therapy for involuntary facial movement. *Eye* 2:12, 1988.
Jordan DR, Anderson RL, Thiese SM: Intractable orbicularis myokymia: Treatment alternatives. *Ophthalmic Surg* 20:280, 1989.
Nielsen VK: Pathophysiology of hemifacial spasm. 1. Ephaptic transmission and ectopic excitation. *Neurology* 34:418, 1984.
Patrinely JR, Whiting AS, Anderson RL: Local side effects of botulinum toxin injections. *Adv Neurol* 49:493, 1988.
Vrabec TR, Levin AV, Nelson LB: Functional blinking in childhood. *Pediatrics* 83:967, 1989.
Wang FM, Chryssanthou G: Monocular eye closure in intermittent exotropia. *Arch Ophthalmol* 106:941, 1988.
Wiggins RE, von Noorden GK: Monocular eye closure in sunlight. *J Pediatr Ophthalmol Strabismus* 27:16, 1990.
Wirtschafter JD: Clinical doxorubicin chemomyectomy: An experimental treatment for essential blepharospasm and hemifacial spasm. *Ophthalmology* 98:357, 1991.

Diplopia

Baker RS, Epstein AD: Ocular motor abnormalities from head trauma. *Surv Ophthalmol* 35:245, 1991.
Balkan R, Hoyt CS: Associated neurologic abnormalities in congenital third nerve palsies. *Am J Ophthalmol* 97:315, 1984.
Ball JB Jr: Direct oblique sagittal CT of orbital wall fractures. *AJR* 148:601, 1987.
Buncic JR: Pediatric neuro-ophthalmology and ocular emergencies. *Ophthalmic Pract* 8:146, 1990.
Burger LJ, Kalvin NH, Smith JL: Acquired lesions of the fourth cranial nerve. *Brain* 93:567, 1970.
Eyster EF, Hoyt WF, Wilson CB: Ocular motor palsy from minor head trauma: An initial sign of basal intracranial tumor. *JAMA* 220:1083, 1972.
Fisher M: An unusual variant of acute idiopathic polyneuritis (syndrome of ophthalmoplegia, ataxia and areflexia). *N Engl J Med* 255:57, 1956.
Grunnet ML, Lubow, M: Ascending polyneuritis and ophthalmoplegia. *Am J Ophthalmol* 74:1155, 1972.
Harley RD: Paralytic strabismus in children. Etiologic incidence and management of the third, fourth and six nerve palsies. *Ophthalmology* 87:24, 1980.
Kahana E, Leibowitz U, Alter M: Brainstem and cranial nerve involvement in multiple sclerosis. *Acta Neurol Scand* 49:269, 1973.
Kirkham TH, Bird AC, Sanders MD: Divergence paralysis with raised intracranial pressure: An electrooculographic study. *Br J Ophthalmol* 56:776, 1972.
Leigh RJ, Zee DS: *The Neurology of Eye Movement*. Philadelphia, FA Davis Co, 1981.
Lessell S, Van Dalen JTW (eds): *Myasthenia Gravis in Neuro-Ophthalmology*. Amsterdam, Elsevier, 1984.
Lesser RL, Kornmehl EW, Pachner AR, et al: Neuro-ophthalmologic manifestations of Lyme disease. *Ophthalmology* 97:699, 1990.
Lewis MA, Goldstein S, Baker RS: Magnetic resonance imaging of the posterior fossa in ocular motility disorders. *J Clin Neuro-ophthalmol* 7:235, 1987.
Lindenberg R: Significance of the tentorium in head injuries from blunt forces. *Clin Neurosurg* 12:129, 1966.
Miller NR: Solitary oculomotor nerve palsy in childhood. *Am J Ophthalmol* 83:106, 1977.
Richards R: Ocular motility disturbances following trauma. *Adv Ophthalmic Plast Reconstr Surg* 7:133, 1987.
Robertson DM, Hines JD, Rucker CW: Acquired sixth nerve paresis in children. *Arch Ophthalmol* 83:574, 1970.
Rucker CW: The causes of paralysis of the third, fourth and sixth cranial nerves. *Am J Ophthalmol* 61:1293, 1966.
Schwartz BS, Goldstein MD, Riberio JMC, et al: Antibody testing in Lyme disease. *JAMA* 262:3431, 1989.
Seybold ME: Myasthenia gravis. *JAMA* 250:2516, 1983.
Smith JL: Lyme disease appears to have many ocular manifestations. *Arch Ophthalmol* 108:337, 1990.
Victor DI: The diagnosis of congenital unilateral third nerve palsy. *Brain* 99:711, 1976.
Weber RB, Daroff RB, Mackey EA: Pathology of oculomotor nerve palsy in diabetics. *Neurology* 20:835, 1970.
Werner DB, Savino PJ, Schatz NJ: Benign recurrent sixth nerve palsies in children. *Arch Ophthalmol* 101:607, 1983.
Winward KE, Smith JL, Culbertson WW, Paris-Hamelin A: Ocular Lyme borreliosis. *Am J Ophthalmol* 108:651, 1989.
Younge BR, Sutula F: Analysis of trochlear nerve palsies: Diagnosis, etiology and treatment. *Mayo Clin Proc* 52:11, 1977.

Hallucinations

Brust JCM, Behrens MM: "Release hallucinations" as the major symptom of posterior cerebral artery occlusion. A report of 2 cases. *Ann Neurol* 2:432, 1977.
Gittinger, JW Jr, Miller NR, Keltner JL, Burde RM: Sugarplum fairies. Visual hallucinations. *Surv Ophthalmol* 27:42, 1982.

Jacobs L, Karpik A, Bosian D, Gothgen S: Auditory-visual synthesis. *Arch Neurol* 38:211, 1981.
Lessell S: Higher disorders of visual function. In Glaser JS, Smith JL (eds): *Neuro-Ophthalmology*, vol 8. St. Louis, CV Mosby Co, 1975.
Levine AM: Visual hallucinations and cataracts. *Ophthalmic Surg* 11:95, 1980.
Newmark ME: Visual hallucinations. *JAMA* 257:82, 1987.
Siegal RK: Hallucinations. In *The Mind's Eye: Readings from Scientific American*. New York, WH Freeman and Co, 1986, pp 109–116.
White NJ: Complex visual hallucinations in partial blindness due to eye disease. *Br J Psychiatry* 136:284, 1980.

Headaches

Corbett JJ, Savino PJ, Thompson HS, et al: Visual loss in pseudotumor cerebri. *Arch Neurol* 39:461, 1979.
Cornblath WT: Ocular and systemic migraine. *Ophthalmic Pract* 8:125, 1990.
Crowell GF, Carlin L: Neurologic complications of migraine. *Am Fam Phys* 26:139, 1982.
Diamond S: Management of headaches: Focus on new strategies. *Postgrad Med* 87:181, 1990.
Diamond S, Medina JL: Review article: Current thoughts on migraine. *Headache* 20:208, 1980.
Drexler ED: Severe headaches. *Postgrad Med* 87:164, 1990.
Gabai I, Spierings E: Prophylactic treatment of cluster headaches with Verapamil. *Headache* 29:167, 1989.
Keltner JL: A red eye and high intraocular pressure. *Surv Ophthalmol* 31:328, 1987.
Keltner JL, Miller NR, Gittinger JW, et al: Pseudotumor cerebri. *Surv Ophthalmol* 23:315, 1979.
Miller NR, Fine SL: *The Ocular Fundus in Neuro-Ophthalmologic Diagnosis*. St. Louis, CV Mosby Co, 1977.
Raskin N: *Headache*. 2d ed. New York, Longman (Churchill Livingstone), 1988.
Sarkies NJC, Sanders MD, Gautier-Smith PC: Episodic unilateral mydriasis and migraine. *Am J Ophthalmol* 99:217, 1985.
Spector RH: Migeraine. *Surv Ophthalmol* 29:193, 1984.

Metamorphopsia

Glaser JS, Savino PJ, Sumers KO, et al: The photostress recovery testing in the clinical assessment of visual function. *Am J Ophthalmol* 83:255, 1970.

Oscillopsia

Alves WM, Colohan ART, O'Leary TJ, et al: Understanding posttraumatic symptoms after minor head injury. *J Head Trauma Rehabil* 1:1, 1986.
Keltner JL: The monocular shimmers—your patient isn't deluded. *Surv Ophthalmol* 27:313, 1983

Painful Ophthalmoplegia

Barricks ME, Traviesa DB, Glaser JS, Levy IS: Ophthalmoplegia in cranial arteritis. *Brain* 100:209, 1977.
Barrow DL, Spector RH, Braun IF, et al: Classification and treatment of spontaneous carotid-cavernous fistulas. *J Neurosurg* 64:724, 1985.
Berenstein A, Scott J, Choi IS, Persky M: Percutaneous embolization of arteriovenous fistulas of the external carotid artery. *AJNR* 7:937, 1986.
Clune JP: Septic thrombosis within the cavernous chamber: Review of the literature with recent advances in diagnosis and treatment. *Am J Ophthalmol* 56:33, 1963.
Fiore PM, Latina MA, Shingleton BJ, et al: The dural shunt syndrome. I. Management of glaucoma. *Ophthalmology* 97:56, 1990.
Grove AS Jr: The dural shunt syndrome: Pathology and clinical course. *Ophthalmology* 91:31, 1984.
Keane JR: Aneurysms and third nerve palsies. *Ann Neurol* 14:696, 1983.
Keltner JL, Satterfield D, Dublin AB, Lee BCP: Dural and carotid cavernous sinus fistulas. *Ophthalmology* 94:1585, 1987.

Kuppersmith MJ, Berenstein A, Choi IS, et al: Management of nontraumatic vascular shunts involving the cavernous sinus. *Ophthalmology* 95:121, 1988.
Levine SR, Twyman RE, Gilman S: The role of anticoagulation in cavernous sinus thrombosis. *Neurology* 38:517, 1988.
O'Dwyer JA, Moscow N, Trevor R, et al: Spontaneous dissection of the carotid artery. *Neuroradiology* 137:379, 1980.
Phelps CD, Thompson HS, Ossoinig KC: The diagnosis and prognosis of atypical carotid-cavernous fistulas (red-eyed shunt syndrome). *Am J Ophthalmol* 93:423, 1982.
Price CD, Hameroff SB, Richards RD: Cavernous sinus thrombosis and orbital cellulitis. *South Med J* 64:1243, 1971.

Photophobia

Marmor MA, Beauchamp GR, Maddox SF: Photophobia, epiphora, and torticollis: A masquerade syndrome. *J Pediatr Ophthalmol Strabismus* 27:202, 1990.
Smith RE, Nozik RA: *Uveitis: A Clinical Approach to Diagnosis and Management*. 2d ed. Baltimore, Williams and Wilkins, 1989.

Photopsia

Davis FA, Bergen D, Schauf C, et al: Movement phosphenes in optic neuritis: A new clinical sign. *Neurology* 26:1100, 1976.
Hoyt WF, Knight CL: Comparison of congenital disc blurring and incipient papilledema in red-free light, a photographic study. *Invest Ophthalmol* 12:241, 1973.
Morse PH, Scheie HG: Light flashes as a clue to retinal disease. *Arch Ophthalmol* 91:179, 1974.

Pupillary Abnormalities

Axelrod FB: Familial dysautonomia. In Gellis SS, Kagan BM: *Current Pediatric Therapy 10*. Philadelphia, WB Saunders, 1982, pp 80–82.
Corbett JJ, Thompson HS: Pupillary function and dysfunction. In Asbury AK, McKhann GM, McDonald WI (eds): *Diseases of the Nervous System: Clinical Neurobiology*. Philadelphia, WB Saunders Co, 1986, pp 606–617.
Grimson BS, Thompson HS: Drug testing in Horner's syndrome. In Glaser JS, Smith JL (eds): *Neuro-Ophthalmology*. St Louis, CV Mosby Co, 1974, 8:265–270.
Grimson BS, Thompson HS: Raeder's syndrome: A clinical review. *Surv Ophthalmol* 24:199, 1980.
Kase M, Nagata R, Yoshida A, et al: Pupillary light reflex in amblyopia. *Invest Ophthalmol Vis Sci* 25:467, 1984.
Loewenfeld IE: "Simple, central" anisocoria: A common condition, seldom recognized. *Trans Am Acad Ophthalmol Otolaryngol* 83:832, 1977.
Miller NR: Disorders of pupillary function, accommodation and lacrimation. In Miller NR (ed): *Walsh and Hoyt's Clinical Neuro-ophthalmology*. 4th ed. Baltimore, Williams and Wilkins Co, 1985, 2:469–528.
Myers GA, Barricks ME, Stark L: Paradoxical pupillary constriction in a patient with congenital stationary night blindness. *Invest Ophthalmol Vis Sci* 26:736, 1985.
Plum F, Posner JB: *The Diagnosis of Stupor and Coma*. Philadelphia, FA Davis and Co, 1972.
Portnoy JZ, Thompson SH, Lennarson L, et al: Pupillary defects in amblyopia. *Am J Ophthalmol* 96:609, 1983.
Thompson HS: Adie's syndrome. Some new observations. *Trans Am Ophthalmol Soc* 75:587, 1977.
Thompson HS: The pupil. In Lessell S, van Dalen JTW (eds): *Current Neuro-ophthalmology*. Chicago, Yearbook Medical Publishers, 1988, pp 201–216.
Thompson HS, Corbett JJ, Cox TA: How to measure the relative afferent pupillary defect. *Surv Ophthalmol* 26:39, 1981.
Thompson HS, Pilley SFJ: Unequal pupils: A flowchart for sorting out the anisocorias. *Surv Ophthalmol* 21:45, 1976.
Thompson HS, Zackon DH, Czarnecki JSC: Tadpole-shaped pupils caused by segmental spasm of the iris dilator muscle. *Am J Ophthalmol* 96:467, 1983.

Trobe JD: Third nerve palsy and the pupil. *Arch Ophthalmol* 106:602, 1988.
Van der Wiel HL, van Ginj J: Localization of Horner's syndrome: Use and limitations of the hydroxyamphetamine test. *J Neurol Sci* 59:229, 1983.
Weinstein JM, Zweifel TJ, Thompson HS: Congenital Horner's syndrome. *Arch Ophthalmol* 98:1074, 1980.

Visual Field Abnormalities

Anderson DR: *Testing the Field of Vision.* St. Louis, CV Mosby Co, 1982.
Fujino T, Kigazawa K, Yamada R: Homonymous hemianopsia: A retrospective study of 140 cases. *Neuro-ophthalmology* 6:17, 1986.
Musarella MA, Chan HSL, DeBoer G, et al: Ocular involvement in neuroblastoma: Prognostic implications. *Ophthalmology* 91:936, 1984.
Newman SA, Miller NR: Optic tract syndrome: Neuro-ophthalmologic considerations. *Arch Ophthalmol* 101:1241, 1983.
Savino PJ, Paris M, Schatz NJ, et al: Optic tract syndrome. *Arch Ophthalmol* 96:656, 1978.
Thompson HS, Montague P, Cox TA, et al: The relationship between visual acuity, pupillary defect in visual field loss. *Am J Ophthalmol* 93:681, 1982.
Trobe JD, Acosta PC, Krischer JP, et al: Confrontation visual field techniques in detection of anterior visual pathway lesions. *Ann Neurol* 10:28, 1981.
Trobe JD, Lorber ML, Schlezinger NS: Isolated homonymous hemianopsia: A review of 104 cases. *Arch Ophthalmol* 89:377, 1973.

14

Sudden and Unexpected Loss of Vision

Robert A. Catalano

The sudden and unexpected loss of vision is a catastrophic event. The affected individual may be overwhelmed with anxiety and disorientation and unable to answer historical or descriptive questions regarding the event. The physician should direct the history by asking the following three questions:

1. Was the visual loss transient (fleeting, lasting seconds to minutes) or sustained (still affected, or lasting more than a few minutes)?
2. Were (are) any ocular symptoms or signs present (e.g., pain, photopsia, tearing, injection, proptosis, reduced motility)?
3. Was (is) the visual loss unilateral or bilateral?

Occasionally the physician will find that the loss of vision could not have been sudden, but because of the mental state or age of the patient, it was purported as such. Examples include the elderly patient with a unilateral optic neuropathy, who discovers his visual loss when the contralateral seeing eye develops a problem, or the young child with dominant optic atrophy who fails his yearly vision screening test at school. While they do not occur acutely, discovery of the visual loss represents an acute, unexpected emergency to the affected individual. Entities that can present this way will be included in this chapter. In contrast, visual loss is expected with severe ocular trauma or infection. Except for the few conditions where there are no obvious external ocular findings, these disorders are discussed elsewhere in this book.

Table 14-1 outlines the discussion of sudden loss of vision as presented in this chapter. Table 14-2 presents the complete differential for each of these categories.

SUSTAINED, UNILATERAL LOSS OF VISION WITH EXTERNAL OCULAR SIGNS

Angle closure glaucoma (Chapter 11), acute corneal (Chapter 10) and orbital disorders (Chapter 12), and ocular inflammation (Chapter 16) present with external ocular signs and symptoms. These signs and symptoms allow the physician to narrow the investigation quickly and direct treatment. Readers are directed to the discussion of these entities in their respective chapters.

SUSTAINED, UNILATERAL LOSS OF VISION WITHOUT EXTERNAL OCULAR SIGNS

In the absence of external ocular signs, rapid and unexpected unilateral loss of vision usually indicates an optic neuropathy or an abnormality of the central retina (the macula). Less frequently, a vitreous hemorrhage, retinal detachment, or abnormality of the choroid can present this way. Several signs are helpful in distinguishing an optic neuropathy from a macular abnormality. The presence of an afferent pupillary defect (see Chapter 1), an acquired dyschromotopsia (abnormality of color vision), or a visual field abnormality that involves more than just central vision suggests an optic nerve disease. The presence of metamorphopsia (the curvilinear distortion of lines and angles as tested with an Amsler grid) and a prolonged photostress recovery time suggest a macular disease. The photostress test involves "bleaching" the macula for 10 seconds with a bright light. The normal recovery time is 60 seconds. Prolongation of this time or an intraocular difference of greater than 15 seconds is abnormal. This test may not be accurate, however, when vision is reduced below 20/80.

Because many disorders are included under this category (see Table 14-2), Figure 14-1 was constructed to help narrow the differential diagnosis. This flowchart uses historical, optic nerve, and retinal findings and broadly outlines the discussion that follows. Each of the categories listed is discussed separately.

TABLE 14-1. SUDDEN AND UNEXPECTED LOSS OF VISION DIFFERENTIAL CATEGORIES

Sustained and unilateral	Sustained and bilateral
With ocular signs and symptoms	**Transient and unilateral** (amaurosis fugax)
Without ocular signs and symptoms	**Transient and bilateral**

Special Considerations with Cranial or Other Trauma

The loss of vision that accompanies a penetrating ocular injury is discussed in Chapter 8. Severe visual loss can also accompany a blunt ocular injury. Most of these injuries are accompanied by visible signs in the retina, optic nerve, or ocular lens and are discussed in Chapters 5 and 6. Two traumatic disorders, however, can present with minimal or delayed clinical findings. Posterior indirect traumatic optic neuropathy can present with a normal-appearing fundus, and the damage in solor maculopathy may not be apparent for several days. Three additional disorders—Terson's syndrome, Purtscher's retinopathy, and traumatic fat embolus—accompany trauma to other parts of the body. In these disorders, involvement of the eye is usually obvious on ophthalmoscopy, but the absence of visible ocular injury may cause a delay in diagnosis.

The optic nerve or its vascular supply can be torn, thrombosed, or compressed by a blunt injury to the orbit. Damage that occurs to the intraorbital (anterior) segment of the optic nerve presents with retinal vascular occlusion, with or without optic disk edema, and vitreous hemorrhage (see Chapter 6). Disruption of the intracanalicular segment, however, may present with subtle, if any, findings. Occasionally, visual loss may occur after a brief period of vision, further obscuring the diagnosis of *posterior indirect traumatic optic neuropathy.* In these cases, an afferent pupillary defect and neuroradiographic evidence of an optic canal fracture would be suggestive. The treatment of this disorder (high-dose intravenous corticosteroids and/or surgical decompression of the optic canal) is reviewed in Chapter 6.

Solar maculopathy, or light damage to the retina, can occur with sun or eclipse viewing. It is most frequently encountered in psychotics and military personnel. One day or 2 days may elapse before blurred central vision (a central scotoma), mild discomfort, or retinal findings are noted. By this time, a small yellow, nodular swelling in the fovea is noted. This resolves after about 2 weeks, leaving a tiny foveal or parafoveal defect resembling a cyst. The final acuity is often better than 20/50 (see also Chapter 7).

Retinal hemorrhages occur in 10% to 20% of patients with a sudden massive hemorrhage in the subarachnoid space, whether due to trauma or a ruptured aneurysm. The hemorrhages can be seen a few hours to days following the subarachnoid hemorrhage and typically occur near the disc margin. They are located in the nerve fiber or preretinal layer. Blood may break through the internal limiting membrane into the vitreous, at which time the name *Terson's syndrome* is applied. Extension into the vitreous, with a resultant decrease in vision, usually occurs days after the subarachnoid event. Findings are often bilateral and preceded by a severe headache or coma.

Purtscher's retinopathy is an uncommon disorder; it results from a sudden increase in intravascular pressure due to a crushing injury of the chest or severe head trauma. Cases have also been reported following chest compression for

Text continues on page 401

TABLE 14–2. SUDDEN, UNEXPECTED VISUAL LOSS

SUSTAINED, UNILATERAL WITH EXTERNAL OCULAR SIGNS	SUSTAINED, UNILATERAL WITHOUT EXTERNAL OCULAR SIGNS	SUSTAINED, BILATERAL	TRANSIENT, UNILATERAL	TRANSIENT, BILATERAL
Ocular trauma Angle closure glaucoma **Corneal disorders** Corneal hydrops Contact lens overwear **Ocular inflammation** Acute iridocyclitis Posterior uveitis Scleritis **Orbital disorders** Pseudotumor Posterior cellulitis Cavernous sinus thrombosis Carotid-cavernous fistula Orbital tumor	**Due to cranial or other trauma** Posterior indirect optic neuropathy Solar maculopathy Terson's syndrome Purtscher's syndrome Traumatic fat embolism **Considerations in AIDS patients** Retinopathy Optic neuropathy **Retinal vascular abnormalities** Retinal artery occlusion Retinal vein occlusion Retinal hemorrhage Retinal tear/detachment Vitreous hemorrhage Central serous retinopathy **Posterior vitreous detachment**	**Central nervous system abnormality** Cerebral vascular accident Pituitary tumor/apoplexy Cortical visual impairment from ischemia, anoxia, or hematoma **Optic nerve abnormality** Postinfectious optic neuritis Toxic/metabolic/ nutritional optic neuropathy Hereditary optic neuropathy Leber's optic neuropathy (often presents unilaterally)	**Vascular** Carotid artery disease Carotid emboli Ocular ischemic syndrome Structural cardiac defects Temporal arteritis Impending vascular occlusion of the retina Uniocular migraine **Papilledema (usually bilateral)**	Papilledema **Vascular** Vertebrobasilar artery insufficiency Vasomotor collapse Cardiac arrhythmia Severe hypertension Migraine **Seizure activity**

Optic nerve abnormalities
Optic neuritis
Ischemic optic neuropathy
  Temporal arteritis
  Nonarteritic
  Associated with systemic lupus erythematosis (SLE)
Acute disc swelling in diabetes
Migrainous optic neuropathy
Radiation optic neuropathy
Compressive optic neuropathy
Leber's optic neuropathy
Lyme disease
Macular abnormalities
Subretinal neovascularization
Macular edema
Stellate retinopathy
Macular hole
Macular pucker
Choroidal abnormality
Hemorrhagic choroidal detachment
Choroidal effusion syndrome
Functional visual loss

Endogenous endophthalmitis
Functional visual loss

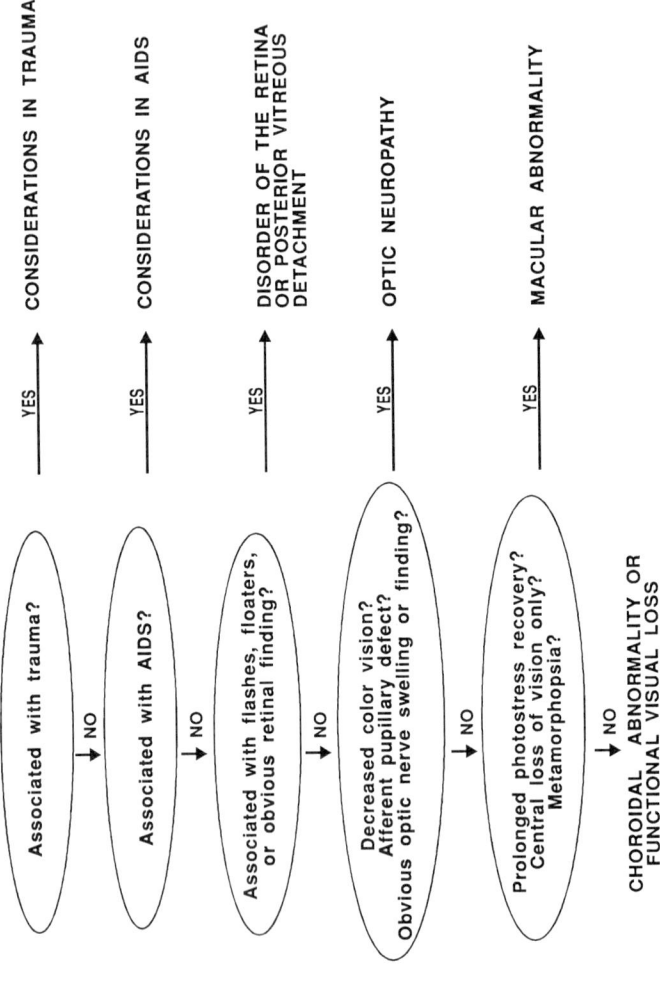

FIGURE 14–1. Algorithm to narrow differential in sustained, unilateral loss of vision without external signs.

cardiopulmonary resuscitation and with seatbelt injury. Retinal hemorrhages, macular edema, peripapillary nerve fiber layer infarcts (distributed along the temporal arcades), and optic disk edema occur acutely. Vision is variably reduced, and an afferent pupillary defect may be present. The condition may occur unilaterally, bilaterally, or asymmetrically. Retinal changes regress over 3 months to 4 months, but a visual deficit and afferent pupillary defect may persist.

Posttraumatic fat embolism presents similar to Purtscher's but has a delayed onset. It most frequently occurs 2 days to 3 days after a fracture involving a long bone (usually the tibia or femur). Fat emboli can also accompany acute pancreatitis. The fat is recognized as hard, yellow-white exudates (Figure 14–2). Occasionally, widespread retinal edema gives the appearance of a pseudo-cherry red spot.

Special Considerations in Patients with AIDS

The most common ocular manifestation of the acquired immune deficiency syndrome (AIDS) is a retinal microvasculopathy, recognized as cotton wool spots (Figure 14–3). These do not cause a reduction in vision. The sudden loss

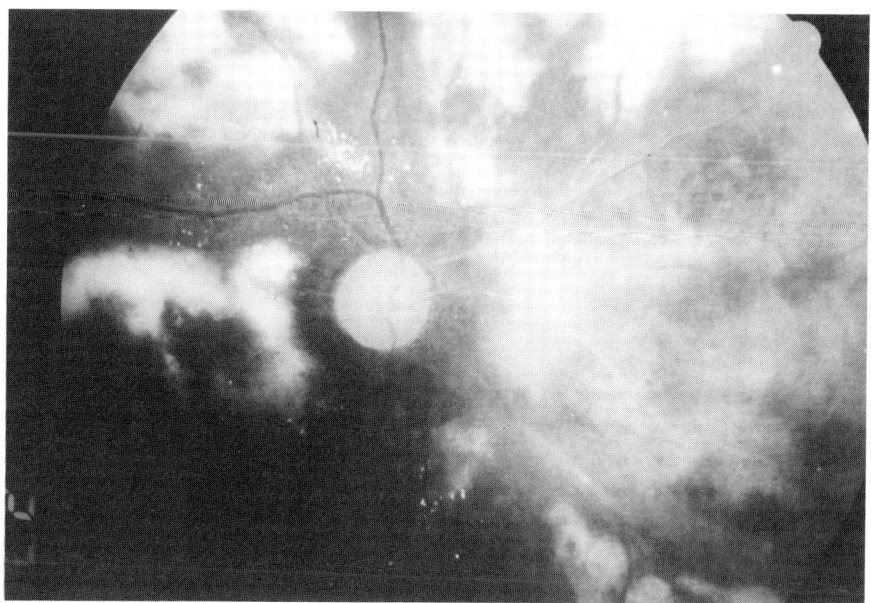

FIGURE 14–2. Central retinal artery occlusion with massive nerve fiber layer infarcts and fat emboli following a femur fracture.

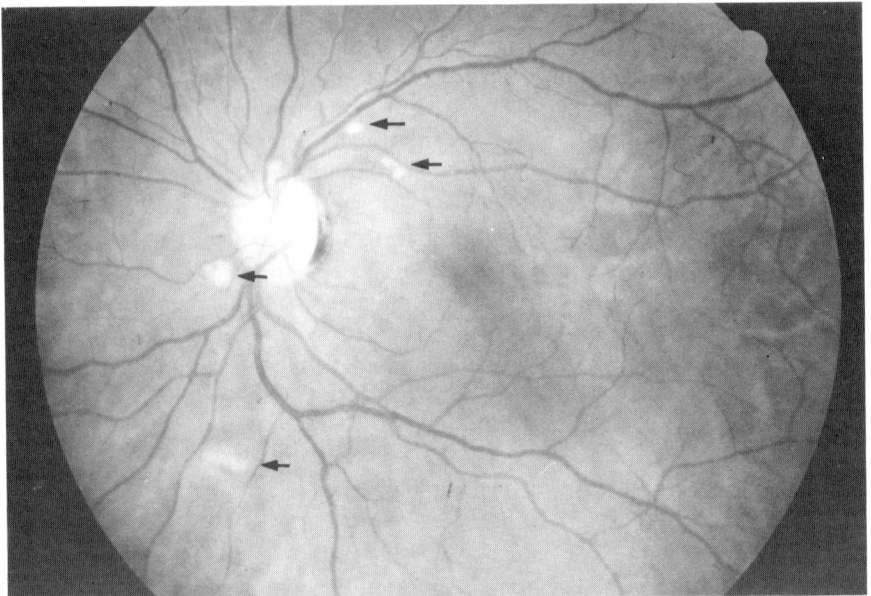

FIGURE 14-3. Retinal microvasculopathy (cotton wool spots) in AIDS (arrows).

of vision in AIDS is usually due to cytomegalovirus (CMV) or toxoplasmosis retinopathy. Rarer causes include other infectious retinopathies, acute retinal necrosis, and an infectious optic neuropathy.

Cytomegalovirus retinopathy presents with painless loss of vision. It is characterized by multiple areas of white retinal opacification, with indistinct borders, intermixed with retinal hemorrhages. Areas along the major vascular arcades are preferentially involved (Figure 14-4). The eye typically appears otherwise quiet, without evidence of anterior chamber or vitreous cells. If the macula is threatened or involved, ganciclovir 2.5 mg/kg can be given intravenously every 8 hours for 10 days to 20 days, followed by a maintenance dose of 5 mg/kg to 6 mg/kg per day, given indefinitely 5 of every subsequent 7 days. Ganciclovir causes bone marrow suppression in up to 40% of AIDS patients; patients who cannot tolerate systemic administration may benefit from intravitreal injections (200 μg in 0.1 mL delivered via the pars plana to the midvitreous, twice weekly until the infection is under control, followed by a maintenance dose of one injection per week). Ganciclovir should not be used with systemic azidothymidine (AZT). A second antiviral, Foscarnet (trisodium phosphonoformate hexahydrate), has similar activity as ganciclovir but also must be continued indefinitely to prevent reactivation of the virus. Because CMV retinopathy is due to a direct infection of retinal cells by the virus, corticosteroids have no role in this disorder.

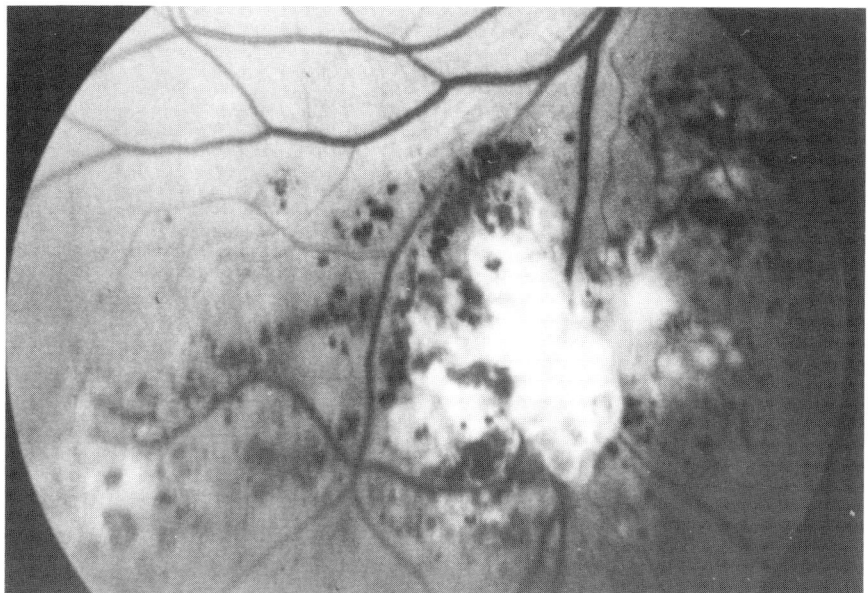

FIGURE 14-4. Periphlebitis and hemorrhagic cytomegalovirus retinitis in AIDS.

Toxoplasmosis can also cause a sudden decrease in vision in individuals with AIDS. It is recognized as a large, yellow-white chorioretinal lesion, without hemorrhage (Figure 14-5). Haziness of the vitreous, due to cells and debris, results in an ophthalmoscopic view that has been described as seeing "a headlight in a fog." Treatment includes pyrimethamine (75 mg by mouth loading dose followed by 25 mg each day for 6 weeks) plus clindamycin (300 mg by mouth 4 times a day for 4 weeks to 6 weeks); sulfadiazine (2 g to 4 g by mouth loading dose followed by 1 g 4 times a day for 6 weeks); or tetracycline (2 g loading dose followed by 250 mg 4 times a day). If anterior segment inflammation is concomitant, topical steroids and cycloplegics are used (see Chapter 16).

Candida retinitis is recognizable as one or more small, white retinal lesions with overlying vitreous debris (Figure 14-6). Systemic antifungal agents do not penetrate the vitreous well. Some clinicians advocate vitrectomy and intravitreal injection of amphotericin B (5 µg) or miconazole (40 µg) for Candida endophthalmitis, but the safety and efficacy of these treatments have not been proved. Other fungal infections, and *Mycobacterium tuberculosis,* and *Herpes simplex* retinitis can also rarely occur.

Acute retinal necrosis is a syndrome in which the retina shows widespread necrosis, with or without overlying vitreous cells or keratitic precipitates (deposits on the endothelial surface of the cornea). Distinctive zones of retinal

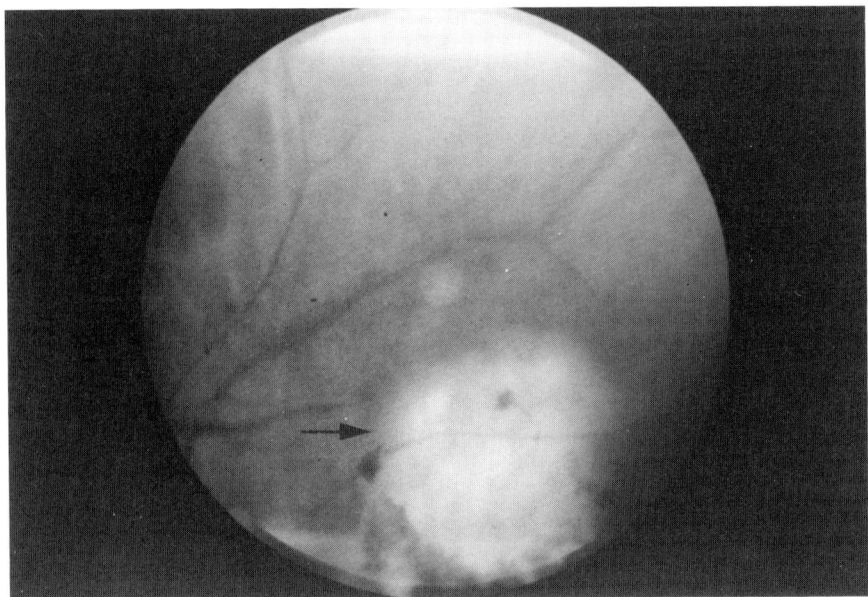

FIGURE 14-5. Toxoplasmosis in AIDS (arrow).

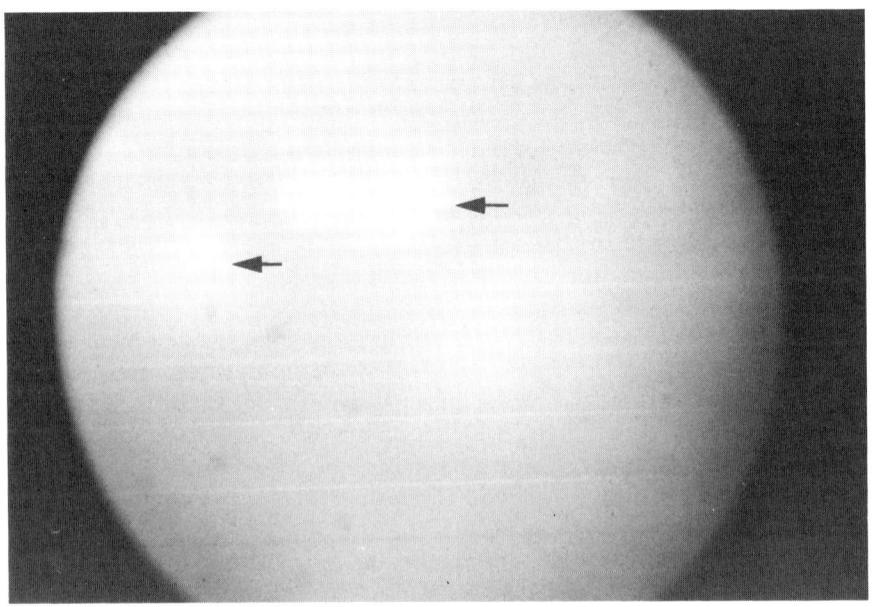

FIGURE 14-6. Candida retinopathy in AIDS (arrows).

necrosis especially surround veins. Intravenous ganciclovir may retard progression; intravenous acyclovir does not appear efficacious. The condition is usually unilateral and rapidly progressive; as many as 25% of affected patients progress to develop a rhegmatogenous (due to a retinal tear) retinal detachment. The etiologic agent may be cytomegalovirus or an acyclovir-resistant herpes simplex or zoster virus.

Syphilis, cytomegalovirus, cryptococcus, herpes zoster, tuberculosis, and the acute retinal necrosis syndrome can all be associated with an *acute optic neuritis* in a patient with AIDS. The optic neuropathy may be the initial symptom of HIV infection. Some causes (particularly syphilis) are responsive to treatment. Therapy for other etiologies has had variable results. Once initiated, herpes zoster optic neuritis can have a fulminant course in the AIDS patient and is usually unresponsive to intravenous acyclovir or corticosteroids.

Due to a Retinal Disorder

The following retinal disorders can cause a rapid loss of vision:

Central retinal artery occlusion
Branch retinal artery occlusion
Ischemic central retinal vein occlusion
Venous stasis retinopathy
Branch retinal vein occlusion
Retinal hemorrhage
Vitreous hemorrhage
Retinal tear or detachment
Central serous retinopathy
Retinal pigment epithelium detachment

A *central retinal artery occlusion* (CRAO) causes an immediate total loss of vision and abolition of pupillary constriction to light (an afferent pupillary defect). Occasionally some retina may be spared (usually in the macular area) if a cilioretinal artery is present. The infarcted retina becomes pale, and the retinal arteries become narrowed. Even in the absence of a cilioretinal artery, the macular area, which is supplied by the choroid, remains perfused. This is often described as a *cherry-red spot* (Figure 14-7). Despite perfusion of the central macula, visual acuity is poor because of infarction of the nerve fiber layer between this area and the optic disc. Inspection of the retinal arteries may reveal sludging of blood and segmentation of the blood column; this is called railway trucking.

CRAO typically occurs in atherosclerotic and hypertensive individuals. Occlusion by an embolus or thrombus is the most frequently presumed cause. Another cause is giant cell (temporal) arteritis of the central retinal artery. Rarely, vasospasm from migraine may be sustained long enough to cause

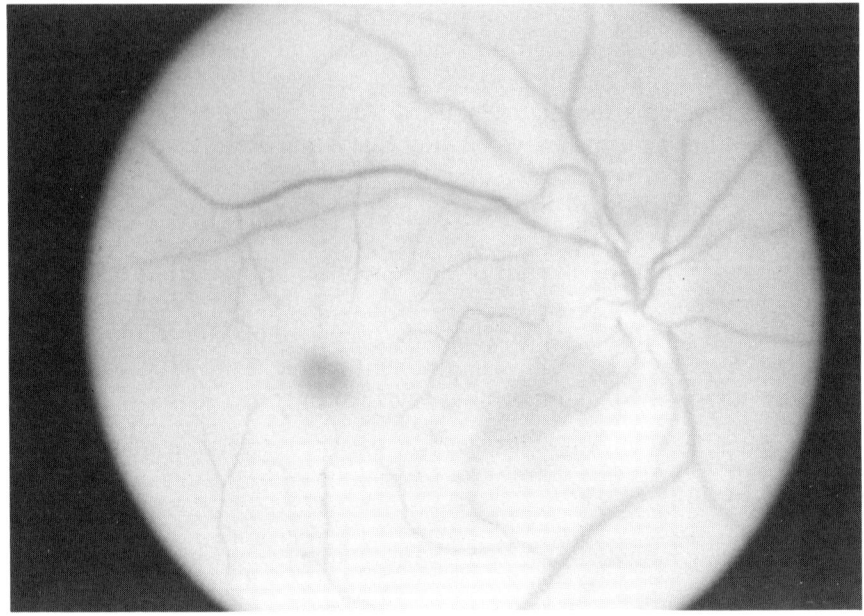

FIGURE 14-7. Central retinal artery occlusion.

infarction of the inner retinal neurons. Other rare causes include collagen vascular diseases (systemic lupus erythematosis and polyarteritis nodosa), hypercoagulation disorders (seen in association with polycythemia and with oral contraceptive use), syphilis, sickle cell disease, and Behcet's disease.

The treatment of CRAO is directed toward dislodging a potential embolus to a more peripheral vessel or relieving vasospasm. If the CRAO originated within 24 hours of presentation, several measures are instituted simultaneously:

1. The patient is placed in a recumbent position without pillows to increase retinal perfusion.

2. Ocular massage is performed by applying firm pressure on the eye, using two fingers, for 20 seconds to 30 seconds as the patient looks down, alternating with 20 seconds to 30 seconds of no pressure.

3. Anterior chamber paracentesis is performed under topical anesthesia and with an eyelid speculum in place. A small incision is made at the limbus with a knife or 30-gauge needle (bevel up) on a TB syringe. The needle or knife is directed over the iris and away from the lens. Fluid is allowed to escape, or 0.1 cc to 0.2 cc is withdrawn. The anterior chamber shallows slightly, and the eye softens. The magnification of a slit lamp or operating microscope is helpful.

4. Carbogen (95% oxygen, 5% carbon dioxide) is inhaled by face mask for 5 minutes to 10 minutes every 2 hours. This may induce retinal vasodilation

and can be continued for up to 48 hours. Breathing into a paper bag similarly increases respiratory levels of carbon dioxide.

5. Acetazolamide 500 mg is given intravenously or by mouth, with or without a topical beta-blocker to lower intraocular pressure.

6. Occasionally, heparin or low-molecular-weight dextrans (Rheomacrodex) are administered intravenously.

7. High-dose steroids are administered urgently if the sedimentation rate and symptoms suggest temporal arteritis.

Individuals with a history of *classic migraine* (typically females between ages 21 and 65 years) may develop an acute central retinal artery occlusion due to vasoconstriction. There is often a history of recurrent episodic monocular visual loss, usually occurring in the absence of headache or scintillating scotoma. The prophylactic use of propranolol, tricyclic antidepressants, or calcium channel blockers for females with a history of classic migraine and episodic monocular visual loss should be considered.

A *branch retinal artery occlusion* causes a sectoral visual field defect. If the superior or inferior retinal artery is involved, an altitudinal visual field defect results (Figure 14-8). Ocular massage and, rarely, paracentesis may be performed, but no therapy has been proved effective.

Ischemic central retinal vein occlusions (CRVO) occur more commonly than

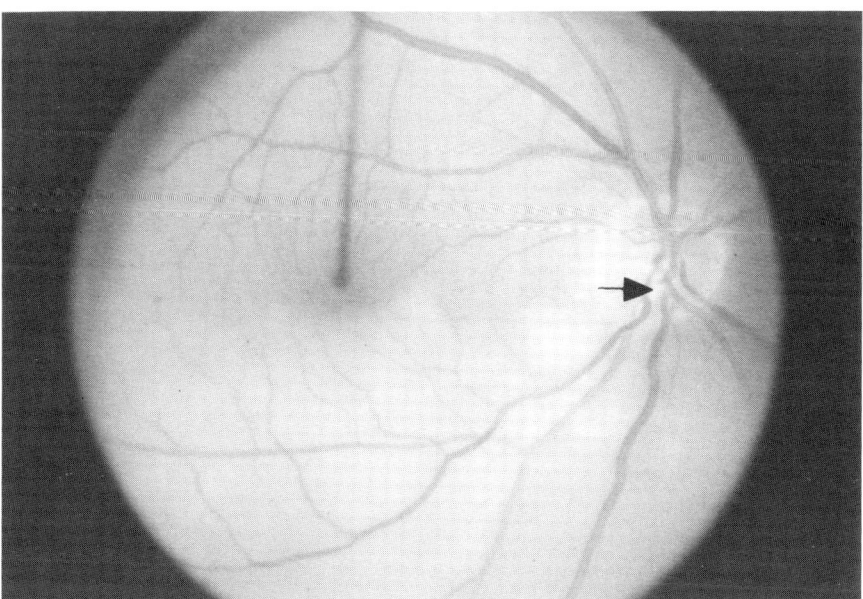

FIGURE 14-8. Inferior branch retinal artery occlusion. Note the calcific emboli in the inferior retinal artery at the disk (arrow).

CRAO. Because the occlusion is often partial, the symptoms are less dramatic, and complete loss of vision is rare. Superficial and deep retinal hemorrhages occur throughout the territory drained by the affected vein (Figure 14-9). Affected veins become distended, tortuous, and dark. Cotton wool spots, which signify an infarcted nerve fiber layer, disk hemorrhages, and slight to moderate disk edema, may also be present. The presence of multiple (>10) cotton wool spots and widespread capillary nonperfusion on fluorescein angiography signifies an ischemic CRVO. This is associated with a greater likelihood of the subsequent development of iris neovascularization. Macular edema may also occur after the onset of CRVO and is heralded by a decrease in central vision.

Vein occlusions usually occur at arteriovenous crossings or within the lamina cribosa. At these sites, veins share an adventitial coat with an adjacent artery. It is believed that atherosclerosis or hypertensive arteriolar sclerosis of the artery impedes flow in the adjacent vein. Nonatherosclerotic associations of CRVO include optic disc edema and drusen, glaucoma, retinal phlebitis (sarcoid, syphilis, or SLE), hyperviscosity states (polycythemia, leukemia, sickle cell disease, multiple myeloma, and cryoglobulinemia, compression of the optic nerve from an orbital tumor or thyroid ophthalmopathy, and certain drugs, most notably diuretics and oral contraceptives.

A complete medical evaluation to rule out cardiovascular disease or dysproteinemia is usually indicated. Ophthalmodynamometry (see Chapter 1) may

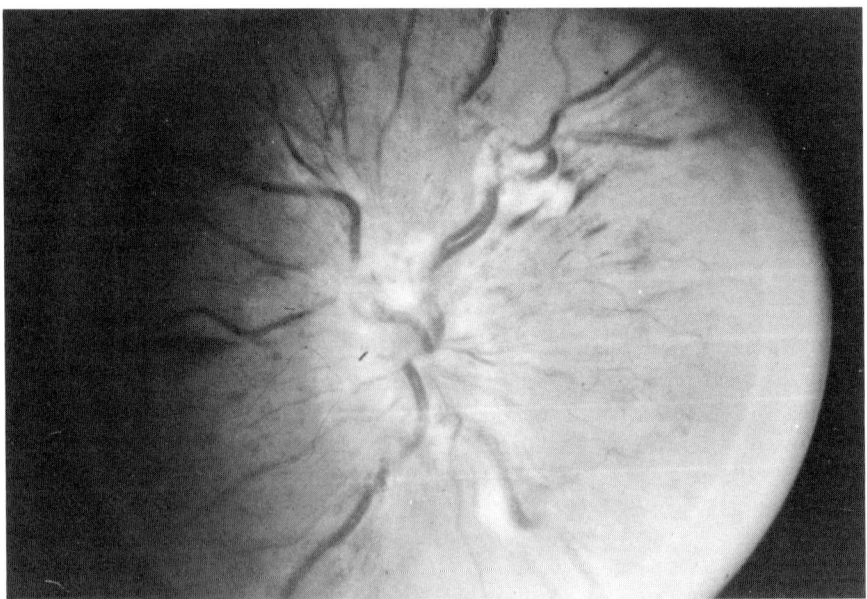

FIGURE 14-9. Central retinal vein occlusion.

help distinguish CRVO from carotid occlusive disease (ocular ischemic syndrome). In CRVO, the ophthalmic artery pressure is normal or elevated; in carotid disease, it is low. The treatment of a CRVO is often palliative. Intraocular pressure elevation is reduced with medications; if diuretics or oral contraceptives are presumed causative, they are changed or discontinued. Aspirin 60 mg to 360 mg per day is often advocated. Retinal photocoagulation may be needed to forestall or treat preretinal or iris neovascularization, especially if the CRVO is ischemic.

Venous stasis retinopathy is a category of central retinal vein occlusion associated with occlusive disease of the carotid artery. It is more common in the third and fourth decades and is characterized by blurred central vision, which improves somewhat as the day progresses. The blurred vision is often accompanied by metamorphopsia and occasionally by floaters. In contrast to patients with ischemic CRVO, 90% of patients with venous stasis retinopathy have good visual acuity—often 20/40 or better. The central field may contain small scotomas that are detectable on Amsler grid testing, and the blind spot may be enlarged. A mild afferent pupillary defect may be noted. Ophthalmoscopically, the optic disc is hyperemic and swollen, and the retinal veins are dilated and tortuous. Small punctate retinal hemorrhages and mild macular edema are common. Cells in the vitreous can occur, corresponding to the complaint of floaters. Approximately 50% of these patients have systemic vasculopathies, including diabetes, hypertension, carotid artery disease, peripheral vascular disease, hyperlipidemia, hyperviscosity, and cryofibrinogenemia. There may be an association with estrogen-containing oral contraceptive agents. If the vision is poor or vitreous cells are present, some clinicians advocate systemic corticosteroids in tapering doses (initially prednisone 0.5 mg/kg to 1.0 mg/kg per day). Deterioration of vision and the presence of unremitting cystoid macular edema of 3 months duration are relative treatment indications. Anticoagulants are generally not recommended.

A *branch retinal vein occlusion* (BRVO) is diagnosed by the sectoral involvement of one vein (Figure 14-10). Unless macular edema or nonperfusion causes a reduction in visual acuity, a BRVO may be asymptomatic. The BRVO Study Group (1986) recommended that peripheral scatter photocoagulation be applied if visual acuity is reduced to 20/40, or worse, and secondary to sustained macular edema (not due to macular nonperfusion). This study also suggested that patients with more than 5 disc diameters of retinal involvement be followed for the development of neovascularization at 4-month intervals. Peripheral scatter laser photocoagulation was recommended only after the development of neovascularization.

Retinal hemorrhages are seen in a variety of conditions. They are often not the cause of a sudden decrease in vision; rather, associated pathology is responsible. In *malignant hypertension* (Figure 14-11), flame-shaped hemorrhages occur concomitant with optic nerve head edema, arteriovenous crossing changes, retinal arteriolar narrowing, nerve fiber layer infarcts (cotton wool

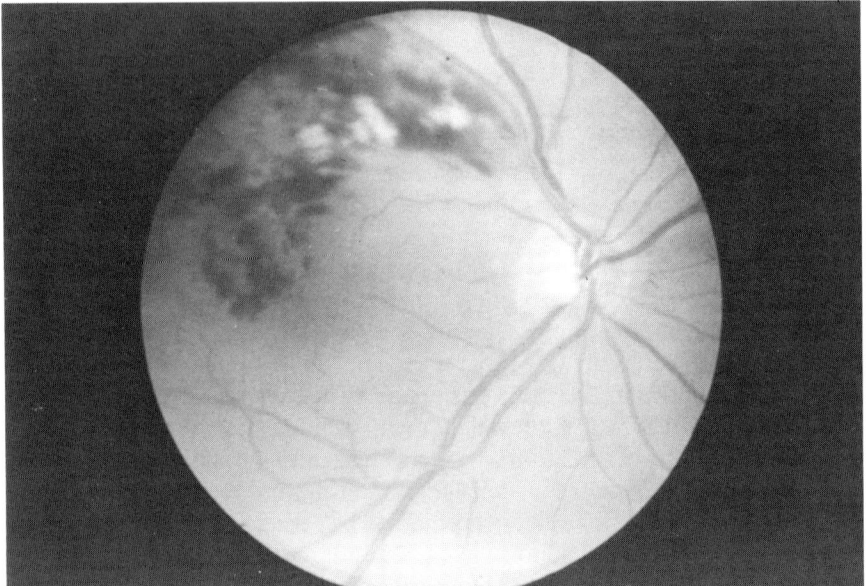

FIGURE 14–10. Superior branch retinal vein occlusion.

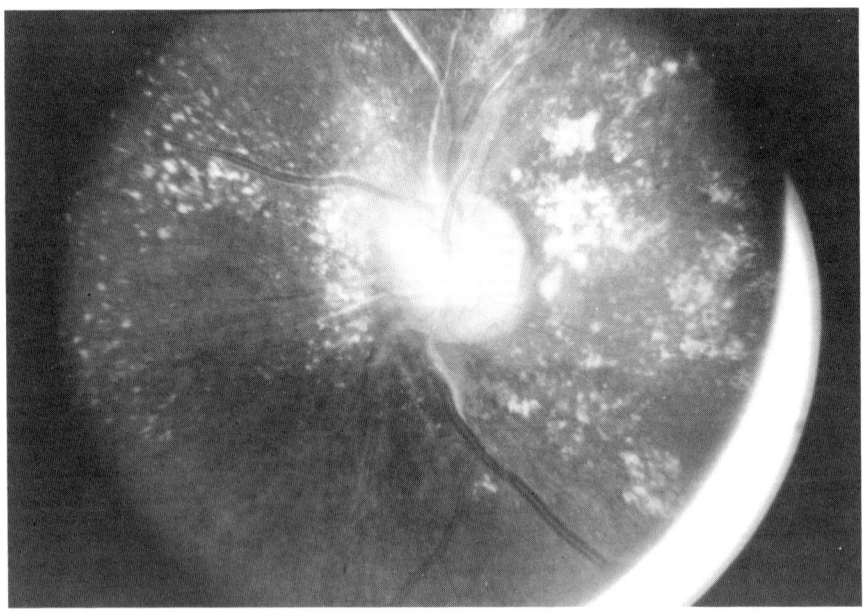

FIGURE 14–11. Malignant hypertension (end stage).

spots), and hard exudates (often in a "macular star" configuration). The macular and optic nerve head changes are responsible for the decreased vision. Similarly, in *diabetic retinopathy,* vitreous hemorrhage, retinal detachment, and macular edema are the principal causes of rapid loss of vision (Figure 14–12).

Common causes of *vitreous hemorrhage* and their associated findings are outlined in Table 14–3. If the vitreous hemorrhage is very dense, a subtle afferent pupillary defect may be present in addition to the decreased vision. If the retina cannot be viewed, examination of the other eye may give clues to the diagnosis. Many conditions are bilateral (e.g., diabetic and sickle cell retinopathy). B-scan ultrasonography should be performed to rule out a retinal detachment or intraocular tumor (see Chapter 2).

The treatment of vitreous hemorrhage depends on the etiology. Bed rest for 2 days to 3 days, with elevation of the head, may permit settling of the blood, as well as reduce the chance of recurrent bleeding. Aspirin and other anticlotting agents are contraindicated. The surgical removal of blood (vitrectomy) is indicated when there is an accompanying retinal detachment or glaucoma due to the breakdown of blood products. This may also be indicated in cases of chronic vitreous hemorrhage (more than 6 months). The indications for vitrectomy in diabetic retinopathy are listed in Table 14–4. The underlying etiology is always treated as soon as possible.

Retinal tears and detachments are common causes of vitreous hemorrhage

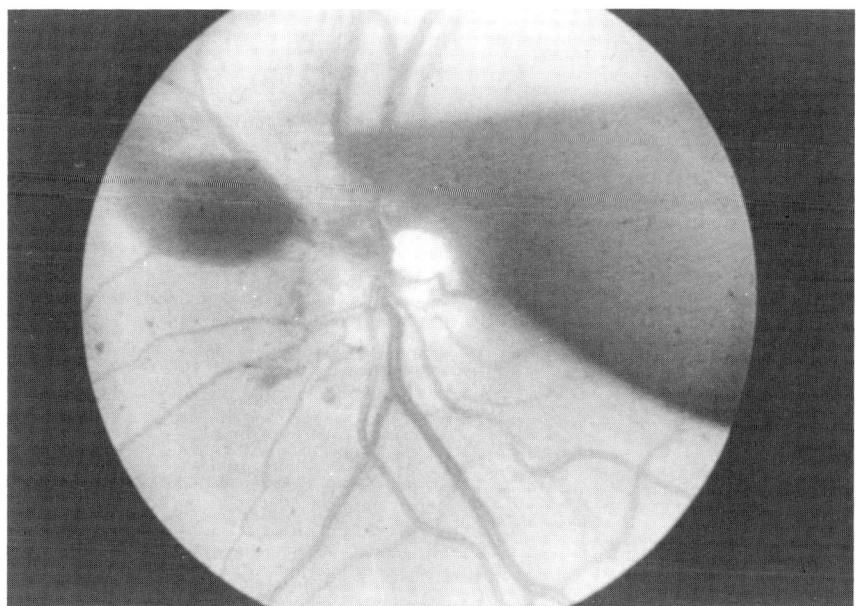

FIGURE 14–12. Preretinal hemorrhage in diabetic retinopathy.

TABLE 14-3. ETIOLOGY OF VITREOUS HEMORRHAGE

CAUSE	ASSOCIATED FINDINGS
Retinal break	Floaters and flashes of light, myopia, trauma
Retinal detachment	Floaters and flashes of light, myopia, trauma; increasing area of darkness like a curtain being drawn
Posterior vitreous detachment	Floaters and flashes of light; black, spider web or threads always present and move with eye; middle aged and elderly
Diabetic retinopathy	Diabetic retinopathy seen in other eye
Retinal vein occlusion	Usually a branch retinal vein occlusion—often months to years previously; older patients with hypertension
Sickle cell disease	Particularly SC disease; blacks; may have "sea fan" peripheral neovascularization
Eales's disease	Males, between third and fourth decades, bilateral with peripheral retinal ischemia
Von Hipple-Lindau	Retinal capillary hemangioma with dilated tortuous feeding artery and draining vein, cerebellar hemangioblastoma, visceral cysts
Intraocular tumor	Malignant melanoma more common in Caucasians; may have proptosis from orbital extension, subretinal fluid and retinal detachment; may need ultrasound to view
Trauma	Terson's syndrome (often bilateral)

TABLE 14-4. INDICATIONS FOR TREATMENT IN DIABETIC RETINOPATHY

Vitrectomy	Dense vitreous hemorrhage causing decreased vision present and unchanging for several months Tractional retinal detachment of the macula Severe proliferative retinopathy when photocoagulation has not been followed by substantial regression of new vessels
Focal laser photocoagulation for macular edema	Hard exudates at or within 500 microns (⅓ disk diameter) of the center of the macula, if associated with thickening of the adjacent retina Retinal thickening at or within 500 microns of the center of the macula Retinal thickening ≥ 1 disk diameter in size (1500 microns), if any part is within 1 disk diameter of the center of the macula
Panretinal retinal photocoagulation	Neovascularization of the disc greater than ¼–⅓ disc diameter in size Neovascularization of the disc (any degree) when associated with vitreous hemorrhage Neovascularization other than at the disk greater than ½ disk diameter in size when associated with vitreous hemorrhage Neovascularization of the iris

and rapid loss of vision. A retinal detachment (RD) is often heralded by symptoms of a retinal break, including flashes of light (photopsias) and floaters, the latter sometimes described as cobwebs that move with the eye. In addition to these symptoms, the patient may notice the appearance of a curtain or shadow in the visual field. If the macula becomes detached, visual acuity drops precipitously. Ocular signs of an acute RD include the presence of pigmented cells (tobacco dust) in the vitreous and an intraocular pressure lower than the fellow eye.

Three types of retinal detachment are described (Table 14-5). Rhegmatogenous and tractional detachments require immediate surgical attention if the macula is threatened. Exudative detachments due to metastatic tumors (usually breast), choroidal melanomas, and inflammatory lesions (e.g., posterior scleritis) may resolve with successful treatment of the underlying condition. Exudative detachments due to colobomas and congenital optic nerve head anomalies (e.g., optic pits) are difficult to treat. Acute retinal tears without detachment may be treated with laser photocoagulation or cryotherapy.

A specific type of retinal detachment, *central serous retinopathy* (CSR) occurs most frequently as a unilateral condition in middle-aged males. A relationship to emotional stress has long been suspected. Ophthalmoscopically, the macular retina is elevated by clear serous fluid. Fluorescein angiography demonstrates leakage through a break in Bruch's membrane, often in a smokestack pattern (see Chapter 2). Distortion and displacement of the macula (Figure 14-13) cause the symptoms of blurred, distorted, and minified vision. Colors may appear less intense, and the patient may note a central blind spot. The detachment may be difficult to appreciate and is best seen using a fundus contact lens

TABLE 14-5. TYPES OF RETINAL DETACHMENT

TYPE	SYMPTOMS	SIGNS	ASSOCIATIONS
Rhegmatogenous (due to a hole)	Flashes, floaters, curtain drawing	Convex elevation of retina next to retinal tear or break, pigment cells and hemorrhage in vitreous, lower IOP, clear subretinal fluid that does not shift	Myopia, trauma, previous ocular surgery
Exudative	Mild to severe vision or field loss	Clear fluid elevation of the retina, subretinal fluid shifts with head movement	Neoplasia, uveal effusion syndrome, retinal coloboma, inflammation, congenital optic nerve anomaly
Tractional	Vision or field loss, may be asymptomatic	Concavely detached retina, fibrous membranes pulling on retina, smooth surface to retina	Diabetes, sickle cell disease, retinopathy of prematurity, toxocariasis

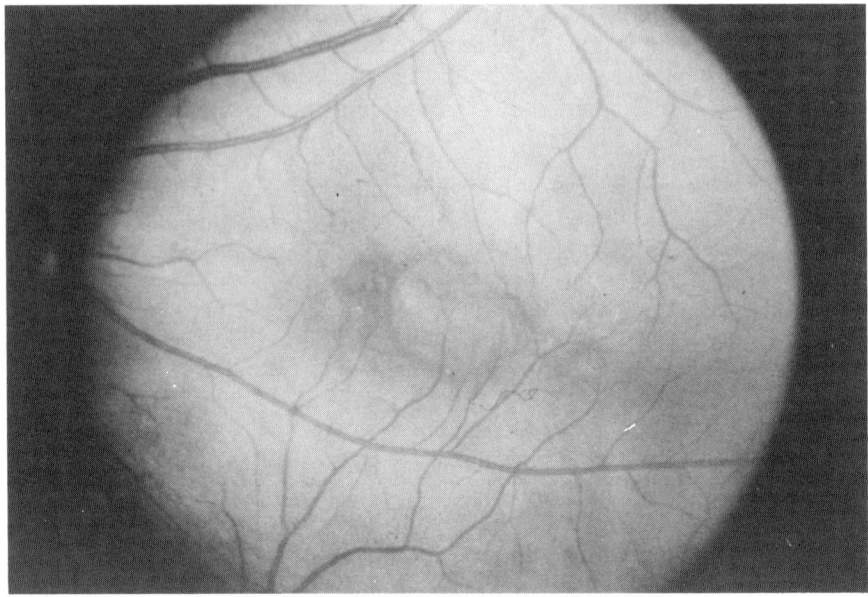

FIGURE 14-13. Central serous retinopathy.

at the slit lamp. Laser photocoagulation can restore vision rapidly, but the final visual outcome has not been shown to be affected by such treatment. This therapy is usually reserved for persistent detachment—lasting more than 4 months to 6 months—or for recurrent CSR with previous permanent visual deficit.

In CSR the sensory retina is detached from the underlying retinal pigment epithelium. In *retinal pigment epithelium detachments,* all layers of the retina are detached from the underlying choroid by serous fluid. The latter appear as nearly inconspicuous grayish mounds and range in size from one-quarter up to two to three disk diameters in size. Rarely, a fluid level can be seen (Figure 14-14); this is better demonstrated by fluorescein angiography. If the macula is involved, vision is reduced. In approximately one-third of affected elderly patients, an underlying choroidal neovascular membrane is present that can lead to disciform macular degeneration.

Due to Posterior Vitreous Detachment

A posterior vitreous detachment (PVD) by itself does not cause a decrease in vision. It can, however, be associated with a retinal break or vitreous hemorrhage. The principal symptom is a floating cobweb, fly (muscae volitantes), or speck in the field of vision. Flashes of light can be noted as the vitreous detaches from the optic nerve head. The opacity moves with eye movement and is best

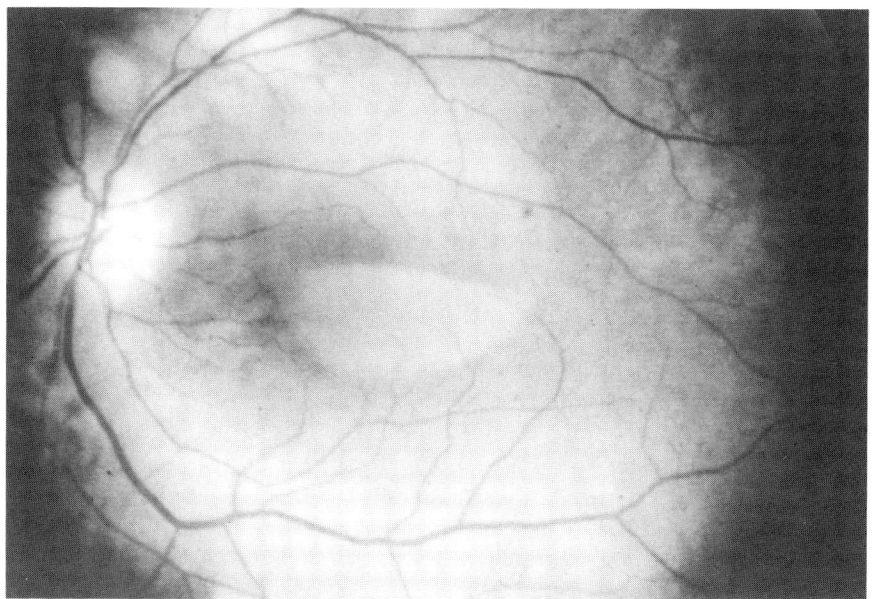

FIGURE 14-14. Retinal pigment epithelium detachment, with fluid level.

appreciated by the patient when their gaze is directed against a bright background. With the ophthalmoscope focused to a plane in front of the retina, the physician should be able to see the opacity. Usually it is in the shape of a thin, clear or black, open ring. Peripheral retinal and disc margin hemorrhages may also be seen. The presence of pigmented cells or vitreous hemorrhage suggests a coexisting retinal break.

In the absence of a retinal break, no treatment is needed for a PVD. A repeat examination, including the peripheral retina, should be performed in 1 week to 3 weeks and again in several months, searching for retinal breaks or a detachment.

Due to an Optic Neuropathy

A number of optic nerve conditions can be associated with a sudden loss of vision. Attention should be directed to the following list when the examination detects a color vision abnormality, afferent pupillary defect, or optic disc swelling:

Optic neuritis
Ischemic optic neuropathy: temporal arteritis, anterior ischemic optic neuropathy, or posterior ischemic optic neuropathy

Optic neuropathy and systemic lupus erythematosis
Diabetic papillopathy
Migrainous optic neuropathy
Sarcoid granuloma within the optic nerve
Radiation optic neuropathy
Leber's optic neuropathy
Other hereditary neuropathies (usually bilateral)
Nutritional or metabolic neuropathy (usually bilateral)
Optic neuropathy and Lyme disease (see also Chapter 13)
Compressive orbital disorders (see Chapter 12)

The history of an "acute onset" of visual loss given by a patient with an optic neuropathy may be misleading. Because of the absence of other symptoms and at times slow progression of pathology, visual loss due to an optic nerve disorder may not be detected until an unrelated incident causes an individual to cover the nonaffected eye. A truly acute onset suggests a vascular or inflammatory etiology. A subacute onset would be characteristic of an inflammatory, toxic, or hereditary optic neuropathy. Slowly progressive loss suggests a compressive disorder. The most common diagnoses are optic neuritis and ischemic optic neuropathy. Table 14–6 lists some of the distinguishing signs between these, papilledema, and pseudopapilledema.

Optic neuritis is an inflammatory disorder of the optic nerve secondary to demyelinating, viral, or autoimmune disease. The history often reveals an antecedent upper respiratory or gastrointestinal viral syndrome. The disorder occurs in individuals between ages 18 and 50 years and is characterized by an acute or subacute, usually unilateral, visual loss. It may be preceded or accompanied by retrobulbar discomfort (especially medially and superiorly), which is aggravated by eye movement. Affected patients may be sensitive to light (photophobic) and may report bright flashes of light (photopsia) with eye movement, especially in dim illumination. A reduction in visual acuity, called Uhtoff's sign, may occur with exercise or an increase in body temperature.

Visual acuity deterioration ranges from minimal loss to "no light perception" over several hours to days; acuity reaches its nadir 1 week to 2 weeks after onset. Colors appear desaturated, and there is a reduced perception of light intensity. Examination reveals an afferent pupillary defect, a central scotoma with or without connection to the blind spot, or a nerve fiber bundle (arcuate) defect. The optic disk is swollen and often surrounded by flame hemorrhages (Figure 14–15). A normal-appearing optic disk suggests *retrobulbar optic neuritis.*

Laboratory investigations should include collagen vascular studies and serologic tests for syphilis. Neuroimaging is controversial but should be performed if the history is atypical or if there is a history of sinus disease to rule out a neoplastic infiltration or a compressive optic neuropathy. In optic neuritis, the optic nerve may appear thickened on magnetic resonance imaging (MRI), but demyelinating plaques are rarely, if ever, appreciated (see Chapter 2).

TABLE 14-6. CHARACTERISTICS OF OPTIC NEURITIS, ISCHEMIC OPTIC NEUROPATHY, PAPILLEDEMA, AND PSEUDOPAPILLEDEMA

SYMPTOMS	OPTIC NEURITIS	ISCHEMIC NEUROPATHY	PAPILLEDEMA	PSEUDO-PAPILLEDEMA
Visual loss	Rapidly progressive, loss of central vision, acuity rarely spared	Acute field defect, commonly altitudinal, acuity variable	No acuity loss until late, may have transient obscurations of vision	+/− enlarged blind spot, arcuate defects, transient obscurations rare
Bilaterality	Rarely bilateral except in children; may alternate in multiple sclerosis	Unilateral acutely, second eye involved subsequently with Foster-Kennedy syndrome	Almost always bilateral, may be asymmetric	Approximately 70% with optic nerve drusen, bilateral, may be asymmetric
Signs				
Visual acuity	Diminished central vision and color vision	Variable acuity loss, worse with temporal arteritis	Normal except when chronic	Normal
Pupillary responses	Decreased reaction, afferent defect when unilateral	Decreased reaction, afferent defect when unilateral	Normal	Normal
Optic nerve	With papillitis: variable disk swelling, cotton wool spots, flame hemorrhages	Pale segmental disk edema with flame hemorrhages	Variable disk swelling and flame hemorrhages	Disk elevation, margin blurred, cup obliterated, no hemorrhages or edema, +/− hyaline bodies
Prognosis				
Vision	Excellent	Poor, especially with temporal arteritis	Good with lowering of intracranial pressure	Good, usually not progressive

Without treatment, visual acuity gradually recovers to 20/20 in 70% of patients; 87% of patients recover to at least 20/40 vision. The prognosis is worse if visual acuity is reduced to no light perception. As many as 25% of patients with this degree of involvement are left with a dense central scotoma and visual acuity of less than 20/400. Even when the acuity is reduced to no light perception, if no improvement occurs by 4 weeks, the diagnosis should be reconsidered. Abnormalities in contrast sensitivity, depth perception, color vision, light intensity perception, pupillary reaction, and Uhtoff's phenomenon may persist for years.

The Optic Neuritis Treatment Trial recently found that oral prednisone (prescribed in a dosage of 1 mg/kg/day for 14 days) was not only ineffective in speeding recovery or in improving the visual outcome after optic neuritis, but actually increased a patient's risk for future attacks in either the affected or fel-

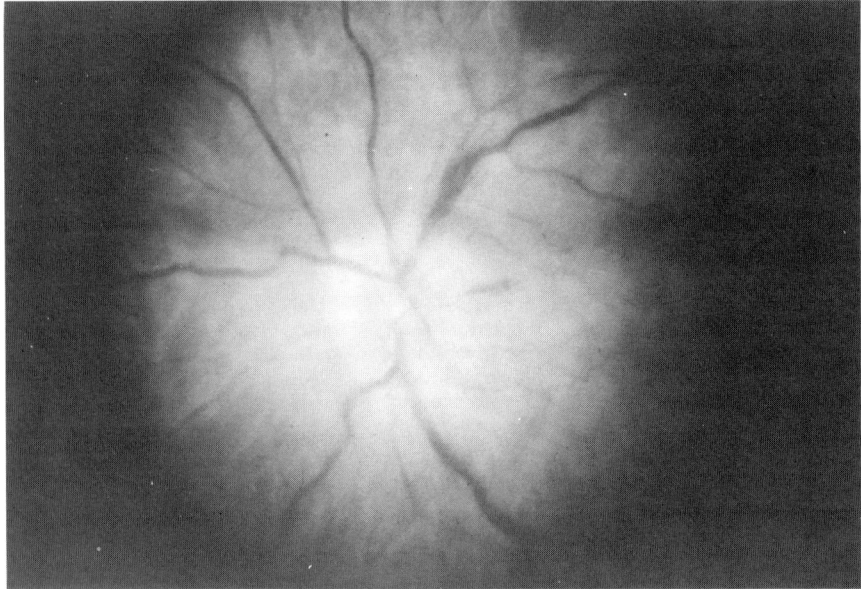

FIGURE 14-15. Optic neuritis.

low eye (NIH, January 1992). Based on these findings there is no role for oral prednisone alone in standard dosages in the treatment of patients with initial episodes of optic neuritis.

Other signs of neurologic dysfunction, separated in time and space from the episode of optic neuritis, suggest multiple sclerosis (MS). As many as 50% of patients with MS develop clinical optic neuritis, and 17% to 80% of patients with isolated optic neuritis develop clinical MS. Female sex, winter onset, recurrence, and age of onset between age 21 and 40 years are correlated with the eventual development of MS. Several tests are available that can support the diagnosis of MS. MRI has been used to detect demyelinating abnormalities elsewhere in the brain to confirm the diagnosis. In addition, the presence of oligoclonal bands in the spinal fluid is suggestive that a patient with optic neuritis may develop MS; the absence of these bands, however, is not protective. Whether either of these tests should be performed with a single episode of isolated optic neuritis is a highly controversial, bioethical issue.

Temporal arteritis, also known as *giant cell arteritis,* is a generalized vasculopathy affecting large and medium-sized arteries. It occurs in patients over age 55 years, generally in northern climates. In addition to involvement of the posterior ciliary arteries (affecting the blood supply to the optic nerve), hepatic, renal, mesentery, coronary, and intracranial arteries may be involved. Systemic symptoms include malaise, fever, weight loss, pain and tenderness of large muscle masses and joints (polymyalgia rheumatica), tenderness over the temporal arteries, and jaw claudication. Although visual loss is usually due to ischemic optic neuropathy, temporal arteritis can cause central retinal artery occlusion or ocular ischemic syndrome.

The condition is bilateral in 50% to 65% of untreated cases, with the second eye usually becoming involved within 10 days of the first eye. Some degree of permanent visual loss is the rule, and blindness occurs in 15% to 40% of untreated cases. Granulomatous inflammation on a temporal artery biopsy, associated with an elevated Westergren erythrocyte sedimentation rate (W-ESR), is diagnostic. A normal W-ESR in males is approximately one-half the individual's age. For females, 5 mm per hour is added to that calculation. Treatment consists of oral prednisone 60 mg to 100 mg per day. Intravenous corticosteroids (1 g methylprednisolone every 12 hours for 5 days) should be considered if visual loss occurred within 48 hours of presentation. The pathologic findings in the temporal artery remain positive for 2 weeks after corticosteroid treatment. Treatment should be instituted immediately if the symptoms are suggestive and the W-ESR is elevated; treatment should never be withheld pending temporal artery biopsy. Steroids are tapered based on the W-ESR and associated signs and symptoms.

Anterior ischemic optic neuropathy occurs in younger individuals than does temporal arteritis. The mean age of affected individuals is age 55 years. Although diabetes and hypertension are risk factors, patients with this disorder are generally in good health, and life expectancy is not shortened. The diagnosis is made if there is no history suggestive of temporal arteritis and the W-ESR is normal. The optic disk, or part of it, is swollen, and the edematous area is usually surrounded by nerve fiber layer hemorrhages (Figure 14–16). An absent or minimal central cup is often noted in the uninvolved eye. Visual loss is less severe than with temporal arteritis, but the lack of recovery is the same, distinguishing these disorders from optic neuritis. Approximately 40% of affected individuals have a visual acuity better than 20/60. Altitudinal visual field defects, especially inferior field defects, and an afferent pupillary defect are common. The second eye becomes involved in 40% of patients within 20 years, and no treatment is believed efficacious. *Posterior ischemic optic neuropathy* is a diagnosis of exclusion in patients of the vasculopathic age group who present with sudden visual loss, a normal W-ESR, and a normal fundus examination.

Females between ages 11 and 40 years with *systemic lupus erythematosis* may develop sudden, unilateral or bilateral visual loss associated with a mild ischemic disk edema. Other neurologic or systemic signs of lupus usually develop within 1 year, if not already present. The diagnosis is based on the findings of antinuclear and anti-DNA antibodies, decreased complement factor C_3, and a cardiolipin assay for lupus anticoagulant factors. Treatment consists of high-dose corticosteroids. One suggested regimen is intravenous prednisolone 1000 mg over 20 minutes every 12 hours for 5 days. This is followed by 100 mg per day oral prednisone, tapered each week by 10 mg per day. Cyclophosphamide 1 mg/kg to 2 mg/kg per day may also be used, with or without systemic steroids.

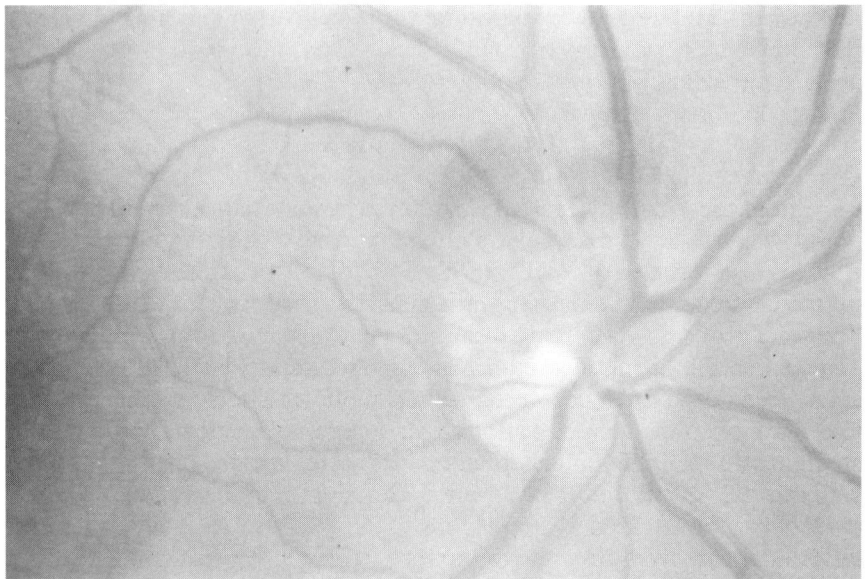

FIGURE 14-16. Ischemic optic neuropathy involving the superior half of the optic disk. (The patient had an inferior altitudinal field defect.)

Insulin-dependent diabetics, 5 to 30 years after the onset of diabetes (often in their second or third decade of life), may present with a unilateral mild decrease in visual acuity (acuity better than 20/50), with or without an afferent pupillary defect, and an enlarged blind spot on visual field testing. The full spectrum of *diabetic papillopathy* is characterized by optic disk edema with prominent surface telangiectatic changes but without neovascularization. The papillopathy is self-limited; improvement of vision begins in 2 weeks to 3 months, and resolution of disk swelling occurs by 3 months. Often the condition is bilateral, suggesting underlying microvascular changes in the optic nerves. Substantial optic atrophy does not follow, and the disorder does not appear to be related to other diabetic retinopathic changes. No treatment is necessary, but the diagnosis is always one of exclusion.

Migrainous optic neuropathy is a rare form of complicated migraine that occurs in patients with a history of classic migraine. Unlike retinal migraine, migrainous optic neuropathy usually occurs in association with a headache. Visual acuity ranges from 20/20 to 20/200, and an afferent pupillary defect is usually present. Visual field testing may detect a nerve fiber bundle, central, or altitudinal defect, and the optic disk may show a pallid swelling.

Sarcoidosis is a systemic inflammatory disorder characterized by noncaseating granulomas in the lungs, liver, spleen, skin, parotid and lacrimal glands, hilar lymph nodes, and eyes. Ocular findings include a chronic granulomatous anterior uveitis, dacryoadenitis, retinal perivasculitis, and orbital granulomas. Granulomas can also develop within the conjunctiva, iris, choroid, vitreous, and optic nerve. The last is associated with a markedly reduced visual acuity (Figure 14-17). Diagnostic studies in suspected sarcoidosis are reviewed in Chapter 2. Anterior uveitis is treated with topical corticosteroids (prednisolone acetate 1%, every 1 hour to 2 hours, gradually tapered), cycloplegics (atropine 1% twice a day; or scopolamine ¼% 3 to 4 times per day). In severe cases, a subtenon steroid injection of triamcinolone 40 mg can be helpful. The effect from a steroid injection lasts 2 weeks to 3 weeks; injections can be repeated in 3 weeks to 4 weeks. Posterior segment and neuro-ophthalmologic complications, such as an optic nerve granuloma, require systemic steroids. Prednisone 60 mg to 80 mg per day is the most efficacious; chlorambucil, azathioprine, methotrexate, and cyclosporine may be of benefit, either additionally or alone. Nonclearing vitreous granulomas and retinal traction may require vitrectomy.

Radiation optic neuropathy has a delayed onset of 6 months to 3 years. It most commonly occurs when the total radiation dose was greater than 5000 rads or when radiation was applied at greater than 250 rads per day.

Leber's optic neuropathy presents as a unilateral sudden decrease in central vision in individuals in their late teens to early twenties. Because it is transmitted through the mitochondria of the egg, it occurs four times more often in males and is transmitted only through maternal lines. Decreased visual acuity

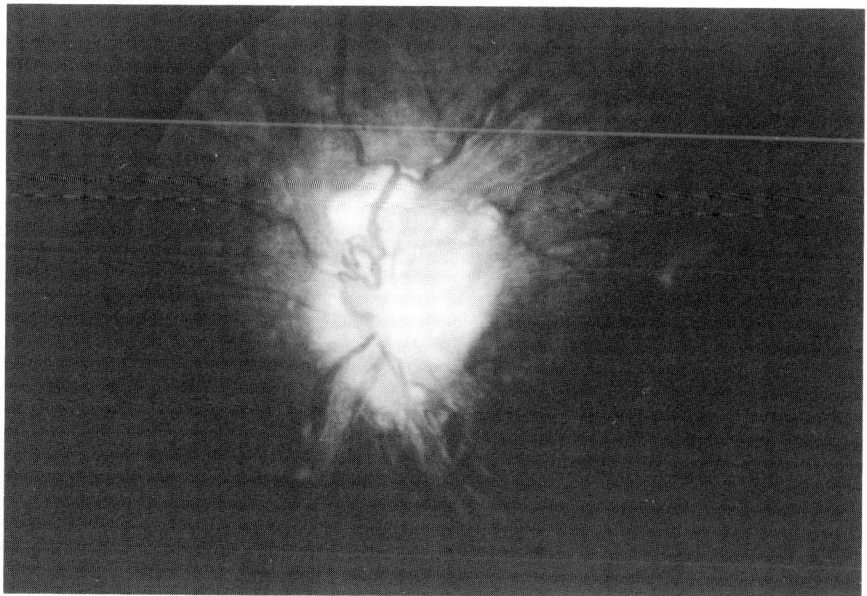

FIGURE 14-17. Sarcoid granuloma of the optic nerve.

to less than 20/200 with a 20° to 30° central field defect is common. The second eye usually develops a similar disorder within days to weeks. If it does not become involved within 1 year, a different diagnosis should be suspected. A peripapillary microangiopathy may be present premorbidly in asymptomatic eyes, and fluorescein angiography may show arteriovenous shunts at the disk without leakage of dye. Partial recovery may occur in 12% to 30% of those affected but may be delayed 1 year to 20 years. Although a deficiency of cyanide detoxification has been noted, Phillips and Gosden (1991) report that treatment with intramuscular hydroxocobalamin and/or oral cystine, even in the acute phase, is unlikely to be of any value. Other hereditary optic neuropathies usually present bilaterally and are discussed below.

Lyme disease is a tick-borne illness caused by the spirochete *Borrelia burgdorferi*. Optic neuritis, papilledema, and neuroretinitis can occur during the second or third stage of the disease. Neurologic manifestations usually present approximately 4 weeks after the first-stage skin rash and are associated with signs of meningitis. Treatment involves intravenous ceftriaxone, cefotaxime, or penicillin (see Chapter 13). *Compressive optic neuropathy* comprises a large category of disorders; included are primary and metastatic tumors, thyroid ophthalmopathy, and orbital inflammation and infections. These disorders are reviewed in Chapter 12.

Due to a Macular Disorder

Abnormalities that cause edema, hemorrhage, or hard exudates in the macula and result in an abrupt decrease in vision include the following:

Exudative age-related macular degeneration.

Hemorrhage from a subretinal neovascular membrane due to another cause (e.g., ocular histoplasmosis, high myopia, angioid streaks, choroidal tumor, traumatic choroidal break).

Macular edema associated with diabetic or hypertensive retinopathy, branch retinal vein occlusion, uveitis, retinal telangectasia (Coats's disease), and the Irvine-Gass syndrome.

Stellate retinopathy associated with optic disk edema, hypertension, and systemic and ocular infections.

Macular hole and macular pucker.

Nonexudative and exudative *age-related macular degeneration* occurs in patients age 50 years or older. The former is characterized by the presence of white concretions, called *drusen,* in the posterior retina, and is associated with a gradual loss of vision. The latter is characterized by the presence of a subretinal (choroidal) neovascular membrane (SRNM) and is associated with a rapid loss of central vision if the SRNM hemorrhages (Figure 14–18). If not obscured by hemorrhage, the neovascular membrane can be visualized by fluorescein

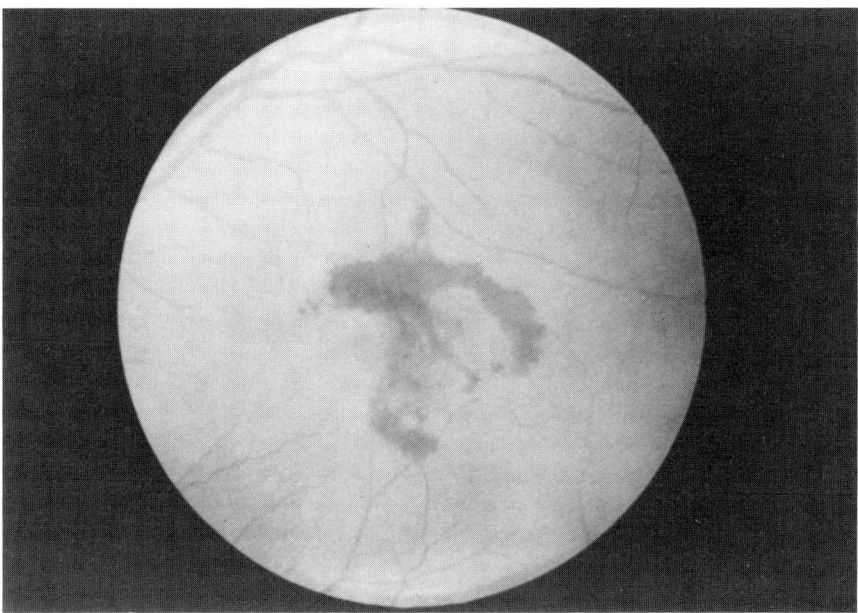

FIGURE 14-18. Subretinal hemorrhage due to rupture of a choroidal neovascular membrane in age-related macular degeneration.

angiography. End-stage macular scarring takes on a disciform appearance (Figure 14-19).

Laser photocoagulation of an SRNM is reserved for cases where there is hope of preserving central vision. The essential indications are separation by at least 200 microns of the SRNM from the center of the foveal avascular zone, and the absence of hemorrhage or exudate in the foveola. Table 14-7 lists other causes of a SRNM and their associated findings. The indications for treatment are the same as those for age-related degeneration.

Macular edema occurs when the capillary bed surrounding the fovea becomes abnormally permeable and leaks fluid, which accumulates deep within or beneath the retina. Proteinaceous exudate is visible as hard, yellow concretions. Serous exudate is visible (using contact lens magnification and slit lamp retroillumination) as multiple cystoid spaces, usually located within the outer plexiform layer of the retina. In certain cases, fluorescein angiography can demonstrate leakage of the dye into the macula (Figure 14-20). Visual acuity is often reduced to 20/200, and the foveal light reflex is blurred.

Causes of macular edema include diabetic or hypertensive retinopathy, branch retinal vein occlusion, uveitis, retinal telangiectasia (Coats's disease), and the Irvine-Gass syndrome (macular edema following cataract surgery). Although the treatment of macular edema is not well established, laser photo-

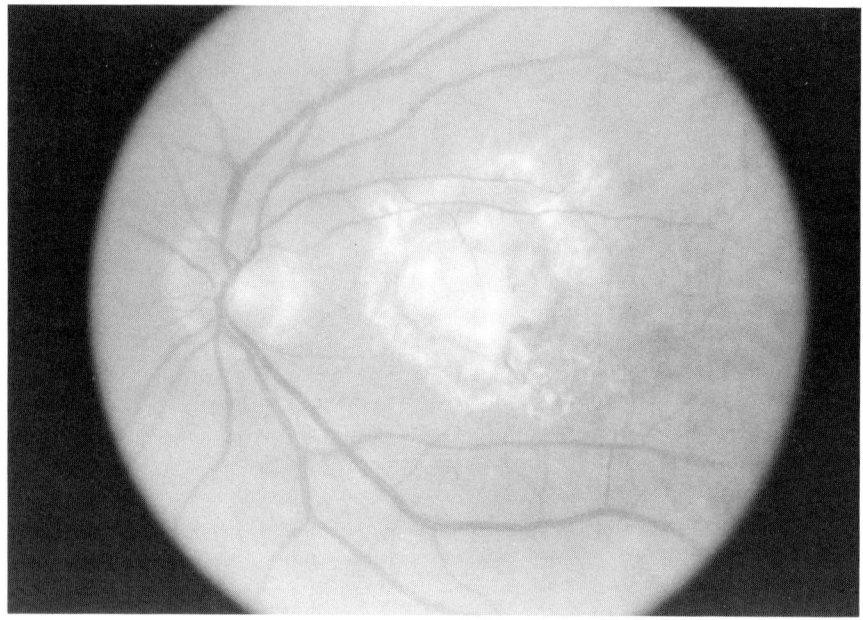

FIGURE 14-19. Disciform age-related macular degeneration (end stage).

coagulation may be efficacious in diabetic macular edema and macular edema due to a branch retinal vein occlusion. The indications for the former are presented in Table 14-4; the indication for the latter is a reduction in visual acuity below 20/40, persisting more than 3 months to 6 months. When macular edema is associated with vitreous incarcerated in a cataract wound, an anterior

TABLE 14-7. CAUSES OF SUBRETINAL NEOVASCULAR MEMBRANES

ETIOLOGY	ASSOCIATED FINDINGS
Age-related macular degeneration	Age > 50 years, retinal drusen; may have only "dry" or atrophic form
Ocular histoplasmosis syndrome	White-yellow, atrophic chorioretinal scars (< 1 mm in size) in the mid-peripheral and posterior retina; chorioretinal scarring adjacent to optic disk; age 20–50 years; residence near Ohio–Mississippi River valley; exposure to chickens, pigeons
High myopia	> 6 diopters of myopia, myopic disc changes (tilted disk, myopic crescent), Fuch spot = hyperpigmentation of the foveola following resorption of foveal hemorrhage
Angioid streaks	Bilateral, reddish-brown; radiate from the peripapillary area in spokelike fashion; distinct tendency to involve macula; seen with pseudoxanthoma elasticum, Paget's disease, Marfan's, Ehlers-Danlos, sickle cell anemia

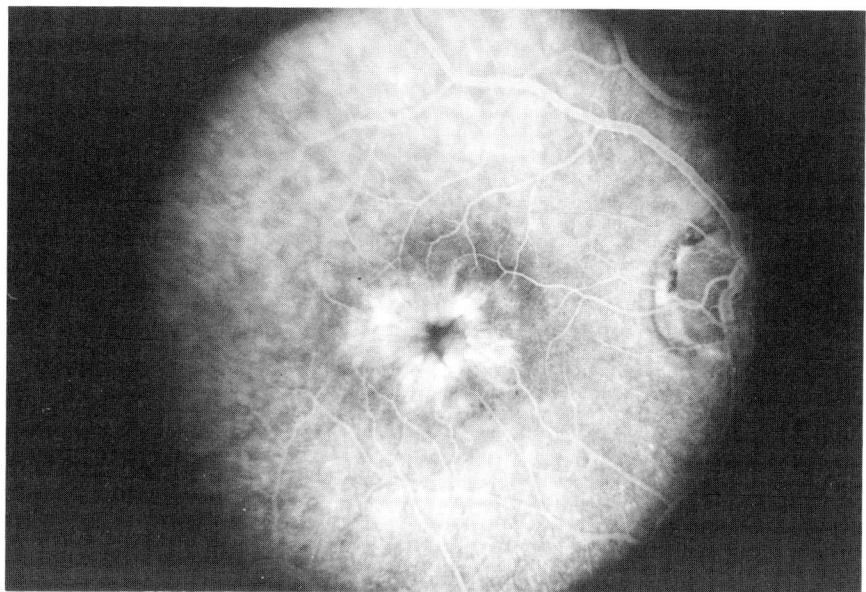

FIGURE 14-20. Fluorescein angiography demonstrating cystoid macular edema.

vitrectomy or lysis of the incarcerated vitreous strand with the YAG laser may be efficacious.

Cystoid macular edema following cataract surgery often resolves spontaneously within 6 months. Some treatments that are used in this setting, as well as for macular edema associated with uveitis, follow (none has been scientifically proved efficacious):

Acetazolamide: 250 mg by mouth each day (used especially for postoperative patients and patients with retinitis pigmentosa).
Indomethacin: 25 mg by mouth 3 times a day for 6 weeks.
Prednisolone acetate 1%: topically 4 times a day for 3 weeks, tapered over 3 weeks.
Prednisone: 40 mg by mouth each day for 5 days, tapered over 2 weeks.
Periocular repository methylprednisolone: 40 mg subtenons, repeated every 1 month or 2 months until no further improvement and then tapered (used particularly for pars planitis).

Stellate retinopathy refers to the star-shaped pattern formed when exudates accumulate within the nerve fiber layer surrounding the fovea. A "macular star" can occur during the acute phase of measles, influenza, psittacosis, Behcet's disease, or the chronic phase of tuberculosis or syphilis. It can also occur with papilledema, papillitis, Coats's disease, and hypertension or following branch retinal artery or vein occlusion. Involvement of only the nasal macula can help localize the source of edema to an inflamed optic nerve (Figure 14–21).

A *macular hole* and *macular pucker* represent two additional macular disorders responsible for a sudden decrease in vision. Full-thickness macular holes occur predominantly in late middle-aged to elderly women and cause a sudden decrease in vision to 20/200. The disorder is recognized ophthalmoscopically as a round red spot in the center of the macula, less than one disc diameter in size, and surrounded by a gray halo. Occasionally, a small operculum above the hole and small yellow deposits within it are visible (Figure 14–22). Macular holes are usually due to epiretinal macular traction or subsequent to trauma or cystoid macular edema. No treatment is effective, but a number of centers are investigating prophylactic vitrectomy for eyes with impending macular holes. Rarely, the presumably early stages of a macular hole have been reported to reverse spontaneously. Usually this occurs with spontaneous separation of the vitreous from the fovea. The risk of subsequent retinal detachment in the presence of a macular hole is surprisingly small, except in patients with high myopia.

Macular pucker (cellophane or surface wrinkling retinopathy) occurs in patients in the same age group as macular holes. The presence of a glistening retinal membrane, and displacement or straightening of the macular retinal vessels, with or without macular edema or detachment, is diagnostic. Macular

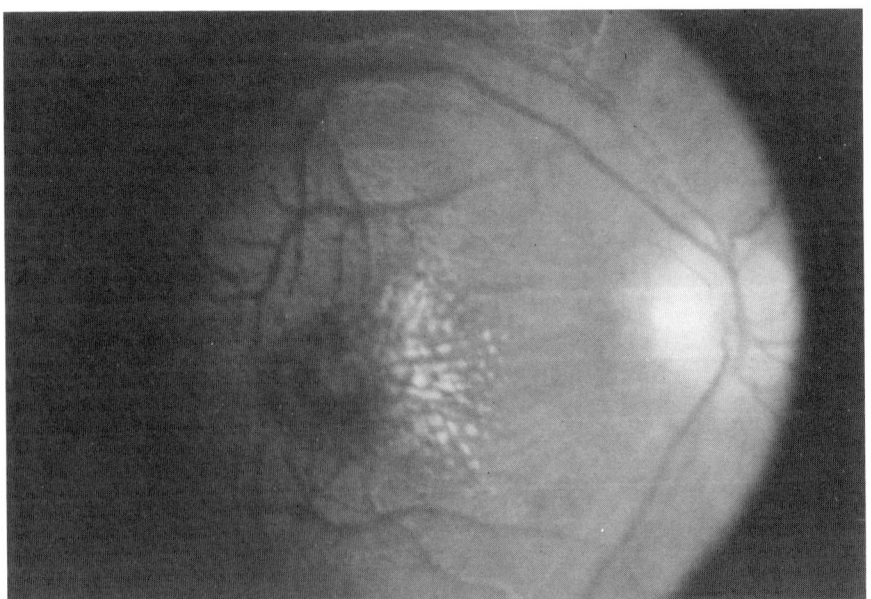

FIGURE 14–21. Stellate retinopathy secondary to optic disk edema.

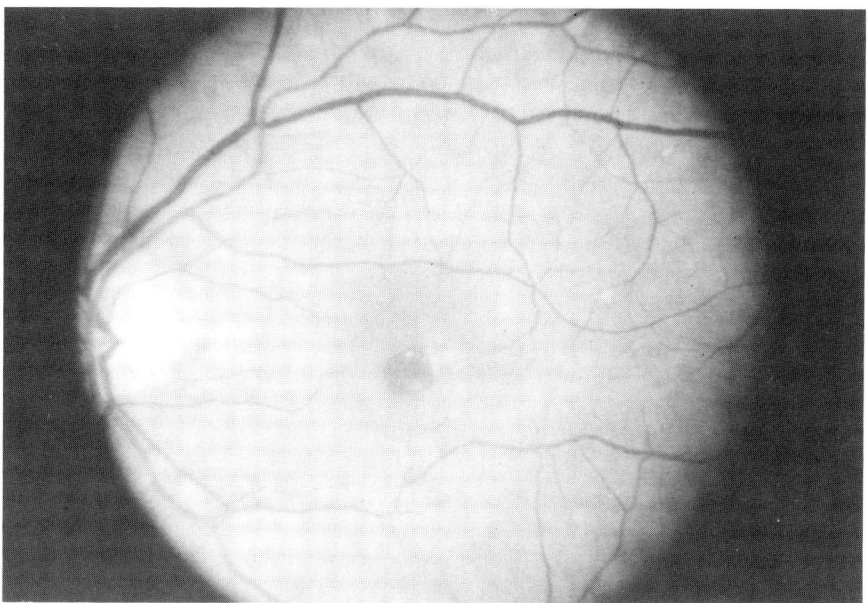

FIGURE 14-22. Macular hole.

pucker can occur idiopathically or may be subsequent to photocoagulation, cyrotherapy, intraocular surgery, uveitis, or retinal vascular disease. If the visual acuity is less than 20/80 to 20/100, surgical peeling of the membrane may be indicated.

Due to a Choroidal Disorder

A *hemorrhagic choroidal detachment* results when a posterior ciliary artery ruptures secondary to a rapid decrease in the intraocular pressure. It most frequently occurs during or after intraocular surgery but can also occur following trauma, spontaneous perforation of a corneal ulcer, or rupture of a subretinal (choroidal) neovascular membrane. A *serous* (clear fluid) *choroidal detachment* may be asymptomatic, but a hemorrhagic detachment is usually associated with severe pain, decreased vision, and a red eye. Additional characteristics include an elevated intraocular pressure and a shallow anterior chamber, which may contain a few inflammatory cells and protein flare. Treatment in severe cases consists of cycloplegic agents, topical steroids, anterior vitrectomy, and/or drainage of the choroidal detachment. Acetazolamide has vasoconstrictive properties, which lessen fluid extravasation from choroidal vessels. Its use has been noted to cause a rapid absorption of suprachoroidal fluid.

The *uveal effusion syndrome* affects males almost exclusively and is often eventually bilateral. Serous retinal detachments of the sensory retina occur, and a choroidal detachment may be associated. The principal symptom is a decrease in the superior visual field, secondary to the inferior collection of fluid. For unknown reasons, the cerebrospinal fluid has an increased pressure and protein content but no pleocytosis. The retina reattaches without treatment after months or years. *Nanophthalmos,* a condition in which the eye but not the ocular lens fails to achieve a normal size is especially associated with the uveal effusion syndrome. In this condition, a thickened scleral wall may impede flow through the vortex veins, and decompression of these veins may relieve the effusion. Because of the disproportionately large lens, this syndrome is also associated with a high incidence of angle closure glaucoma.

SUSTAINED BILATERAL LOSS OF VISION

A. Central nervous system abnormality

1. Cerebral vascular accident
2. Pituitary tumor, apoplexy, parasellar disorder
3. Cortical blindness from ischemia, anoxia, or hematoma

B. Optic nerve abnormality

1. Postinfectious optic neuritis
2. Toxic, metabolic, nutritional optic neuropathy
3. Hereditary optic neuropathy
4. Leber's optic neuropathy (usually presents unilaterally)

C. Endogenous endophthalmitis

D. Functional visual loss (see Chapter 15)

Hemorrhagic and nonhemorrhagic *cerebral vascular accidents* result in acute neurologic dysfunction, bilateral visual field deficits, and occasionally death. *Pituitary and other parasellar abnormalities* can cause acute or slowly progressive neurologic and visual field abnormalities. The visual field examination can help localize the site of the lesion (Chapter 13). Computed tomography (CT) often does not demonstrate any abnormality for the first 48 hours following acute, nonhemorrhagic infarct. MRI, however, can demonstrate cerebral edema within hours of the event. Parasellar abnormalities are better appreciated with MRI than with CT (see Chapter 2).

Cortical blindness, also known as cerebral blindness, is characterized by a complete loss of all visual sensation, including a lack of appreciation for light or dark and loss of reflex lid closure to threatening gestures. The pupils may still constrict to light and accommodation due to brain stem pathways. The ophthalmic examination is otherwise normal, but there may be associated hemiplegia, sensory disorders, aphasia, and disorientation. A denial of blindness, *Anton's syndrome,* and the *Riddoch phenomenon* (the perception of moving but not static targets) may be seen if only the occipital lobe is involved. In adults, cortical blindness may be caused by trauma or space-occupying, inflammatory, infectious, vascular, and degenerative lesions. In infants, hydrocephalus, meningoencephalitis, cerebral dysgenesis, traumatic subdural and cerebral hemorrhages, and degenerative disorders are causative.

Postinfectious optic neuritis is a condition that occurs predominantly in children and is frequently associated with a systemic viral infection or immunization. It differs from optic neuritis in adults in being typically bilateral and associated with a meningoencephalitis. Marked neurologic deficits, including seizure activity and cerebellar dysfunction, may or may not be present. MRI (but not CT) often demonstrates enhancing intracranial lesions in the acute phase, consistent with demyelinated plaques. The etiology is believed to be postviral and not related to multiple sclerosis. Cat-scratch disease has been implicated in a few children. Treatment for the acute visual loss is controversial because the usual outcome without treatment is good. Intravenous methylprednisolone 0.25 mg/kg to 4.8 mg/kg every 6 hours for 5 days has been used.

Toxic, metabolic, and nutritional optic neuropathies generally cause a gradual rather than an acute visual loss, but patients often present with "acute" symptoms. Many drugs can cause an optic neuropathy, particularly antitubercular agents, chloramphenicol, digoxin, barbiturates, lithium, chlorpropamide (Diabinese), disulfiram (Antabuse), nitrosureas, oral contraceptives, D-penicillamine, amiodarone, methanol, and vincristine. Toxic damage to the optic nerves can also be produced by the ingestion of various heavy metals, including arsenic, lead, and mercury; and the inhalation of organophosphate pesticides, organic chemicals, Lysol, organic glues, and Jamaican tea. Thiamine, vitamin B_{12}, and zinc deficiencies, or abnormalities in their metabolism, can cause similar findings. Another term used for patients with nutritional deficiency (often alcoholics) is *tobacco/alcohol amblyopia.* The visual loss is symmetric and often involves the central visual field with a connection to the blind spot (cecocentral visual field deficit; see Chapter 13). Visual acuity may be reduced to 20/200, and the optic nerve may be atrophic. The prognosis, however, is not always poor. Even patients with focal optic atrophy may have a substantial improvement in visual acuity with treatment. Therapy consists of discontinuing a causative medication, intramuscular hydroxycobalamin (1 cc intramuscularly every day for 3 days and then weekly), and oral thiamine (50 mg by mouth twice a day), if nutritionally deficient. The latter can also be supplied by over the counter preparations, or in brewer's yeast tablets.

Dominant optic neuropathy has an insidious onset between 4 years and 8 years of age, with a moderately reduced visual acuity of typically between 20/30 to 20/80 at presentation. Because it occurs in young children, it may be heralded as a sudden loss of vision. The optic nerve often shows a wedge-shaped temporal pallor; visual field testing reveals a central scotoma connected to the blind spot, and color vision testing demonstrates a loss of blue-sensitive cones (acquired tritan dysfunction). The visual acuity may eventually diminish to 20/200. The condition is inherited as an autosomal dominant trait, and examination of the parents may confirm a subtle abnormality. *Recessive optic atrophy* has an earlier onset and an eventual reduction of acuity to less than 20/300.

Endogenous (metastatic) endophthalmitis is a rare, usually bilateral condition that occurs in extremely ill, often immunologically comprised individuals. It can be associated with subacute bacterial endocarditis. In developing countries, a disproportionate number of children are affected, likely due to malnutrition. In every case, a hematogenous spread of bacteria or fungi is presumed. Identified organisms have included *Pseudomonas aeruginosa, Streptococcus pneumonia, Mycobacterium tuberculosis, Escherichia coli, Neisseria meningitides, Streptococcus pyogenes,* and *Candida albicans.* The treatment is similar to postsurgical endophthalmitis (see Chapters 16 and 17). Many cases respond poorly to medical management, in which case a vitrectomy, with the injection of intravitreal antibiotics, is necessary.

TRANSIENT UNILATERAL LOSS OF VISION *(AMAUROSIS FUGAX)*

The differential diagnosis for a transient unilateral loss of vision includes:

A. Vascular
   1. Carotid artery disease
      a. Carotid emboli
      b. Ocular ischemic syndrome
   2. Structural cardiac defects
   3. Temporal arteritis
   4. Impending vascular occlusion of retina
   5. Retinal migraine (see Chapter 13)
B. Papilledema (usually bilateral)
C. Functional visual loss (see Chapter 15)

Carotid vascular disease is the most common cause of *amaurosis fugax,* or transient monocular blindness, in the elderly. Embolic causes should especially be suspected when the visual loss is altitudinal, or monocular and lateralized. The diagnosis becomes more certain when the attacks are associated with hemiparesis, hemisensory loss, or aphasia. Episodes frequently last between 2 minutes and 10 minutes and can occur as frequently as 10 to 20 times per day. During an attack, a dimming or a complete darkening of vision is noted; the return of vision can be sectoral or altitudinal. Examination of the retina during an attack may show migratory calcific or cholesterol emboli traversing the arterial system or a complete arterial occlusion. Often, however, the retina appears normal. Experimentally, the retina can withstand only about 100 minutes of total central retinal artery occlusion before irreversible damage occurs.

Some patients with carotid artery disease note blurring of vision, lasting several minutes, when going from a dark to a bright room. Other patients are asymptomatic and retinal microemboli are found incidentally. Cholesterol emboli, also called *Hollenhorst plaques,* tend to lodge at the bifurcation of medium to small arterioles. They are bright yellow or orange, irregular in shape, and larger than the blood column (Figure 14-23). Platelet-fibrin emboli are grayish-white, amorphous structures, similar in size to the blood column (Figure 14-24). Calcific emboli are grayish-white and the same size or larger than the arteriole, and they are usually found near the optic disk (Figure 14-8). The first two types of emboli are associated with carotid artery disease; the latter is associated with aortic or valvular heart disease. Patients with emboli from the carotid system have an increased death rate due to cardiovascular disease but not strokes.

The *ocular ischemic syndrome* is an additional sign of carotid occlusive disease. It may present as amaurosis fugax and occasionally as orbital pain. Patients may also note afterimages or delayed recovery of vision after exposure to a bright light (photostress test). The condition is usually unilateral and occurs in middle-aged and elderly individuals. By ophthalmoscopy, distended but not tortuous veins, narrowed retinal arteries, and mid-peripheral retinal hemorrhages are seen. Disk edema and hemorrhages are not usually present, but neovascularization of the disk occurs in up to one-third of cases. Occasionally, retinal artery pulsations in concert with the systolic pulse, and cotton wool

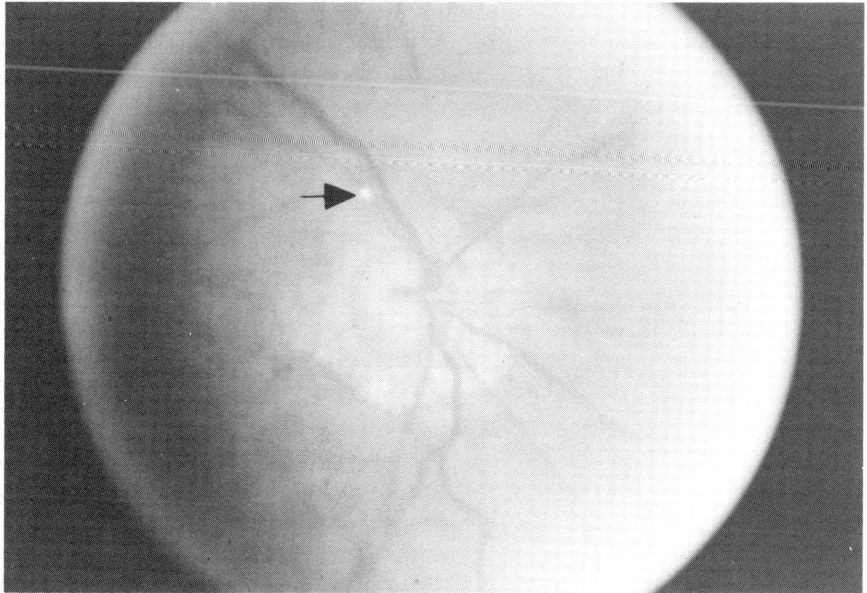

FIGURE 14-23. Hollenhorst plaque (arrow).

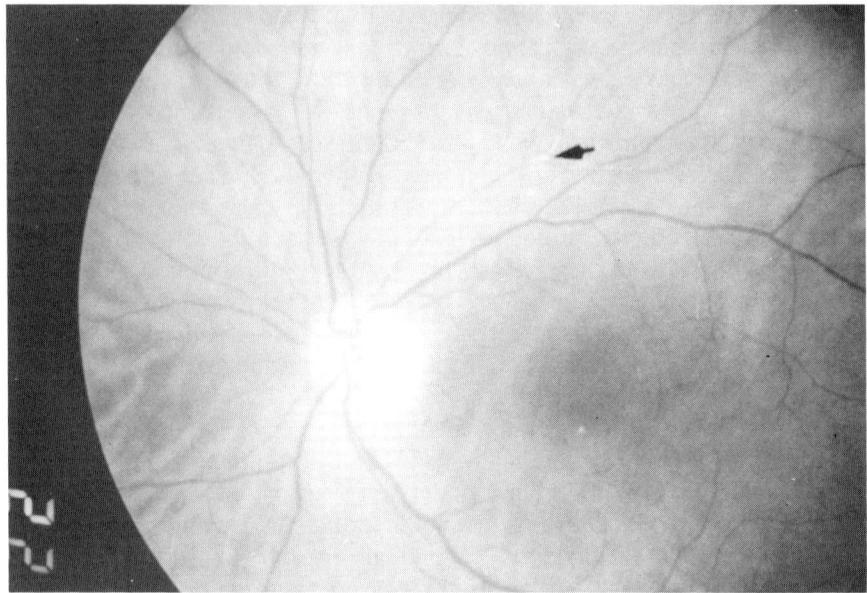

FIGURE 14-24. Platelet fibrin emboli in superior branch retinal artery.

spots, due to retinal ischemia, are seen. Additional signs include injection of the episcleral vessels (red eye), edema of the cornea, cells in the anterior chamber (anterior uveitis), neovascular glaucoma, cataract, and iris atrophy. A central retinal artery occlusion may imminently occur. Aortic arch disease due to atherosclerosis, aneurysm, syphilis, or Takayasu's disease may present similarly—it is distinguished from ocular ischemic syndrome by the absence of radial pulses, and the presence of exertional pain in proximal arm muscles, and bilaterality in aortic disease.

Several noninvasive tests exist to screen for carotid artery disease, but generally they do not detect a stenosis of less than 80%. Carotid angiography and intra-arterial digital subtraction angiography best visualize the arterial system (see Chapter 2). Ophthalmodynamometry is useful in detecting diminished perfusion of retinal arteries due to carotid occlusive disease (see Chapter 1).

The treatment of carotid vascular disease is controversial. There is insufficient evidence that an endarterectomy will prevent a stroke or death. Furthermore, the morbidity of this procedure may exceed its benefit in patients who never experienced a transient ischemic event. Aspirin, 300 mg per day, may be useful because it inhibits platelet aggregation. In the ocular ischemic syndrome, neovascularization and neovascular glaucoma are treated with panretinal photocoagulation; medications to reduce the intraocular pressure may also be necessary (see Chapter 11).

Atheromatous disease of the ipsilateral extracranial carotid artery is not the only cause of amaurosis fugax. Transient monocular blindness is also seen with temporal arteritis, papilledema (particularly when due to pseudotumor cerebri), ophthalmic artery stenosis or aneurysm, structural (usually valvular) cardiac abnormalities, and migraine.

TRANSIENT BILATERAL LOSS OF VISION

A. Papilledema

B. Vascular

   1. Vertebrobasilar artery insufficiency
   2. Vasomotor collapse, hypotension
   3. Cardiac arrhythmia, heart failure
   4. Severe systemic hypertension
   5. Migraine (see Chapter 13)

C. Seizure activity

Papilledema is a sign of increased intracranial pressure (ICP). In the context of this chapter, it is one of the diagnostic entities that should be considered when a patient presents with the symptom of transient loss of vision. It should be remembered, however, that papilledema is only a sign, not a diagnosis in itself. The discovery of papilledema should lead to a differential of causes of increased ICP (Table 14–8).

TABLE 14–8. ETIOLOGIC CAUSES OF PAPILLEDEMA

Intracranial tumors
Cerebral tumors (especially infratentorial)
Hamartomas
Teratomas

Vascular
Cerebral hematomas
Aneurysms
Subdural hematoma
Epidural hematoma
Subarachnoid hemorrhage
Arteriovenous malformations

Infectious
Granulomas (sarcoid, tubercular, syphilitic)
Paracytic lesions (cysticercus cysts)
Brain abscess (especially occipital lobe) (unilaterality may have localizing value)
Meningitis, encephalitis (due to diffuse cerebral edema)
Lyme disease

Guillain-Barré syndrome

Craniostenoses

Spinal cord tumors (especially ependymomas or neurofibromas)

Mucopolysaccharidoses

The distinguishing features of papilledema, optic neuropathies, and optic disk drusen *(pseudopapilledema)* are listed in Table 14–6. The principal symptom of papilledema is a transient obscuration of vision. Described as a "dimming of vision," obscurations usually last only seconds but can occur several times a day. They can often be incited by orthostatic changes. Initially the visual acuity is normal unless the macula is involved by exudate or edema. Rarely, an acute visual loss can occur due to a superimposed ischemic optic neuropathy. The visual field usually shows only a mild enlargement of the blind spot; the pupillary responses and color vision are also usually normal. Signs of papilledema include hyperemia of the optic disk, obscuration of blood vessels near the optic disk (due to swelling of the peripapillary nerve fiber layer), and flame-shaped hemorrhages at the disk margin (Figure 14–25). With chronicity, the hemorrhages, exudate, and venous dilation decrease, but the disk elevation persists. Chronicity can lead to optic pallor, constriction of the retinal vessels, and calcifications on the surface of the disk. Irreversible loss of vision and an inferior nasal or arcuate visual field defect can result.

Papilledema is a neurologic emergency. It can be accompanied by other signs of increased ICP, including headaches, nausea, and vomiting. Neuroimaging should be performed; if no intracranial masses are detected, a lumbar puncture should follow. In children, posterior fossa tumors are often found. In adults, metastatic and primary cerebral neoplasms are more common.

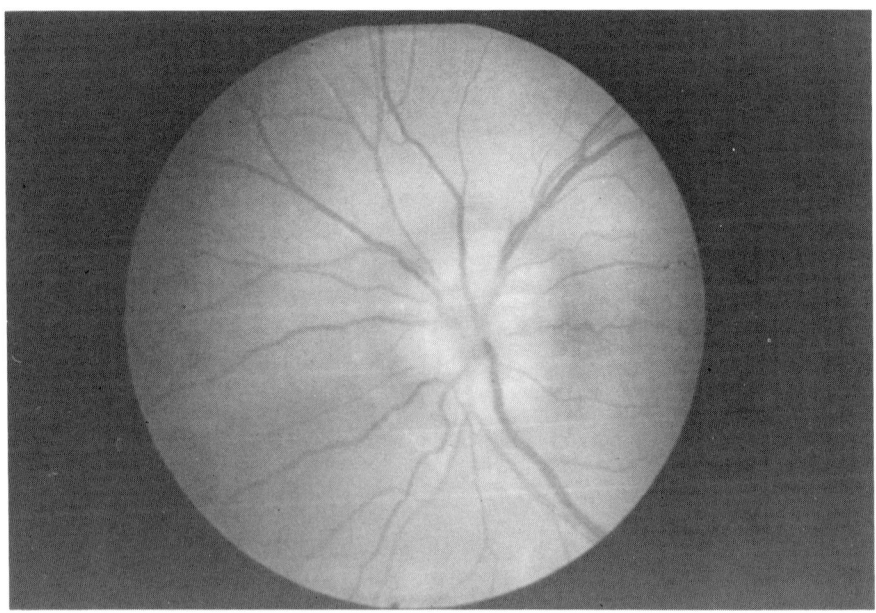

FIGURE 14–25. Papilledema.

Another common cause of papilledema in adults is *pseudotumor cerebri,* a condition seen predominantly in females in their third decade of life who present with headaches, visual disturbances, tinnitus, dizziness, nausea, and/or vomiting. In addition to transient visual obscurations, vague "gray-outs" of vision, lasting minutes to hours, and episodes of horizontal diplopia worse at distance fixation (due to sixth nerve paresis), may be noted. Obesity and pregnancy are often associated. The disorder also occurs with vitamin A, nalidixic acid, oral contraceptive, penicillin, and tetracycline use, corticosteroid use or withdrawal (especially in children), and lead or arsenic poisoning. It can occur with iron deficiency anemia, chronic lung disease (due to polycythemia), systemic lupus erythematosis, or malignant hypertension or following radical neck dissection. Severe intractable headaches and visual field loss are indications for treatment, which may include medical management with acetazolamide (500 mg to 2 g per day) or furosemide (40 mg to 80 mg per day), repeat lumbar punctures, optic nerve sheath decompression, or lumbar peritoneal shunt.

Other common causes of transient, bilateral loss of vision are related to circulatory disturbances. These include vertebrobasilar artery insufficiency, vasomotor collapse due to orthostatic hypotension, caridac arrhythmia, heart failure, and severe systemic hypertension.

REFERENCES

Acquired Immune Deficiency (AIDS)

Caskey PJ, Ai E: Recognition of the ophthalmic manifestations of AIDS. *Ophthalmic Pract* 8:229, 1990.
Duker JS, Blumenkranz MS: Diagnosis and management of the acute retinal necrosis syndrome. *Surv Ophthalmol* 35:327, 1991.
Duker JS, Shakin EP: Rapidly progressive outer retinal necrosis in the acquired immunodeficiency syndrome. *Am J Ophthalmol* 111:254, 1991.
Forster DJ, Dugel PU, Frangieh PE, et al: Rapidly progressive outer retinal necrosis in the acquired immune deficiency syndrome. *Am J Ophthalmol* 110:341, 1990.
Heinemann MH, Bloom AF, Horowitz J: Candida albicans endophthalmitis in a patient with AIDS. *Arch Ophthalmol* 105:1172, 1987.
Holland GN, Engstrom RE Jr, Glasgow BJ, et al: Ocular toxoplasmosis in patients with the acquired immune deficiency syndrome. *Am J Ophthalmol* 106:653, 1988.
Holland GN, Sidikaro Y, Kreiger AE, et al: Treatment of cytomegalovirus retinopathy with ganciclovir. *Ophthalmology* 94:815, 1987.
Jabs DA, Green WR, Fox R, et al: Ocular manifestations of acquired immune deficiency syndrome. *Ophthalmology* 96:1092, 1989.
Jabs DA, Newman C, De Bustros S, Pold BF: Treatment of cytomegalovirus retinitis with gancyclovir. *Ophthalmology* 94:824, 1987.
Litoff D, Catalano RA: Herpes zoster optic neuritis in human immunodeficiency syndrome. *Arch Ophthalmol* 108:782, 1990.
Morse PH: Cytomegalovirus retinitis and its treatment. *Ophthalmic Pract* 8:251, 1990.
Schuman JS, Orellana J, Friedman AH, Teich SA: Acquired immunodeficiency syndrome (AIDS). *Surv Ophthalmol* 31:384, 1987.
Sidikaro Y, Silver L, Holland GN, Kreiger AE: Rhegmatogenous retinal detachments in patients with AIDS and necrotizing retinal infections. *Ophthalmology* 98:129, 1991.

Walmsley SL, Chew E, Read SE, et al: Treatment of cytomegalovirus retinitis with trisodium phosphonoformate hexahydrate (Foscarnet). *J Infect Dis* 157:569, 1988.

Winward KE, Hamed LM, Glaser JS: The spectrum of optic nerve disease in human immunodeficiency virus infection. *Am J Ophthalmol* 107:373, 1989.

Carotid and Cerebral Vascular Disorders

Brown GC: Anterior ischemic optic neuropathy occurring in association with carotid artery obstruction. *J Clin Neuro-ophthalmol* 6:39, 1986.

Bruno A, Corbett JJ, Biller J, et al: Transient monocular visual loss patterns and associated vascular abnormalities. *Stroke* 21:34, 1990.

Burde RM, Savino PJ, Trobe JD: *Clinical Decisions in Neuro-Ophthalmology.* St Louis, CV Mosby Co, 1985.

Trobe JD: Carotid endarterectomy: Who needs it? *Ophthalmology* 94:725, 1987.

Vine AK, Maguire PT, Martonyi C, Kincaid MC: Recombinant tissue plasminogen activator to lyse experimentally induced arterial thrombi. *Am J Ophthalmol* 105:266, 1988.

Warlow C: Carotid endarterectomy: Does it work? *Stroke* 15:1068, 1984.

Choroidal Disorders

Bellows AR, Chylack LT Jr, Hutchinson BT: Choroidal detachment. Clinical manifestations, therapy and mechanism of formation. *Ophthalmology* 88:1107, 1981.

Brubaker RF, Pederson JE: Ciliochoroidal detachment. *Surv Ophthalmol* 27:281, 1983.

Ruiz RS, Salmonsen PC: Expulsive choroidal effusion: A complication of intraocular surgery. *Arch Ophthalmol* 94:69, 1976.

Endophthalmitis (Metastatic)

Farber BP, Weinbaum DL, Dummer JS: Metastatic bacterial endophthalmitis. *Arch Intern Med* 145:62, 1985.

Garg SP, Talwar D, Verma LK: Metastatic endophthalmitis: A reappraisal. *Ann Ophthalmol* 23:74, 1991.

Greenwald MJ, Wohl LG, Sell CH: Metastatic bacterial endophthalmitis: A contemporary reappraisal. *Surv Ophthalmol* 31:81, 1986.

Macular Abnormalities

Akiba J, Yoshida A, Trempe CL: Risk of developing a macular hole. *Arch Ophthalmol* 108:1088, 1990.

Bressler NM, Bressler SB, Fine SL: Age-related macular degeneration. *Surv Ophthalmol* 32:375, 1988.

De Bustros S: Early stages of macular holes: To treat or not to treat. *Arch Ophthalmol* 108:1085, 1990.

Early Treatment Diabetic Retinopathy Study Research Group: Photocoagulation for diabetic macular edema. ETDRS Report 1. *Arch Ophthalmol* 103:1796, 1985.

Gass JDM: Idiopathic sensile macular hole: Its early stages and pathogenesis. *Arch Ophthalmol* 106:629, 1988.

Macular Photocoagulation Study Group: Argon laser photocoagulation for neovascular maculopathy: Three year results from randomized clinical trials. *Arch Ophthalmol* 104:694, 1986.

Macular Photocoagulation Study Group: Argon laser photocoagulation for ocular histoplasmosis: Results of a randomized clinical trial. *Arch Ophthalmol* 101:1347, 1983.

Wiznia RA: Reversibility of the early stages of idiopathic macular holes. *Am J Ophthalmol* 107:241, 1989.

Optic Nerve Disorders

Beck RW: The optic neuritis treatment trial. *Arch Ophthalmol* 106:1051, 1988.

Beck RW, Servais G, Hayreh SS: Anterior ischemic optic neuropathy: IX. Cup to disc ratio and its role in pathogenesis. *Ophthalmology* 94:1503, 1987.

Boghen DR, Glaser JS: Ischemic optic neuropathy. The clinical profile and natural history. *Brain* 98:689, 1975.

Cohen MM, Lessell S, Wolf PA: A prospective study of the risk of developing multiple sclerosis in uncomplicated optic neuritis. *Neurology* 29:208, 1979.

Cowan CL, Knox DL: Migraine optic neuropathy. *Ann Ophthalmol* 14:164, 1982.

Cox TA: Prognostic factors in optic neuritis. *Ann Neurol* 11:324, 1982.

Dutton JJ, Burde RM, Klingele TG: Autoimmune retrobulbar optic neuritis. *Am J Ophthalmol* 94:11, 1982.

Ebers GC: Optic neuritis and multiple sclerosis. *Arch Neurol* 42:702, 1985.

Farris BK, Pickard DJ: Bilateral postinfectious optic neuritis and intravenous steroid therapy in children. *Ophthalmology* 97:339, 1990.

Fleishman JA, Beck RW, Linares OA, et al: Deficits in visual function after resolution of optic neuritis. *Ophthalmology* 94:1029, 1987.

Francis DA, Compston DAS, Batchelor JR, McDonald WI: A reassessment of the risk of multiple sclerosis developing in patients with optic neuritis after extended follow-up. *J Neurol Neurosurg Psychiat* 50:758, 1987.

Gebarski SS, Gabrielson TO, Gliman S, et al: The initial diagnosis of multiple sclerosis: Clinical impact of magnetic resonance imaging. *Ann Neurol* 17:469, 1985.

Guyer DR, Miller NR, Auer CL, et al: The risk of cerebrovascular and cardiovascular disease in patients with anterior ischemic optic neuropathy. *Arch Ophthalmol* 103:1136, 1985.

Hackett ER, Martinez RD, Larsen PF, Paddison RM: Optic neuritis in systemic lupus erythematosis. *Arch Neurol* 31:9, 1974.

Hall S, Persellin S, Lie JT, et al: The therapeutic impact of temporal artery biopsy. *Lancet* 2:1217, 1983.

Hayreh SS, Zahourk RM: Anterior ischemic optic neuropathy: VI. In juvenile diabetics. *Ophthalmologica* 182:13, 1981.

Hedges TR, Gieger GL, Albert DM: The clinical value of negative temporal artery biopsy specimens. *Arch Ophthalmol* 101:1251, 1983.

Hess RF, Plant GT (eds): *Optic Neuritis.* Cambridge, Cambridge University Press, 1986.

Huston KA, Hunder GG, Lie JT, et al: Temporal arteritis. A 25 year epidemiologic, clinical and pathologic study. *Ann Intern Med* 88:162, 1978.

Johns K, Lavin P, Elliot JH, Partain CL: Magnetic resonance imaging of the brain in isolated optic neuritis. *Arch Ophthalmol* 104:1486, 1986.

Katz B: Disc swelling in an adult diabetic patient. *Surv Ophthalmol* 35:158, 1990.

Keltner JL: Giant cell arteritis: Signs and symptoms. *Ophthalmology* 89:1101, 1982.

Kline LB, Glaser JS: Dominant optic atrophy: The clinical profile. *Arch Ophthalmol* 97:1680, 1979.

Link H, Stendahl-Brodin L: Optic neuritis and multiple sclerosis. *N Engl J Med* 308:1294, 1983.

Lubow M, Makley TA Jr: Pseudopapilledema of juvenile diabetes mellitus. *Arch Ophthalmol* 85:417, 1971.

Mehler ME, Rabinowich L: The neuro-ophthalmologic spectrum of temporal arteritis. *Ann Neurol* 22:147, 1987.

Nikoskelainen E, Frey H, Salmi A: Prognosis of optic neuritis with special reference to cerebrospinal fluid immunoglobulins and measles virus antibodies. *Ann Neurol* 9:545, 1981.

Nikoskelainen E, Hassinen IE, Paljarvi L, et al: Leber's hereditary optic neuropathy, a mitochondrial disease? *Lancet* 2:1474, 1984.

Nikoskelainen E, Hoyt WF, Nummelin K, Schatz H: Fundus findings in Leber's hereditary optic neuropathy. III. Fluorescein angiographic studies. *Arch Ophthalmol* 102:981, 1984.

O'Hara M, O'Connor PS: Migrainous optic neuropathy. *J Clin Neuro-ophthalmol* 4:85, 1984.

Ormerod IEC, McDonald WI, du Boulay GH, et al: Disseminated lesions at presentation in patients with optic neuritis. *J Neurol Neurosurg Psychiat* 49:124, 1986.

Perkins GD, Rose FC: *Optic Neuritis and Its Differential Diagnosis.* Oxford, Oxford Medical Publications, 1979.

Phillips CI, Gosden CM: Leber's hereditary optic neuropathy and Kearns-Sayre syndrome: Mitochondrial DNA mutations. *Surv Ophthalmol* 35:463, 1991.

Repka MX, Savino PJ, Schatz NL, et al: Clinical profile and long-term implications of anterior ischemic optic neuropathy. *Am J Ophthalmol* 96:478, 1983.

Rizzo JF, Lessell S: Risks of developing multiple sclerosis after uncomplicated optic neuritis: A long term prospective study. *Neurology* 38:185, 1988.

Salmon JF, Pan EL, Murray ADN: Visual loss with dancing extremities and mental disturbances. *Surv Ophthalmol* 35:299, 1991.
Sanders EACM, Reulen JPH, Hogenhuis LAH: Central nervous system involvement in optic neuritis. *J Neurol Neurosurg Psychiat* 47:241, 1984.
Sedwick LA: The perils of Pauline: Visual loss in a tippler. *Surv Ophthalmol* 35:454, 1991.
Sergott RC, Cohen MS, Bosley TM, et al: Optic nerve decompression may improve the progressive form of nonarteritic ischemic optic neuropathy. *Arch Ophthalmol* 107:1743, 1989.
Shults WT: Ischemic optic neuropathy. Still the ophthalmologist's dilemma. *Ophthalmology* 91:1338, 1984.
Slamovits TL, Rosen CE, Cheng KP, Striph GC: Visual loss in patients with optic neuritis and visual loss to no light perception. *Am J Ophthalmol* 111:209, 1991.
Spoor TC, Rockwell DL: Treatment of optic neuritis with intravenous megadose corticosteroids: A consecutive series. *Ophthalmology* 95:131, 1988.
Weinstein JM, Feman SS: Ischemic optic neuropathy in migraine. *Arch Ophthalmol* 100:1097, 1982.
Weiss AH, Beck RW: Neuroretinitis in childhood. *J Pediatr Ophthalmol Strabismus* 26:198, 1989.

Papilledema

Brourman ND, Spoor TC, Ramocki JM: Optic nerve sheath decompression for pseudotumor cerebri. *Arch Ophthalmol* 106:1378, 1988.
Corbett JJ: Problems in the diagnosis and treatment of pseudotumor cerebri. *Can J Neurol Sci* 10:221, 1983.
Corbett JJ, Savino PJ, Thompson HS, et al: Visual loss in pseudotumor cerebri. *Arch Neurol* 39:461, 1982.
Miller NR, Fine SL: *The Ocular Fundus in Neuro-opthalmologic Diagnosis.* St Louis, CV Mosby Co, 1977.
Orcutt JC, Page NGR, Sanders MD: Factors affecting visual loss in benign intracranial hypertension. *Ophthalmology* 91:1303, 1984.
Smith CA, Orcutt JC: Surgical treatment of pseudotumor cerebri. *Int Ophthalmol Clin* 20:265, 1986.
Wall M, Hart WM, Burde RM: Visual field defects in idiopathic intracranial hypertension (pseudotumor cerebri). *Am J Ophthalmol* 96:654, 1983.

Retinal Vascular Disorders

Branch Vein Occlusion Study Group: Argon laser scatter photocoagulation for prevention of neovascularization and vitreous hemorrhage in branch vein occlusion. *Arch Ophthalmol* 104:34, 1986.
Diabetic Retinopathy Study Research Group: Photocoagulation treatment of proliferative diabetic retinopathy: The second report of the diabetic retinopathy study findings. *Ophthalmology* 85:82, 1978.
Diabetic Retinopathy Vitrectomy Study Research Group: Early vitrectomy for proliferative diabetic retinopathy in eyes with useful vision: Results of a randomized trial—Diabetic retinopathy vitrectomy study report 3. *Ophthalmology* 95:1307, 1988.
Dodson PM, Kritzinger EE: Underlying medical conditions in young patients and ethnic differences in retinal vein occlusion. *Trans Ophthalmol Soc UK* 104:114, 1985.
Frucht J, Yanko L, Merin S: Central retinal vein occlusions in young adults. *Acta Ophthalmol* 62:780, 1984.
Gittinger JW: Unilateral blurred vision and dilated retinal veins. *Surv Ophthalmol* 31:270, 1987.
Hayrey SS: Classification of central retinal vein occlusion. *Ophthalmology* 90:458, 1983.
Kearns TP: Differential of central retinal vein obstruction. *Ophthalmology* 90:475, 1983.
Parr J: Sudden loss of vision. In Parr J: *Introduction to Ophthalmology.* Oxford, Oxford University Press, 1989, pp 216–221.
Servais GE, Thompson HS, Hayrey SS: Relative afferent pupillary defect in central retinal vein occlusion. *Ophthalmology* 93:301, 1986.

Sarcoidosis

Aaberg TM: The role of the ophthalmologist in the management of sarcoidosis. *Am J Ophthalmol* 103:99, 1987.
Jabs DA, Johns CJ: Ocular involvement in chronic sarcoidosis. *Am J Ophthalmol* 102:297, 1986.
James DG: Ocular sarcoidosis. *Ann NY Acad Sci* 465:551, 1986.
Karma A, Huhti E, Poukkula A: Course and outcome of ocular sarcoidosis. *Am J Ophthalmol* 106:467, 1988.
Palestine AG, Nussenblatt RB, Chan CC: Treatment of intraocular complications of sarcoidosis. *Ann NY Acad Sci* 465:564, 1986.

Traumatic Disorders

Anderson RL, Panje WR, Gross CE: Optic nerve blindness following blunt forehead trauma. *Ophthalmology* 89:445, 1982.
Feist RM, Kline LB, Morris RE, et al: Recovery of vision after presumed direct optic nerve injury. *Ophthalmology* 94:1567, 1987.
Joseph MP, Lessell S, Rizzo J, Momose J: Extracranial optic nerve decompression for traumatic optic neuropathy. *Arch Ophthalmol* 108:1091, 1990.
Kline LB, Morowetz RB, Swaid SN: Indirect injury to the optic nerve. *Neurosurgery* 14:756, 1984.
Lam BL, Weingeist TA: Corticosteroid-responsive traumatic optic neuropathy. *Am J Ophthalmol* 109:99, 1990.
Lessell S: Indirect optic nerve trauma. *Arch Ophthalmol* 107:382, 1989.
Miller NR: The management of traumatic optic neuropathy. *Arch Ophthalmol* 108:1086, 1990.
Spoor TC, Mathog RH: Restoration of vision after optic canal decompression. *Arch Ophthalmol* 104:805, 1985.

15

Functional and Psychotic Ophthalmologic Disorders

Robert A. Catalano

He who knows hysteria knows medicine.—Osler

Several ophthalmologic abnormalities that are seen as acute emergencies have a nonorganic or functional basis. The term *functional* is often not immediately clear to patients, families, and even some health care workers. It is used to suggest that the disorder is one of function rather than structure. In this context, it means that the physical structure is undamaged and presumably capable of full function. Older terms for these disorders—*hysteria, conversion reaction,* and *pithiatism*—should be avoided, because their meaning and relationship to the psyche is even less lucid than *functional.* Furthermore, the term *functional* does not, in itself, indicate whether the apparent loss is feigned or fancied. Patients who deliberately and knowingly feign loss *(malingerers),* as well as highly suggestive individuals, without malicious intent, comprise the extremes of any functional disorder. Most patients fall within these extremes.

In every case, the challenge to the ophthalmologist or emergency physician is to determine whether the alleged loss has an organic basis. Because the physician often sets out to disprove the patient's claim of impairment, dealing with these patients and the distorted physician-patient relationship is often frustrating. The most difficult patients to examine and treat are those with organic disease but symptoms exaggerated out of proportion to the underlying pathology. For a variety of reasons, these patients often do not voluntarily divulge previous diagnoses to their new physician caretakers. A careful check of old records for existing disease is prudent when symptoms outweigh findings on examination. These patients are usually classified as having disease "with a functional overlay."

The most commonly encountered functional ophthalmologic disorder is loss of visual field or acuity. Less common disorders are visual hallucinations, photophobia, and headache. A few disorders of ocular motility, including accommodative spasm and voluntary nystagmus, are almost always functional. Disorders such as functional blinking and eyelid pulling occur predominantly in children. Table 15–1 lists commonly encountered functional disorders.

Whether functional losses should be classified as psychiatric disorders is controversial. These patients often report considerable situational stress but generally do not need psychiatric evaluation or treatment. This cannot be said of individuals who self-induce ocular injuries. Included in this group are patients with *ocular Munchausen's syndrome* and those with delusional psychosis. Most clinicians would agree that self-infliction of injury separates functional from psychotic patients. The latter need urgent psychiatric care.

FUNCTIONAL LOSS OF VISUAL FIELD OR ACUITY

Functional visual loss, also known as retinal anesthesia, ocular hysteria, hysterical amblyopia, visual conversion reaction, and "ophthalmic flake syndrome," has been reported to comprise 1% to 5% of a typical ophthalmology practice. There is a 2:1 predominance of females and a clustering of children between ages 9 and 12 years. In children, the disorder is somewhat different than it is in adults, but the diagnostic techniques are the same.

In both children and adults, the burden of proof rests with the examiner. The examiner must demonstrate that the patient with a suspected functional loss of vision is capable of normal vision and has no underlying organic disease. Disorders that may be misdiagnosed as functional loss include mild amblyopia, keratoconus, central serous retinopathy, retinitis pigmentosa without pigment, and early Stargardt's disease. If a relative afferent pupillary defect is present, functional visual loss is at most only part of the diagnosis. It is not uncommon for patients with organic disease to have a functional overlay. Whenever there

TABLE 15–1. OPHTHALMOLOGIC DISORDERS THAT CAN BE FUNCTIONAL

Loss of visual acuity or visual field	Headache
Spasm of the near reflex	Blinking
Voluntary nystagmus	Eyelid pulling
Visual hallucinations	Eyelash and eyebrow plucking
Pupillary abnormalities	Propulsion of the eyeballs
Photophobia	

is reasonable doubt or if good visual acuity cannot be confirmed with certainty, reexamination is prudent. The diagnosis of malingering should be made with even greater caution because it implies that the patient is consciously feigning disability for secondary gain.

Suggested Techniques to Disprove Visual Loss

Observation of Behavior

Malingerers are often visibly agitated, terse, and unpleasant. They may give themselves away by trying too hard to prove their loss. They might wildly search (in vain) when asked to try to look at their hand (even the blind can align their hands in front of their face when asked). The truly blind are also able to sign their name without difficulty; malingerers will not. Malingerers go out of their way to walk into obstacles placed slightly out of their path.

The *"suggestible innocent"* (Thompson, 1985) may have already seen several physicians and may be primed to describe a homonymous or other field loss in addition to visual loss. This person's visual acuity or visual field may improve with suggestion. Suggesting that pupillary dilation allows more light to enter the eyes from the sides often eliminates peripheral field constriction. The suggestible patient will glide undauntedly through an obstacle course as if using radar and may exhibit indifference to the alleged visual disability.

Visual Acuity Testing

If the visual loss is binocular, the following methods are used:

1. Test visual acuity binocularly starting with the 20/15 line, and express astonishment when the patient cannot read this. Next, offer the 20/20 line as a major concession and call the 20/25 line "huge."
2. Set up an obstacle course and observe how the patient follows you into another room.
3. Make grimaces at the patient and watch his or her reaction.
4. Move a hand-held mirror in front of the patient's face. It will be difficult for the seeing patient not to move their eyes (tracking his or her face) as the mirror moves.
5. Rotate an O.K.N. drum in front of the patient. Conscious inattention is necessary to avoid the development of optokinetic nystagmus.
6. Check for saccadic accuracy. Quickly and innocuously ask patients to "look here"; accuracy suggests good vision.

If the visual loss is monocular, use the following techniques:

1. Using a trial frame or phoropter, fog the seeing eye with a high plus lens and place a plano or -0.12 lens in front of the "nonseeing" eye.

2. Test for near stereovision using the Titmus or random dot E test. Excellent stereopsis is inconsistent with poor vision in one eye.
3. Test distance visual acuity with the vectograph stereo slide while the patient wears polarizing glasses.
4. Test visual acuity using the duochrome filter in the projector while the patient wears red-green glasses. The green lens should be placed over the good eye because the red letters are more difficult to see.
5. Test color vision using Ishihara color plates while the patient wears red-green glasses with the green lens over the good eye. The plates cannot be viewed through the green filter. Reading the plates indicates visual acuity of at least 10/200 in the suspected eye.
6. Test visual acuity with $+2.00$ and -2.00 diopter cylinders placed in front of each eye in a trial frame. Rotate them to neutralize each other in the "bad" eye, and add to each other in the "good" eye.
7. While the patient is reading, place a $+10.00$ diopter sphere in front of the "good" eye.
8. While the patient is reading aloud, place a 10 diopter base-out prism in front of the suspected eye. If it is being used, the eye will turn in; it will turn out again when the prism is removed.
9. While the patient is reading aloud, place a 10 diopter base-up or base-down prism in front of the suspected eye. This prism power exceeds vertical fusional ability. If the eye is being used reading will immediately become difficult or impossible.

Visual Field Abnormalities Suggestive of Functional Disorder

Visual field testing for functional visual loss should be performed using the following techniques with a tangent screen or Goldmann perimeter. Automated perimetry, as currently practiced, may not be able to differentiate functional from organic disorders.

1. *Spiraling fields:* Start the testing in one quadrant in the peripheral field. Mark a dot, and move to the next quadrant. Continue in a circular fashion; functional patients often constrict their visual field as the test progresses.
2. *Tubular fields:* Test the patient in front of a tangent screen at 1 m. Then move the patient back to 2 m. The visual field should widen the farther the patient sits from the tangent screen. The field of the functional patient may constrict as he or she is moved backward. Remember to increase the size of the test object when going to 2 m to keep the subtended arc the same.
3. *Enlargement of field following pupillary dilation:* Retest the visual field after dilating the pupils. The peripheral field may enlarge in suggestive patients.
4. *Monocular temporal hemianopsia:* When this occurs, recheck for the presence of a relative afferent pupillary defect or the persistence of the hemi-

anopsia on binocular testing. Check for saccadic accuracy by having the patient first look in the direction opposite the alleged hemianopsia and request that he or she then look at an object in the primary position, which should be the hemianopic field. Rule out chiasmal compression; look for junctional scotoma in opposite eye.

5. *Loss of previously defined blind spot:* The physiologic blind spot should be consistently reproduced.

6. *Geometric fields:* Suggestive patients may be talked into demonstrating triangular-, square-, or star-shaped visual fields. The use of pins on the tangent screen may be helpful.

Functional Visual Loss in Adults

Unlike children who present with a moderate reduction in visual acuity, adults with nonorganic visual disorders often present with "blindness" of one or both eyes. Similar to children, however, an array of associated signs and symptoms, including telltale nonorganic patterns of visual field loss, voluntary nystagmus, and spasm of the near reflex, is often present.

It is generally not advisable to confront the patient with the inconsistencies of the examination or to act in an accusatory fashion. Emphasis of positive findings is better than explanations of inconsistencies. The patient who directly confronts the physician regarding these generally needs reassurance. If substantial conflict remains, this patient may be the rare individual with functional visual loss in need of psychiatric assistance. Placebo treatments, including unnecessary glasses or eye exercises, should be avoided because they send mixed signals to the patient.

Similar to children, reassurance usually results in acceptance that the eyes are healthy. Unlike children, however, formal reexamination several years later may reveal repeated visual complaints and similar old patterns of visual loss or field constriction.

Functional Visual Loss in Children

Most children with this disorder demonstrate a moderate reduction in visual acuity ranging from 20/30 to 20/100. The symptoms are more often bilateral than unilateral, and associated symptoms, including voluntary nystagmus, spasm of the near reflex, and even bitemporal hemianopsia, can often be elicited.

Several studies have demonstrated that many affected children have significant family and/or school-related conflict. Initial attempts to elicit this connection may be met with frank parental denial or disbelief. It is often only months after resolution that this is recognized. Many children are of above-average intelligence and previously "A" students. Stressful home situations are also common, and several cases of physically or sexually abused children with this disorder have been reported.

The disorder is self-limited, but the duration of symptoms can be prolonged prior to diagnosis. Upon diagnosis and with reassurance to both the parents and child, symptoms resolve rapidly. Symptoms resolve in 25% of children within 1 day and 75% of affected children within 2 months (Catalano et al., 1986). There does not appear to be any correlation between the duration of symptoms prior to diagnosis and subsequent recovery time. Multiple anecdotal reports of resolution with hypnosis, plano glasses, placebo eyedrops or pills, and prayer meetings exist, but none has been proved more efficacious than reassurance alone. Furthermore, reassurance and parental support may lead to a more rapid resolution than benign neglect or punishment.

There is substantial disagreement in the literature regarding the need for and efficacy of psychiatric intervention. Referral is usually indicated when the complex of symptoms is indicative of a severe psychiatric disturbance, but often reassurance by a concerned ophthalmologist and parent(s) is the only treatment necessary. Recurrence of symptoms or the late onset of other somatic complaints is rare.

SPASM OF THE NEAR REFLEX

The near-synkinetic response physiologically and unconsciously occurs to correct the otherwise blurred retinal image of near objects. It can also occur secondary to a conscious awareness of near. The response consists of the triad of convergence of the eyes, pupillary constriction, and accommodation of the ocular lens (an increase in the thickness and surface curvature of the lens to increase the focusing power of the eye).

Spasm of the near reflex, also known as accommodative spasm, consists of an excessive or inappropriate near response for the visual fixation distance. Characteristically, both pupils are miotic (small), the eyes are turned in up to 50°, and the accommodative power of the eye is increased up to 10 diopters (Figure 15–1). The latter is confirmed by demonstrating less need for minus requirement (less myopia) on cycloplegic refraction (refraction using drops that paralyze the ability to accommodate) as compared to dry refractions. Invariably, it is difficult to maintain this spasm, and the typical patient presents with episodic or intermittent spasms lasting seconds to minutes. An occasional patient, however, may be able to maintain this for longer periods.

Patients with this disorder usually complain of headache, eye strain, blurred vision, and/or diplopia. Adults often give a history of head trauma. On examination, the spasm can often be precipitated by having the patient fixate an interesting (accommodative) near object, by manipulating the eyelids, or by requesting the patient gaze in a given direction. The most common misdiag-

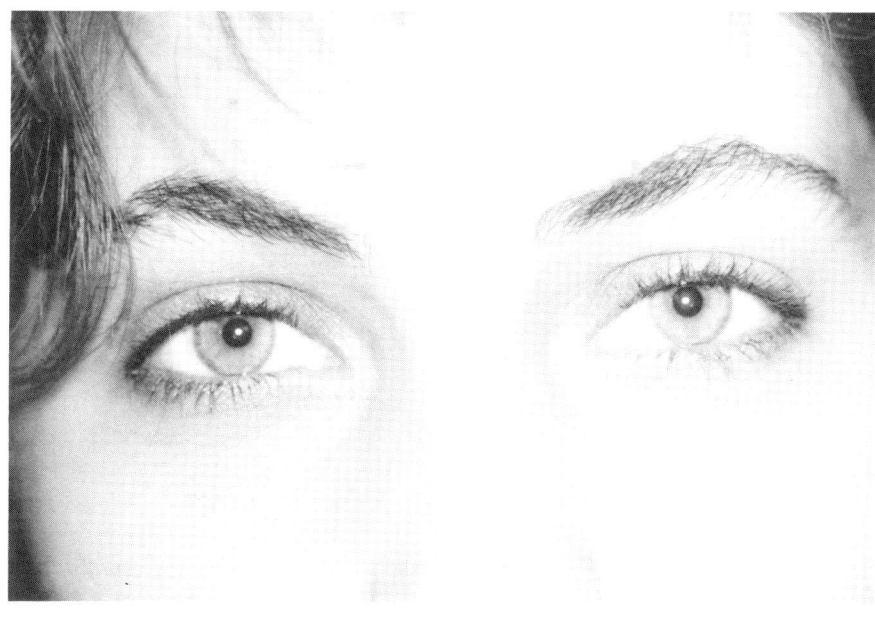

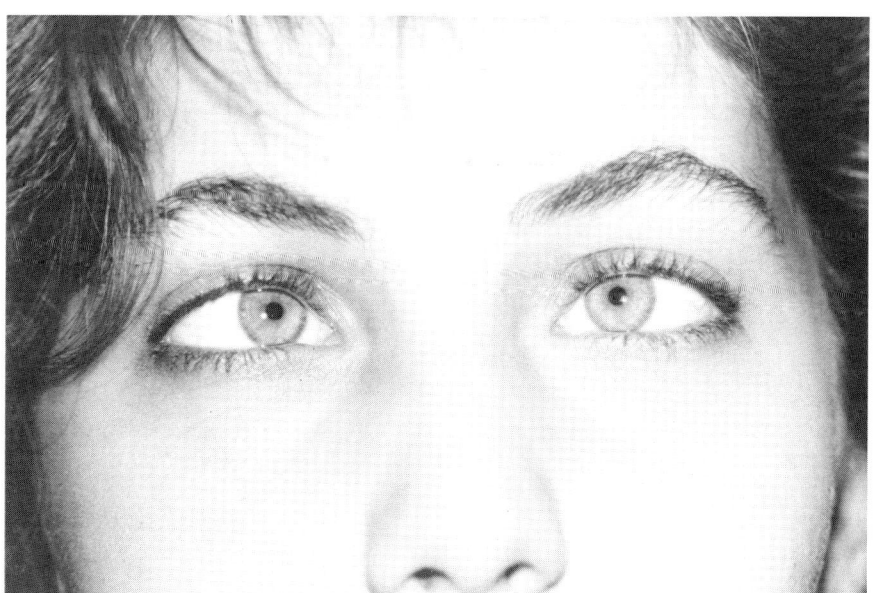

FIGURE 15–1. Spasm of the near reflex. Top: baseline state; bottom: miosis and esotropia (inward turning of the eyes) during spasm.

nosis in these patients is bilateral sixth nerve palsy. The intermittence of this condition, as well as the associated miosis and increased accommodation with these spasms, is suggestive against a sixth nerve disorder.

Organic spasms of the near reflex have rarely been reported (Table 15-2). Usually patients with organic etiologies have associated neurologic problems or are unaware of their symptoms because of depressed consciousness. Convergence spasm related to an accommodative factor can also rarely occur in children and even more rarely in adults. Treatment for a latent hyperopia resolves this problem.

VOLUNTARY NYSTAGMUS

Voluntary nystagmus is a rapid, high-frequency, small-amplitude, difficult-to-maintain, horizontal oscillation of the eyes. It gives the appearance of a fine rapid pendular nystagmus but actually consists of rapid right-to-left saccades. It can be recognized by its extreme rapidity (approximately 20 hertz) and the brevity of each episodic burst. Most subjects cannot sustain the oscillation for more than 10 seconds, and the maximum duration is estimated at less than 30 seconds. As many as 1% to 5% of the population may be able to generate these oscillations to some degree. There appears to be some hereditary influence, and it may be more common in individuals of British descent.

Unlike some of the other disorders discussed in this chapter, voluntary nystagmus is not a trait that develops or is seen in suggestive individuals. The subject has full appreciation of its occurrence and generates it either as a party trick or in a conscious effort to feign illness. Individuals with this ability were commonly seen in circus side shows of the past, and the medical literature cites many individuals who used this to be relieved from activities ranging from military duty to coal mining. It is now believed that "coal miner's nystagmus" commonly seen in British miners in the eighteenth and nineteenth centuries was, in fact, voluntary nystagmus.

The disorder can usually be easily recognized by its rapidity and the inability of the individual to maintain the oscillation for longer than a few seconds. Individuals who appear to be able to maintain this for prolonged periods should be observed closely. Usually they turn away from the observer, grimace, or intermittently close their eyes to rest their eyes between oscillatory bursts.

TABLE 15-2. ORGANIC CAUSES OF SPASM OF THE NEAR REFLEX

Accommodative factor	Pituitary tumor
Cerebellar tumor	Vestibulopathy
Arnold-Chiari malformation	Previous head trauma

FUNCTIONAL VISUAL HALLUCINATIONS

Visual hallucinations can be the result of lesions anywhere in the visual pathway. They can also accompany complicated migraine attacks, drug use or withdrawal, poisoning, psychosis, or sensory deprivation. Organic visual hallucinations are generally characterized as being secondary to either release or irritative phenomena. *Release hallucinations* typically last long periods of time (minutes to hours) and vary in pattern. They usually occur in the absence of other sensory or motor phenomena and typically in an area where the visual field is blind. *Irritative hallucinations* are briefer, stereotypically repetitive, and associated with other sensory or motor symptoms or signs. Chapter 13 reviews the organic causes of visual hallucinations.

Unlike most of the other disorders discussed in this chapter, *functional hallucination* is not a well-defined entity. The term has been used to describe any isolated, well-formed visual hallucination. The only nonpsychotic, non-drug related hallucinations that may appropriately be classified as functional (in concert with the other disorders in this chapter) are the occasional hallucinations reported by some children with behavioral problems associated with situational stress. Even this entity, however, overlaps with psychotic hallucinations.

Hallucinations secondary to sensory deprivation (sundowning) are generally well recognized in the context of the situation. They are described further in Chapter 13; they represent transient psychotic episodes associated with agitation, confusion, and hyperactivity.

The physician treating emergency patients must recognize common descriptions of hallucinogenic drug use. These generally induce one of four types of images or forms:

1. Well-defined patterns such as gratings, lattices, honeycombs, or chessboards.
2. Cobwebs.
3. Tunnels, alleys, or cones.
4. Spirals.

Images are often reported as located at a reading distance. They may vary in color saturation and often are described as intensely bright and symmetrical. During the peak hallucinatory period, individuals frequently report becoming part of the imagery and being dissociated from their bodies. Rapid changes in imagery (as many as 10 changes per second) may occur at the peak, during which time individuals may believe the images are real.

It is also important to recognize some additional organic causes of formed visual hallucinations, which are distinguished by accompanying signs and symptoms. Hallucinations due to temporal lobe disease may be accompanied by the sensation of smelling foul odors or seizure activity. The hallucinations of complicated migraine headaches often involve the distortion of body parts and may follow a typical headache or be accompanied by olfactory, gustatory, or auditory hallucinations. Hallucinations from insulin hypoglycemia are similar to sensory deprivation hallucinations in being associated with disorientation and agitation and are accompanied by signs of epinephrine release, including shakiness, sweating, palpatation, anxiety, nausea, and vomiting. They are alleviated promptly with correction of the hypoglycemia.

Ocular motility testing may be helpful in distinguishing functional from organic hallucinations when the alleged hallucination moves. Patients with organic hallucinations can usually generate smooth pursuit movements (usually horizontal) to follow the movement of the hallucination. Functional patients cannot and usually execute a series of repeating saccades (often vertical) when asked to follow the movement.

FUNCTIONAL PUPILLARY ABNORMALITIES

Functional pupillary abnormalities consist of the dilation or constriction of one or both pupils. They occasionally occur innocuously in individuals who care for others and inadvertently instill miotic or mydriatic eyedrops in their own eyes. The disorder is functional only when it occurs secondary to malingering or when a highly suggestive individual believes this represents a pathologic condition.

The workup of individuals with pupillary abnormalities is given in Chapter 13. Attention should be especially directed to the flowchart used for patients with anisocoria (Figure 13–8). The small pupil that follows miotic instillation dilates poorly, if at all, in dim illumination. The large pupil that follows mydriatic instillation does not constrict to light or the near reflex. It constricts asymmetrically, if at all, to the instillation of pilocarpine 1%.

PHOTOPHOBIA

A variety of ocular conditions can cause scattering of light rays and glare. Physiologically, this causes squinting or blepharospasm, as well as pupillary constriction. Organic causes of the sudden onset of photophobia are discussed in Chapter 13 and include abnormalities of the cornea, lens, retina, or optic nerve. Central nervous system diseases or disorders and toxic or drug-induced punctate corneal erosions can also induce photophobia.

Photophobia, or light-sensitive eyes, is a common complaint. Bright lights and glare are annoying to any individual with good vision. An individual's tolerance for discomfort is typically the deciding factor between those who complain of photophobia and those who recognize its physiologic significance. It is also not unusual for parents to have their child examined solely for the complaint of photophobia. True ocular pathology is usually not found, but particular attention should be paid to cone degenerations or dystrophies and strabismus. Many children with an intermittent strabismus close one or both eyes (usually always the same one) upon going from indoors to outdoors. Additionally, a few children with posterior fossa tumors have been reported as presenting with photophobia, epiphora (tearing), and torticollis (head tilt).

FUNCTIONAL HEADACHES

Organic causes of headache are discussed in Chapter 13. The term *functional headaches* is used by some clinicians to refer to "tension" or situational stress-induced headaches. "Tension" are the most commonly encountered headaches; they tend to occur in multiple family members. A history of inescapable unpleasant circumstances is often elicited.

Even young children can develop tension headaches. Usually there is a family history of one or both parents reacting in a similar fashion to situational stress. To distinguish tension from more serious organic causes of headache, it is helpful to observe the child's activity level during the headache episode. Tension headaches do not usually prevent a child from participating in activities that he or she normally finds enjoyable (such as watching television). Furthermore, the pain in tension headaches is not usually severe enough to cause the child to cry.

FUNCTIONAL BLINKING

Organic causes of excessive blinking are discussed in Chapter 13. These include ocular conditions associated with pain, photophobia, systemic conditions (e.g., hypoparathyroidism, Gilles de la Tourette syndrome, and tardive dyskinesia) and facial musculature syndromes (e.g., essential blepharospasm and hemifacial spasm).

Some clinicians use the term *functional blinking* to describe the benign episodic twitches of facial myokymia that are related to situational stress. Others reserve it for children who present with the isolated symptom of excessive blinking without other ocular or systemic signs or symptoms and without baseline undulations of the orbicularis oculi muscle. Functional blinking is seen in young children, with an increased incidence in those age 3 to 7 years. Unlike functional visual loss, females are not predominantly affected. Furthermore, a temporally related stressful event can be identified in fewer than half of these children. In the majority of cases, the main secondary gain for the child is increased attention from the caretaker. Similar to functional visual loss and eyelid pulling (Table 15–3), complete resolution of symptoms occurs within 1 day to 3 months in most children given reassurance only. Placebo treatments and psychiatric intervention are seldom, if ever, warranted. Recurrence of blinking or the development of other functional disorders is rare. The latter usually take the form of nose wrinkling, nose rubbing, or ear pulling.

TABLE 15-3. FUNCTIONAL VISUAL DISORDERS OF CHILDREN

	FUNCTIONAL VISUAL LOSS	FUNCTIONAL BLINKING	FUNCTIONAL EYELID PULLING
Associated stresses	Conflict at home or school, abuse	None usually identified	None usually identified
Other symptoms	Common	Rare	Rare
Affected sex	Female > male	Female = male	Female = male
Average age	9–12 years	3–7 years	5–9 years
Resolution with reassurance	Within 2 months in 75%	Usually rapid (day to weeks)	Usually rapid (day to weeks)
Recurrences	Rare	Rare	Rare

FUNCTIONAL EYELID PULLING

Individuals pull on their eyelids for several reasons. Usually they are trying to relieve ocular irritation secondary to misdirected eyelashes, a foreign body, or an inflammatory disorder of the eyelid. Occasionally, they are trying to create a stenopeic slit to reduce an uncorrected refractive error or relieve diplopia related to a strabismic disorder. On rare occasions, children may pull on their eyelids in the absence of an underlying ocular or systemic disease (Figure 15–2).

The mean age of children who do this is 7 years, and, like functional blinking, there is no female predominance. Children appear to do this to gain attention or because their eyes were initially irritated and they developed the habit. When questioned, children may say they do this to "look funny" or because their "eyes are not opening enough." They often cite other children who do the same. Similar to functional blinking but again unlike functional visual loss in children, there is usually no temporally related or recognized stressful event.

Resolution of symptoms occurs quickly (usually within 2 weeks) upon the physician's reassurance. Recurrences of this, as with other functional disorders in children, are rare.

FUNCTIONAL EYELASH AND EYEBROW PLUCKING

Eyelash and eyebrow plucking is a common habit. Often it is done cosmetically, and commonly it occurs as a neurotic bad habit. It should be considered functional only when the patient is not consciously aware of the habit or when

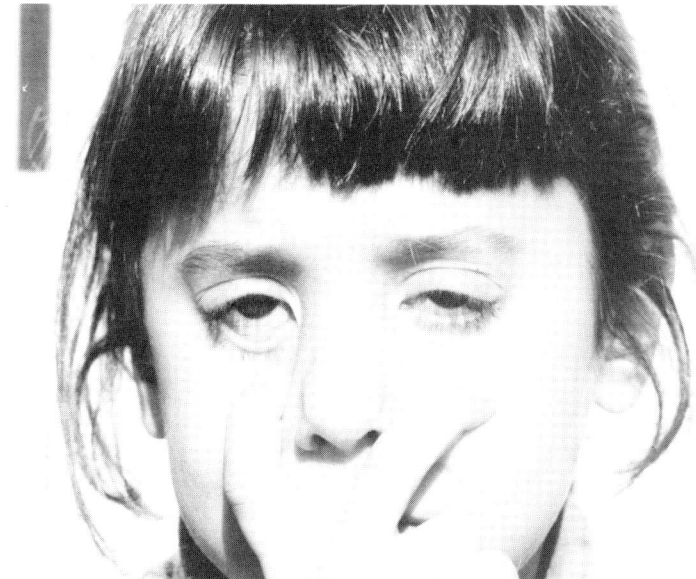

FIGURE 15-2. Functional eyelash and eyebrow pulling.

the vigor with which it is done suggests a severe underlying systemic or emotional disorder (Figure 15-3). Severely affected individuals also tend to pull out their scalp hair. Counseling may be required.

VOLUNTARY PROPULSION OF THE EYEBALLS

Voluntary propulsion of the eyeballs (eye popping) is often pseudo-propulsion due to an exaggerated ability to raise the upper eyelid and depress the lower eyelid, creating the appearance of forward movement of the eye. It is more easily performed by individuals with shallow orbits and rarely can be induced iatrogenically by physicians who flip the upper eyelid of a patient to search for a foreign body. As with patients who can volitionally induce nystagmus, individuals with this ability were often seen in circus side shows of the past.

Rarely, an individual is described who can truly propulse his or her eyes. Repetitive performance of this dangerous practice is highly suggestive of a psychotic or borderline personality disorder. It may be a forme fruste of autoenucleation. Usually the patient performs the maneuver by squeezing the globe from above and below with finger pressure. Reports of patients who do this have noted the development of extremely high intraocular pressures, dilated pupils, and anterior and posterior segment ischemia in the propulsed eye. Optic nerve damage and blindness can result.

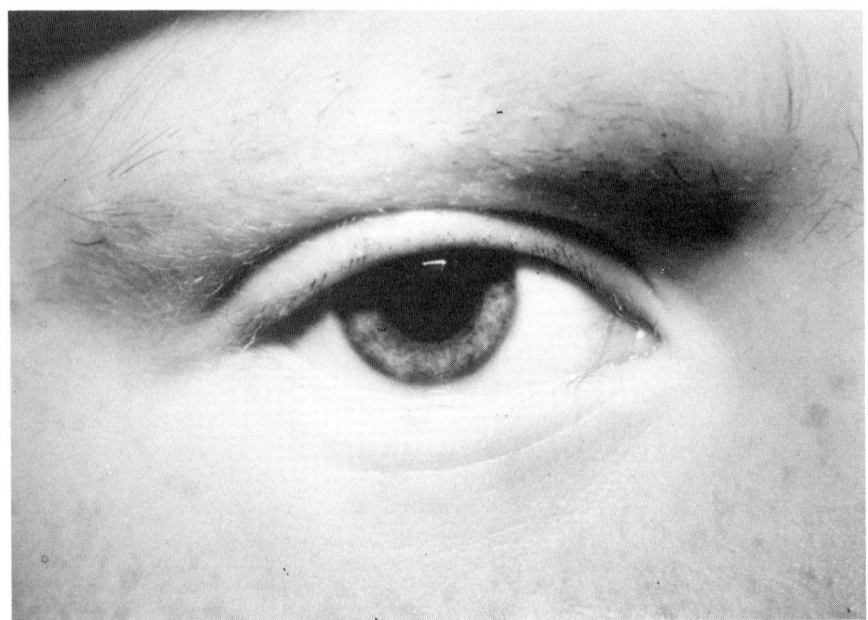

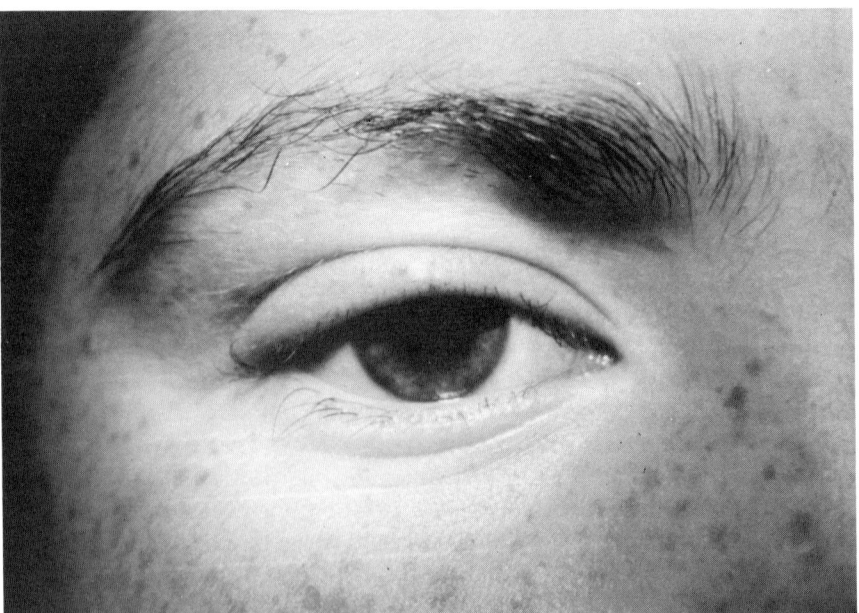

FIGURE 15-3. Functional eyelash and eyebrow plucking. Top: self-epilation of eyelashes and eyebrows; bottom: three months later after counseling. (Photographs courtesy of Maury A. Marmor, M.D.)

OCULAR MUNCHAUSEN'S SYNDROME

Munchausen's syndrome is used to describe individuals who deliberately attempt to deceive physicians through fictitious or misrepresented signs and symptoms. They often successfully simulate true disease states and subject themselves to numerous inappropriate medical and surgical interventions before the diagnosis of Munchausen's syndrome is made. As opposed to malingerers, the potential secondary gain of patients with this disorder is not readily apparent. Furthermore, these patients commonly self-inflict injuries. In contrast, the malingerer may accentuate the claim of disability from an existing condition but will not self-inflict further injury. Munchausen patients may knowingly deceive but appear unable to control their actions.

Reported self-induced injuries include subconjunctival hemorrhages, injection of air, fecal material, or other foreign bodies into the orbit, alkali burns to the cornea, autoenucleation, and retinal detachments induced by eye rubbing. In addition to ocular signs and symptoms, these patients often feign or cause other illness, such as deafness and aspiration pneumonia.

Psychiatric remediation in Munchausen's syndrome is often disappointing. Over the course of their lives, these patients often resort to further self-mutilation. It is noteworthy that prior to the development of ocular symptoms, many of these patients will have been previously diagnosed as having schizophrenia or a borderline personality disorder. Additionally, these individuals may commonly be employed as health professionals. Familiarity with the health care system and easy access to medical instruments may enable them to carry out their deceptions more successfully.

PSYCHOTIC SELF-MUTILATION (AUTOENUCLEATION)

> . . . if thy right eye offend thee, pluck it out and cast it out from thee.—Matthew 5:29.

Individuals who self-mutilate their eyes are always suffering from a severe psychosis. They often give Matthew's admonishment as the reason for their action. The disorder is also called *Oedipism,* from the Greek tragedy in which Oedipus tore out his eyes upon learning that the oracle's prediction that he would kill his father and marry his mother had come true.

Krauss, Yee, and Foos (1984) historically reviewed the disorder and found that the age range of reported patients was age 15 to 53 years, with a peak incidence in the third and fourth decades. It occurred as often in males as females, and approximately 40% of reported cases were bilateral. In 75% of cases, the act was committed by patients already under psychiatric care. The majority carried the diagnosis of chronic psychotic depression or schizophrenia, and auditory and visual hallucinations were common in these individuals. Self-enucleation was predominantly carried out using only one's own fingers.

Numerous reports also exist of individuals who self-mutilated but fell short of autoenucleation. Descriptions of injuries similar to those induced by individuals with ocular Munchausen's syndrome exist. The two disorders may overlap, but those who readily admit their action (usually for delusional reasons) are generally diagnosed as having an acute psychosis.

REFERENCES

Blinking

Vrabec TR, Levin AV, Nelson LB: Functional blinking in childhood. *Pediatrics* 83:967, 1989.

Eyelid Pulling

Catalano RA, Trevisani MG, Simon JW: Functional eyelid pulling in children. *Am J Ophthalmol* 110:300, 1990.

Hallucinations

Gittinger JW Jr: Sugarplum fairies. Visual hallucinations. *Surv Ophthalmol* 27:42, 1982.
Lessell S, Currie JN: Ocular motility testing in the evaluation of visual hallucinations. *Am J Ophthalmol* 95:772, 1983.
Lukianowicz N: Hallucinations in non-psychotic children. *Psychiatr Clin* 2:321, 1969.
Siegel RK: Hallucinations. In *The Mind's Eye: Readings from Scientific American.* New York, WH Freeman and Co, 1986, pp 109–116.

Photophobia

Marmor MA, Beauchamp GR, Maddox SF: Photophobia, epiphora, and torticollis: A masquerade syndrome. *J Pediatr Ophthalmol Strabismus* 27:202, 1990.
Wiggins RE, von Noorden GK: Monocular eye closure in sunlight. *J Pediatr Ophthalmol Strabismus* 27:16, 1990.

Propulsion of the Eyeballs

Berma B: Voluntary propulsion of the eyeballs. *Arch Intern Med* 117:648, 1966.
Slamovits T: Popping eyes. *Surv Ophthalmol* 33:273, 1989.
Tamai M, Mizuno K, Okuyama S: Self-inflicted proptosis misdiagnosed as orbital malignancy. *Am J Ophthalmol* 96:812, 1983.

Psychotic Self-mutilation

Ananth J, Kaplan HS, Lin KM: Self-inflicted enucleation of an eye: Two case reports. *Can J Psychiatry* 29:145, 1984.
Duke-Elder S: Self-inflicted injuries. In Duke-Elder S: *System of Ophthalmology.* St Louis, CV Mosby, 1972, 14:56–58.
Khan JA, Buescher L, Ide CH, et al: Medical management of self-enucleation. *Arch Ophthalmol* 103:386, 1985.
Krauss HR, Yee RD, Foos RJ: Autoenucleation. *Surv Ophthalmol* 29:179, 1984.
MacLean G, Robertson BM: Self enucleation and psychosis. *Arch Gen Psychiatr* 33:242, 1976.
Moskovitz RA, Byrd T: Rescuing the angle within: PCP-related self enucleation. *Psychosomatics* 24:402, 1983.

Noel LP, Clarke WN: Self-inflicted ocular injuries in children. *Am J Ophthalmol* 94:630, 1982.
Rosenberg PN, Krohel GB, Webb RM, Hepler RS: Ocular Munchausen's syndrome. *Ophthalmology* 93:1120, 1986.
Stannard K, Leonard T, Holder G, et al: Oedipism reviewed: A case of bilateral ocular self-mutilation. *Br J Ophthalmol* 68:276, 1984.
Whitherspoon CD, Feist FW, Morris RE, Feist RM: Ocular self-mutilation. *Ann Ophthalmol* 21:255, 1989.
Winans JM, House LR, Robinson HE: Self-induced orbital emphysema as a presenting sign of Munchausen's syndrome. *Laryngoscope* 93:1209, 1983.
Yang HK, Brown GC, Margargal LE: Self-inflicted ocular mutilation. *Am J Ophthalmol* 91:658, 1981.

Spasm of the Near Reflex

Cogan DG, Freese CG Jr: Spasm of the near reflex. *Arch Ophthalmol* 54:752, 1955.
Dagi LR, Chrousos GA, Cogan DC: Spasm of the nerve reflex associated with organic disease. *Am J Ophthalmol* 103:582, 1987.
Guiloff RJ: Organic convergence spasm. *Acta Neurol Scandinav* 61:252, 1980.
Herman P: Convergence spasm. *Mt Sinai J Med* 44:501, 1977.
Jeanrot N: Convergence spasms in the adult. *J Fr Ophthalmol* 10:135, 1987.

Visual Loss

Catalano RA, Simon JW, Krohel GB, Rosenberg PN: Functional visual loss in children. *Ophthalmology* 93:385, 1986.
Costenbader FD, Mousel DK: Functional amblyopia in early adolescence. *Clin Proc Child Hosp* 20:49, 1964.
Donin JF: The ophthalmic flake syndrome. In Smith JL (ed): *Neuro-ophthalmology 1982.* New York: Masson, 1981, pp 89–98.
Drews RC: Organic versus functional ocular problems. *Inter Ophthalmol Clinics* 7:666, 1967.
Gittinger JW Jr: Functional monocular temporal hemianopsia. *Am J Ophthalmol* 101:226, 1986.
Gittinger JW Jr: Functional hemianopsia: A historical perspective. *Surv Ophthalmol* 32:427, 1988.
Kathol RG, Cox TA, Corbett JJ, Thompson HS: Functional visual loss; follow-up of 42 cases. *Arch Ophthalmol* 101:729, 1983.
Keltner JL, May WN, Johnson CA, Post RB: The California syndrome: Functional visual complaints with potential economic impact. *Ophthalmology* 92:427, 1985.
Kramer KK, LaPiana FG, Appleton B: Ocular malingering and hysteria: Diagnosis and management. *Surv Ophthalmol* 24:89, 1979.
Miller BW: A review of practical tests for ocular malingering and hysteria. *Surv Ophthalmol* 17:241, 1973.
Rada RT, Meyer GG, Kellner R: Visual conversion reaction in children and adults. *J Nerv Ment Dis* 166:580, 1978.
Savir H, Segal M: A simple test for detection of monocular functional visual impairment. *Am J Ophthalmol* 106:500, 1988.
Smith TJ, Baker RS: Perimetric findings in functional disorders using automated techniques. *Ophthalmology* 94:1562, 1987.
Thompson HS: Functional visual loss. *Am J Ophthalmol* 100:209, 1985.
Weintraub MI: *Hysterical Conversion Reactions.* Jamaica, NY, Spectrum Publications, 1983.

Voluntary Nystagmus

Aschoff JC, Becker W, Rettelbach R: Voluntary nystagmus, saccadic suppression, and stabilization of the visual world. *Vision Res* 20:717, 1980.
Shults WT, Stark L, Hoyt WF, et al: Normal saccadic structure and voluntary nystagmus. *Arch Ophthalmol* 95:1399, 1977.
Zahn JR: Incidence and characteristics of voluntary nystagmus. *J Neurol Neurosurg Psychiatry* 41:617, 1978.

IV

Infections/ Antibiotics/ Corticosteroids/ Tetanus

16

Ocular Infections and Inflammation

David Litoff
Michael W. Belin

OPHTHALMIA NEONATORUM

Ophthalmia neonatorum is conjunctivitis that occurs within the first month of life. It presents as diffuse conjunctival injection, swelling (chemosis), lid edema, and a purulent or watery discharge. (Figure 16-1). Its multiple etiologies include silver nitrate, *Chlamydia trachomatis, Neisseria gonorrhea, Herpes simplex,* and other bacteria. Prompt diagnosis is essential to prevent visual loss or a life-threatening systemic infection.

Evaluation

When evaluating ophthalmia neonatorum, a complete history is essential, including: time of onset, presence of venereal disease in the parents, contact with any other individuals with conjunctivitis, bilateral or unilateral presentation, and overall general health of the neonate. The initial workup includes conjunctival scrapings for Gram's and Giemsa stains; blood, chocolate, Thayer-Martin, and viral cultures; and a Chlamydia rapid identification test (Table 16-1). Table 16-2 presents differential clinical findings in ophthalmia neonatorum.

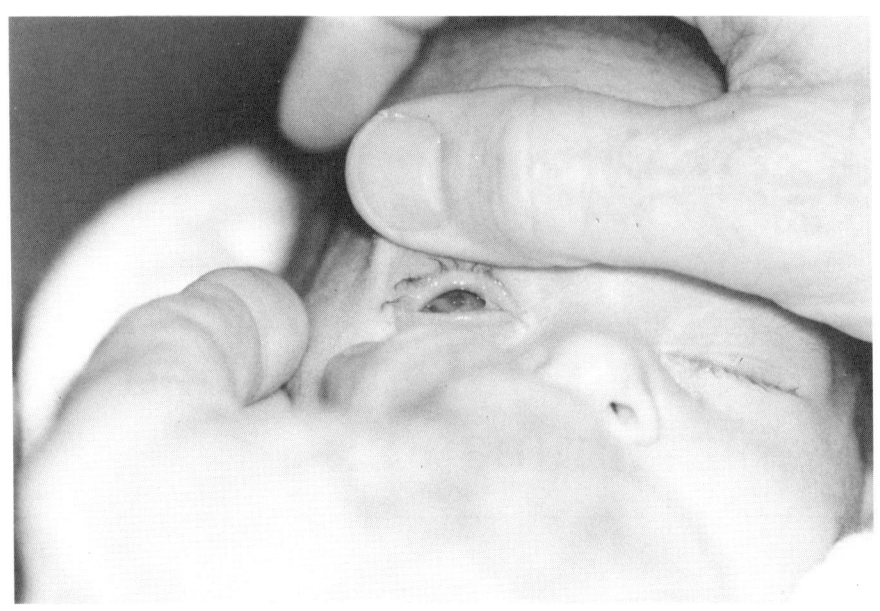

FIGURE 16-1. Ophthalmia neonatorum due to Chlamydia infection.

TABLE 16-1. MICROBIOLOGIC MEDIA AND STAINS FOR INVESTIGATION OF OPHTHALMIA NEONATORUM

MEDIA	USE
Blood agar	All-purpose medium useful for most bacteria and fungi
Chocolate agar	Neisseria and Hemophilus
Thayer-Martin	Neisseria
Viral culture	Viruses
Chlamydia test	Chlamydia
Gram's stain	Bacteria and fungi
Giemsa stain	Chlamydia

TABLE 16-2. DIFFERENTIAL CLINICAL FINDINGS IN OPHTHALMIA NEONATORUM

DIAGNOSIS	TIME OF ONSET	DISCHARGE	GRAM'S STAIN/GIEMSA STAIN	RAPID TEST CHLAMYDIA
Silver nitrate	2–36 hr	Minimal	No cells or bacteria	Negative
Chlamydia	1–2 wk	Mucopurulent	Inclusion bodies	Positive
Bacterial	3–30 days	Purulent	Bacteria	Negative
Gonococcal	2–5 days	Purulent	Gram-negative diplococci	Negative
Herpes	1–14 days	Mucopurulent	Giant cells	Negative

Silver Nitrate

Silver nitrate 1% solution is commonly used at birth as a prophylaxis against ophthalmia neonatorum. Its use is required by law in some states. Recently, there has been a trend toward using erythromycin ointment because the latter also covers Chlamydia. While silver nitrate has dramatically reduced the incidence of *N. gonorrhea* from approximately 10% to 0.3%, it may cause a toxic conjunctivitis. This usually presents as a diffuse bilateral conjunctivitis occurring several hours after birth and lasting up to 36 hours. This is the most common cause of ophthalmia neonatorum at institutions where silver nitrate is used; it has no significant sequela and resolves rapidly. The neonate should be reevaluated every 12 hours until resolution; if this has not resolved within 36 hours, an alternate diagnosis should be considered.

Infectious Conjunctivitis

Chlamydia trachomatis is the most common cause of infectious ophthalmia neonatorum. It usually occurs 1 week to 2 weeks after birth, most commonly during the second week. Chlamydia conjunctivitis typically presents as a mild unilateral or bilateral mucopurulent conjunctivitis. Unlike adults, neonates cannot develop a follicular reaction; a papillary reaction, however, can be seen. The diagnosis of Chlamydia can be made by culture, the identification of intracytoplasmic paranuclear inclusion bodies on a Giemsa stain of a conjunctival scraping (Figure 16-2), a positive immunofluorescent test using monoclonal antibodies, or an enzyme-linked immunoassay.

Systemic antibiotics are required because 10% to 30% of untreated neonates develop Chlamydia pneumonitis, which is potentially fatal. The recommended treatment is erythromycin syrup 50 mg/kg per day in four divided doses with topical erythromycin or sulfacetamide ointment four times daily for 2 weeks to 3 weeks. In addition, the mother and her sexual partner(s) should be treated with erythromycin 250 mg to 500 mg 4 times daily or tetracycline 250 mg to 500 mg 4 times daily for 7 days. Tetracycline should not be given to nursing mothers.

Common causes of nongonococcal bacterial conjunctivitis in the neonate include *Staphylococcus aureus, Streptococcus pneumonia, Escherichia coli, Pseudomonas aeruginosa, Klebsiella pneumonia, Proteus mirabilis, Enterobacter species, Serratia marscens,* and *Hemophilus influenza*. Bacterial conjunctivitis occurs 3 days to 30 days after delivery. Risk factors for its development include lacrimal duct obstruction and corneal abrasions. The diagnosis is made with Gram's stain and culture. Initial treatment for gram-positive organisms includes erythromycin or bacitracin ointment, and for gram-negative organisms, gentamicin or tobramycin ointment, 4 times daily for 7 days. The final antibiotic selection is based on culture and sensitivity results.

Gonococcal infections are contracted when the neonate is exposed to

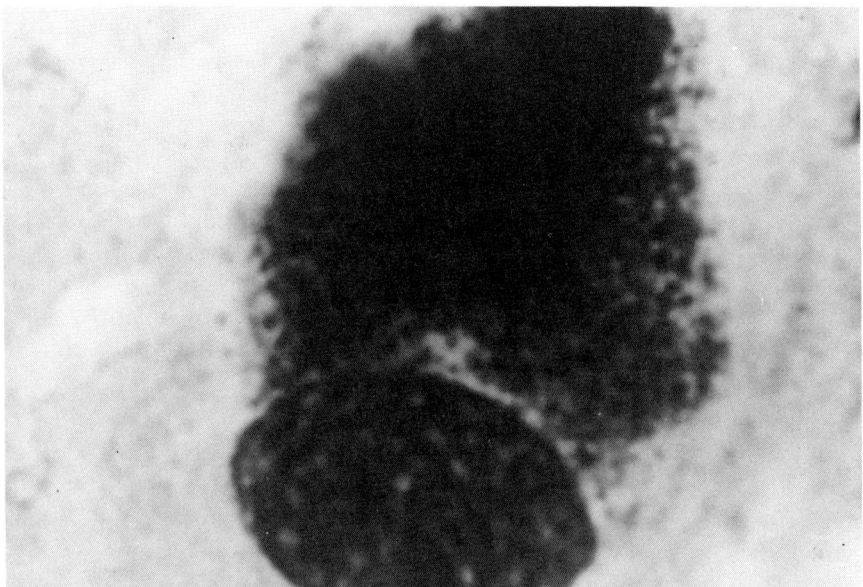

FIGURE 16-2. Intracytoplasmic paranuclear inclusion bodies seen on a Giemsa stain of conjunctival scraping in a patient with Chlamydia conjunctivitis.

infected maternal vaginal discharge. Infants born by cesarean section are at risk if premature rupture of the membranes has occurred. Gonococcal ophthalmia neonatorum usually presents as a hyperacute conjunctivitis with a thick purulent discharge 2 days to 5 days after birth (Figure 16-3). In rare instances, the presentation is delayed until up to 3 weeks following delivery. Gonococcal ophthalmia neonatorum is a severe infection; without prompt treatment, corneal perforation and blindness may result. The diagnosis is made by Gram's stain smears of the conjunctival exudate, which reveal multiple polymorphonucleocytes with gram-negative intracellular diplococci (Figure 16-4). Culture on chocolate agar or Thayer-Martin is mandatory for the definitive diagnosis and antibiotic sensitivities. An immunoassay is also available for rapid diagnosis. Infants with suspected *N. gonorrhea* should be hospitalized and isolated. The current recommended treatment is ceftriaxone 50 mg/kg to 100 mg/kg per day intravenously (IV) in two divided doses for 1 week or a single dose of 125 mg intramuscularly (IM). Additional therapy should include topical bacitracin ointment 4 times daily and periodic topical saline irrigation. If corneal involvement is present, scopolamine ¼% 3 times daily should be added. In addition, all neonates with gonococcal ophthalmia neonatorum should be prophylaxed for Chlamydia with erythromycin syrup 50 mg/kg per day in four divided doses for 2 weeks. A serological test for syphilis should also be performed.

Herpes simplex ophthalmia neonatorum often presents within the first 2

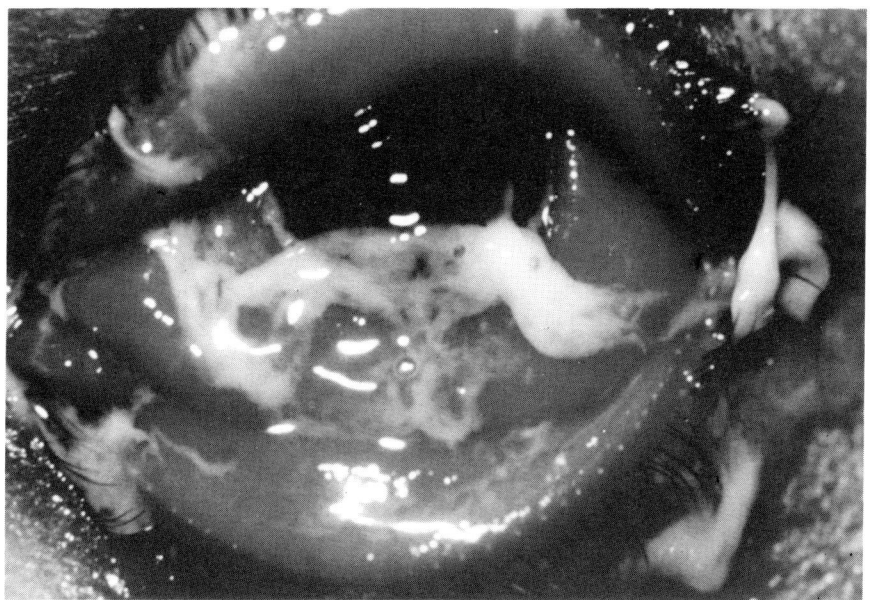

FIGURE 16-3. Neisseria gonococcal conjunctivitis.

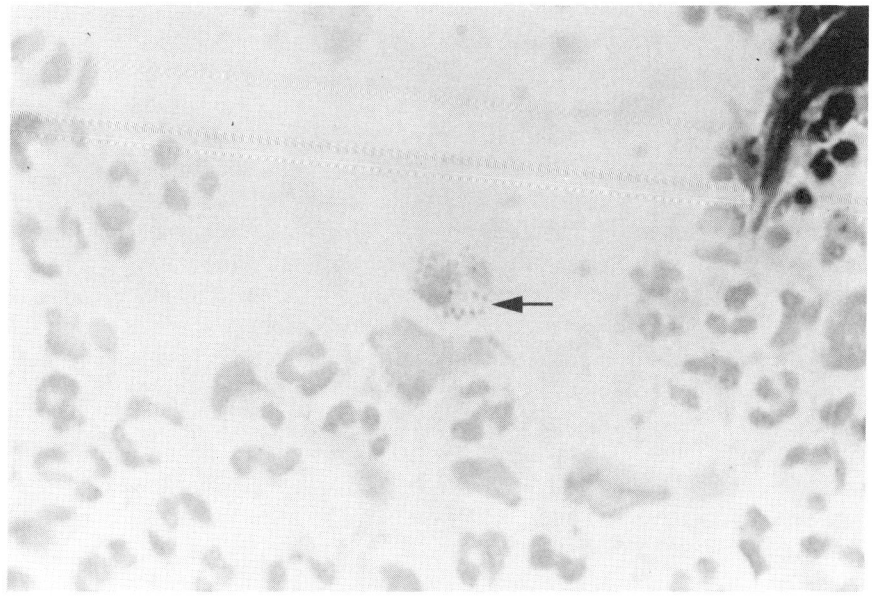

FIGURE 16-4. Gram-negative diplococci (gonococci).

weeks of age as keratoconjunctivitis with a mucupurulent discharge, lid edema, and chemosis. There may also be a typical herpetic vesicle on the eyelid. Diagnosis can be made by identifying multinucleated giant cells on a Giemsa stain of a conjunctival scraping or by direct viral cultures. Systemic involvement may occur with herpetic ophthalmia neonatorum, and the mortality rate of disseminated neonatal *H. simplex* infections approaches 50%. The diagnosis is made by viral culture, and the treatment consists of topical trifluridine (Viroptic) beginning at 9 times per day with a gradual taper. Systemic involvement requires concomitant intravenous acyclovir managed by a pediatric infectious disease consultant.

INFECTIOUS DISORDERS

Orbital Infections

Preseptal cellulitis, an infection that involves the eyelids and periorbital area anterior to the orbital septum, is often preceded by facial trauma, local skin infections, and/or upper respiratory tract or middle ear infections. The patient presents with erythema, swelling, and tenderness of the eyelids and periorbital area. Conjunctivitis and chemosis may be present. Abnormal pupillary reaction, proptosis, ophthalmoplegia, and decreased visual acuity are indicative of orbital involvement (orbital cellulitis).

Preseptal cellulitis in children usually occurs secondary to an upper respiratory tract or middle ear infection with subsequent spread to the preseptal area via blood vessels or lymphatics. *H. influenza, S. aureus,* and *S. pneumoniae* are the most common bacterial causes of preseptal cellulitis in this age group. Blood cultures are positive in 4% to 58%, and conjunctival cultures are occasionally helpful when blood cultures are negative.

Posttraumatic preseptal cellulitis follows periorbital puncture wounds and lacerations. The common etiologic agents are *S. aureus* and *S. pyogenes.* Other causes include anaerobic bacteria, *S. epidermidis,* and polymicrobial infections. The diagnosis is principally clinical. A computed tomography (CT) scan should be obtained, however, if the globe cannot be adequately examined or if there is any suspicion of penetration of the orbital septum. In cases of suppurative preseptal cellulitis, incision and drainage of the abscess should be performed and Gram's stain and cultures obtained. Selection of the initial antibiotic coverage is based on the Gram's stain.

Preseptal cellulitis can be associated with skin infections, including impetigo, erysipelas, and secondary bacterial infections of other dermatologic disorders (e.g., viral exanthems and allergic dermatitis). The principal organisms are *S. aureus, S. pyogenes,* other streptococci, anaerobes, and, rarely, gram-negative bacilli.

Patients over age 5 years can be treated on an outpatient basis. Hospitalization with IV antibiotics is recommended in children under age 5 years because in infants preseptal cellulitis can rapidly progress to orbital cellulitis or meningitis. For patients over age 5 years, Augmentin or Ceclor for 10 days (children: 20 mg/kg-40 mg/kg per day in three divided doses; adults: 500 mg 3 times daily) is recommended. In penicillin-allergic patients, Bactrim (children: 8/40 mg/kg per day in two divided doses; adults: 160/800 mg 2 times daily) or erythromycin (children: 30 mg/kg to 50 mg/kg per day in four divided doses; adults: 500 mg 4 times daily) is recommended. If the patient is under age 5 years or the preseptal cellulitis is not responding to outpatient therapy, hospitalization with intravenous nafcillin or oxacillin (children: 150 mg/kg per day in four divided doses; adults: 1 g to 2 g IV every 4 hours) with ceftazidime (children: 90 mg/kg to 150 mg/kg per day in three divided doses; adults: 1 g to 2 g IV every 8 hours) for 10 days to 14 days is recommended. Warm compresses and broad-spectrum topical antibiotics may also be helpful. In traumatic cases, tetanus prophylaxis should be given as outlined in Chapter 17.

Orbital cellulitis is an infection that involves structures posterior to the orbital septum (Figure 16-5). In addition to the signs and symptoms of preseptal cellulitis, proptosis, ophthalmoplegia (reduced eye movements), pain, abnormal pupillary reaction, decreased vision, diplopia, and fever may be present. Immediate diagnosis and treatment is essential because cavernous sinus thrombosis, meningitis, or brain abscess can occur. The most common etiol-

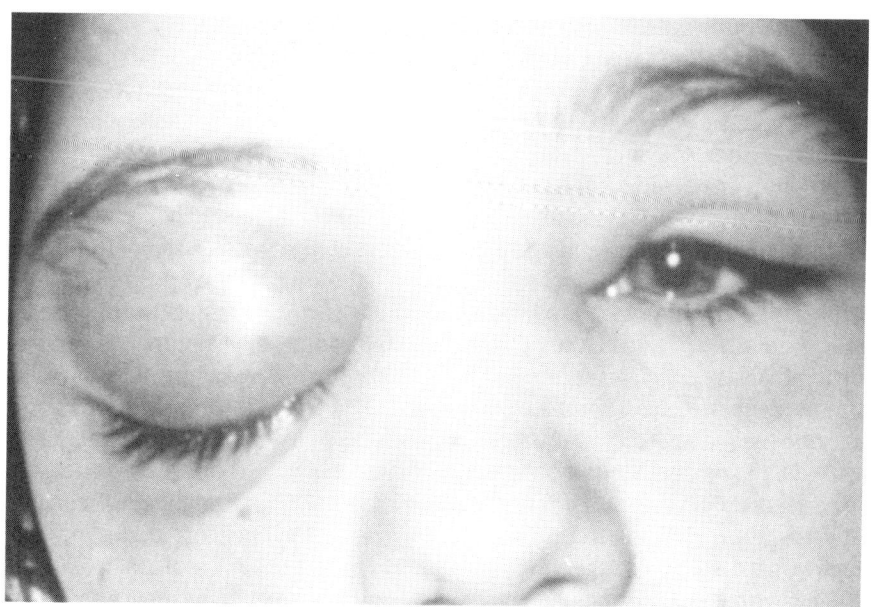

FIGURE 16-5. Orbital cellulitis.

ogy is direct extension from sinusitis, most commonly ethmoiditis. This is responsible for 75% of cases of orbital cellulitis. Infection related to trauma is responsible for 5% of orbital cellulitis, and the remaining 20% is idiopathic. The most common bacteria are *S. aureus,* streptococci, *H. influenza,* and *S. pneumonia.*

The indications for orbital CT in orbital cellulitis are discussed in Chapter 12. Blood and nasal cultures, followed by immediate high-dose IV antibiotics, are mandatory. A multispecialty approach with involvement of an ophthalmologist, otolaryngologist, internist or pediatrician, and neurosurgeon (if a brain abscess is present) is necessary. The treatment of orbital cellulitis in children includes hospitalization with intravenous nafcillin (150 mg/kg per day divided every 4 hours) or vancomycin (40 mg/kg per day in two divided doses) with ceftazidime (150 mg/kg per day in three divided doses). For adults, ceftazidime (3 g to 6 g 3 times daily) or gentamicin (1.75 mg/kg loading dose and then 1 mg/kg every 8 hours) with nafcillin (1 g to 2 g every 4 hours). If an anaerobic infection is suspected, clindamycin or metronidazole (Flagyl) should be added. Patients with orbital cellulitis must be followed with frequent monitoring of vision and pupillary response.

A subperiosteal abscess, which lies between the periorbita and the bone, can develop in orbital cellulitis. The diagnosis must be suspected when there is lack of improvement with appropriate antibiotic treatment of orbital or preseptal cellulitis. CT scans can be helpful in making this diagnosis; however, there have been reports of false-positive and false-negative scans. Treatment recommendations are controversial, especially regarding surgical intervention. Antibiotic treatment alone is often successful in the management of subperiosteal orbital abscesses in children (see Chapter 12).

Mucormycosis is a rare but life-threatening fungal infection involving the orbit. It usually occurs in patients with diabetes, particularly those with ketoacidosis. Other risk factors are renal failure, tumors, and therapy with antimetabolites or steroids. It is caused by ubiquitous fungi such as Mucor and Rhizopus. Mucormycosis typically begins with a unilateral headache, orbital pain, fever, decreased vision, and rhinorrhea. Its presentation is similar to orbital cellulitis, with lid edema, proptosis, and ophthalmoplegia as prominent features. There is often rapid progression with loss of consciousness, multiple cranial nerve palsies, and necrosis of periorbital and nasal structures. If mucormycosis is suspected, an immediate CT scan of the sinuses, orbits, and brain should be performed. In addition, biopsies should be obtained from the necrotic tissue to confirm the diagnosis. Because of its rapid, fulminant course, early diagnosis is essential. Even with early diagnosis, mortality approaches 50%. Treatment recommendations include an otorhinolaryngological consultation and intravenous amphotericin B. If systemic side effects are not prominent with a test dose, intravenous amphotericin 0.3 mg/kg dissolved in 500 mL of 5% dextrose solution over 1 hour to 3 hours is recommended every day. The dose can be advanced to 0.5 mg/kg to 0.6 mg/kg. Other treatment modalities such as hyperbaric oxygen and exenteration may be necessary if progressive infection occurs.

Inflammation of the Eyelids

A chalazion is a chronic inflammatory reaction involving the secretory glands of the eyelid (Figure 16-6). It typically presents as an inflamed nodule following an acute focal infection (stye) of a meibomian gland or a gland of Moll or Zeis. Blockage of these glands results in their contents being forced into the surrounding tissue, causing a localized inflammatory response. Patients present with pain, tenderness, erythema, and a lid nodule.

Treatment consists of warm compresses for 5 minutes to 10 minutes 4 to 6 times daily and topical ophthalmic antibiotic ointment. If the patient has significant blepharitis, treatment with lid scrubs is beneficial. If the chalazion does not resolve after several weeks of conservative treatment, an incision and curettage can be performed. An alternative form of treatment is to inject 0.2 mL to 0.5 mL triamcinolone 40 mg/ml into and around the lesion; however, permanent depigmentation of the overlying skin, atrophy of the subcutaneous tissue, and granuloma formation can occur. Tetracycline (250 mg 4 times daily) has been reported to be successful for the treatment of chronic chalazions.

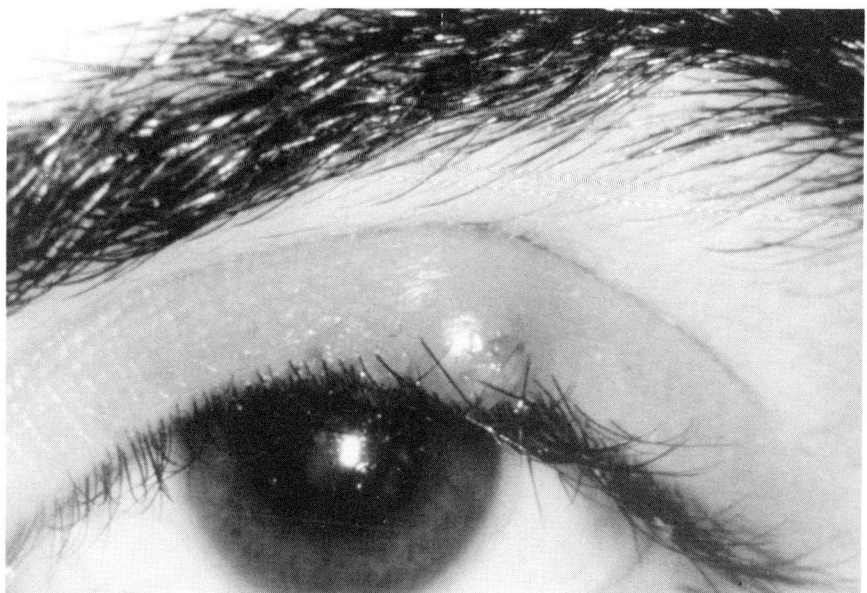

FIGURE 16-6. Chalazion.

Recurrent chalazions must be examined histologically to rule out sebaceous cell carcinoma.

Lacrimal Infections

Acute dacryoadenitis is an infection of the lacrimal gland. It typically presents with unilateral swelling, erythema, and localized tenderness of the lacrimal gland. Chemosis and conjunctival injection with a mucopurulent discharge may also be present. There may be ptosis with a characteristic S-shaped deformity of the upper eyelid (Figure 16–7). In addition, proptosis may be present with displacement of the globe inferiorly and medially. Ipsilateral preauricular lymphadenopathy, fever, and an elevated white blood cell count with a left shift are often present.

The etiology of acute dacryoadenitis is usually bacterial or viral. Bacterial causes include Staphylococcus, Streptococcus, and *N. gonorrhea.* Viral causes, which are more common, include mumps, influenza, Epstein-Barr, and herpes. A complete workup includes cultures of any ocular discharge, complete blood count, and a CT scan of the orbit. These should be performed when proptosis or ophthalmoplegia is present. Acute bacterial dacryoadenitis can usually be successfully treated with oral antibiotics such as Augmentin (children: 20 mg/kg to 40 mg/kg per day in three divided doses; adults: 250 mg to 500 mg

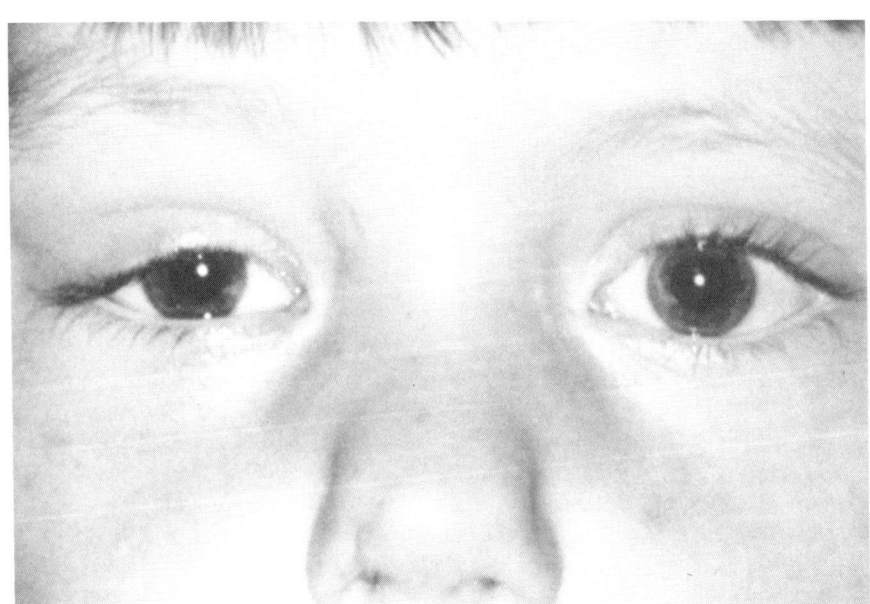

FIGURE 16–7. Dacryoadenitis. Note the S-shaped lid deformity.

3 times daily), or Keflex (children: 25 mg/kg to 50 mg/kg per day in four divided doses; adults: 250 mg to 500 mg 4 times daily) for 7 days to 10 days. In the rare cases of abscess formation, surgical drainage may be necessary. For viral dacryoadenitis, symptomatic treatment with cool compresses and analgesics is helpful.

Acute dacryocystitis is a bacterial infection of the lacrimal sac. In newborns, it usually occurs secondary to congenital nasolacrimal duct obstruction; in adults, it is usually secondary to localized inflammation of the lacrimal system from an upper respiratory infection. Dacryocystitis can develop rapidly; the patient presents with pain, erythema, and swelling over the lacrimal sac (Figure 16-8). On examination, a mucopurulent discharge may be expressed from the punctum. Augmentin or Ceclor (20 mg/kg to 40 mg/kg per day in three divided doses) is recommended in children and Dicloxacillin or Keflex (500 mg in four divided doses) in adults. In pediatric cases with systemic manifestations (e.g., fever), hospitalization with intravenous cefuroxime (50 mg/kg to 100 mg/kg per day in three divided doses) is recommended. In addition, topical antibiotics such as sulfacetamide or erythromycin 4 times daily and warm compresses with gentle massage to the inner canthal region are recommended.

Chronic dacryocystitis is an indolent infection of the lacrimal drainage system. Symptoms include epiphora, blepharitis, and a mild chronic conjunctivitis; there may be mild tenderness over the lacrimal sac. In infants, chronic

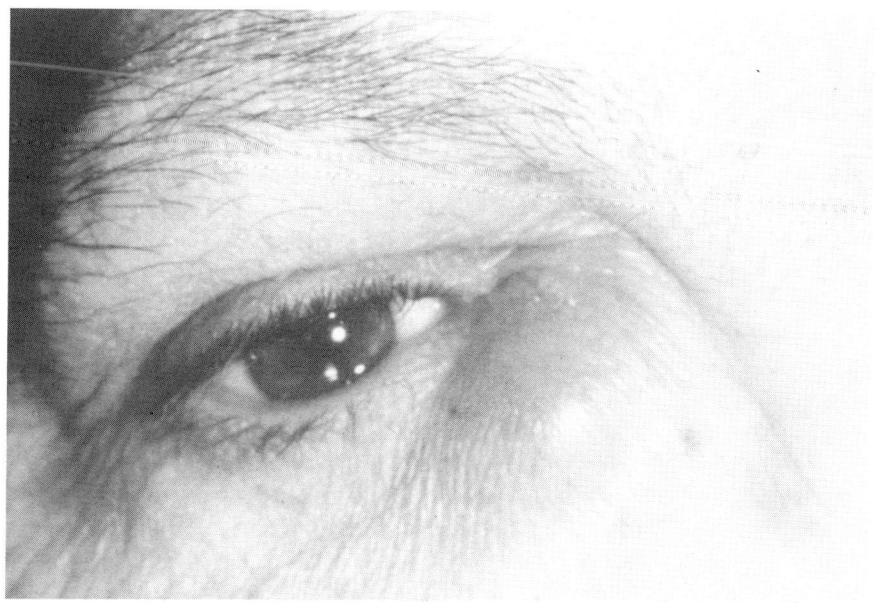

FIGURE 16-8. Dacryocystitis.

dacryocystitis can be treated with lid hygiene, topical antibiotics, and lacrimal sac massage. Occasionally it is necessary to instill 1 drop of a topical antibiotic (sulfacetamide 10% or Polytrim) daily to prevent purulent dacryocystitis. When this occurs, early probing and irrigation to relieve an obstructed nasolacrimal duct should be considered. In over 90% of infants with congenital nasolacrimal duct obstruction, the obstruction and chronic infection will spontaneously resolve within the first year of life. In adults, medical treatment is usually unsuccessful, and a dacryocystorhinostomy is necessary.

Conjunctival Infections

The differential diagnosis of a "red" eye includes viral, bacterial, chlamydial, allergic, and toxic conjunctivitis; ocular inflammation; and glaucoma. Conjunctivitis is characterized by inflammation of the conjunctiva and discharge. Figure 16–9 presents a flowchart helpful in narrowing the differential diagnosis.

Viral Conjunctivitis

Viral conjunctivitis frequently follows an upper respiratory tract infection or exposure to someone with a red eye. Clinical signs include a watery discharge, subconjunctival hemorrhages, membranes or pseudomembranes, subepithelial infiltrates, follicles, a palpable preauricular node, and edematous eyelids (Figure 16–10). The normal incubation period is from 5 days to 10 days; however, viral shedding persists for 10 days to 12 days. Viral conjunctivitis can be unilateral or bilateral, with many cases starting as unilateral and progressing to bilateral in several days. Corneal involvement secondary to adenovirus generally occurs within 1 day to 5 days of onset as a diffuse superficial punctate keratitis. This will either resolve or progress to deeper corneal involvement with subepithelial infiltrates (Figure 16–11). These subepithelial infiltrates typically resolve within 2 months to 4 months but occasionally persist for years. Although viral conjunctivitis is usually a clinical diagnosis, laboratory tests can be helpful. A Gram's stain of the conjunctival scrapings usually shows a predominance of polymorphonuclear leukocytes during the first several days, followed by a lymphocytic predominance. An adenovirus antigen detection immunoassay and an enzyme immunofluorescent assay (Adenoclone, Cambridge Bioscience) for rapid detection of adenovirus are available. Viral cultures can be used to confirm the diagnosis. Viral conjunctivitis often becomes progressively worse over the first several days and may not resolve for up to 2 weeks to 3 weeks. Patients should be considered contagious for the first 10 days to 12 days from the day of onset, and care should be taken to prevent transmission in the office. Supportive treatment consists of artificial tears and cool compresses several times per day, which may be effective in alleviating symp-

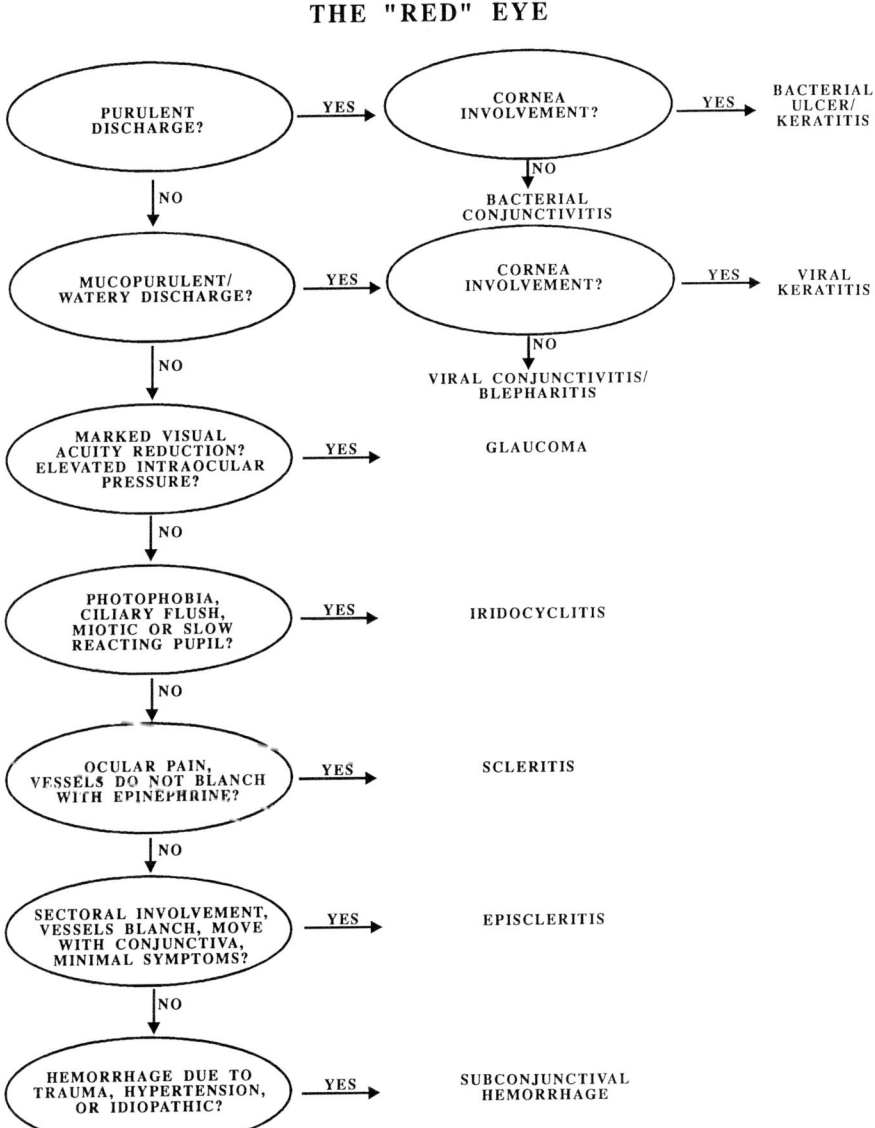

FIGURE 16-9. Flowchart to narrow the differential diagnosis of a "red" eye.

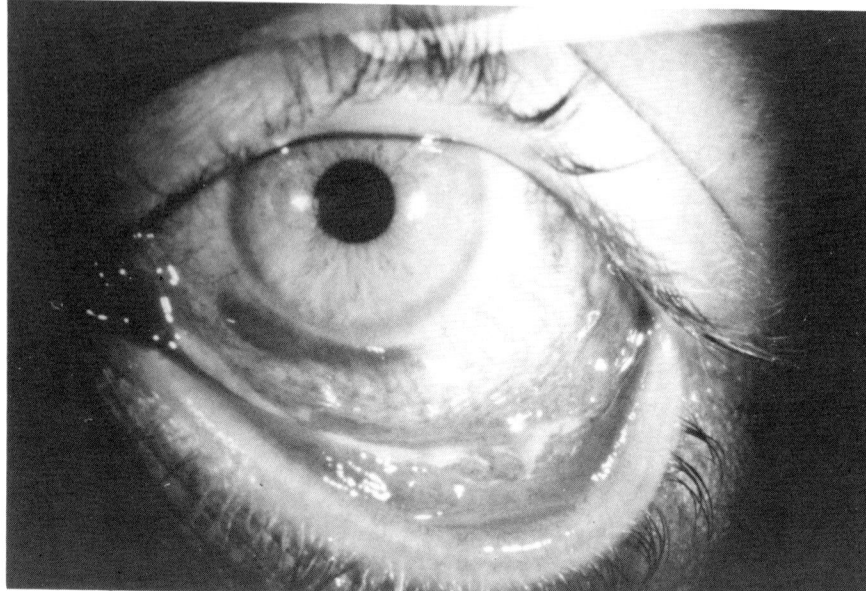

FIGURE 16-10. Adenovirus conjunctivitis (epidemic keratoconjunctivitis) with pseudomembrane.

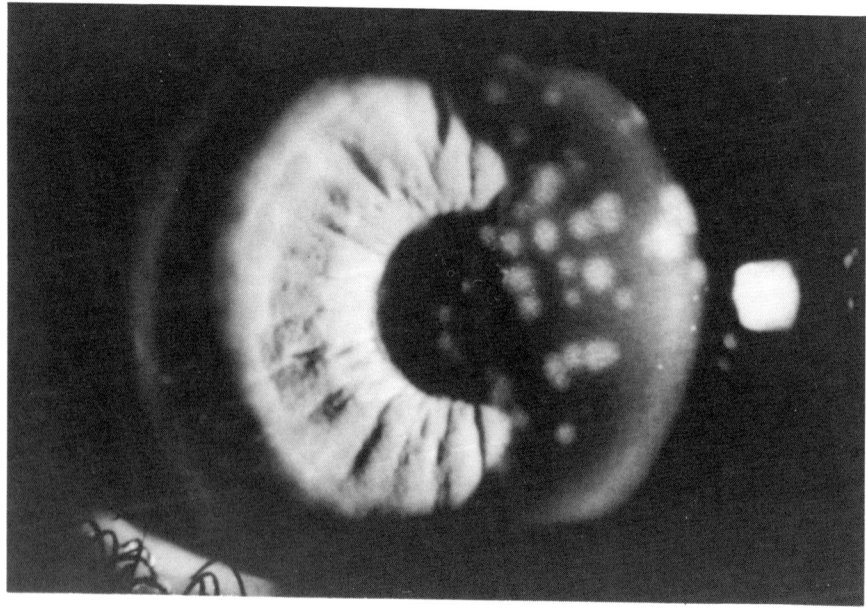

FIGURE 16-11. Subepithelial infiltrates seen in viral conjunctivitis.

toms in some patients. Topical antihistamine/vasoconstrictor (Vasocon-A) drops may be helpful in reducing the itching and burning. The role of topical corticosteroids is reserved for treatment of significant subepithelial infiltrates or severe conjunctivitis with scarring or pseudomembrane formation. Topical corticosteroids are not without risk, and their use mandates close ophthalmologic follow-up. Topical steroids should never be used if there is a possibility of herpetic infection.

Bacterial Conjunctivitis

The principal causes of acute bacterial conjunctivitis are Staphylococcus, Streptococcus, Neisseria, and Hemophilus. Most cases of acute bacterial conjunctivitis are self-limiting. An exception is Neisseria, which can progress to corneal perforation. Conjunctival cultures are useful in identifying the specific bacteria and determining the antibiotic sensitivities. Acute bacterial conjunctivitis presents with a mucopurulent discharge with unilateral or bilateral involvement. A major difference between bacterial and viral conjunctivitis is that preauricular lymphadenopathy does not occur with bacterial conjunctivitis; Neisseria is again an exception. The initial management of bacterial conjunctivitis includes bilateral conjunctival cultures and Gram's stain. A broad-spectrum topical antibiotic (e.g., Polytrim 4 times daily) is often selected prior to culture results. In documented *N. gonorrhea* or *meningitis* conjunctivitis, treatment consists of a single intramuscular injection of 1.0 g ceftriaxone. In addition, topical therapy such as erythromycin ointment may be used. Patients with Neisseria conjunctivitis should also be treated for suspected concomitant chlamydial disease. Because of the risk of corneal perforation, patients with potentially poor compliance should be hospitalized.

Adult Chlamydial Conjunctivitis

Adult chlamydial conjunctivitis is a sexually transmitted ocular disease. There is often a history of accompanying cervicitis or urethritis. The ocular findings usually present from several days to weeks after contact with infected genital secretions. Patients typically present with hyperemia, a mild mucopurulent discharge, a papillary conjunctivitis that progresses to chronic follicular conjunctivitis, and an associated preauricular lymphadenopathy. Corneal involvement is common with a micropannus of 1 mm to 2 mm along the superior limbus (Figure 16-12). In addition, a superficial punctate epithelial keratitis may be present with subepithelial infiltrates that begin near the superior pannus. Untreated chlamydial conjunctivitis can lead to conjunctival scarring. The diagnosis should be suspected in any sexually active individual with a chronic conjunctivitis and can usually be confirmed with laboratory testing. A conjunctival scraping stained with Giemsa can reveal cytoplasmic paranuclear inclusion bodies in epithelial cells (Figure 16-2). Antigen detection assays with

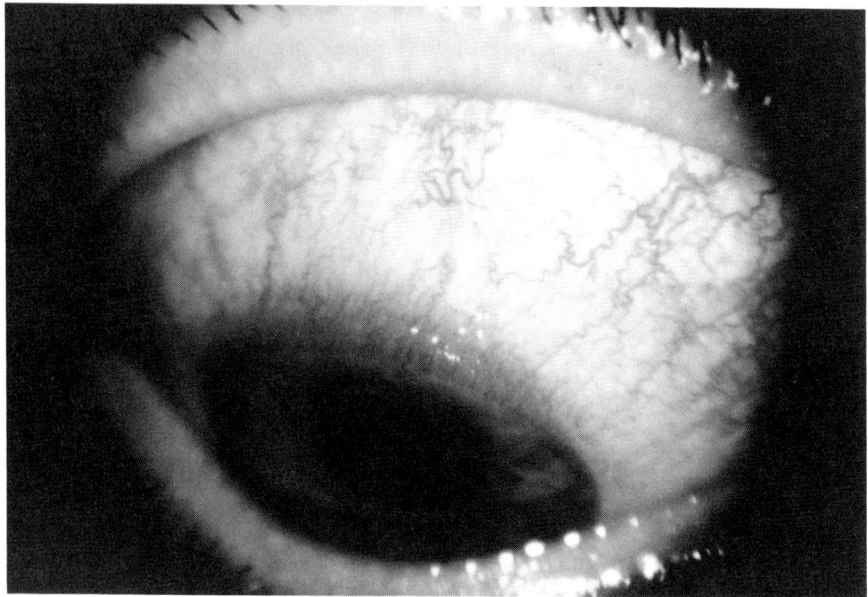

FIGURE 16-12. Adult chlamydial conjunctivitis with superior pannus.

fluorescent monoclonal antibodies or enzyme immunoassays can aid in the rapid diagnosis of chlamydial disease. The majority of these assays are not designed for conjunctival scraping; however, their use in ocular disease has gained wide acceptance. Treatment consists of oral doxycycline 100 mg twice daily for 3 weeks, tetracycline 250 mg to 500 mg 4 times daily, or erythromycin 250 mg to 500 mg 4 times daily for 3 weeks. Topical tetracycline or erythromycin ointment 2 times daily is useful if an abundant mucopurulent discharge is present. The patient's sexual partner(s) need to be treated concurrently to prevent reinfection.

Allergic Conjunctivitis

Allergic conjunctivitis results when a specific allergen (such as pollen) mediates a local IgA or circulating IgE antibody response. It presents with chemosis, erythema, conjunctival hyperemia, lid swelling, and a mucoid discharge. Approximately 15% of the population is affected at some time with allergic conjunctivitis. The diagnosis is clinical; however, the presence of eosinophils on conjunctival scrapings is helpful in confirming the diagnosis. Treatment consists of oral antihistamines (e.g., Seldane 2 times daily), cool compresses, topical vasoconstrictor/antihistamine drops (e.g., Vasocon-A four times daily), topical 4% cromolyn sodium, and, if severe, mild topical steroids.

Corneal Infections

Bacterial corneal infections are caused by a variety of organisms. Because the corneal epithelium is an effective barrier to microbial penetration, bacterial keratitis is usually preceded by an epithelial defect. Only three species of bacteria can directly penetrate an intact corneal epithelium: Neisseria, *Corynebacterium diphtheriae,* and Shigella. Risk factors for bacterial keratitis include traumatic corneal injury, corneal injury secondary to contact lens wear, an epithelial defect, viral keratitis, and surgical procedures of the cornea. The typical presentation is conjunctivitis, pain, photophobia, mucopurulent discharge, and decreased vision. An infiltrate of the corneal stroma associated with an overlying epithelial defect is called a corneal ulcer. There is usually evidence of surrounding inflammation with folds in Descemet's membrane, an anterior uveitis, and a hypopyon in severe cases (Figure 16-13).

While the history and examination may suggest the etiologic diagnosis, a corneal scraping for Gram's stain and culture is mandatory. A Kimura spatula (Figure 16-14) is used for obtaining material from the ulcer floor and margins where the yield is highest. The spatula is sterilized between cultures by flaming using an alcohol lamp. A sterile 23-gauge needle can be substituted if a Kimura spatula is unavailable. Culture media, including blood and chocolate agars, nutrient broth, thioglycolate broth, and Sabouraud's agar, should be plated

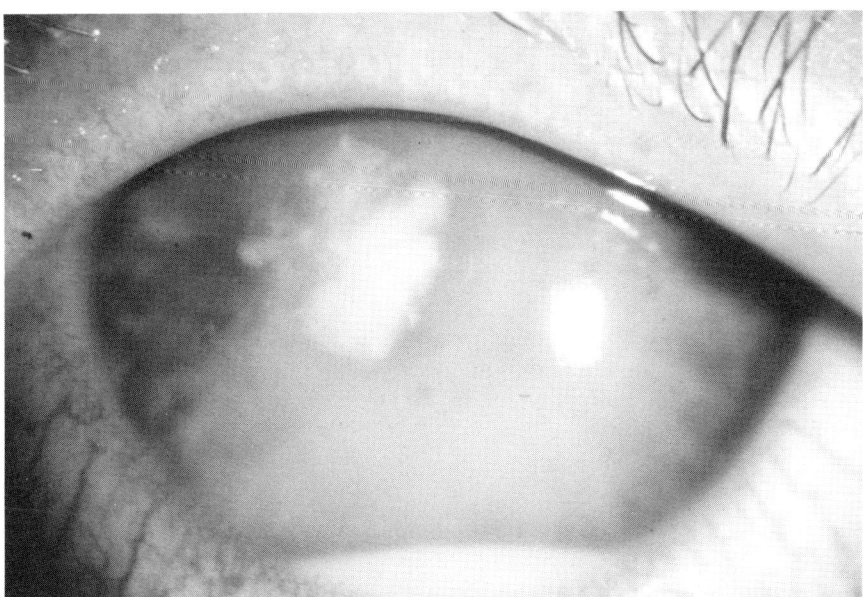

FIGURE 16-13. Corneal ulcer with hypopyon.

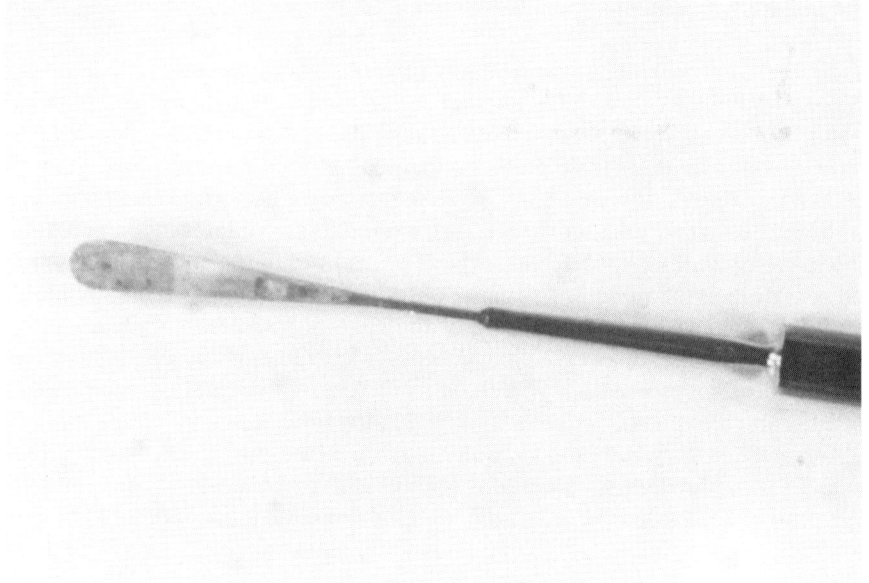

FIGURE 16-14. Kimura spatula.

before therapy is initiated (see Chapter 2). Fresh media must be used and taken directly to the microbiology laboratory.

The treatment regimen varies depending on the clinical severity and geographic location where the patient becomes infected. Small, superficial infiltrates without epithelial disruption may be treated with a broad-spectrum topical antibiotic (e.g., Polytrim, gentamicin, tobramycin, or neosporin 4 to 6 times daily). Significant corneal ulcers are treated with fortified cefazolin (33 mg/mL to 50 mg/mL) alternating with a fortified aminoglycoside (gentamicin, tobramycin 10 mg/mL to 15 mg/mL) hourly. In the presence of resistant gram-positive organisms, vancomycin (33 mg/mL to 50 mg/mL) may be substituted for cefazolin. The final decision is based on the clinical response of the patient, as well as the culture and sensitivities. Newer antibiotics, such as ciprofloxin, may also play a role in the initial treatment of bacterial keratitis. Further antibiotic considerations are discussed in Chapter 17.

Herpes Simplex Infections

Herpes simplex viruses can be subdivided into two types: HSV-I, which is responsible for most ocular infections in adults, and HSV-II, which causes most neonatal ocular infections. Primary ocular herpes infections typically occur between the ages of 6 months and 5 years and present with unilateral eyelid vesicles, which are often accompanied by a follicular conjunctivitis (Figure 16–15). Other findings are epithelial keratitis, corneal anesthesia, and mild iritis. Following the primary infection, the herpes virus can remain dormant in the trigeminal ganglion until a precipitating factor such as stress, trauma, fever, or bright sunlight reactivates the virus. Recurrent infections most commonly present as epithelial keratitis. Other manifestations are stromal keratitis, disciform keratitis, and metaherpetic keratitis.

Herpes simplex epithelial keratitis usually presents with a unilateral red eye, pain, photophobia, tearing, and decreased vision. On examination, an epithelial dendritic ulcer with an associated conjunctivitis and iritis is usually present (Figure 16–16). Recurrent epithelial disease may present as a superficial punctate keratitis, which progresses to a dendritic keratitis. The differential diagnosis includes varicella-zoster, which can present with a dendritic keratitis, and a healing epithelial defect in which a pseudodendrite can be seen. A third form of recurrent epithelial keratitis presents as geographic ulceration. This often develops with corticosteroid enhancement of epithelial keratitis or in an immunocompromised individual. Diagnosis is usually clinical, but viral cultures can be useful for confirmation. Immunofluorescence assays can be used to identify herpes antigens on corneal or conjunctival scrapings. Treatment consists of topical antivirals such as trifluridine (Viroptic) every 2 hours while awake with a gradual taper. If an anterior uveitis is present, a cycloplegic agent (e.g., Cyclo-

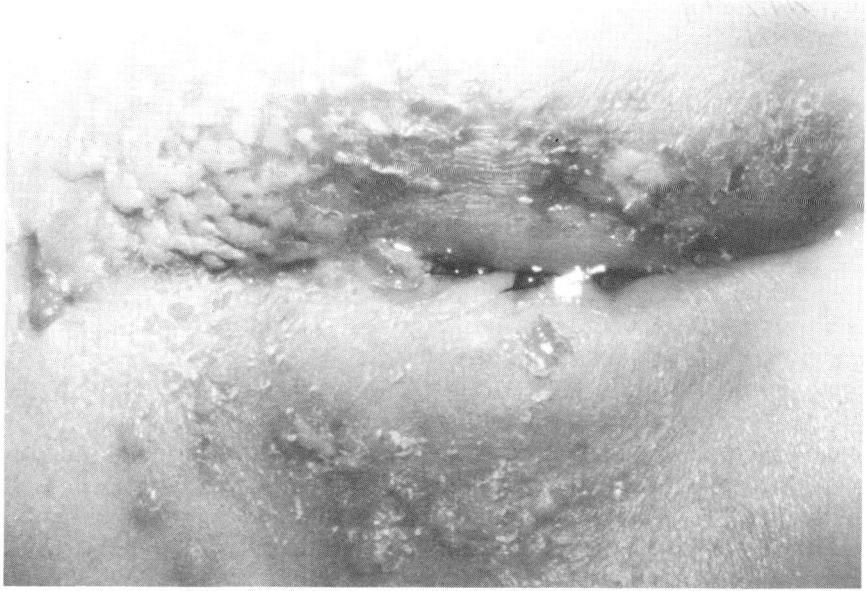

FIGURE 16–15. Primary herpes simplex ocular infection.

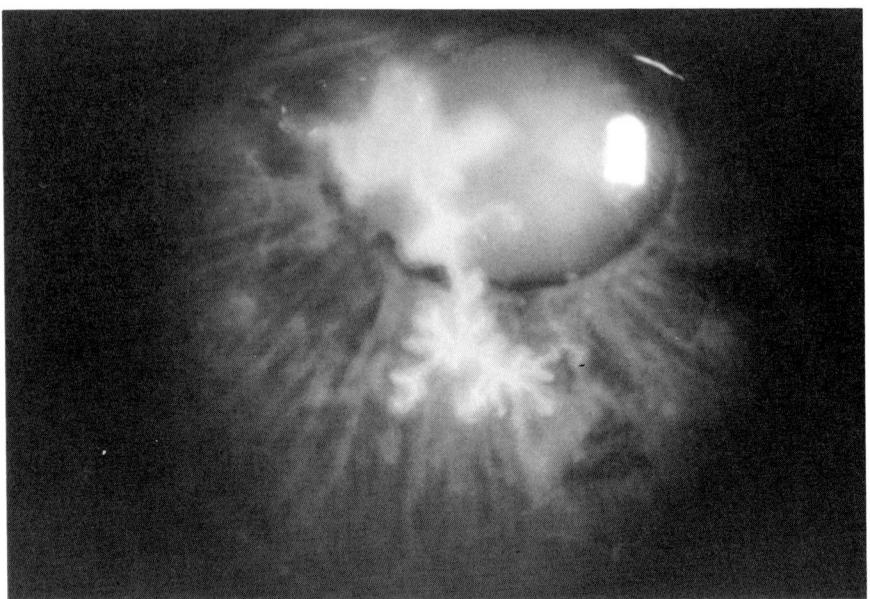

FIGURE 16-16. Herpes simples dendritic keratitis.

gyl 1%) 3 times daily is also useful. Concurrent prophylactic topical antibiotics are not indicated.

Herpes simplex stromal keratitis has various clinical forms, including disciform keratitis (Figure 16–17), infiltrative stromal keratitis, and metaherpetic keratitis. Disciform keratitis may present with localized stromal edema, Descemet's folds, keratic precipitates, and an iridocyclitis. The stromal edema is often disc-shaped and central or paracentral in location without epithelial involvement. Disciform keratitis is believed to represent a cell-mediated immune response to viral antigens.

Infiltrative stromal keratitis presents with diffuse corneal and stromal edema, often with an accompanying epithelial ulceration. In chronic cases, lipid or cholesterol crystals may be deposited in the cornea. Other late findings are deep corneal vascularization, posterior synechiae, and trabeculitis—the last associated with increased intraocular pressure.

Metaherpetic keratitis is characterized by indolent stromal and epithelial edema. The corneal lesion is typically oval in shape, without evidence of an overlying epithelial defect. Other findings are anterior uveitis, hypopyon, corneal anesthesia, corneal thinning with descemetocele formation, and perforation.

Treatment of stromal keratitis consists of topical antivirals (Viroptic) 6 times daily. Concomitant corticosteroid use is controversial. While steroids clearly reduce the amount of inflammation and associated discomfort, recurrences

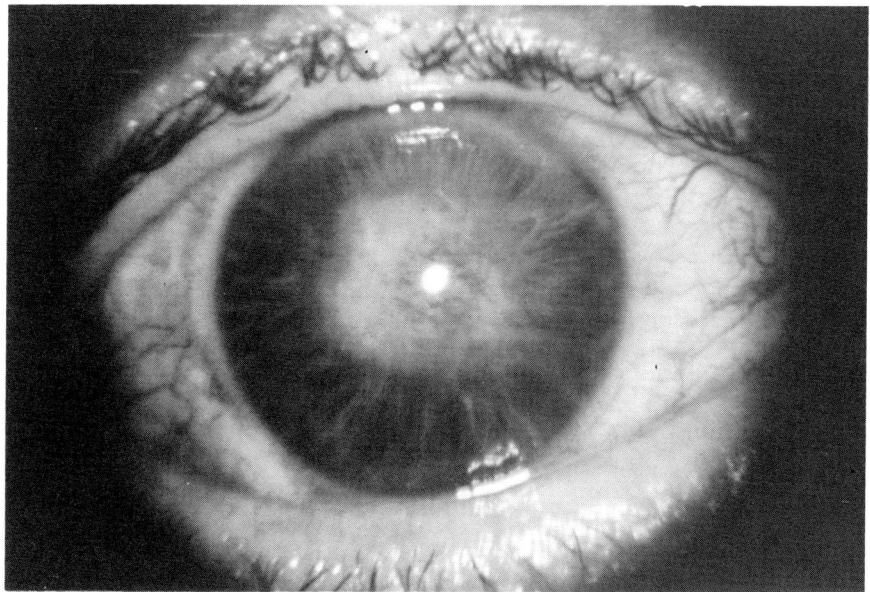

FIGURE 16-17. Disciform herpes simplex stromal infiltrate.

may be more frequent and severe. Recently, systemic acyclovir (200 mg 5 times daily) has been advocated for the treatment of stromal keratitis in adults. If significant corneal scarring is present, penetrating keratoplasty may be indicated.

Fungal Keratitis

Fungal keratitis is more commonly encountered in the southern and southwestern United States. Septate fungi such as Fusarium or Aspergillus are the most common pathogens; inoculation often occurs after trauma with vegetable matter. Nonseptate fungi such as Mucoraceae are rarely responsible for keratitis, and nonfilamentous fungi such as Candida are more commonly seen in northern climates and in immunocompromised individuals. Risk factors for fungal keratitis include corneal injury by organic material, soft contact lens wear, immunosuppression, and prolonged use of topical antibiotics. Fungal keratitis often presents as a primary infiltrate with satellite lesions (Figure 16-18). Cultures should be performed on the available fungal media (without inhibitors), as well as room-temperature blood agar. The laboratory must be informed of the suspected fungal keratitis because many of the saprophytes will be disregarded as contaminants. If the culture is negative and fungal keratitis is suspected, a corneal biopsy should be performed for a higher yield. Natamycin (Natacyn) is the drug of choice against filamentous fungi. Initially, the

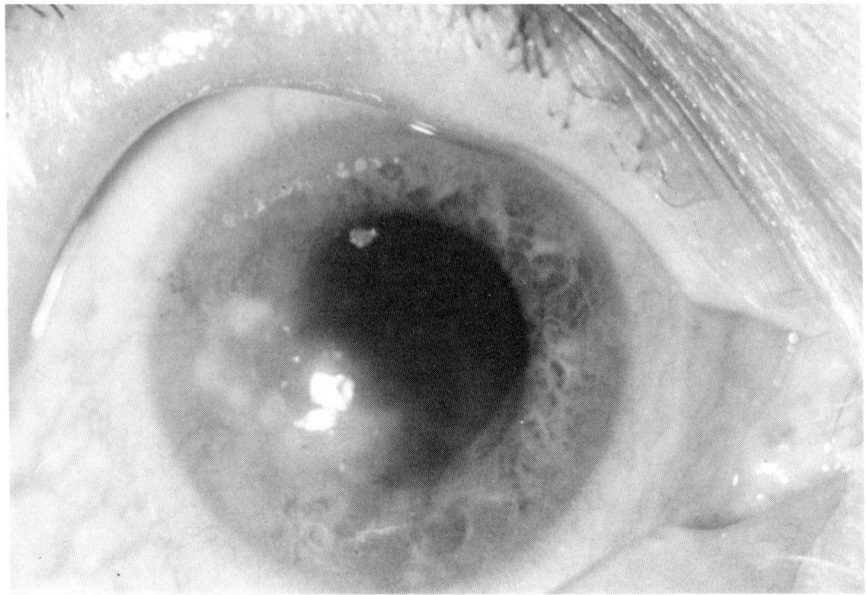

FIGURE 16-18. Fungal keratitis.

agent should be administered hourly, around the clock, for several days, with a gradual taper. Amphotericin B 0.15% appears more effective against Candida and other yeasts. Other topical antifungals, including miconozole and clotrimazole, may be considered in resistant cases. Oral antifungals, ketoconazole and fluconozole, may also be effective in resistant cases.

Acanthamoeba Keratitis

Acanthamoeba keratitis should be considered in any patient with a history of contact lens wear. Acanthamoeba is a potentially devastating protozoan corneal infection that has only recently been described. The organism is a ubiquitous protozoan that has been isolated from drinking water, swimming pools, hot tubs, and as a normal flora of humans. The use of homemade saline is a common finding in many cases of Acanthamoeba keratitis, and for this reason contact lens wearers should use only commercially prepared saline solutions. Acanthamoeba exists in a trophozoite and a cystic form. In the cystic form, the Acanthamoeba is highly resistant to antibiotics or chemical disinfectants. Diagnosis requires a positive identification of the organism.

Early clinical signs of infection are corneal ulceration, conjunctivitis, uveitis, and pain out of proportion to the amount of corneal and anterior segment inflammation. Often the epithelial or subepithelial infiltrates progress to a corneal stromal ring infiltrate (Figure 16-19). Corneal scraping should be per-

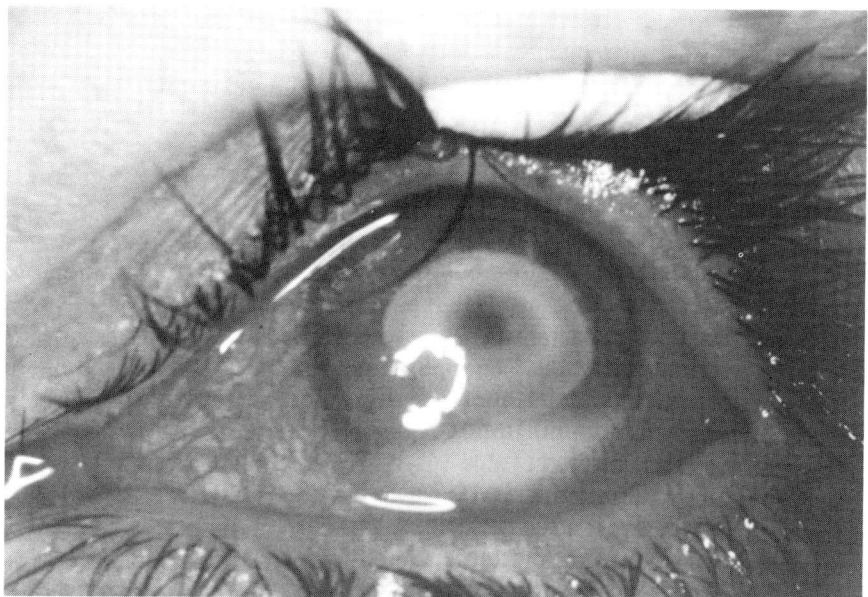

FIGURE 16-19. Acanthamoeba keratitis with hypopyon.

formed whenever Acanthamoeba is suspected. A Giemsa stain may show the cysts. The Calcofluor white stain can show both the trophozoite and the cysts, but it requires the use of a fluorescent microscope. Culture of Acanthamoeba requires a nonnutrient agar with an *E. coli* overlay. If corneal scrapings and cultures are negative, a corneal biopsy may yield positive results.

Treatment is difficult and controversial. Many cases progress despite intensive medical treatment. Propamidine isethionate 0.1% (Brolene) has been shown to have in vitro activity against Acanthamoeba. Brolene, an over-the-counter medication in Great Britain, is currently not available in the United States except through the Centers for Disease Control (CDC). Neosporin has also been shown to have in vitro activity against Acanthamoeba. Other agents such as clotrimazole, ketoconazole, itraconazole, miconazole, and paramomycin have been found effective in some cases. Patients should be started on a multidrug regimen such as topical Brolene and Neosporin with or without a concurrent antifungal. Drops are usually instituted hourly for the first several days and slowly tapered but often must be maintained for a minimum of 6 months.

Endophthalmitis

Postoperative endophthalmitis is an infrequent complication of intraocular surgery that requires immediate treatment. The incidence of endophthalmitis following intraocular surgery ranges from 0.1% to 0.5%. Patients typically present with conjunctivitis, chemosis, increasing eye pain, and decreasing vision beginning 1 day to 2 days following surgery. On examination, there is more inflammation than expected. There may be a hypopyon, marked eyelid edema, or significant vitreous debris (Figure 16–20). Often the cellular reaction in the anterior chamber and vitreous precludes a red reflex. The most common source of the bacteria is the normal flora of the periocular area. The most common organism is *S. epidermidis,* followed by *S. aureus* and streptococcal species (except pneumococcus). Less common organisms include gram-negative and anaerobic bacteria. Organisms that have previously been considered nonpathogenic (e.g., propiobacterium) have recently been identified as causes of late-onset "chronic infectious" endophthalmitis. Fungal endophthalmitis is usually more indolent with its onset, occurring 3 or more weeks after surgery. In cases of suspected endophthalmitis, aqueous and vitreous samples should be Gram's stained and cultured (Table 16–3). Treatment consists of intravitreal antibiotics, topical antibiotics, and intravenous antibiotics. A diagnostic and therapeutic vitrectomy is often performed. The current intravitreal antibiotics of choice are vancomycin and amikacin. Intravenous imipenem is a good choice because of its good ocular penetration and broad-spectrum coverage. Chapter 17 details the antibiotic treatment of postoperative and posttraumatic endophthalmitis.

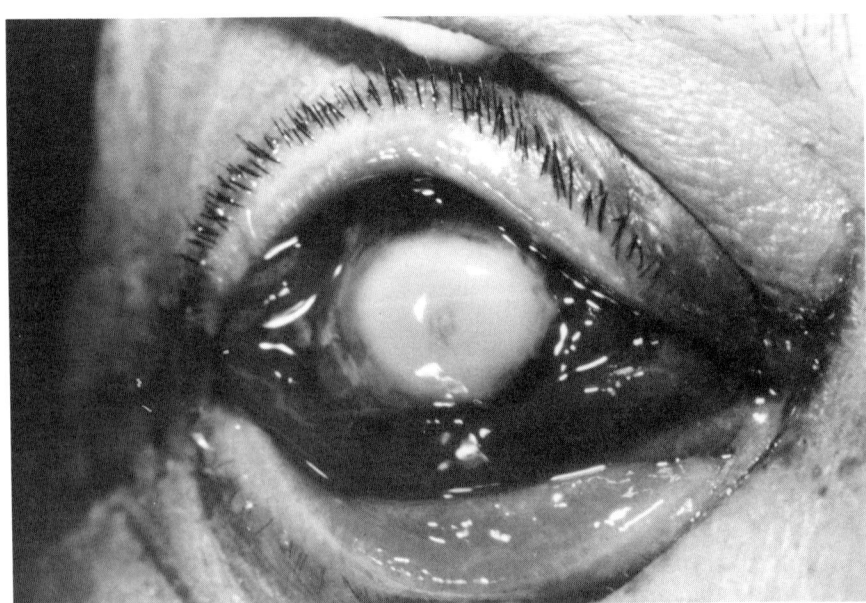

FIGURE 16–20. Endophthalmitis.

TABLE 16-3. CULTURE MEDIA AND STAINS FOR SUSPECTED ENDOPHTHALMITIS

MEDIA OR STAIN	USE
Blood agar (25° and 37°)	Most bacteria and fungi
Chocolate agar	Hemophilus and Neisseria
Thioglycolate	Anaerobic bacteria (P. acnes)
Sabouraud's agar	Fungi and yeast
Gram's stain	Bacteria and fungi
Calcofluor stain	Fungi

*Culture specimen should be undiluted specimen from both anterior chamber and vitreous.

Herpes Zoster Ophthalmicus

Herpes zoster ophthalmicus (HZO) is caused by the Varicella zoster virus. The initial contact with the virus results in chicken pox. The virus is not eliminated from the body but remains in the gasserian ganglion in a latent state. Viral reactivation that involves any of the branches of the ophthalmic nerve is referred to as herpes zoster ophthalmicus. HZO is more common in young children and adults over age 50 years. Most elderly patients with HZO are healthy, with no known precipitating factors. There is an increased incidence in immunosuppressed patients and a marked increase in patients with AIDS. Adults under age 40 years presenting with herpes zoster should be considered harborers of HIV infection until proved otherwise.

The usual presentation begins with a prodrome of fever, malaise, chills, and a burning or tingling sensation in the involved dermatome. Erythematous skin lesions appear within 2 days and gradually progress to vesicular lesions. These skin lesions often become confluent and form pustules and crusted lesions (Figure 16-21). In immunocompromised patients, the skin lesions are more severe. Ocular findings include vesicles on the lids, conjunctivitis, keratitis, uveitis, scleritis, retinitis, choroiditis, optic neuritis, and glaucoma. The cutaneous lesions of zoster heal within 3 weeks, although ocular features can persist for months. Treatment for the skin lesions of herpes zoster is oral acyclovir, 800 mg 5 times per day for 7 days to 10 days. To reduce the incidence of postherpetic neuralgia in patients over age 60 years consider adding prednisone 60 mg per day with a rapid taper over 10 days. For the treatment of herpes zoster ophthalmicus, begin oral acyclovir 800 mg 5 times per day. The exact duration of therapy and whether delayed therapy is efficacious remains unknown. For conjunctivitis, cool compresses and artificial tears are helpful. If uveitis is present, a cycloplegic agent with topical steroids is warranted. Pain may be severe during the first several weeks, and analgesics may be required. Multiple medications have been anecdotally reported useful for the treatment of postherpetic neuralgia. These include amitriptyline, cimetidine 400 mg twice daily, and Zostrix cream applied to the affected area 4 times daily.

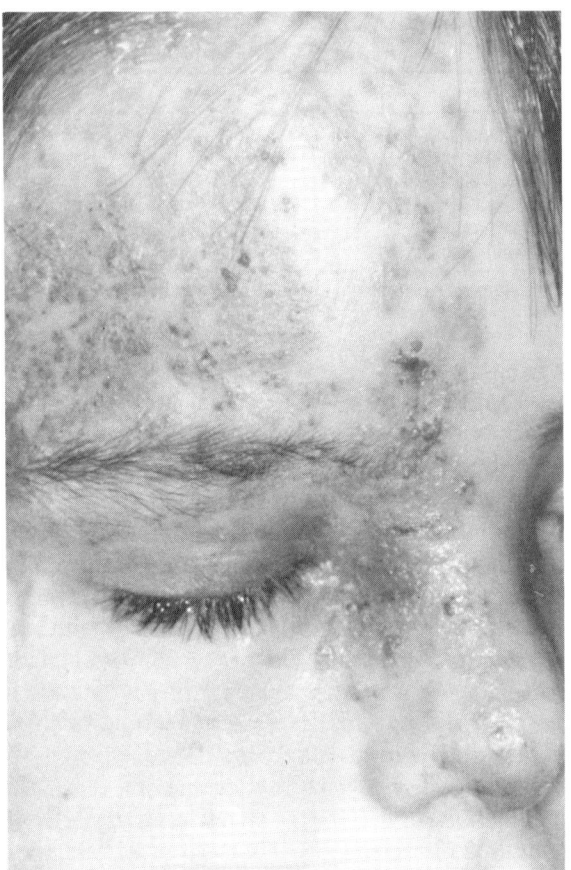

FIGURE 16-21. Herpes zoster. Note involvement at tip of nose (Hutchinson's sign).

OCULAR INFLAMMATION

Episcleritis

Episcleritis is a transient, usually self-limited, inflammatory disease of the episclera. Most cases are idiopathic. Episcleritis presents as either diffuse (Figure 16-22) or nodular episcleral inflammation. Most patients with episcleritis are asymptomatic; however, some experience mild to moderate pain. Bilateral involvement is present in approximately 30% of patients. On examination, there are prominent, inflamed radial superficial episcleral vessels. The episcleral tissue often appears salmon-pink to red and is movable over the underlying sclera. A topical vasoconstrictor such as phenylephrine decreases the redness of episcleritis in contrast to scleritis, where the deeper scleral vessels will

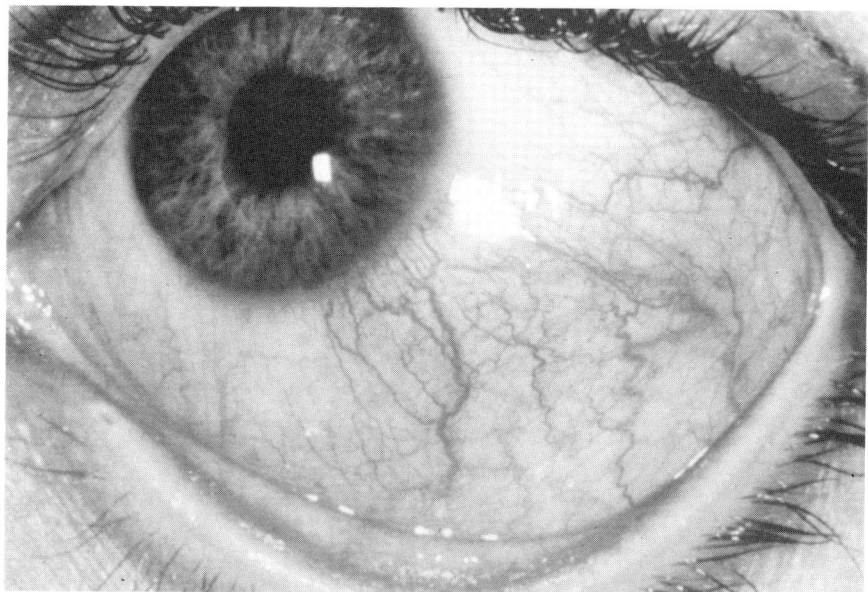

FIGURE 16-22. Diffuse episcleritis.

remain engorged. Laboratory tests are generally not necessary, but in recurrent or prolonged episodes, an FTA-ABS, rheumatoid factor, antinuclear antibody, or uric acid level may be helpful. Because most cases resolve within several weeks, treatment is supportive. In recurrent episodes or very symptomatic individuals, weak topical steroids or topical or systemic nonsteroidal antiinflammatory agents can be used to suppress inflammation.

Scleritis

Scleritis is a severe inflammatory disease of the sclera and overlying episclera. Approximately one-third of all cases of scleritis are associated with long-standing rheumatoid arthritis. Other associated conditions are syphilis, herpes zoster, herpes simplex, tuberculosis, Wegener's granulomatosis, Crohn's disease, and systemic lupus erythematosis. Scleritis is bilateral in slightly more than half of all cases. The vast majority of cases are anterior, with only 2% of cases presenting as posterior scleritis. Anterior scleritis can be divided into nodular (40%), diffuse (45%), or necrotizing (15%). In nodular anterior scleritis, there are red, tender, immobile nodules that do not blanch with topical vasoconstrictors (Figure 16-23). Diffuse anterior scleritis is the most benign, as well as the most common, form of scleritis. Necrotizing anterior scleritis is the most destructive form of this disease, with 60% of patients developing complications

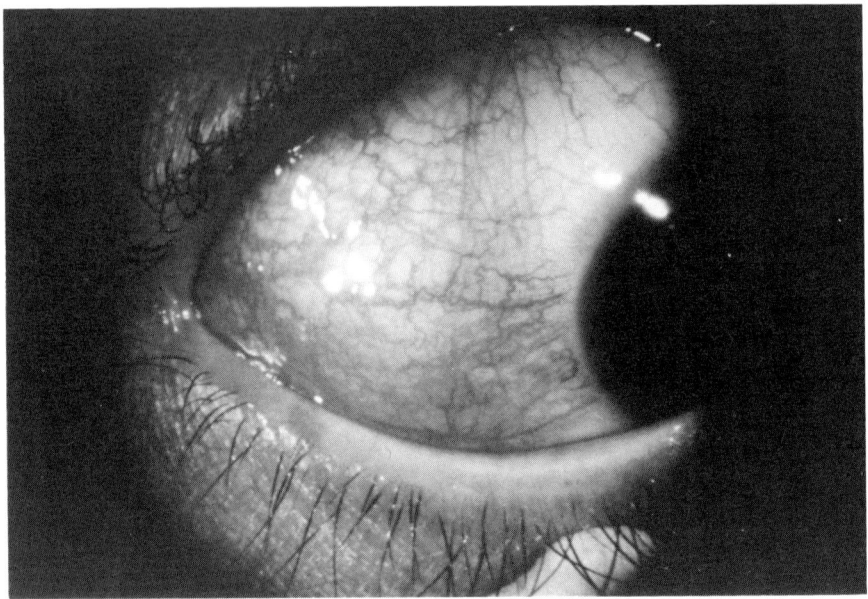

FIGURE 16-23. Nodular scleritis.

in addition to scleral thinning. Inflammatory necrotizing scleritis presents with inflammation and is a severe, destructive form of scleritis. Ischemia develops, and progressive necrosis can lead to exposure of the underlying uveal tissue with perforation (Figure 16-24). In necrotizing anterior scleritis without inflammation (scleromalacia perforans), progressive scleral thinning develops. This is frequently associated with long-standing rheumatoid arthritis and often presents asymptomatically (Figure 16-25). Posterior scleritis is a rare form of scleritis characterized by pain, proptosis, exudative retinal detachments, papilledema, choroidal folds, and uveal effusion syndrome.

Patients with scleritis usually present with deep, throbbing pain, often referred to the forehead or periocular area. Examination reveals scleral edema and engorged episcleral vessels, which produce a purplish-red color of the sclera. Corneal changes are present in up to 50% of patients with scleritis. Other frequent complications are cataracts, uveitis, and glaucoma. Because many systemic disorders are associated with scleritis, a complete workup and appropriate consultations are important. The initial investigation in patients with scleritis should include sedimentation rate, FTA-ABS, rheumatoid factor, antinuclear antibody, PPD skin test, and chest X rays.

Treatment is directed primarily at the underlying disorder if it is identifiable. Topical corticosteroids are usually inadequate in controlling the inflammation seen with scleritis; however, they can be useful as adjunctive therapy to systemic anti-inflammatory agents. Oral nonsteroidal anti-inflammatory agents

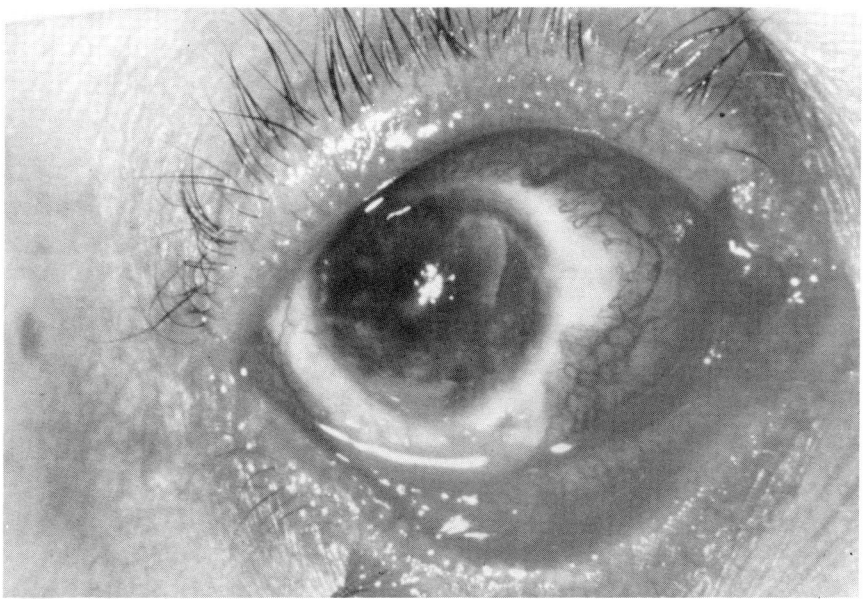

FIGURE 16-24. Necrotizing scleritis.

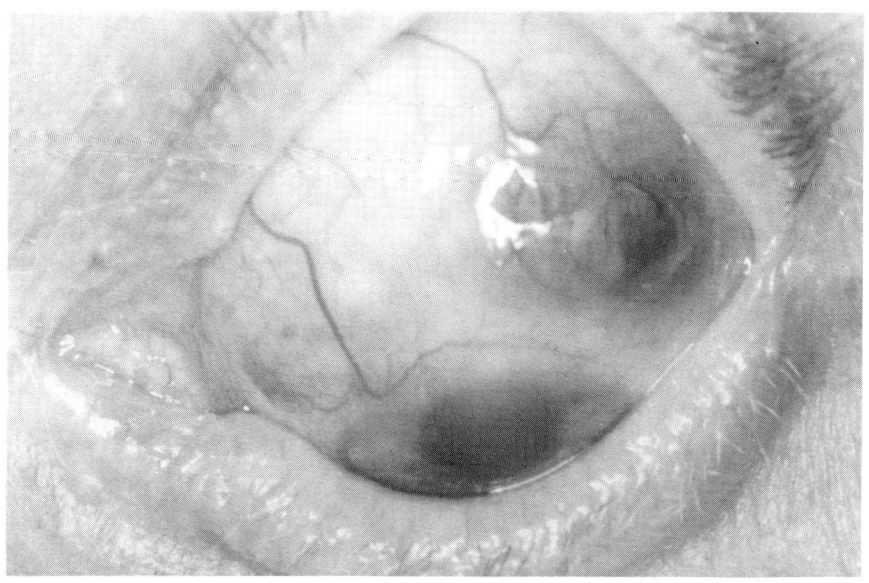

FIGURE 16-25. Patient with scleromalacia perforans.

such as fluribiprofen (Ansaid) 100 mg 3 times daily or indomethacin (Indocin) 75 mg twice daily are a good choice for the initial treatment of scleritis. In severe nonnecrotizing scleritis and in all cases of necrotizing scleritis, high-dose (80 mg to 160 mg daily) oral prednisone should be used. Other immunosuppressive agents such as cyclophosphamide, azathioprine, or methotrexate may be considered for selected patients. Cyclosporine A has been reported useful in treating patients with necrotizing scleritis who were unresponsive to other immunosuppressive agents. Surgical treatment is rarely indicated; however, in specific cases such as corneal or scleral perforation, a scleral patch graft may be necessary.

Anterior Uveitis

Inflammation of the uveal tissue (iris, ciliary body, and choroid) is called uveitis. Anterior uveitis (commonly called iritis) is inflammation limited to the anterior segment of the eye (iris and ciliary body). Patients with iritis present with pain, erythema, photophobia, and decreased vision. On examination, cells and flare are present in the anterior chamber. Keratitic precipitates (KPs), the most common corneal finding in anterior uveitis, are aggregates of inflammatory cells that accumulate on the corneal endothelium. Other ocular findings are posterior synechiae, miosis, hypopyon (Figure 16–26), cataracts, and

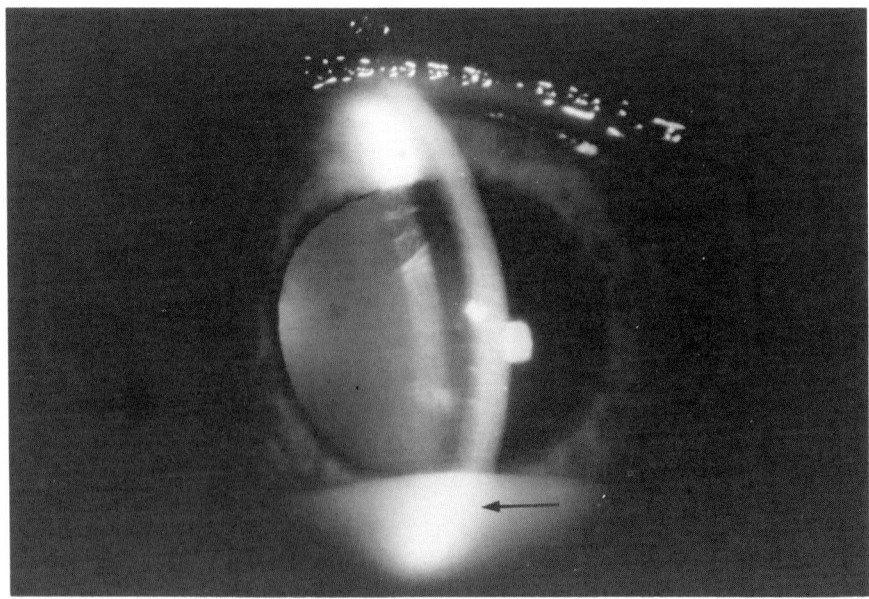

FIGURE 16–26. Hypopyon in a patient with uveitis.

cystoid macular edema. While the vast majority of cases of iritis are idiopathic, the differential diagnosis includes trauma, connective tissue disease, viruses, and sarcoidosis. An extensive medical workup is usually performed only in bilateral or recurrent cases. Laboratory testing includes complete blood count (CBC), angiotensin-converting enzyme (ACE), sedimentation rate (ESR), antinuclear antibody (ANA), FTA-ABS, PPD, HLA-B27 antigen test, sacroiliac X rays, and lyme titer. In selected cases, suspicious of sarcoidosis, a chest X ray and gallium scan is recommended (see Chapter 2).

Treatment of mild to moderate iritis includes a cycloplegic agent (e.g., scopolamine) to relieve ciliary spasm and prevent posterior synechiae (inflammatory adhesions of iris to lens capsule) and topical steroids to suppress inflammation. The frequency of instillation of the topical steroid is dependent on the severity of inflammation, with a gradual taper necessary to prevent rebound inflammation. A typical starting dose is scopolamine ¼% 3 times daily and prednisolone acetate 1% every 2 hours while awake. Severe iritis not responding to topical therapy may require systemic steroids.

Pars Planitis

Pars planitis is a variant of uveitis in which the primary focus of inflammation occurs in the anterior vitreous and peripheral retina. Pars planitis has no sexual or racial predilection but is more common in teenagers and young adults. The etiology is unknown; however, an immune reaction at the vitreous base has been suggested. Seventy percent to 80% of patients have bilateral involvement at presentation, although it is often more active in one eye than the other. Patients typically present with blurred vision or floaters with minimal pain or photophobia. The characteristic presentation of pars planitis is that of a quiet, external eye with minimal or absent anterior chamber reaction. An accumulation of a yellow-gray exudate at the ora serrata, termed snowbanking, is often seen. Other abnormalities are a perivasculitis (Figure 16–27), cystoid macular edema, optic disc edema, and occasionally peripheral neovascularization, which may result in fibrovascular contraction and progress to retinal detachment. Because the disease tends to have a long and protracted course and to minimize the risks involved with prolonged steroid therapy, treatment is usually withheld until vision decreases to below 20/40. Topical steroids are usually inadequate to control acute exacerbations but have a role as maintenance therapy. Periocular and/or systemic steroids are often required to suppress the acute inflammatory response. Because of the chronic recurring nature of pars planitis, periocular depot injections may prevent some of the long-term sequela of long-term steroid therapy. A suggested dose is 0.5 cc of 80 mg/cc methylprednisolone. An alternate agent is 0.55 cc of triamcinolone 40 mg/cc. Injections may be given every 2 weeks to 26 weeks depending on the patient's condition. Severe cases not responding to systemic steroids may require immunosuppressive agents or antimetabolites.

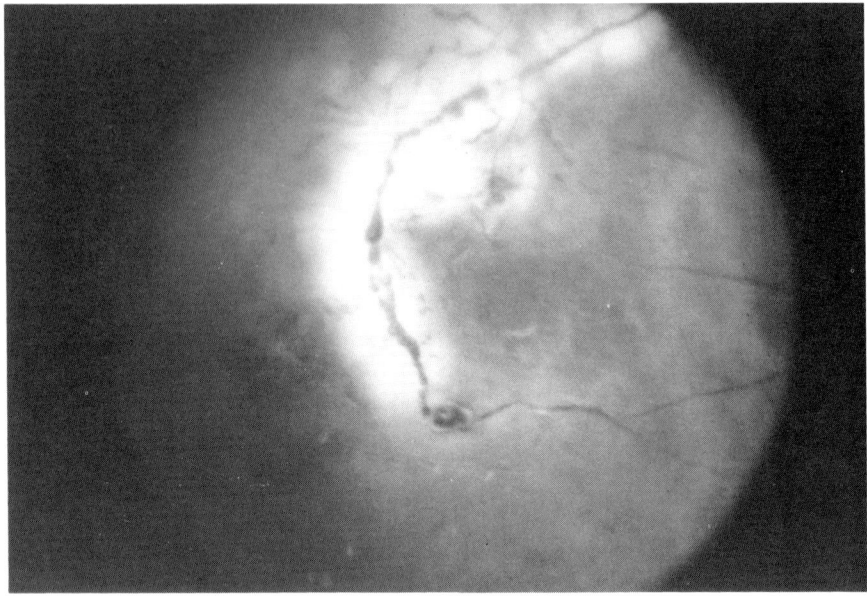

FIGURE 16-27. Perivasculitis in posterior uveitis.

Ocular Toxoplasmosis

Posterior uveitis is inflammation limited to the choroid. Ocular toxoplasmosis, the most common cause of posterior uveitis in humans, is caused by an obligate intracellular protozoan, *Toxoplasma gondii*. The finding of an inactive atrophic pigmented chorioretinal scar is presumptive evidence of previous exposure (Figure 16-28). Acute cases probably represent a late reactivation, and patients usually present with floaters and decreased vision. On examination, vitreous inflammation with a whitish-yellow chorioretinal lesion is noted in the posterior pole. Additional findings are perivasculitis and satellite scars. The diagnosis is usually made on clinical appearance; however, serum antibody levels are useful in demonstrating previous contact with toxoplasmosis. Other laboratory tests include the indirect hemagglutination test, enzyme-linked immunoabsorbent assays, and immunofluorescent assays. Not all patients with ocular toxoplasmosis require treatment; most heal spontaneously. Treatment is recommended if the chorioretinitis threatens the macula or optic nerve. The recommended treatment includes sulfadiazine and pyrimethamine with folinic acid as first-line therapy. Prednisone is often added if the lesion is threatening the macula or optic nerve. Clindamycin has also been shown to be effective for the treatment of toxoplasmosis (Table 16-4). In rare cases, significant vitreous debris requires a vitrectomy to improve vision. While

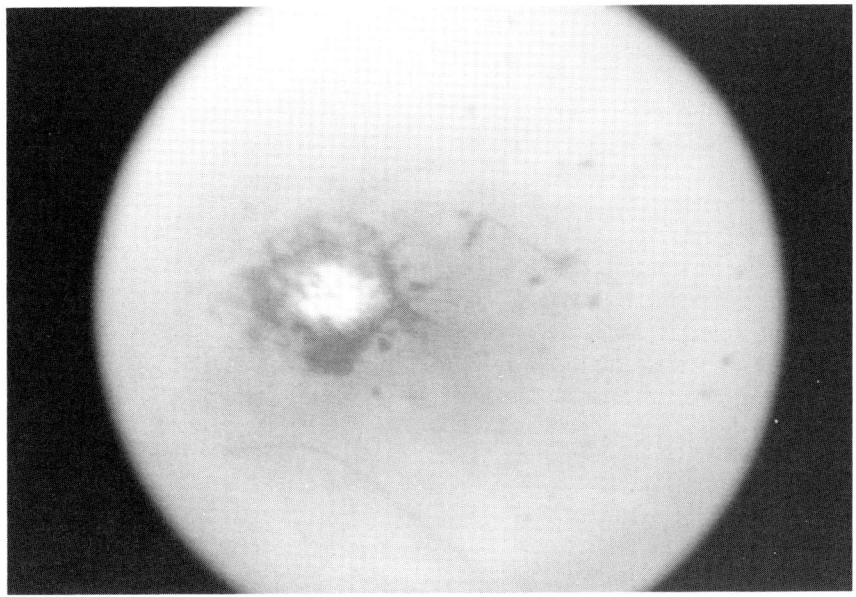

FIGURE 16-28. Toxoplasmosis scar.

the most common cause of posterior uveitis is toxoplasmosis, other common causes are sarcoidosis, syphilis, ocular histoplasmosis, cytomegalovirus, toxocariasis, and Candida.

Sympathetic Ophthalmia

Sympathetic ophthalmia is a rare bilateral panuveitis that occurs following a unilateral penetrating injury, either accidental or surgical. It is believed to

TABLE 16-4. RECOMMENDED TREATMENT FOR OCULAR TOXOPLASMOSIS (ORAL DOSES)

DRUG	LOADING DOSE	MAINTENANCE	DURATION
Pyrimethamine*	50 mg	25 mg daily	4–6 wks
Sulfadiazine†	2–4 g	1 g 4 times a day	4–6 wks
Prednisone‡		40–80 mg daily (tapered)	3–4 wk
Folinic acid		3–5 mg daily	4–6 wks
Clindamycin§		300 mg 4 times a day	4–6 wks

*Whole blood count and platelets should be monitored weekly. Folinic acid should be used concurrently.
†Fluid intake should be maximized to decrease the possibility of sulfadiazine renal crystallization.
‡Contraindicated if tuberculosis, AIDS, or systemic infection is suspected.
§Observe for pseudomembranous colitis.

represent a hypersensitivity or autoimmune response to exposed uveal pigment. This condition can begin as early as 10 days or as long as 50 years following the original injury. The incidence is reported as 0.2% following trauma and 0.01% following surgery. The usual presentation of sympathetic ophthalmia includes bilateral granulomatous uveitis with small depigmented retinal pigment epithelial nodules called Dalen-Fuchs nodules. Although the total number of patients that develop sympathetic ophthalmia is very small, the potential for significant visual loss in the nontraumatized eye exists. Prevention of sympathetic ophthalmia by enucleation of the injured eye before the sympathizing eye becomes involved is the only known way to prevent this disease. Once diagnosed, enucleation is not always curative, and aggressive treatment with topical, periocular, and systemic steroids is recommended. Cyclosporine has been used with some success in the treatment of sympathetic ophthalmia.

Acknowledgment: Photographs for Figures 16.1, 2, 4, 7, 8, 9, 10, 12, 13, 14, 15, 17, 18, 19, 20, 21, 22, and 28 courtesy of Robert A. Catalano.

REFERENCES

Aaberg TM: The expanding ophthalmologic spectrum of Lyme disease. *Am J Ophthalmol* 107:77, 1989.
Auran JD, Starr MB, Jakobiec FA: Acanthamoeba keratitis. A review of the literature. *Cornea* 6(1):2–26, 1987.
Balfour HH Jr, Bean B, Laskin OL, et al: Acyclovir halts progression of herpes zoster in immunocompromised patients. *N Engl J Med* 308:1448, 1983.
BenEzra D: Immunosuppressive treatment of uveitis. *Int Ophthalmol Clin* 30(4):309, 1990.
Copeland RA: Lyme uveitis. *Int Ophthalmol Clin* 30(4):291, 1990.
Driebe WT, Stern GA, Epstein RJ: Acanthamoeba keratitis. Potential role for topical clotrimazole in combination chemotherapy. *Am J Ophthalmol* 106:1196, 1988.
External disease and cornea. *Basic and Clinical Science Course.* American Academy of Ophthalmology, sec 7, 1988–1989.
Ferry AP, Abedi S: Diagnosis and management of rhinoorbitalcerebral mucormycosis (phycomycosis). *Ophthalmology* 90:1096, 1983.
Ficker LA, Kirkness CM, Rice NSC, Steele AM: The changing management and improved prognosis for corneal grafting in herpes simplex keratitis. *Ophthalmology* 96:1587, 1989.
Forster RK: Etiology and diagnosis of bacterial postoperative endophthalmitis. *Ophthalmology* 85:320, 1978.
Goto H, Rao NA: Sympathetic ophthalmia and Vogt-Koyanagi-Harada syndrome. *Int Ophthalmol Clin* 30(4):279, 1990.
Hagler WG, Walters PV, Nahmias AJ: Ocular involvement in neonatal herpes simplex virus infection. *Arch Ophthalmol* 82:169, 1969.
Hammerschlag MR, Chandler JW, Alexander ER, et al: Erythromycin ointment for ocular prophylaxis of neonatal chlamydial infection. *JAMA* 244:2291, 1980.
Hutchison DS, Smith RE, Haughton PB: Congenital herpetic keratitis. *Arch Ophthalmol* 93:70, 1975.
Intraocular inflammation, uveitis and ocular tumors. Basic and Clinical Science Course. American Academy of Ophthalmology, sec 3, 1988.
Jabs DA: Ocular toxoplasmosis. *Int Ophthalmol Clin* 30(4):264, 1990.
Jabs DA, Green WR, Fox R, et al: Ocular manifestation of acquired immune deficiency syndrome. *Ophthalmology* 96:1092, 1989.

Krick JA, Remington JS: Toxoplasmosis in the adult–an overview. *N Engl J Med* 298:550, 1978.

Lawless M, Martin F: Orbital cellulitis and preseptal cellulitis in children. *Aust N Z J Ophthalmol* 14:211, 1986.

Liesegang TJ: Corneal complications from herpes zoster ophthalmicus. *Ophthalmology* 92:316, 1985.

McGill J, Fraunfelder FT, Jones BR: Current and proposed management of ocular herpes simplex. *Surv Ophthalmol* 20:358, 1976.

Mandelbaum S, Forster RK: Late onset endophthalmitis associated with filtering blebs. *Ophthalmology* 92:964, 1985.

Mayers M: Ocular sarcoidosis. *Int Ophthalmol Clin* 30(4):257, 1990.

Nassenblatt RB, Palestine AG, Chan CC: Cyclosporine A therapy in the treatment of intraocular inflammatory disease resistant to systemic corticosteroids and cytotoxic agents. *Am J Ophthalmol* 96:275, 1983.

Orbit, eyelids, and lacrimal system, section 9. In Basic and Clinical Science Course. San Francisco, American Academy of Ophthalmology, 1988.

Pavesio CE, Nozik RA: Anterior and intermediate uveitis. *Int Ophthalmol Clin* 30(4):244, 1990.

Portnoy SL, Insler MS, Kaufman HE: Surgical management of corneal ulceration and perforation. *Surv Ophthalmol* 34:47, 1989.

Rapoza PA, Quinn TC, Kiesslling LA, et al: Epidemiology of neonatal conjunctivitis. *Ophthalmology* 93:456, 1986.

Rapoza PA, Quinn TC, Kiessling LA, et al: Assessment of neonatal conjunctivitis with a direct immunofluorescent monoclonal antibody stain for Chlamydia. *JAMA* 255:3369, 1986.

Reynard M, Riffenburgh RS, Maes EF: Effect of corticosteroid treatment and enucleation in the visual prognosis of sympathetic ophthalmia. *Am J Ophthalmol* 96:290, 1983.

Rosenbaum JT, Wernick R: Selection and interpretation of laboratory tests for patients with uveitis. *Int Ophthalmol Clin* 30(4):238, 1990.

Schanzlin DJ: Herpes simplex eye infections. Focal Points 1981. Clinical Modules for Ophthalmologists.

Schwartz JN, Donnelly EH, Klintworth GK: Ocular and orbital phycomycosis. *Surv Ophthalmol* 22:3, 1977.

Stamper RL: Ophthalmology Clinics of North America : Corneal and External Disease. December 1990.

Steinkuller PG, Jones DB: Preseptal and orbital cellulitis and orbital abscess. In Linberg JV: *Oculoplastic and Orbital Emergencies.* Norwalk, CT, Appleton & Lange 1990, pp 51–66.

Stenson S, Newman R, Redukowicz: Conjunctivitis in the newborn. *Ann Ophthalmol* 13:329, 1981.

Tabbara KF, O'Connor GR: Treatment of ocular toxoplasmosis with clindamycin and sulfadiazine. *Ophthalmology* 87.129, 1980.

Watters EC, Wallar PH, Hiles DA, et al: Acute orbital cellulitis. *Arch Ophthalmol* 94:785, 1976.

Wilhelmus KR: Common Venereal Diseases and the Eye. Focal Points 1987. Clinical Modules for Ophthalmologists.

Winterkorn J: Lyme disease: Neurologic and ophthalmic manifestations. *Surv Ophthalmol* 35:191, 1990.

Womack LW, Liesegang TJ: Complications of herpes zoster ophthalmicus. *Arch Ophthalmol* 101:42, 1983.

17

Antibiotics, Steroids, and Tetanus Immunization

Peter Zloty
Michael W. Belin

ANTIBIOTIC PROPHYLAXIS

Lid Lacerations

Trauma to the eyelids and periocular structures rarely results in infection. The lids and adnexal structures are endowed with an excellent blood supply, as evidenced by their brisk bleeding after trauma, which assists the healing process and helps to prevent infection. Except in cases of bite wounds or with soil, fecal, or other contaminated objects, antibiotic prophylaxis other than a topical ointment (e.g., bacitracin ointment) is usually unnecessary. When antibiotics are needed, the choice is simplified because of the good penetration of antibiotics into the lids and surrounding tissues. The use of antibiotics does not obviate the need for meticulous cleansing of the wound and removal of all foreign material. Additionally, the tetanus immunization status should be assessed in all patients with lid lacerations.

When a wound infection occurs, the proper antibiotic choice is dictated by the characteristics of the wound and the offending microorganism. Wound drainage, if present, should be cultured. Results of culture and sensitivity testing help to guide therapy. It is important to note, however, that routine culture swabs will not readily support the growth of anaerobes, and this must especially be considered in "sterile" infections.

Most superficial infections of the skin after lacerating trauma are due to streptococci and *Staphylococcus aureus.* These are well covered by oral amoxicillin/clavulanic acid (Augmentin), cephalexin (Keflex), or erythromycin (for penicillin-allergic patients). Wounds with anaerobic bacteria or *Bacillus cereus* infection, which may result from soil or fecal contamination, are treated with oral clindamycin 150 mg to 300 mg 4 times daily. Clindamycin covers most pathogenic *Staphylococcus aureus* and streptococci, many *S. epidermidis,* and many anaerobic bacteria and bacillus species. Unfortunately, clindamycin, like the cephalosporins, has poor activity against enterococci (Sanford, 1991). Pseudomembranous colitis, a lower intestinal infection due to *Clostridium difficile,* may develop in patients taking clindamycin. The most prominent symptom is severe diarrhea. A stool assay readily detects the toxin produced by *C. difficile.* The treatment is prompt discontinuation of clindamycin and administration of oral vancomycin, 125 mg PO every 6 hours for 10 days. While *C. difficile* is associated to a greater degree with clindamycin than with other antibiotics, it can occur secondary to the use of any antibiotic, even penicillin.

Frank infections of the eyelids and surrounding structures in young children, especially under age 5 years, should be treated with intravenous therapy. The orbital septum is not well developed in this age group and may have been violated by the trauma. Extension of the preseptal infection to the orbit may result.

Animal and Human Bites

Special consideration should be given to lid injuries secondary to bite wounds (Table 17–1). Complications of dog and cat bites include recurrent abscesses and cellulitis. In some susceptible individuals, bacteremia and death have resulted. Children are especially prone to animal bites of the face and periocular tissues. Dogs account for approximately 80% of these, with cats a distant second at about 10%. The remaining percentage of bites to the ocular structures are produced by rats, raccoons, ferrets, monkeys, and humans. The bacteriology of the oral flora of these animals is important in determining the infections that may result.

Animal bites should be vigorously cleansed, irrigated, and, when necessary, debrided. High-pressure irrigation with a syringe and small catheter is advantageous to high-volume, low-pressure irrigation. In general, the use of prophylactic antibiotics to cover oral flora is controversial. Dog bites to the face that present within 6 hours to 8 hours are usually sutured. Because suturing increases the risk of abscess and infection, prophylactic antibiotics are probably warranted (see Chapter 4).

The oral flora of animals include streptococci, *Pasteurella multocida, Staphylococcus aureus* and *S. epidermidis, Eikenella corrodens, Dysgonic fermenter*

TABLE 17-1. ANTIBIOTIC PROPHYLAXIS IN ANIMAL BITES

SCENARIO	PROPHYLAXIS
Animal bite (Domestic dog or cat)	Augmentin 40 mg/kg/day in 3 divided doses Not to exceed 500 mg 3 times a day; Suspension and chewable tablets 125 mg and 250 mg are available.
	OR
	Cefuroxime (Ceftin tablets) 20 mg/kg/day in 2 divided doses Not to exceed 500 mg twice daily; Tablets of 125 mg, 250 mg, and 500 mg are available. Cefuroxime (intravenous) 75 mg/kg/day in three divided doses given every 8 hours; Not to exceed 3 g daily.
	OR
	Ceftriaxone 50 mg/kg/day as a single IM dose or intravenously in 2 divided doses, not to exceed 2 g daily for children or 4 g daily for adults.
If frank preseptal cellulitis develops, intravenous therapy is preferred over oral dosing. This is especially true for children. Computed tomography scanning should be performed to rule out orbital extension of the injury and of the infection. Treatment with intravenous cefuroxime or ceftriaxone will cover most of the bite wound flora well; however, the best therapy in actual infection is probably still penicillin and either nafcillin or oxacillin. The latter is preferred because of less peripheral phlebitis. This combination is also prudent when DF-2 is of concern (the penicillin dose however, should be doubled).	
Aqueous penicillin G	75,000 units/kg/day IV (25,000 units/kg every 8 hours) Double this dose if DF2 infection.
Oxacillin	250 mg/kg/day IV (62.5 mg/kg every 6 hours).

type 2 (DF2), and Bacteroides. Feder, Stanley, and Barbara (1987) found that *P. multocida* was the most commonly isolated bacteria cultured from patients hospitalized with animal bites. A good broad-spectrum oral antibiotic recommended for animal bite prophylaxis, with good activity against *S. aureus, P. multocida,* and streptococci, is amoxicillin/clavulanic acid (Augmentin, 40 mg/kg in three divided doses by mouth; up to 500 mg per dose). It should be noted that two 250 mg tablets are not interchangeable with a single 500 mg tablet, in that two 250 mg tablets have twice the clavulanic acid as a single 500 mg tablet, and this increased dosage is not recommended. The addition of clavulanic acid to amoxicillin renders it beta lactamase stable. Augmentin is therefore active against beta lactamase, producing *S. aureus, S. epidermidis,* and *H. influenzae.* Augmentin (amoxicillin/clavulanic acid) covers nearly all bacteria that Keflex (cephalexin) does, plus the enterococci; no cephalosporin covers enterococci.

A single intramuscular (IM) dose of the third-generation cephalosporin ceftriaxone (Rocephin), given once every 24 hours, also gives adequate coverage for most of the bacteria of concern (Table 17-1). Most of the first-generation cephalosporins (i.e., cefazolin) and many second-generation cephalosporins (i.e., cefoxitin) do not cover *P. multocida* consistently. However, cefuroxime, a second-generation agent with good activity against *P. multocida,* is an acceptable alternative agent, which can be given both orally and intravenously (Goldstein and Citron, 1988).

Dysgonic fermenter type 2 (DF2) is a gram-negative rod found in the oral flora of dogs and cats. Bite wounds infected with DF2 can induce a fatal septicemia in splenectomized individuals or those with altered cellular immunity, such as alcoholics or patients on chronic steroids. Severe tissue necrosis, disseminated intravascular coagulation, and cardiovascular collapse can occur. A high index of suspicion and prompt treatment with antibiotics can be life saving. Treatment of DF2 infection is usually with intravenous penicillin G, 2 million to 4 million units every 4 hours (adults) or 75,000 units/kg per day divided every 4 to 6 hours (children).

Rabies prophylaxis is reviewed in Chapter 4.

Orbital Fractures

Routine blowout orbital fractures of the ethmoid and maxillary sinuses probably do not need special antibiotic coverage. But if the patient has a concurrent sinus infection, a fracture of the sinus walls with laceration of the sinus mucoperiosteum could result in seeding of the orbit with bacteria. Patients are frequently advised to avoid nose blowing since this can result in orbital emphysema. Such an occurrence clearly demonstrates communication between the sinuses and the orbit after fracture. Typical bacterial pathogens in sinusitis are *Streptococcus pneumoniae* (pneumococcus), *H. influenza,* and group A streptococcus. It is reasonable to cover for these bacteria in patients with orbital fractures and documented or suspected sinusitis. Cephalexin, 40 mg/kg per day in 4 divided doses, or Augmentin, 40 mg/kg per day in 3 divided doses, is suggested. Chronic sinusitis, particularly in diabetics, may contain anaerobes. With the development of penicillin-resistant bacteroides strains, penicillin is no longer suggested. Clindamycin, 150 mg to 300 mg by mouth 4 times daily, should be used.

Orbital fractures with exposed bone are compound fractures at risk for developing osteomyelitis. Cefazolin 1 g intravenously every 6 hours should be given until surgical repair. After repair, an additional four doses followed by several days of an oral cephalosporin should cover most commonly encountered organisms.

ENDOPHTHALMITIS

Ocular infections that arise from bloodborne infections are termed *endogenous endophthalmitis.* This group is distinguished from ocular infections that arise due to external environmental pathogens that enter the eye with penetrating trauma and surgery and are termed *exogenous endophthalmitis.* The two exogenous types are postoperative and posttraumatic endophthalmitis.

Postoperative Endophthalmitis and Antibiotic Prophylaxis of Elective Surgery

Postoperative endophthamitis following elective surgical cases is rare (less than 0.1% of cases). *S. epidermidis* is the most common pathogen. Other bacteria recovered from culture are *S. aureus, S. viridans,* and various gram-negative rods such as *Pseudomonas* and *Proteus.* The anaerobe *Propionobacterium acnes* has been associated with late-onset infection. For comparative purposes, Table 17-2 lists the mean time to diagnosis in posttraumatic endophthalmitis. Rare instances of fungal infection have been reported, many due to contaminated intraocular irrigation solutions. The causative microorganisms are often skin flora that are carried into the eye during the operative procedure. The regimens and rationale for treatment of postoperative endophthalmitis are beyond the scope of this book; readers are referred to Peyman, Raichand, and Bennett (1980); Mandlebaum and Forster (1987); Talley, D'Amico, Talamo, et al. (1987); and Oum, D'Amico, and Wong (1989). The treatment, however, shares some similarities to posttraumatic infection (see Tables 17-3 and 17-4).

Antibiotic prophylaxis is a controversial subject in most surgical fields. Controlled studies have demonstrated decreased wound infections in cardiovascular and gynecologic surgery with preoperative administration of a first-generation cephalosporin. Cefazolin is often used. These data have been extrapolated to other fields, where their application is less clear. In ophthalmology, cefazolin and gentamicin are often used in potentially contaminated cases. In elective eye surgery, however, the low incidence of postoperative infection, as well as the inability of most systematically administered antibiotics to enter the eye (Barza, 1989; Cunha-Vaz, 1979), argues against the use of prophylaxis. Additionally, cefazolin has been shown to be ineffective against more than half of the *S. epidermidis* isolated, the most common organism iso-

TABLE 17-2. CLINICAL DIAGNOSIS OF ENDOPHTHALMITIS AFTER TRAUMA

Staphylococcus epidermidis	4 days
Bacillus cereus	24–36 hours
Streptococcus viridans	48 hours
Various fungi	> 2 weeks

(Adapted from: Affeldt JC, Flynn HW Jr, Forster RK, et al: Microbial endophthalmitis resulting from ocular trauma. *Ophthalmology* 94:407, 1987. Brinton GS, Topping TM, Hyndiuk RA, et al: Posttraumatic endophthalmitis. *Arch Ophthalmol* 102:547, 1984.)

lated in postoperative as well as posttraumatic endophthalmitis, and systemic gentamicin has significant renal toxicity.

Posttraumatic Endophthalmitis

Posttraumatic endophthalmitis is a serious complication of penetrating ocular injury. Infection can follow severe disorganizing trauma to the eye, as well as seemingly benign self-sealing corneal perforations. The incidence of posttraumatic ocular infection is reported as 2% to 7%, with a higher risk associated with retained intraocular foreign bodies.

The causative organisms are as varied as the mechanisms of injury. In addition, every penetrating object is colonized with its own flora. The environment the patient was in prior to the injury is also important. Van Bijsterveld and Richards (1965) were able to culture *Bacillus cereus* from the normal, uninflamed eyes of farmworkers. It is presumed that conjunctival flora can be carried into the intraocular tissues by missile-type injuries; therefore, this colonization is probably significant. Farm implements are also heavily contaminated with *B. cereus,* as well as anaerobic bacteria. Injuries occurring in or associated with stream or lake water may be contaminated with *Aeromonas hydrophila*, a gram-negative rod similar to pseudomonas. Exogenous fungal (not bloodborne) endophthalmitis, though rare, has also been reported (Pflugfelder, Flynn, Zwickey, et al., 1988).

The offending organisms found in posttraumatic endophthalmitis (in descending order of frequency) are: *S. epidermidis, B. cereus, S. aureus,* streptococci (pneumoniae, viridans, enterococci), various gram-negative rods (enterobacteraciae, pseudomonas), various anaerobes (Clostridia, Bacteroides), and various fungi (Fusarium, Candida) (Parrish and O'Day, 1987; Pflugfelder et al., 1988).

Most ophthalmologists reserve the term *endophthalmitis* for infections with vitreous involvement. In late infection, the vitreous takes on characteristics of an abscess cavity, with a low pH, low oxygen tension, and toxic enzymes. It is important to remember that an entire class of antibiotics, the aminoglycosides, is rendered relatively ineffective in this environment (Braude, 1986). Bacterial absorption of aminoglycosides requires oxygen and near-normal pH. Treatment of a purulent vitreous cavity based heavily on the activity of aminoglycosides is hampered by this often-overlooked characteristic.

Experimental studies have demonstrated vitreous sterilization in experimentally induced endophthalmitis if treatment is begun early with appropriate drugs. Delay in treatment beyond 36 hours, however, resulted in lack of vitreous sterilization and subsequent poor retinal function, in spite of maximally tolerated antibiotic levels (Oum et al., 1989). Prompt diagnosis and therapy is therefore essential for functional recovery. Posttraumatic inflammation and the attendant signs and symptoms of infection, however, depend greatly on the degree of disorganization of the eye, the virulence of the organism, and the size of the innoculum.

Bacillus cereus is present in dust, water, soil, fecal, and vegetable matter. It is not killed by alcohol or detergents; rather, it requires 10 minutes of boiling or autoclaving to destroy. The normally produced heat of dissociation of metal on metal splintering does not destroy the spores. In the eye, *Bacillus* produces rapid retinal necrosis with vascular sheathing. Like clostridial endophthalmitis, it produces a systemic leukocytosis and fever even if infection is isolated to the eye. It may also produce intraocular gas. There have been only a few reported cases of functional visual recovery after *B. cereus* endophthalmitis (Schemmer and Driebe, 1987; Beer, Ludwig, and Packer, 1990). It is uniformly resistant to cefazolin and is resistant to the levels of gentamicin that penetrate the eye after systemic administration (Braude, 1986; Davey and Tauber, 1987).

Treatment Rationale in Traumatic Endophthalmitis

Trauma is associated with the introduction of foreign bodies and microorganisms into the eye. Prudence therefore dictates a more liberal use of prophylactic antibiotics in these cases than for routine elective surgery. The degree of inflammation and signs and symptoms of infection depend greatly on such factors as the degree of disorganization of the eye, the virulence of the organism, and the size of the inoculum. Organisms such as *B. cereus* are particularly devastating, with onset of clinical infection as early as 4 hours after injury (Beer et al., 1990). Infections with other pathogens are less virulent. The eye can harbor *S. epidermidis* without frank inflammation for over 72 hours. This is an important consideration since commonly used systemic antibiotics given as prophylaxis for penetrating ocular injuries (e.g., cefazolin and gentamicin) rely on the inflammatory breakdown of the blood ocular barrier for penetration (Martin, Ficker, Aguilar, et al., 1990). Commonly used systemic, topical, and periocular antibiotics do not penetrate the uninflamed cye well, yet this is often the state the minimally traumatized eye is in before frank supperation begins. These agents are either inconsistently effective against the more likely offending bacteria or ineffective at the doses typically administered. Realizing this, some experienced investigators advocate direct intravitreal antibiotic injections in the case of retained intraocular foreign bodies without signs of infection due to the twofold higher incidence of infection in these cases (particularly *B. cereus*).

The ideal approach to antibiotic prophylaxis suggests the use of relatively nontoxic agents that have good ocular penetration and a high level of activity against the most likely encountered organisms. Clearly this is not achieved with systemic cefazolin and gentamicin, which are frequently used for this purpose. Gentamicin has excellent activity in vitro but has limited intraocular penetration. Cefazolin has good gram-positive coverage except for *S. epidermidis,* the most common cause of endophthalmitis. It too has poor intraocular penetration except in a markedly inflamed eye. This combination arose when little else was available. Systemic vancomycin, unlike cefazolin, has uniformly excellent staphylococcal coverage, but it does not penetrate the aqueous in sufficient concentration to be effective when it is given systemically, and it potentiates the nephrotoxicity of gentamicin and other aminoglycosides (Sanford, 1991).

Antimicrobials for exogenous endophthalmitis should be chosen based on their ability to penetrate blood ocular barriers and their microbial sensitivities. Some general principles to help guide ophthalmologists in selecting and using antibiotics are listed below and in Tables 17-3 and 17-4. An exhaustive review of microbial sensitivities is beyond the scope of this chapter. Interested readers are referred to the excellent handbook by Sanford (1991).

Primaxin (imipenem-cilastatin) is a carbapenem (penicillin type) bactericidal antibiotic that covers a wide variety of gram-positive, gram-negative, and anaerobic infections. Imipenem, the active drug, is a potent agent best known for its ability to retain superb gram-positive coverage while being effective against a host of gram-negative bacteria, including Pseudomonas. It also covers *Propionobacterium acnes* and other anaerobes. A review of the ophthalmologic literature of the last 20 years reveals very few bacterial isolates from endophthalmitis patients that would not be susceptible to imipenem. Additionally, Primaxin gains access into the aqueous and vitreous humor without inflammation in concentrations above the minimum inhibitory concentration (MIC) for most bacteria of concern (Axelrod, Newton, Klein, et al., 1987; Braude, 1986). Cilastatin is an agent that interferes with the renal excretion of imipenem, the active drug, enhancing the drug level. Cilastatin, however, does not directly enhance imipenem's antibacterial activity as clavulanic acid does for amoxicillin. Additionally, probenecid does not have an additive effect on serum or ocular levels for Primaxin as it does for other beta lactams.

Ciprofloxacin is an excellent antistaphylococcal and antipseudomonal agent. A quinolone antibiotic available for intravenous, oral, and topical use, it has good intraocular penetration with oral administration and excellent penetration with intravenous dosing. Unlike imipenem, it is not especially good against streptococci and does not cover anaerobes. It does, however, cover *B. cereus,* aeromonas, and the enterobacteraciae. It too achieves concentrations in both the aqueous and vitreous well above its minimal inhibitory concentration for *S. aureus* and *epidermidis* (Fern, Sweeney, Doig, et al., 1986; Behrens-Baumann and Martell, 1987).

Third-generation cephalosporin antibiotics have enhanced gram-negative coverage but typically have less gram-positive activity compared to the first-generation cephalosporins. The third-generation antipseudomonal agent ceftazidime (Fortaz), however, may be a better agent than cefazolin against gram-positive bacteria in ocular infections because it has far greater intraocular penetration than cefazolin (Tables 17-5 and 17-6). Cefazolin's aqueous drug level is less than 1% of the serum concentration, whereas ceftazidime's aqueous level is 14% of the serum level. Cephradine (Velosef) is a first-generation

Text continues on page 508

TABLE 17-3. POSTTRAUMATIC ENDOPHTHALMITIS TREATMENT PROPHYLAXIS RECOMMENDATIONS

SCENARIO	PROPHYLAXIS
Corneal perforation without lens or iris trauma and without IOFB*†	
Adults	Ciprofloxacin 500–750 mg by mouth twice daily PLUS Topical vancomycin 3.3–5% solution or topical fortified aminoglycoside or topical trimethoprim/polymyxin B (Polytrim): 1 drop every 5 minutes × 6 and then every hour
Children, pregnant, and nursing women	Cephradine (Velosef) 10 mg/kg by mouth 4 times a day, not to exceed 500 mg QID PLUS Topical Ciprofloxacin (Ciloxan) or topical vancomycin 3.3–5% solution: 1 drop every 5 minutes × 6 and then every hour
Penicillin-allergic children	Trimethoprim/sulfamethoxazole 5 mL of suspension per every 10 kg by mouth, 2 times a day, not to exceed 20 mL twice daily PLUS Topical ciprofloxacin (Ciloxan) or topical vancomycin 3.3–5% solution: 1 drop every 5 minutes × 6 and then every hour
Deep, penetrating ocular injury with probable contamination	
Adults	Primaxin 1 g intravenously ASAP and every 6 hours × 48 hours
Children	Primaxin 12 mg/kg intravenously ASAP and every 6 hours × 48 hours; not to exceed 4 g daily‡
Penicillin-allergic adults (*not* pregnant or nursing)	Ciprofloxacin 400 mg intravenously ASAP and every 12 hours
Mildly penicillin-allergic children (not anaphylaxis), and pregnant or nursing women	Ceftazidime 30 mg/kg intravenously ASAP and every 8 hours × 48 hours; not to exceed 6 g daily PLUS *(if fecal/soil contamination)* Clindamycin 10 mg/kg intravenously ASAP and every 8 hours × 48 hours; not to exceed 2 g daily
Severely penicillin allergic children, pregnant or nursing women	Tobramycin 1.5 mg/kg intravenously ASAP and every 8 hours. *Must check serum trough and peak levels at third dose and every 36 hours thereafter* PLUS *(if fecal/soil contamination)* Clindamycin 8 mg/kg intravenously ASAP and every 8 hours × 48 hours
Corneal perforation with lens/iris trauma or if contamination likely	Above plus topical agents†
Intraocular foreign body	Above plus consider intravitreal injections (Table 17–4)†

The suggestions in this table are specifically designed to provide well-tolerated, broad-spectrum coverage against organisms typically found in cases of ocular trauma. These regimens are not intended for use in routine, noncontaminated, elective surgical cases, where there is a typically low infection rate. It would not be medically justifiable or cost effective to use these antibiotics for routine surgical prophylaxis. There is a danger that these antibiotics may lose their effectiveness due to the emergence of resistant strains of bacteria if widely and inappropriately used.

*IOFB: intraocular foreign body.

†Topical agents, particularly ointments, should not be used on an eye that is not self-sealing or that has not been surgically closed.

‡We have noted less pain at IV site if dissolved in 150 cc D5W instead of the usual 50 cc to 100 cc.

TABLE 17-4. TREATMENT OF ENDOPHTHALMITIS

Table 17-3 suggests recommendations for *prophylactic therapy* only. If during the observation period, while on these regimens, frank infection develops, immediate alternate management is begun. Signs of exogenous endophthalmitis are pain, turbidity of the aqueous and/or vitreous, retinal vascular sheathing, intraocular fibrin, corneal clouding, or infiltrate, and hypopyon. The presentation initially may be mild with only persistent iritis and decreased vision (often attributed to cystoid macular edema). Once endophthalmitis is in the differential diagnosis, however, treatment must be given for this until proved otherwise. The usual management consists of diagnostic aqueous and vitreous taps and intracameral antibiotic injections.

Specimen Retrieval

1. Perform an anterior chamber paracentesis with an MVR blade or 27-gauge needle and withdraw approximately .05 cc to .1 cc fluid. Directly inoculate onto the following:
    a) Chocolate agar (*not* Thayer Martin). This is the single most important plate to inoculate if only a small sample is retrieved. It will support the growth of most of the bacteria of concern.
    b) Glass slide. This is the next most important step. A second slide held flat should be drawn over the first to create two thin smears. One slide is Gram stained, the second is for Giemsa stain if fungal infection is suspected.
    c) Blood agar. Both bacteria and most ocular pathogenic fungi will grow on this medium. The laboratory must be alerted not to disregard fungi as contaminants (they will unless instructed not to) and to hold all eye specimens for at least 5 days.
    d) Thioglycolate (anaerobic media). Medium must be inoculated deeply. Do not use a cotton swab to push the specimen into medium as the air in the swab is also inserted and is toxic to the anaerobes. Use a sterile instrument (57 blade) or a hypodermic needle.
    e) Sabouraud's agar (fungal media). If unavailable or if insufficient specimen, tell the laboratory to hold the blood agar plate for 3 weeks and observe for fungi.
2. A conjunctival dissection, sutured closed at the end of the procedure, is suggested. Through the pars plana (3.5 mm from the limbus), a 22-gauge hypodermic needle is directed toward the center of the vitreous. The operating microscope ensures accurate placement, although in a turbid eye the indirect ophthalmoscope may provide a better view of the needle tip. Approximately .15 mL to .25 mL is aspirated, and cultures are handled as above. Some surgeons favor removing the syringe from the needle at this point and changing to the syringe containing the antibiotics and injecting. An advantage of this technique is that vitreous strands are forced out of the needle and are less likely to be pulled out of the eye. Some surgeons find that changing the syringes while the needle is in the eye is cumbersome and risks retinal injury. The technique for injection is left up to the individual surgeon. The value of limited vitrectomy with injection of retrieved material into blood culture bottles is not determined. Loss of red reflex is almost always an indication for formal vitrectomy.

Treatment

1. Using nonbacteriostatic .9% saline, have the pharmacy prepare sterile, filtered solutions of vancomycin 10 mg in 1 mL and amikacin 4 mg in 1 mL.
2. Through the paracentesis, with a 30-gauge cannula, inject the following into the anterior chamber: vancomycin 0.5 mg (0.05 mL) and amikacin .2 mg (0.05 mL).
3. Through the vitreous tap site, inject the following into the vitreous cavity: vancomycin 1.0 mg (0.1 mL) and amikacin .4 mg (0.1 mL).
    Earlier studies suggested that the addition of clindamycin was prudent in cases of retained intraocular foreign bodies or when *Bacillus cereus* was suspected. Recently *B. cereus* species resistant to clindamycin have been reported. Vancomycin and amikacin provide excellent coverage against *B. cereus,* as well as for all of the likely causes of traumatic (as well as postoperative) endophthalmitis. Therefore, the addition of clindamycin is probably superfluous.
4. Subconjunctival injections will enhance corneal and anterior chamber antibiotic levels. Based on animal studies, the following is recommended: vancomycin 12.5 mg in .2 mL* and amikacin 25–50 mg in .2 mL. If steroids are favored, consider Decadron 4–12 mg in .2 to .5 mL.

TABLE 17-4. TREATMENT OF ENDOPHTHALMITIS (continued)

Treatment

5. Systemic therapy will probably enhance antimicrobial levels significantly only after the intracameral antibiotics begin to diffuse out of the eye in 24 to 48 hours. If culture reports reveal a resistant organism to the initially given antibiotics or if there is no clinical improvement, some investigators suggest repeat antibiotic injections. In any case, systemic therapy will be only an adjunct to and not the curative factor in acute endophthalmitis. Systemic therapy with both vancomycin and amikacin has additive ototoxicity and nephrotoxicity, and close monitoring of both of their serum levels is essential. Additionally, as the inflammation lessens over time, their penetration will decrease for the same reasons they were not suggested for prophylaxis. From an infectious disease standpoint, their use systemically is not justifiable. For example, infectious disease specialists usually do not treat pneumoccocal meningitis with penicillin, even though it is the best antipneumococcal drug available and it penetrates into the inflamed meninges, because its absorption into the central nervous system becomes variable as the disease progresses. Similarly, ophthalmologists should probably not use poorly penetrating drugs to treat intraocular disease. For these reasons we suggest the use of the agents listed in Table 17-3 for systemic therapy to augment intracameral endophthalmitis therapy.
6. Though rare, exogenous fungal endophthalmitis must be considered in cases of late-onset infection after trauma (Table 17-2). If fungi are seen on Gram's or Giemsa stain or if a positive fungal culture is obtained, then the following antifungal therapy is recommended: intravitreal: amphotericin B 5 μg (.005 mg) in .1 mL; subconjunctival: amphotericin B 1 mg in .5 mL.

Though systemic antifungal therapy has not been shown to be effective in the treatment of vitreous infection, ketoconazole is often recommended (Pflugfelder et al., 1988). It is given as three 200 mg tablets, once daily.

*Doses of subconjunctival vancomycin higher than this have been associated with anecdotal reports of conjunctival necrosis and should be avoided.

TABLE 17-5. DIFFUSION OF ANTIBIOTIC INTO AQUEOUS HUMOR

	DOSE	CONCENTRATION (μg/ml)
Cefazolin	1 g IV	<.6
Gentamicin	1 mg/kg IV	<.8
Tobramycin	1 mg/kg IV	3.4
Amikacin	7.5 mg/kg IV	0
Imipenem	1 g IV	2.99
Ciprofloxacin	400 mg IV	.8
Ceftazidime	2 g IV	3.4–11.0
Cefuroxime	1 g IV	1.7
Vancomycin	500 mg IV	<.8
Cephradine	1 g PO	1.99

(Adapted from: Sanford JP: *Guide to Microbial Therapy 1991.* West Bethesda, MD, Antimicrobial Therapy, 1991; Barza M: Antibacterial agents in the treatment of ocular infections. *Infect Dis Clin NA* 3(3):533, 1989. Axelrod JL, Kochman RS: Cephradine levels in human aqueous humor. *Arch Ophthalmol* 99:2034, 1981. Fern AI, Sweeney G, Doig M, Lindsay G: Penetration of ciprofloxacin into aqueous humor. *Transactions of the Ophthalmological Societies of the United Kingdom* 105:650, 1986. Behrens-Baumann W, Martell J: Ciprofloxacin concentrations in human aqueous humor following intravenous administration. *Chemotherapy* 33(5):328, 1987. Martin DF, Flicker LA, Aguilar HA, et al: Vitreous cefazolin levels after intravenous injection: Effects of inflammation, repeated antibiotic doses, and surgery. *Arch Ophthalmol* 108:411, 1990. Axelrod JL, Newton JC, Klein RM, et al: Penetration of imipenem into human aqueous and vitreous humor. *Am J Ophthalmol* 104:649, 1987. Lesar TS, Fiscella RG: Antimicrobial drug delivery to the eye. *Drug Intel Clin Pharm* 19:642, 1985.)

TABLE 17-6. ANTIBIOTIC PENETRATION (μg/mL)

		AQUEOUS	VITREOUS
Ciprofloxacin	400 mg IV	.80	.40
	750 mg oral	.18	.06
Imipenem	1 gram IV	2.99	2.53
Tobramycin	1 mg/kg	2–3.0	—
Cefazolin	1 g IV	<.6	—

(Adapted from: Sanford JP: *Guide to Microbial Therapy 1991*. West Bethesda, MD, Antimicrobial Therapy, 1991. Fern AI, Sweeney G, Doig M, Lindsay G: Penetration of ciprofloxacin into aqueous humor. *Transactions of the Ophthalmological Societies of the United Kingdom* 105:650, 1986. Behrens-Baumann W, Martell J: Ciprofloxacin concentrations in human aqueous humor following intravenous administration. *Chemotherapy* 33(5):328, 1987. Axelrod JL, Newton JC, Klein RM, et al: Penetration of imipenem into human aqueous and vitreous humor. *Am J Ophthalmol* 104:649, 1987. Lesar TS, Fiscella RG: Antimicrobial drug delivery to the eye. *Drug Intel Clin Pharm* 19:642, 1985.)

cephalosporin with essentially the same spectrum as cefazolin; however, it has significantly better intraocular penetration, with a peak aqueous level of approximately 8% of the serum level, even with oral administration. Unlike cefazolin, cephradine is available in both oral and intravenous form.

Currently, only approximately 50% of *S. epidermidis* are sensitive to the first-generation cephalosporins, and only approximately 60% are sensitive to gentamicin (Braude, 1986; Sanford, 1991). In contrast, imipenem, ciprofloxacin, and vancomycin retain high activity. This does not take into account the different rates of ocular penetration but only the actual sensitivities under ideal conditions. If these penetration differences were considered, imipenem fares best, followed by ciprofloxacin (Axelrod et al., 1987; Fern et al., 1986; Behrens-Baumann et al., 1987).

Specific Treatment Recommendations for Exogenous Endophthalmitis

We suggest the use of systemic therapy with Primaxin (imipenem/cilastatin) for traumatized eyes that are highly suspicious for intraocular contamination (Table 17–3). It has excellent penetration into the uninflamed aqueous and vitreous humors and is highly effective against *S. epidermidis* and *S. aureus*. It also covers *B. cereus, H. influenzae,* a wide variety of streptococci, and anaerobes, and has activity against Pseudomonas, Aeromonas, and *P. acnes.*

For penicillin-allergic patients, we recommend ciprofloxacin intravenously. Its coverage is similar to imipenem except for streptococci and anaerobic coverage. Prophylaxis may be augmented with clindamycin for anaerobic coverage if fecal or soil contamination is suspected. The addition of clindamycin to ciprofloxacin also covers streptococci (except for enterococci) that are missed by ciprofloxacin.

Children under age 12 years and pregnant women SHOULD NOT receive ciprofloxacin as it has been associated with cartilage growth abnormalities in animal studies. These patients should receive ceftazidime (Fortaz) (Table 17-3). Ceftazidime has good ocular penetration and covers many gram-positive bacteria in the concentrations it achieves in the eye. It should be augmented with clindamycin for coverage of *B. cereus* and to enhance gram-positive and anaerobic coverage. Another third-generation cephalosporin, cefotaxime, is an alternative to ceftazidime. It has better gram-positive coverage than ceftazidime, but its ocular penetration is less, reducing both its gram-positive coverage and its gram-negative activity.

For suspected endophthalmitis, rapid evaluation with aqueous and vitreous tap for culture and Gram's stain and injection of antibiotics is mandatory. Vitrectomy in these cases has the theoretic advantage of removing toxic debris and decreasing the bacterial load. The NIH Endophthalmitis Vitrectomy Study is being conducted to establish guidelines concerning the timing of vitrectomy. Most vitreous surgeons opt for vitrectomy in cases where the red reflex is lost. When the red reflex is preserved, a vitreous tap for culture and injection of antibiotics is usually preferred (Table 17-4).

The intravenous treatment of ocular infections is expensive (Table 17-7). It should be noted that gentamicin may be relatively inexpensive, but close monitoring of serum blood levels and renal function tests to avoid renal and ototoxicity can make the administration of this drug more expensive than it initially appears.

TABLE 17-7. COST ANALYSIS OF DAILY IV THERAPY

Imipenem	$152.80
Ceftazidime	$84.00
Gentamicin	$23.00†
Cefazolin	$24.00
Vancomycin*	$78.00†
Clindamycin*	$32.00
Ciprofloxacin (oral)	$8.00
Ciprofloxacin (IV)	$50.00

*Poor ocular penetration.
†Cost of the antibiotic only. Add approximately $50.00 per day if renal function tests are done every 36 hours.
(Costs are derived from product references appearing in Drug Topics Redbook 1990. Oradell, NJ, Medical Economics Co., 1990.)

OCULAR STEROIDS IN THE ACUTE SETTING

We do not favor the use of steroids in cases of acute penetrating ocular trauma. From an infectious disease perspective, the use of steroids serves only to reduce the ability of the eye to sterilize the inoculum of microorganisms it has encountered. While inflammation due to the release of proteolytic and collagenolytic enzymes from leukocytes is harmful, the release of toxins and enzymes from enhanced bacterial growth is much worse. The eye should be treated with antibiotics, cycloplegic agents, and close monitoring. If infectious endophthalmitis develops, intraocular antibiotics must be administered. Steroid injection into the vitreous at the time of tap or vitrectomy is at the discretion of the surgeon.

TETANUS IMMUNIZATION

Recommendations for tetanus prophylaxis are based on the condition of the wound, the mechanism of injury, and the presence of contaminants. A tetanus-prone wound is typically a crush or projectile injury. The presence of devitalized tissue and soil, saliva, or fecal contamination is a risk factor. Wounds left untreated for more than 6 hours to 8 hours are also more likely to develop tetanus infection.

Adequate immunization must be determined for any patient with a traumatic injury. A useful guide is the routine immunization schedule, as follows: An infant receives a combination vaccine of pediatric diphtheria, pertussis, and tetanus (DPT) at ages 2, 4, 6, and 18 months. A booster dose at age 4 to 6 years is required by most states prior to a child's entering school. An additional booster of adult tetanus, diphtheria (Td) is given at approximately age 14 to 16 years. Thereafter, Td is given every 10 years for the remainder of the patient's life. This general guideline is useful when one is concerned about a child with a bite who has recently "received his shots for school." Table 17–8 will guide

TABLE 17–8. TETANUS IMMUNIZATION AND PROPHYLAXIS

HISTORY OF ADSORBED TETANUS TOXOID (DOSES)	TETANUS-PRONE WOUNDS		NONTETANUS-PRONE WOUNDS	
	Td[1]	TIG*	Td[1]	TIG*
Unknown, or fewer than 3	Yes	Yes	Yes	No
3 or more[2]	No[4]	No	No[3]	No

[1] Under age 7: administer diphtheria pertussis tetanus (DPT) .5 cc IM. Over age 7, use tetanus diphtheria (Td) "For adult use" .5 cc IM.
[2] If only three doses of fluid toxoid have been received, a fourth dose of toxoid, preferably an adsorbed toxoid, should be given.
[3] Yes, if more than 10 years since last dose.
[4] Yes, if more than five years since last dose. (More frequent boosters are not needed and can accentuate side effects.)

*TIG = tetanus immune globulin.
(Adapted from: American College of Surgeons, Committee on Trauma: *Prophylaxis Against Tetanus in Wound Management,* 1987.)

the physician in determining if tetanus prophylaxis is required (see also Chapter 4). It is important to note that for children less than age 7 years, DPT is preferred to tetanus toxoid alone. For persons age 7 years and older, Td is preferred to tetanus toxoid alone. In addition to the use of toxoid, tetanus immune globulin (TIG) is essential when the immunization history is unknown or the patient has received only one toxoid vaccine previously. Pertussis-containing vaccine should never be given to anyone over the age of 7 years.

REFERENCES

Affeldt JC, Flynn HW Jr, Forster RK, et al: Microbial endophthalmitis resulting from ocular trauma. *Ophthalmology* 94:407, 1987.
Axelrod JL, Kochman RS: Cephradine levels in human aqueous humor. *Arch Ophthalmol* 99:2034, 1981.
Axelrod JL, Newton JC, Klein RM, et al: Penetration of imipenem into human aqueous and vitreous humor. *Am J Ophthalmol* 104:649, 1987.
Baile WE, Stowe EC, Schmitt AM: Aerobic bacterial flora of oral and nasal fluids of canines with reference to bacteria associated with bites. *J Clin Microbiol* 7:223, 1978
Barza M: Antibacterial agents in the treatment of ocular infections. *Infect Dis Clin NA* 3(3):533, 1989.
Beer PM, Ludwig IL, Packer AJ: Complete visual recovery after *Bacillus cereus* endophthalmitis in a child. *Am J Ophthalmol* 110(2):212, 1990.
Behrens-Baumann W, Martell J: Ciprofloxacin concentrations in human aqueous humor following intravenous administration. *Chemotherapy* 33(5):328, 1987.
Braude, AI: *Infectious Diseases and Medical Microbiology.* 2d ed. Philadelphia, WB Saunders Company, 1986.
Brinton GS, Topping TM, Hyndiuk RA, et al: Posttraumatic endophthalmitis. *Arch Ophthalmol* 102:547, 1984.
Brook I: Microbiology of human and animal bite wounds in children. *Pediatr Infect Dis J* 6(1):29, 1987.
Cunha-Vaz J: The blood-ocular barriers. *Surv Ophthalmol* 23:279, 1979.
D'Amico DJ, et al: Comparative toxicity of intravitreal aminoglycoside antibiotics. *Am J Ophthalmol* 100:264, 1985.
Davey RT Jr, Tauber WB: Posttraumatic endophthalmitis: The emerging role of Bacillus cereus infection. *Rev Infect Dis* 9:110, 1987.
Drug Topics Redbook 1990. Oradell, NJ, Medical Economics Company 1990.
Endophthalmitis Vitrectomy Study: *Manual of Operations.* Bethesda, MD, National Institutes of Health, 1989.
Feder HM, Shanely JD, Barbara JA: Review of 59 patients hospitalized with animal bites. *Pediatr Infect Dis J* 6:24, 1987.
Fern AI, Sweeney G, Doig M, Lindsay G: Penetration of ciprofloxacin into aqueous humor. *Transactions of the Ophthalmological Societies of the United Kingdom* 105:650, 1986.
Findling JW, Pohlman GP, Rose HD: Fulminant gram negative bacillemia (DF-2) following a dog bite in an asplenic woman. *Am J Med* 68:154, 1980.
Forster RK: Etiology and diagnosis of bacterial postoperative endophthalmitis. *Ophthalmology* 85:320, 1978.
Friedman E, Peyman GA, May DR: Endophthalmitis caused by *Propionibacterium acnes*. *Can J Ophthalmol* 13:50, 1978.
Goldstein EJ, Citron DM: Comparative activities of cefuroxime, amoxicillin-clavulanic acid, ciprofloxacin, enoxacin, and ofloxacin against aerobic and anaerobic bacteria isolated from bite wounds. *Antimicrobiol Agents Chemotherap* 32(8):1143, 1988.
Goldstein EJ, Citron DM, Finegold SM: Dog bite wounds and infection: A prospective clinical study. *Ann Emerg Med* 9:508, 1980.
Goldstein EJ, Citron DM, Richwald GA: Lack of in vitro efficacy of oral forms of certain cephalosporins, erythromycin, and oxacillin against *Pasteurella multocida*. *Antimicrobiol Agents Chemotherap* 32(2):213, 1988.

IV—Infections/Antibiotics/Corticosteroids/Tetanus

Gonnering RS: Ocular adnexal injury and complications in orbital dog bites. *Ophthal Plast Reconstr Surg* 3:231, 1987.

Hemady R, Zaltas M, Paton B, et al: Bacillus-induced endophthalmitis: New series of 10 cases and review of the literature. *Br J Ophthalmol* 74:26, 1990.

Herman DC, Bartley GB, Walker RC: The treatment of animal bite injuries of the eye and ocular adnexa. *Ophthal Plast Reconstr Surg* 3:237, 1987.

Kalb R, Kaplan MH, Tenebaum MJ, et al: Cutaneous infection at dog bite wounds associated with fulminant DF-2 septicemia. *Am J Med* 78:687, 1985.

Kervick GN, Flynn HW Jr, Alfonso E, Miller D: Antibiotic therapy for Bacillus species infections. *Am J Ophthal* 110(6):683, 1990.

Leopold IH: Recent developments in chemotherapy of ocular diseases. *J Ocul Pharmacol* 2(2):185, 1986.

Lesar TS, Fiscella RG: Antimicrobial drug delivery to the eye. *Drug Intel Clin Pharm* 19:642, 1985.

Mandelbaum S, Forster RK: Postoperative endopthalmitis. *Int Ophthalmol Clin* 27:95, 1987.

Martin DF, Ficker LA, Aguilar HA, et al: Vitreous cefazolin levels after intravenous injection: Effects of inflammation, repeated antibiotic doses, and surgery. *Arch Ophthalmol* 108:411, 1990.

Nobe JR, Gomez DS, Liggett P, et al: Post traumatic and postoperative endophthalmitis: A comparison of visual outcome. *Br J Ophthalmol* 71:614, 1987.

O'Day DM, Smith RS, Gregg CR, et al: The problem of Bacillus species infection with special emphasis on the virulence of *Bacillus cereus*. *Ophthalmology* 88:833, 1981.

Oum BS, D'Amico DJ, Wong KW: Intravitreal antibiotic therapy with vancomycin and aminoglycoside: An experimental study of combination and repetitive injections. *Arch Ophthalmol* 107:1055, 1989.

Parrish CM, O'Day DM: Traumatic endophthalmitis. *Int Ophthalmol Clin* 27:112, 1987.

Paton BG, Ormerond LD, Peppe J: Evidence for a feline reservoir for dysgonic fermenter 2 keratitis. *J Clin Microbiol* 26(11):2439, 1988.

Pavan PR, Brinser JH: Exogenous bacterial endophthalmitis treated without sytemic antibiotics. *Am J Ophthalmol* 104:121, 1987.

Peyman GA, Herbst R: Bacterial endophthalmitis: Treatment with intraocular injection of gentamicin and dexamethasone. *Arch Ophthalmol* 91:416, 1974.

Peyman GA, Raichand M, Bennett TO: Management of endophthalmitis with pars plana vitrectomy. *Br J Ophthalmol* 64:472, 1980.

Pflugfelder SC, Flynn HW, Zwickey TA, et al: Exogenous fungal endophthalmitis. *Ophthalmology* 95:19, 1988.

Pflugfelder SC, Hernandez E, Fliesler SJ, et al: Intravitreal vancomycin: Retinal toxicity, clearance, and interaction with gentamicin. *Arch Ophthalmol* 105:841, 1987.

Puliafito CA, Baker AS, Haaf J, et al: Infectious endophthalmitis review of 36 cases. *Ophthalmology* 89:921, 1982.

Sanford JP, *Guide to Antimicrobial Therapy 1991*. West Bethesda, MD, Antimicrobiol Therapy, 1991.

Schemmer GB, Driebe WT Jr: Posttraumatic *Bacillus cereus* endopthalmitis. *Arch Ophthalmol* 105:342, 1987.

Stevenson TR, Thacker JG, Rodeheaver GT, et al: Cleansing of the traumatic wound by high pressure irrigation. *J Am Coll Emerg Phys* 5:17, 1976.

Tabbara KF, O'Connor GR: Ocular tissue absorption of clindamycin phosphate. *Arch Ophthalmol* 93:1180, 1975.

Talamo JH, D'Amico DJ, Kenyon KR: Intravitreal amikacin in the treatment of bacterial endophthalmitis. *Arch Ophthalmol* 104:1483, 1986.

Talley AR, D'Amico DJ, Talamo JH, et al: The role of vitrectomy in the treatment of postoperative bacterial endophthalmitis: An experimental study. *Arch Ophthalmol* 105:1699, 1987.

Van Bijsterveld OP, Richards RD: Bacillus infections of the cornea. *Arch Ophthalmol* 74:91, 1965.

Appendix: Common Abbreviations in Ophthalmology

Abbreviations for Headings Used in the Ten-Part Eye Examination

Robert A. Catalano

1. Ophthalmic history

    CC   = chief complaint
    HPI   = history of present illness
    POH   = past ocular history
    FMH   = family history of ophthalmic disorders

2. Systemic history

    ROS   = review of systems (general medical history)
    MEDS   = current medications
    ALL   = allergies

3–10. Ocular examination

    3. V_A = visual acuity
    4. **EXT**   = external examination
    5. **PUP**   = pupils
    6. **MOT**   = ocular alignment and motility
    7. **VF**   = visual field examination
    8. **SLE**   = slit lamp examination
    9. **T**   = tonometry (measurement of intraocular pressure)
    10. **FUND**   = fundus examination

Notations and Abbreviations Used to Record Visual Acuity

V_A = visual acuity
cc = with correction
sc = without correction
PH = acuity looking through a pinhole
NI = no improvement
W = wears (the patient's spectacle correction)
PC = present correction (spectacle)
J = Jaeger notation (near vision)
+ = convex lens used to treat hyperopia
− = concave lens used to treat myopia
SPH = spherical lens
RE = right eye
LE = left eye
OD = oculus dexter: right eye
OS = oculus sinister: left eye
OU = oculi uterque: both eyes
D = distance acuity
N = near acuity
E = E game
Pics = Allen pictures

Acuity Notations in Infants

F+F = fixate and follow
CSM = central, steady, maintained fixation
C(S)M = central, unsteady, maintained fixation (nystagmus)
CS(M) = central, steady, but not maintained fixation (amblyopia)
GCM = good, central, maintained fixation
G(C)M = eccentric but maintained fixation
GC(M) = good, central, but not maintained fixation (amblyopia)

Acuity Notations in Older Children and Adults

20/50 − 1 = missed one letter on 20/50 line
20/50 + 2 = resolved 20/50 line and two letters on 20/40 line
20/30 Pics = 20/30 on Allen chart
20/25 E = 20/25 on E game

CF at 1′ = count fingers at 1 foot
HM at 3′ = hand motion at 3 feet
LP   = light perception
NLP   = no light perception
LP c proj = light perception with projection

Quadrants:
ST = superotemporal
IT = inferotemporal
SN = superonasal
IN = inferonasal

Example

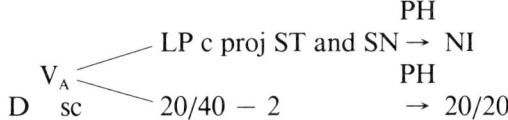

This indicates that without correction, the distance vision in the right eye is light perception with projection in the superotemporal and superonasal quadrants. In the left eye, the patient could read all but two letters on the distant 20/40 line. No improvement in vision of the right eye was obtained looking through a pinhole, but the vision in the left eye improved to 20/20.

Notations and Abbreviations Used to Record Pupillary Responses

RRL = round, reactive to light
RAPD = relative afferent pupillary defect graded from 0 (no RAPD) to 4+ (brisk RAPD)
4 → 2 = 4 mm wide pupils in dim illumination constricting to 2 mm in bright illumination
0 to 4+ = briskness of light and near responses graded from 0 (no response) to 4+ (brisk)

Examples

Pupils: 4 → 2 RRL s RAPD
5 → 3 RRL c RAPD

This indicates that the right pupil is 4 mm wide in dim illumination and constricts to 2 mm in bright illumination. It is also without an afferent pupillary defect. The left pupil is 5 mm wide in dim illumination, constricts to 3 mm, and has a relative afferent pupillary defect.

Pupils: Size	Light response	Near response	RAPD
4 → 2	4+	4+	0
5 → 3	3+	3+	2+
or: 4/5 → 2/3	4+/3+	4+/3+	0/2+

This further indicates that right pupil responds more briskly by both the light and near reflex than the left pupil. This also grades the relative afferent pupillary defect in the left eye as 2+.

Notations and Abbreviations Used to Record Ocular Alignment and Motility

Extraocular Muscles

EOM = extraocular movements
RSR = right superior rectus
RLR = right lateral rectus
RIR = right inferior rectus
RMR = right medial rectus
RSO = right superior oblique
RIO = right inferior oblique

LSR = left superior rectus
LLR = left lateral rectus
LIR = left inferior rectus
LMR = left medial rectus
LSO = left superior oblique
LIO = left inferior oblique

Ocular Alignment

E = esophoria
X = exophoria
DVD = dissociated vertical deviation
ET = esotropia
XT = exotropia
HT = hypertropia

E(T), X(T) = intermittent esotropia, exotropia
E′, X′, ET′, XT′, E(T)′, X(T)′ = the prime (′) indicates that the measurements were taken at near fixation
EX = EX′ = 0 : no ocular misalignment
ortho = orthophoria (no ocular misalignment)

Ocular Measurements

PD = Δ – prism diopters
° = degrees
K = Krimsky test (given in prism diopters)
H = Hirschberg test (given in degrees)
ROTS = ocular rotations
    usually graded from 4− (maximum underaction)
    to 4+ (maximum overaction)
        OA = overaction of a muscle
        UA = underaction of a muscle
A = accommodation
AC = accommodative convergence
NPA = near point of accommodation
AC/A = accommodative convergence to accommodation ratio
NPC = near point of convergence

Notations and Abbreviations Used to Record Findings on Slit Lamp Examination

C,C,S	= cornea, conjunctiva, and sclera
AC	= anterior chamber
D + C	= deep and clear
cells	= presence of red or white blood cells in the anterior chamber of the eye; graded on a scale of 0 to 4+
flare	= presence of proteinaceous material in the anterior chamber
K	= keratometer reading (refractive power of the cornea)
KP	= keratic precipitates (accumulations of inflammatory cells on the posterior (endothelial) surface of the cornea
hyphema	= layering of red blood cells in the anterior chamber (eight ball = complete filling of anterior chamber)
hypopyon	= layering of inflammatory cells in the anterior chamber

Notations and Abbreviations Used to Record Findings on Fundus Examination

D	= optic disk
M	= macula
V	= vessels
C/D	= cup to disc ratio
DD	= disc diameters
F	= fundus
HE	= hard exudate
SE	= soft exudate

Notations and Abbreviations Used to Record Findings on Visual Field Examination and Tonometry

Visual Field

VF   = visual field
Conf = confrontational visual field

Tonometry

T   = tonometry
T_{AP} = applanation tonometry
$T_{SCH\ 5.5}$ = Schiotz tonometry with a 5.5 g weight
FT   = finger tension
TT   = tactile tension (same as above)
IOP = intraocular pressure

Examples

VF ⟨ full to conf / full to conf   indicates that the visual field was full to confrontation in both eyes.

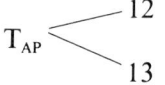   indicates that the intraocular pressure in the right eye measured by applanation tonometry was 12 mm Hg; in the left eye, it was 13 mm Hg.

INDEX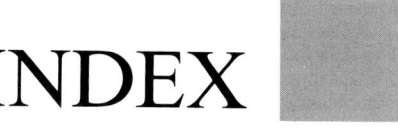

Note: Page numbers in *italics* refer to illustrations; page numbers followed by t refer to tables.

Abduction blindness, 293
Abrasion, corneal, penetrating injury in, 201–203, *203*
  lid, 138
Abscess, orbital, 299
  subperiosteal, 468
Abuse, of child, 99–102, 100t, *101*
Acanthamoeba keratitis, 482–483, *483*
Acetaminophen, in angle-closure glaucoma, 268
  in cluster headache, 370
  in hyphema, 161t
  in migraine, 369
Acetazolamide, in angle-closure glaucoma, 267–268, 269
  in central retinal artery occlusion, 407
  in chemical burns, 185t, 186
  in choroidal detachment, 427
  in hyphema, 161t
  in infantile glaucoma, 281
  in macular edema, 425
  in orbital hemorrhage, 140
  in phacolytic glaucoma, 165
  in pseudotumor cerebri, 435
  in traumatic retrobulbar hemorrhage, 127
N-Acetyl-L-cysteine (Mucomyst). *See* Acetylcysteine (Mucomyst).
Acetylcysteine (Mucomyst), in chemical burns, 185t, 188
  in corneal ulceration, 183, 185t
  in dry eye syndrome, 233
  in filamentary keratopathy, 247–249
Acid burn, 179. *See also* Burn(s).
Acquired immune deficiency syndrome (AIDS), 401–405, *402–404*
Active force generation test, 22–23
Acuity, visual, 6–12
  blunt injury and, 137
  functional loss of, 442–446
  recording of, 10, 12t
Acyclovir, in herpes simplex, 481
  in herpes zoster ophthalmicus, 485
Adenoid cystic carcinoma, 329
Adenovirus conjunctivitis, *474*

Adie's pupil, 355, 362
Adrenergic(s), alpha agonist, 255, 258
  beta blocker. *See* Beta-blocker(s).
  keratoconjunctivitis and, 27
Adriamycin. *See* Doxorubicin (Adriamycin).
Aeromonas hydrophila, 502
Age-related macular degeneration, 422–423
AIDS (acquired immune deficiency syndrome), 401–405, *402–404*
Albright's syndrome, 331
Alcohol, amblyopia and, 429
  cluster headache and, 371
  hallucinations and, 375
  lid injuries and, 109
Algorithm(s), in computed tomography, 52
Alice in Wonderland syndrome, 374, 377
Alkali burn(s), 179. *See also* Burn(s).
  classification of, 180–181, 181t
Allen picture eye chart, 91, *92*
Allergy, in conjunctivitis, 476
  in lid reactions, 128, *129*
  medicinal, 6
Alpha agonists, in dislocated lens, 255
  in phakomorphic glaucoma, 258
Amaurosis fugax, 430–433, *431*, *432*
Amaurotic pupil, 361
Amblyopia, tobacco or alcohol, 429
Amicar (aminocaproic acid), 160, 161t
Amikacin, diffusion of, 507t
  in endophthalmitis, 484, 506t, 507t
Aminocaproic acid (Amicar), 160, 161t
Aminoglycoside(s), in corneal infections, 478
  in endophthalmitis, 502, 505t
  in toxic keratopathy, *247*
  myasthenia gravis and, 353
Amiodarone, 429
Amitriptyline, in herpes zoster ophthalmicus, 485
  in migraine, 369
Ammonium hydroxide, in burns, 179, 180t
Amoxicillin/clavulanic acid (Augmentin), in animal bite, 499t
  in bites, 499
  in dacryoadenitis, 470

523

524 Index

Amoxicillin/clavulanic acid (Augmentin) (*Continued*)
  in dacryocystitis, 471
  in lid injury, 121, 498
  in orbital cellulitis, 299
  in orbital fractures, 500
  in preseptal cellulitis, 467
Amphetamine, mydriasis and, 363
Amphotericin B, in aspergillosis, 320
  in endophthalmitis, 507t
  in fungal keratitis, 482
  in mucormycosis, 319, 346, 468
Amsler grid, *24*, 24–25
Amvisc, in corneal laceration, 205
Anabolic steroid(s), in hereditary angioedema, 128
Anaerobes, in posttraumatic endophthalmitis, 502
Analeptic(s), tardive dyskinesia and, 382
Analgesia, in angle-closure glaucoma, 268
  in corneal ulceration, 184
  in pediatric examination, 103t
  in thermal burns, 191
  in ultraviolet burns, 193
Anatomy, in pupillary abnormalities, 355–356
  of lacrimal drainage system, *218*, 218–219
  of orbit, 131–137, *132*, 133t, *134–136*, 135t
Anesthesia, in corneal ulceration, 184
  in examination, 3
  in filamentary keratopathy, 247
  in infantile glaucoma, 280
  in lid injury, 113–115, 114t, 115, *116*
  in pediatric examination, 102, 103t
  in penetrating injury, 201
  miosis and, 362
  risk with, 104t
Aneurysm(s), differential diagnosis of, 290
  dissecting aortic, 360
  intracranial, 78
Angioedema, hereditary, 128
Angiography, cerebral, 58–59, *61*
  digital subtraction (DSA), 58–59, *61*
  fluorescein, 61, *62*
    complications of, 79
  magnetic resonance, 59–60
Angioneurotic edema, 128
Angle-closure glaucoma. *See* Glaucoma, angle-closure.
Animal bite(s), 120–122, *122*, *123*
  antibiotics in, 498–500, 499t
Aniridia, with dislocated ocular lens, 253, *253*
Anisocoria, 356–362, *358*
Annular keratopathy, traumatic posterior, 155–156
Annulus of Zinn, 133–134
Ansaid (flurbiprofen), 490
Antabuse (disulfiram), 429
Antazoline phosphate with naphazoline (Vasocon-A), 475, 476

Anti-inflammatory agent(s), 488
Antibiotic(s), 497–512
  action of, 6t
  endophthalmitis and, 484, 500–511, 507t
    elective surgery and, 501t, 501–502
    postoperative, 501t, 501–502
    posttraumatic, 502–509, 505t–508t, 509t
  in animal bites, 121, 498, 499t, 499–500
  in bacterial conjunctivitis, 475
  in cavernous sinus thrombosis, 344
  in chalazion, 469
  in chemical burns, 185t
  in corneal abrasion, 202–203
  in corneal infection, 478
  in corneal laceration, 205
  in dacryoadenitis, 470
  in dacryocystitis, 231–232, 471, 472
  in human bites, 498
  in intraocular foreign body injury, 212
  in lid injury, 113, 115, 138, 497
  in nasolacrimal duct probing, 221
  in ophthalmia neonatorum, 463
  in orbital cellulitis, 299
  in orbital emphysema, 142
  in preseptal cellulitis, 467
  in prophylaxis, 497–500
    for bite wounds, 498–500, 499t
    for lid laceration, 497–498
    for orbital fractures, 500
  in recurrent corneal erosions, 245
  in subperiosteal abscess, 468
  in superficial punctate keratopathy, 246
  in thermal burns, 191
  in ultraviolet burns, 193
  tetanus immunization and, 510t, 510–511
  with steroids. *See also* Steroid(s).
    in acute setting, 510
    in superficial punctate keratopathy, 246
Anticholinergic(s), action of, 6t
Anticoagulant(s), in aseptic cavernous sinus thrombosis, 344
  in lid injury, 109, 111–112
Antifibrinolytic(s), in hereditary angioedema, 128
  in hyphema, 160, 161t
Antihistamine(s), in allergic conjunctivitis, 476
  in angle-closure glaucoma, 264
  in pupillary block glaucoma, 272
  in tearing, 227
  with vasoconstrictor (Vasocon-A), in viral conjunctivitis, 475
Antimicrobial(s). *See* Antibiotic(s).
Antipsychotic(s), in angle-closure glaucoma, 264, 272
  in miosis, 362
  in tardive dyskinesia, 382
Antirabies prophylaxis, 113
Antitetanus prophylaxis, 112t, 112–113

Index   525

Antitubercular agent(s), 429
Antiviral(s), 27
Anton's syndrome, 429
Aortic artery aneurysm, dissecting, 360
Aphakic pupillary block, 273
Applanation tonometer, 33, *35*
　for child, 91, *95*
　in infantile glaucoma, 280, *282*
　of Perkins, 91, *95*, 280, *282*
Apraclonidine, 255
Argyll-Robertson pupil, 363
Arsenic, in optic neuropathy, 429
　in pseudotumor cerebri, 435
Arteriovenous fistula(s), orbital, *321*, 321–322
　intra-arterial digital subtraction angiography of, *61*
Arteritis, giant cell. See Temporal arteritis.
Artificial tear(s), action of, 6t
　in dry eye syndrome, 233
　in exposure keratopathy, 249
　in filamentary keratopathy, 247
　in inflammatory corneal ulcers, 239
　in recurrent corneal erosions, 245
　in superficial punctate keratopathy, 246
　in viral conjunctivitis, 472
A-scan, 45–46, *46*, 47
Ascorbic acid, in chemical burns, 185t, 186
　in corneal ulceration, 183
Aspergillosis, in keratitis, 481
　in nontraumatic orbital disorders, 319
Aspirin, in carotid vascular disease, 432
　in cluster headache, 370
　in lid injury, 109
　in migraine, 369, 370
Asthenopia, 371–372
Ativan (lorazepam), 161t
Atresia, of lacrimal puncta, 222–223
Atropine, in chemical burns, 185t, 186
　in contact dermatitis, 128, *129*
　in hyphema, 161t
　in interstitial keratitis, 250
　in keratoconjunctivitis, 27
　in malignant glaucoma, 273
　in sarcoidosis, 421
Attenuation coefficients, 52, 53t
Auditory-induced phosphene, 379
Augmentin. See Amoxicillin/clavulanic acid (Augmentin).
Auscultation, for orbital bruits, 14
Autoenucleation, psychotic, 455–456
Avulsion, of lid skin, 138
　of optic nerve, 172, *173*
　of vitreous base, 170
Axial view, of orbit, 53–55, *54*, *55*
Azathioprine, in myasthenia gravis, 353
　in sarcoidosis, 421
　in scleritis, 490
　in thyroid ophthalmopathy, 317
　in Wegener's granulomatosis, 320

Bacillus cereus, endophthalmitis and, 501t, 506t
　exogenous, 508, 509
　posttraumatic, 502, 503, 504
　in lid laceration, 498
Bacitracin, in infectious conjunctivitis, 463
　in lid abrasions, 138
　in lid burns, 127
　in lid lacerations, 113
　in *Neisseria gonorrhea* infections, 464
　in thermal burns, 191
Bacterial conjunctivitis, 475
Bacteroides infection, in child, 299
Bactrim, 467
Bagolini's striated glass test, 22
Bandage lens, in chemical burns, 188, *189*
　in inflammatory corneal ulcers, 239
　in recurrent corneal erosions, 245
Barbiturate(s), in miosis, 362
　in optic neuropathy, 429
　in oscillopsia, 375
Base view, of orbit, 49
Battle's sign, 342
Bedavanija's formula, for ophthalmodynamometry readings, 41t
Behavior observation, in disproving visual loss, 443–444
Benadryl (diphenhydramine), 79
Benedikt's syndrome, 342, 351
Benign mixed tumor, 328–329
Berlin's edema, 167–168
Beta-blocker(s), action of, 6t
　in angle-closure glaucoma, 267, 269, 274
　in chemical burns, 185t, 186
　in dislocated lens, 255
　in hyphema, 161t
　in orbital hemorrhage, 140
　in phakomorphic glaucoma, 258
　in Posner-Schlossman syndrome, 275
　in pupillary block, 273
　in retinal artery occlusion, 407
　in retrobulbar hemorrhage, 127
Beta lactamase, 499
Beta-methasone acetate, 304
Beta-methasone sodium phosphate, 304
Betadine, 115
Betagan, 185t
Betoptic, 185t
Bilateral ecchymoses, differential diagnosis in, 293
Binocular diplopia, sudden onset of, 336–353. See also Diplopia.
Binocular visual loss, test(s) for, 443
Bite(s), animal, 120–122, *122*, *123*, *125*
　antibiotics in, 498–500, 499t
　human, 120–122, *122*, *123*
Black eye, 138, *139*
Black tissue, 293
Bleeding. See Hemorrhage.

Blephamide (prednisone acetate with sulfacetamide sodium), 246
Blepharitis, superficial punctate keratopathy versus, *247*
Blepharochalasis, 15
Blepharospasm, 381–383, *382*
Blindness, abduction, 293
  cerebral or cortical, 428–429
  functional, 445–446
  legal, definition of, 10–11
  sudden and unexpected. *See* Loss of vision, sudden and unexpected.
Blinking, functional, 451, 542t
  in retinal disorders, 381–383, *382*
Blood pressure elevation with palpation, 292
Blowout fracture(s), of orbital floor, 142–146, *143–145*
Blowout patch technique, in descemetocele, 241
Blunt injury(ies), 131–177
  ocular, 153–177
    choroid in, 166–167, *167*
    conjunctiva and sclera in, 153–155, *154*
    cornea in, 155–157, *156*
    iris in, 157–159, *158*
    lens in, *163*, 163–165, *165*
    optic nerve injury in, 172–173, *173*
    prognosis in, 153, 154t
    retina in, 167–172, *168*, *169*, *171*
    traumatic hyphema in, *159*, 159–162, 160t–162t
    vitreous hemorrhage in, 166
  orbital, 131–151
    anatomy in, 131–137, *132*, 133t, *134–136*, 135t
    evaluation of, *135*, 137–138
    fractures in, 141–150. *See also* Orbital fracture(s).
    hemorrhage in, 138–140, 139t, *140*
    lid abrasions in, 138
    lid ecchymosis and, 110, 138, *139*
    ocular adnexa in, 131–137, *132*, 133t, *134–136*, 135t
    ophthalmoplegia in, 140–141, 141t
    soft tissue injuries in, 138–141
    tests in, 63–67, *66*, *67*
    prognosis in, 153, 154t
Blurring of oblique muscle, as radiographic sign, 293
Bone(s), destruction of, 293
  of orbit, 131–133, *133*, *136*
Bottle top colors, for medications, 5, 6t
Brain stem disorders, 75–76
Branch retinal artery occlusion (BRAO), 407, *407*
Branch retinal vein occlusion (BRVO), 409, *410*
BRAO (branch retinal artery occlusion), 407, *407*

Brevital (methohexital), 103t
Brolene (propamidine isethionate), 483
Bruch's membrane, fluid leakage from, *62*
Bruit(s), 14, 292
BRVO (branch retinal vein occlusion), 409, *410*
B-scan, 46, *47*, 47
Bupivacaine, 114t
Burkitt's lymphoma, 310
Burn(s), 179–196, 180t
  chemical, 179–190, 180t
    acid, 179
    alkali, 180–181, 181t
    chemical mediators in, *182*, 182–184
    clinical manifestations of, 180–182, *181*, 181t
    intraocular pressure in, 184
    treatment of, 184–190, 185t
    ulceration control in, *182*, 182–184
  electrical, 192, *192*
  lid, 127, *128*
  radiation, 192–194, *193–195*
  thermal, 127, *128*, 190–192
  treatment of, 184–190, 185t
    acute phase, 184–187, *187*
    intermediate phase, 188–189, *189*
    late or chronic phase, 189–190, *190*

Calcification, 293
  in retinoblastoma, *68*
  plain film radiography of, 48
Calcium channel blocker(s), 407
Calcium hydroxide, 179, 180t, 186
Caldwell view, of orbit, 49, *49*
  in injury, 63
Caloric test, 22
Canaliculus, 135
  lacerated, repair of, 119–120, *120*
Candida retinitis, in acquired immune deficiency syndrome, 403, *404*
Cantholysis, *119*
Canthotomy, 119
Capillary hemangioma, *303*, 303–304
Carbamazepine, 382
Carbapenem, 504
Carbonic anhydrase inhibitor(s), in angle-closure glaucoma, 267–268, 274
  in chemical burns, 186
  in dislocated lens, 255
  in phakomorphic glaucoma, 258
  in Posner-Schlossman syndrome, 275
  in pupillary block, 273
Carcinoembryonic antigen (CEA), 294
Carcinoma. *See also* Malignant *entries*; Neoplasm(s); *specific neoplasm.*
  adenoid cystic, 329
  differential diagnosis of, 290, 291

Carcinoma (*Continued*)
  nasopharyngeal, 341
  of lacrimal sac, *224*
Carcinomatous meningitis, 341
Cardinal positions of gaze, 19, 134, *135*, 135t
Carotid-cavernous fistula, cranial nerve palsy with, *343*, 343-344
  glaucoma and, 279
  nontraumatic orbital disorders and, *321*, 322
  tests for, 78
  traumatic, 342
Carotid vascular disease, 430-433
Cat scratch disease (CSD), 121, *122*
  of lid, 121
Cataract(s), congenital, 384, *385*
  contusion, 164, *165*
  electrical, 192, *192*
  Glassblower, 193, *194*
  mature, 256, *257*
  Morgagnian, 256, *257*
  nontraumatic acute, 255-256, *256*
  posterior subcapsular, 255-256, *256*
Cavernous hemangioma, 323, 324
Cavernous sinus. *See also* Carotid-cavernous fistula.
  cranial nerve palsy and, *343*, 343-344
  tests in, 75
Cavernous sinus thrombosis, 322-323
  tests for, 75
  traumatic, 342, *343*
CEA (carcinoembryonic antigen), 294
Ceclor. *See* Cefaclor (Ceclor).
Cefaclor (Ceclor), in cellulitis, 299, 467
  in dacryocystitis, 232, 471
Cefazolin, cost of, 509t
  diffusion of, 507t
  in animal and human bites, 499
  in corneal infections, 478
  in endophthalmitis, 501
  in intraocular foreign body injury, 212
  in orbital fractures, 500
  in traumatic endophthalmitis, 503, 504, 508
  penetration of, 508t
Cefotaxime, in exogenous endophthalmitis, 509
  in Lyme disease, 345, 422
Cefoxitin, 499
Ceftazidime (Fortaz), cost of, 509t
  diffusion of, 507t
  in endophthalmitis, 504, 505t
  in exogenous endophthalmitis, 509
  in orbital cellulitis, 299, 468
  in preseptal cellulitis, 467
Ceftin. *See* Cefuroxime (Ceftin, Zinacef).
Ceftriaxone (Rocephin), in bacterial conjunctivitis, 475
  in bites, 499, 499t

Ceftriaxone (Rocephin) (*Continued*)
  in Lyme disease, 345, 422
  in *Neisseria gonorrhea*, 464
Cefuroxime (Ceftin, Zinacef), diffusion of, 507t
  in animal and human bites, 499t, 499-500
  in dacryocystitis, 232, 471
  in orbital cellulitis, 299
Cellulitis, orbital, 297, *297*, 298t, 298-299
  tests for, *73*, 73-74
  preseptal, 466-467
  child with, 297, 298, 298t
Celluvisc, in chemical burns, 189
  in dry eye syndrome, 233
Central retinal artery occlusion (CRAO), 405-407, *406*
Central retinal vein occlusion (CRVO), 407-409, *408*
Central serous retinopathy (CSR), 413-414, *414*
Cephalalgia headache, 368
Cephalexin (Keflex), in bites, 499
  in dacryoadenitis, 471
  in dacryocystitis, 231-232, 471
  in lid lacerations, 113, 498
  in orbital fractures, 500
Cephalosporin(s), in bites, 499
  in dacryocystitis, 231
  in lid injuries, 121, 498
  in orbital cellulitis, 299
  in traumatic endophthalmitis, 504, 508
Cephradine (Velosef), diffusion of, 507t
  in endophthalmitis, 504, 505t, 508
Cerebral angiography, 58-59, *61*
  advantages and disadvantages of, 64t, 65t
Cerebral blindness, 428-429
Cerebral infarction, tests for, 76, *76*
Cerebral vascular accident, 428
Cerebrovascular disease, headaches and, 365t
Chalazion, 16, *469*, 469-470
Chamber angle, anterior, recession of, 162
Chemical burn(s). *See* Burn(s).
Chemical mediator(s), in burns, *182*, 182-184
Chemosis, 155
Child. *See* Infant; Pediatric care.
Chlamydia trachomatis, in conjunctivitis, 463
  in adult, 475-476, *476*
  in ophthalmia neonatorum, *81*, 461, 463-466, *464*, *465*
  versus superficial punctate keratopathy, *247*
Chloral hydrate, 102-103, 103t
Chlorambucil, in sarcoidosis, 421
  in Wegener's granulomatosis, 320
Chloramphenicol, in orbital cellulitis, 299
  optic neuropathy and, 429
Chloroma, 310
Chlorpropamide (Diabinese), 429

528 Index

Cholinergic(s), action of, 6t
  in angle-closure glaucoma, 268
Chorioretinitis proliferans, 168–169
Chorioretinitis sclopetaria, 168–169
Choristoma(s), in child, 295, 302
Choroid, blunt injury of, 166–167, *167*
  in sudden and unexpected loss of vision, 427–428. *See also* Choroidal detachment.
Choroidal detachment, angle-closure glaucoma and, 270–272, *271*
  B-scan ultrasonogram of, *47*
  hemorrhagic, 427–428
  serous, 427
  tests for, 69, *69*
Choroidal disorder(s), 63–70, *69, 70*
  hemangiomas as, 69–70
  hemorrhage as, 69, *70*
  inflammatory diseases as, 70, *70*
  trauma in, 63–67, *66, 67*
  tumors as, 67–69, *68*
Choroidal fold, 293
Cicatricial pemphigoid, ocular, 239
Cigarette smoking, cluster headache and, 371
Ciliary body tumor, angle-closure glaucoma and, 270–272
Ciliary ganglion lesion, 362
Ciloxan. *See* Ciprofloxacin (Ciloxan).
Cimetidine, 485
Ciprofloxacin (Ciloxan), cost of, 509t
  diffusion of, 507t
  endophthalmitis and, 505t
    exogenous, 508, 509
    traumatic, 504, 508
  penetration of, 508t
Clavulanic acid. *See* Amoxicillin/clavulanic acid (Augmentin).
Clindamycin, cost of, 509t
  endophthalmitis and, 505t, 506t
    exogenous, 509
  in intraocular foreign body injury, 212
  in lid lacerations, 498
  in orbital cellulitis, 468
  in orbital fractures, 500
  in toxoplasmosis, 403, 492, 493t
Clivus ridge syndrome, 346–347
Clonidine, 370
Clostridium botulinum toxin, 382, 383
Clostridium difficile, 498
Clotrimazole, in *Acanthamoeba* keratitis, 483
  in fungal keratitis, 482
Cloxacillin, 299
Cluster headache, 370–371
Coat's disease, 387, *387*
Cocaine, hallucinations and, 375
  in lid lacerations, 114
Cocaine test, in Horner's syndrome, 357, 360
Codeine, miosis and, 362

Collagen vascular disease, 239
Coloboma, as pupillary abnormality, 355, *356*
  in child, 70, *70*
Color vision, 11
Color vision plate, *13*
Common canaliculus, 135
Commotio retinae, 167–168, *168*
Compazine (prochloroperazine), 161t, 369
Compressive optic neuropathy, 422
Computed tomography (CT), 51–56, *54–56*
  advantages and disadvantages of, 62, 64t, 65t
  in binocular diplopia, 340
  ocular and orbital trauma and, 63, 66, *67*
Concussion edema, 167–168
Confrontational visual field test, 23
Congenital cataract, 384, *385*
Congenital coloboma, 70, *70*
Congenital glaucoma, 279–283, *280*, 281t, *282*
Congenital lacrimal drainage disorder(s), 219–223, *220, 222, 223*
Congenital syphilis, facies of, *251*
Conjunctiva, degeneration of, 28
  edema of, 155
  fleshy mass under, 292
  follicular reaction of, *28*
  foreign bodies in, 199–201, *200, 202*
  Giemsa stain of, *81, 82*
  infection of. *See* Conjunctival infection.
  laceration of, 155, 198–199
  slit lamp examination of, 27, 28
  specimens from, 79, *81, 82*
  yellow, 292
Conjunctival flap, descemetocele and, 240
Conjunctival infection, 472–476, *473*. *See also* Conjunctivitis.
  allergy and, 476
  bacterial, 475
  chlamydial, 475–476, *476*
    ophthalmia neonatorum in, 463–466, *464, 465*
  viral, 472–475, *474*
Conjunctivitis, allergic, 476
  bacterial, 475
  chlamydial, 475–476, *476*
    Giemsa stain of, *81*
    ophthalmia neonatorum and, 463–466, *464, 465*
  viral, 472–475, *474*
  angle-closure glaucoma versus, 263t
Contact dermatitis, 128, *129*
Contact lens, bandage. *See* Bandage lens.
  in corneal disorders, 242–243, *243, 244*
  in recurrent corneal erosions, 245
  in retinal examination, 39
  overwear of, 242
  superficial punctate keratopathy versus disorders from, *247*

Index 529

Contrast agent(s), iodinated intravascular, 78–79
  sensitivity to, 9–10, *10*
Contusion cataract, 164, *165*
Convergence insufficiency, 372
Conversion reaction, term of, 441
Copious irrigation, in chemical burns, 184, 185t
Corkscrew epibulbar vessel(s), 292
Cornea, blunt injury of, 155–157, *156*
  foreign bodies in, 199–201, *200*, *202*
  infection of, *477*, 477–478, *478*
  noninfectious ulcer of, 237–239, *238*, 238t
  nonpenetrating, noninfectious emergencies of, 237–250
    contact lenses in, 242–243, *243*, *244*
    descemetocele in, *240*, 240–242, *241*
    exposure keratopathy in, 249
    filamentary keratopathy in, 246–249, *248*
    inflammatory ulcers in, 237–239, *238*, 238t
    interstitial keratitis in, 249–250, *251*
    neurotrophic keratopathy in, 249, *250*
    recurrent erosions in, 243–246, *245*
    superficial punctate keratopathy in, 246, 247t, *248*
  pannus of, soft contact lens and, 242, *243*
  penetrating injury of, abrasions and, 201–203, *203*
    lacerations and, 203–207, *204*, *206*
    recurrent erosions of, 243–246, *245*
    slit lamp examination of, 30
    traumatic rupture of, 157
Corneal dystrophy, map-dot-fingerprint, 244, *245*
Corneal scraping(s), 79
Coronal orbital view, *54*, 56
Cortical blindness, 428–429
Corticosteroid(s). *See also* Steroid(s).
  action of, 6t
  floaters and, 381
  in angle-closure glaucoma, 267, 274
  in chemical burns, 185t, 186
  in corneal ulceration, 183
  in iritis, 158
  in myasthenia gravis, 353
  in opthalmoplegia, 141
  in phacolytic glaucoma, 165
  in polyarteritis nodosa, 320
  in pseudotumor, 301, 435
  in sarcoidosis, 421
  in scleritis, 488
  in systemic lupus erythematosis, 419
  in temporal arteritis, 419
  in traumatic optic neuropathy, 172, 173, 397
  in viral conjunctivitis, 475
Cortisol, hallucinations and, 375

Corynebacterium diphtheriae, 477
Cotton applicator, eversion of upper lid with, 199, *200*
Coumadin, 112
COWS, mnemonic, 22
Cranial nerve palsy(ies), 341–347
  cavernous sinus or superior orbital fissure syndromes and, *343*, 343–344
  fourth nerve, 349–350, *350*, *351*
  in neurogenic disorders, 346
  infection in, 345–346
  intracranial pressure and, 346–347
  isolated, 347–352
  neoplasia with, 341–342
  ophthalmoplegic migraine in, 347
  sixth nerve, 347–349, *348*, 349t
  third nerve, 351–352, *352*
  trauma in, 342, *343*
  vascular disorders in, 342–343
Cranial trauma, sudden and unexpected loss of vision in, 397–401, *401*
CRAO (central retinal artery occlusion), 405–407, *406*
Cromolyn sodium, in allergic conjunctivitis, 476
  in vernal keratoconjunctivitis, 246
CRVO (central retinal vein occlusion), 407–409, *408*
Cryoprecipitate(s), 112
CSD (cat scratch disease), 121, *122*
CSR (central serous retinopathy), 413–414, *414*
CT. *See* Computed tomography (CT).
Culture, in endophthalmitis, 485t
Cup-to-disk ratio, 37
  in infantile glaucoma, 280, *282*
Cyanoacrylate, in chemical burns, 188
  in descemetocele, *241*, 241–242
Cyclogyl. *See* Cyclopentolate (Cyclogyl).
Cyclopentolate (Cyclogyl), in herpes simplex, 479–480
  in iritis, 158
  in phacolytic glaucoma, 165
  in pupillary block, 273
  in recurrent corneal erosions, 245
  in superficial punctate keratopathy, 246
Cyclophosphamide, in myasthenia gravis, 353
  in rhabdomyosarcoma, 308
  in scleritis, 490
  in systemic lupus erythematosis, 419
  in thyroid ophthalmopathy, 317
  in Wegener's granulomatosis, 320
Cycloplegia, in angle-closure glaucoma, 268, 269
  in choroidal detachment, 427
  in examination, 3
  in interstitial keratitis, 250
  in iritis, 158

Cycloplegia (*Continued*)
  in phacolytic glaucoma, 165
  in pupillary block, 273
  in recurrent corneal erosions, 245
  in sarcoidosis, 421
  in secondary angle-closure glaucoma, 274
  in superficial punctate keratopathy, 246
  in toxoplasmosis, 403
Cyclosporine, in sarcoidosis, 421
  in scleritis, 490
  in sympathetic ophthalmia, 494
Cyproheptadine, 369
Cyst(s), congenital coloboma with, 70, *70*
  dermoid, 305-306, *306*
  epidermoid, 305-306
L-Cysteine, corneal ulceration and, 183, 185t
Cystic carcinoma, adenoid, 329
Cystine, in Leber's optic neuropathy, 422
Cystoid macular edema, 425, *425*
Cytomegalovirus retinopathy, 402

Dacryoadenitis, *40*, 470-471
  acute, 329
  chronic, 329-331
Dacryocystitis, *471*, 471-472
  acute, 231-232, *232*
Dacryocystography, in child, 60-61
  in epiphora, 229, 230, *230*
Dacryocystorhinostomy, 230-231
Dacryolith(s), 224
Dacryoscintigraphy, 229
Dalmane (flurazepam), 161t
Dalrymple sign, 316
Danazol, 128
Decongestant(s), 299
Demerol (meperidine), 103t
Dendritic ulcer, 479, *480*
Depth perception, 11
Depth perception chart of Titmus, 11, *13*
Dermatitis, contact, 128, *129*
Dermatochalasis, 15
Dermoid cyst, 305-306, *306*
Descemetocele, *240*, 240-242, *241*
Desmarre retractor, 199, *200*
Detachment(s), choroidal. *See* Choroidal detachment.
  of retina. *See* Retina, detachments of.
  posterior vitreous (PVD), 379
    sudden vision loss in, 414-415
Dexamethasone, in chemical burns, 186
  in migraine, 369
  in traumatic optic neuropathy, 173
DF2 (dysgonic fermenter type 2), 498
Diabetes, neuropathy in, 366t
  ocular abnormalities in, 255
  papillopathy in, 420
  retinopathy in, 411, 412t

Diabinese (chlorpropamide), 429
Diagnostic test(s), 45-89
  disorders and, 63-78
    brain, *76*, 76-78, *77*
    brain stem and posterior fossa, 75-76
    choroidal. *See* Choroidal disorder(s).
    nontraumatic, 72t, 72-74, *73*, *74*
    ocular motility, 74
    optic nerve and sheath, *71*, 71-72
    retinal. *See* Retina.
    sella turcica, cavernous sinus and optic chiasm, 75
    traumatic, 63-67, *66*, *67*
    tumor, 64-69, *68*
  imaging techniques in, advantages and disadvantages of, 62, 64t-66t
    cerebral angiography, 58-59, *61*
    computed tomography, 51-56, *54-56*
    costs of, 78t, 78-79
    dacryocystography in, 60-61
    fluorescein angiography in, 61, *62*
    magnetic resonance, 56-57, *58-60*
    magnetic resonance angiography, 59-60
    orbital venography, 60
    plain film radiography in, 48-50, *49-53*
    ultrasound in, 45-48, *46*, *47*
  laboratory studies in, 79-83, 80t-82t, *80-83*
  uveitis and, 83-86, 84t, 85t
  risks of, 78t, 78-79
Dialysis, retinal, 170, *170*
Dicloxacillin, in dacryocystitis, 231, 471
  in lid lacerations, 113
Digital subtraction angiography (DSA), 58-59, *61*
Digital tonometry, 36
Digitalis glycosides, hallucinations and, 375
  optic neuropathy and, 375
Digoxin, 429
Dihydroergotamine, 369
Diopter lens, Volk 90, 39
Diphenhydramine (Benadryl), 79
Diphtheria immunizations, 510, 511
  in diphtheria, pertussis, and tetanus, 103t, 510, 511
  in diphtheria and tetanus, 510, 511
Dipiverin, 280
Diplococcus, Gram-negative intracellular, *80*
Diplopia, 336-353
  cranial nerve palsy and, 341-347
  fourth nerve in, 349-350, *350*, *351*
  infection in, 345-346
  intracranial pressure in, 346-347
  isolated, 347-352
  neoplasia with, 341-342
  neurogenic disorders and, 346
  ophthalmoplegic migraine in, 347
  sixth nerve in, 347-349, *348*, 349t

Diplopia (*Continued*)
    cranial nerve palsy and, third nerve in, 351–352, *352*
    trauma in, 342, *343*
    vascular disorders in, 342–343
    history of, 337–338
    localization of involved muscle or nerve in, 338–339
    muscular disorders in, 352–353
    physical findings and evaluation of, 338–340, 339t, 341t
Dipyridamole, 370
Direct illumination, slit lamp technique of, 26, *26*
Direct ophthalmoscopy, 38, *39*
Direct orbital floor fracture, term of, 142
Disciform keratitis, herpes simplex and, 480, *481*
Disk diameter (DD), 37
Dislocation, traumatic lens, *163*, 163–164
Disodium EDTA, 186
Dissecting aortic artery aneurysm, 360
Dissimilar image test, 21
Dissimilar target test, 22
Distance visual acuity conversions and percentage of loss of central vision, 8t
Distichiasis, 15
Disulfiram (Antabuse), 429
Dog bite(s), lid and, 121, *125*
Doll's head test, 22
Dominant optic neuropathy, 429–430
Doppler technique, 47. *See also* Ultrasonography.
Double vision, 336–353. *See also* Diplopia.
Doxorubicin (Adriamycin), in hemifacial spasm, 382–383
    in rhabdomyosarcoma, 308
Doxycycline, in chemical burns, 185t, 186
    in chlamydial conjunctivitis, 476
    in corneal ulceration, 183
    in Lyme disease, 345
DPT (diphtheria, pertussis, and tetanus), 103t, 510, 511
Drainage system, lacrimal. *See* Lacrimal drainage system.
Drusen, 422
Dry eye syndrome, 233
    diagnosis of, 228
    superficial punctate keratopathy versus, *247*
Duction(s), diplopia in, 339, 339t
    examination of, 19, 22, *23*
Dural sinus fistula, 321
Duratears, 201
Dye test, Jones', 16–17
Dysgonic fermenter type 2 (DF2), 498
Dyskinesia, tardive, 382
Dysplasia, fibrous, orbital, 331
    optic nerve, 293

Ecchymosis, of lid, *110*, 110–111, 138, *139*
    bilateral, 293
Ectopia lentis, 251–255, *252–254*
Ectropion, 15, *225*
Edema, angioneurotic, 128
    Berlin's, 167–168
    concussion, 167–168
    conjunctival, blunt injuries and, 155
    macular, 423–425, *425*
    retinal, 167–168
Eikenella corrodens, 498
Electrical burn, 192, *192*
Electrical cataract, 192, *192*
ELISA (enzyme-linked immunosorbent assay), 345
Embolism, fat, posttraumatic, 401, *401*
    platelet-fibrin, 431, *432*
Emphysema, orbital, fracture in, 141–142, *142*
    plain film radiography of, 48
Encephalitis, 365t
Encephalocele, 297, 312, *312*, *313*
Endophthalmitis, 500–511
    endogenous, term of, 500
    visual loss in, 430
    infectious, 483–484, *484*, 485t
    metastatic, 430, 500
    phacoanaphylactic, 278
    postoperative, 501t, 501–502
    posttraumatic, 505t–508t
    tests for, 79
    treatment for, 508–509, 509t
Endrate with saline, 186
Enophthalmos, 12
Enterobacter, 463
Enterococci, 502
Entropion, 15, *226*
Enzyme-linked immunosorbent assay (ELISA), 345
Eosinophilic granuloma, 310
Epiblepharon, 15–16
Epicanthus, 15
Epidermal growth factor, in corneal ulceration, 183
Epidermoid cyst, 305–306
Epinephrine, in imaging techniques, 79
    in lid injuries, 109
    in Posner-Schlossman syndrome, 275
    lidocaine with, hemangioma and, 304
    lid lacerations and, 114
Epiphora, 217, 225–230, *228*, *230*
    nonobstructive causes of, 225
    term of, 219
Episcleral pressure, glaucoma and, 279
Episcleritis, 486–487, *487*
Epithelial cells, conjunctival, Giemsa stain of, *82*

532 Index

Epithelial detachment, of retinal pigment. *See* Retina, detachments of.
Epithelial downgrowth, of cornea, 270, *270*
Epithelial keratitis, herpes simplex and, 479
Epithelization, in alkali burn, 186, *187*
Ergotamine, in cluster headache, 370, 371
　in migraine, 369
Erosion(s), corneal recurrent, 243–246, *245*
Erythematosus, systemic lupus, 419
Erythrocyte sedimentation rate (W-ESR), Westergren, 340
Erythromycin, in bacterial conjunctivitis, 476
　in chlamydial conjunctivitis, 476
　in dacryocystitis, 471
　in infectious conjunctivitis, 463
　in lid abrasions, 138
　in lid lacerations, 498
　in Lyme disease, 345
　in *Neisseria gonorrhea*, 464
　in orbital emphysema, 142
　in preseptal cellulitis, 467
　in probing of nasolacrimal duct, 221
　in recurrent corneal erosions, 245
　in rosacea, 239
　in superficial punctate keratopathy, 246
Escherichia coli, in *Acanthamoeba* keratitis, 483
　in child, 299
　in infectious conjunctivitis, 463
Essential blepharospasm, blinking and, 382
Estrogen, migraine and, 367
Ethmoid sinus, 136, *136*
　mucocele in, *332*
Excretory system, lacrimal, 134–136
Exogenous endophthalmitis, term of, 501
Exophthalmometer, 12t, *15*
Exposure keratopathy, in cornea, 249
　superficial punctate keratopathy versus, *247*
Extraocular muscle(s), 133–134, *134*
　cardinal positions of gaze to test, 135t
　thickened, 294
Eye, aqueous humor flow in, *262*
　burns of. *See* Burn(s).
　examination of. *See* Ocular examination.
　immobility of, differential diagnosis of, 293
　pediatric. *See* Pediatric care.
　penetrating injuries to. *See* Penetrating injury(ies).
　slit lamp examination of. *See* Slit lamp.
Eye chart, 91, *92*
Eye shield, 111, *112*, *116*
Eyeball, voluntary propulsion of, 453
Eyebrow or eyelash plucking, functional, 452–453, *454*
Eyelid, 109–130
　abrasions of, 138
　bites or scratches in, 120–122, *122*, *123*
　ecchymosis of, *110*, 110–111, 138, *139*
　eversion of upper, 199, *200*

Eyelid (*Continued*)
　examination of, 14–15
　foreign bodies in, 122–123, *124*
　functional pulling of, 452, *453*
　history of injury to, 109
　inflammation of, *469*, 469–470
　lacerations of, 111–120
　　anesthesia in, 113–114, 114t
　　antibiotics in, 113, 497–498
　　anticoagulants and, 111–112
　　antirabies prophylaxis in, 113
　　antitetanus prophylaxis in, 112t, 112–113
　　assessment in, 111, *112*
　　evaluation and considerations for, 111–114
　　operative techniques for, 115–120, *116*, 117t, *118–120*
　　patient preparation for repair in, 109–110
　　recreational drugs and, 109
　　referrals in, 129
　　regional anesthesia for, 114–115, *116*
　　retrobulbar hemorrhage in, 125–127, *126*
　　thermal and chemical burns in, 127, *128*
　　toxic and allergic reactions in, 128, *129*
　　traumatic ptosis in, 123–125, *125*, *126*
　malpositions of, 225, *225*, *226*
　mass in, 16
　retraction and lag of, on downward gaze, 293
　skin discoloration of, 292
　slit lamp examination of. *See* Slit lamp.
　swelling of, 293
　thermal burns of, 127, *128*
　twitching of, 381–383, *382*
Eyewear, protective, 97, *97*, *98*, 98t

Facial asymmetry, differential diagnosis of, 293
Facial myokymia, 383
Family history, 5
Fat embolism, posttraumatic, 401, *401*
Fat suppression, in magnetic resonance imaging, 57, *60*
Fentanyl, 103t
Fever, cat scratch, 121, *122*
　Haverhill, 121–122
　rat bite, 121–122
　Sodoku, 122
Fibronectin, 183
Fibrous dysplasia, in orbit, 331
Fibrous histiocytoma, 326–327
Filamentary keratopathy, 246–249, *248*
Fissure, orbital, inferior, 133
　superior, 132
　　cranial nerve palsy and, 343–44, *343*
Fistula(s), arteriovenous, *321*, 321–322
　carotid-cavernous. *See* Carotid-cavernous fistula.
　dural sinus, 321
　lacrimal sac, 222, *223*

Flagyl. *See* Metronidazole (Flagyl).
Flap, descemetocele and, 240, *240*
  Gundersen, 240
Flick phosphene, 379
Floater(s), in retinal disorders, 380-381
Fluconazole, 482
Flucytosine, 320
Fluorescein angiography, complications of, 79
  in child, 61, *62*
  in external corneal disorders, 30
  in lacrimal drainage assessment, 220, 228-229
  in superficial punctate keratopathy, 246
Fluorometholone (FML), in interstitial keratitis, 250
  in superficial punctate keratopathy, 246
Flurazepam (Dalmane), 161t
Flurbiprofen (Ansaid), 490
FML (fluorometholone), in interstitial keratitis, 250
  in superficial punctate keratopathy, 246
Folinic acid, 492, 493t
Follicle(s), 27
Follicular conjunctival reaction, *28*
Foramen, optic, enlarged, 311, *311*
Forced duction test, 22, *23*
  in diplopia, 340
Forceps injury, obstetrical, *156*, 156-157
Foreign body(ies), 197-213. *See also* Penetrating injury(ies).
  in cornea and conjunctiva, 199-201, *200*, *202*
  in lid and orbit, 122-123, *124*
  intraocular, *209*, *210*, 210-211
  intraorbital, 211-212, *212*
  plain film radiography of, *51*
  retained, failure to diagnose, 63-67
Fortaz. *See* Ceftazidime (Fortaz).
Foscarnet (trisodium phosphonoformate hexahydrate), 402
Fossa, posterior, disorders of, 75-76
Four diopter base-out test, 22
Four dot test of Worth's, 22
Fourth nerve palsy, 349-350, *350*, *351*
Fovea, disk diameters of, 37
Foveola, disk diameters of, 37
Foville's syndrome, 347
Fracture(s), orbital. *See* Orbital fracture(s).
Fresh frozen plasma, in hereditary angioedema, 128
Frontal seizure(s), 381
Frontal sinus, 136, *136*, 137
Functional and psychotic disorder(s), 441-457
  blinking in, 451, 452t
  eyelash and eyebrow plucking in, 452-453, *454*
  headaches in, 451

Functional and psychotic disorder(s) (*Continued*)
  lid pulling in, 452, 452t, *453*
  loss of visual field or acuity in, 442-446
    adult with, 445
    child with, 445-446, 452t
    diagnosis of, 443-445
  Munchausen's syndrome in, 455
  photophobia in, 450-451
  pupillary abnormalities in, 450
  self-mutilation in, 455-456
  spasm of near reflex in, 446-448, *447*, 448t
  visual hallucinations in, 449-450
  voluntary nystagmus in, 448
  voluntary propulsion of eyeballs in, 453
Fundus, 37-42, *38-41*, 40t, 41t
  findings in, notations and abbreviations to record, 40t
Fungi, in endophthalmitis, 501t, 502
  in keratitis, 481-482, *482*
Furosemide (Lasix), in angle-closure glaucoma, 268
  in pseudotumor cerebri, 435
Fusarium, Gomori-methenamine-silver stain of, *83*
  in keratitis, 481

Gadolinium-diethylene triamine pentacetic acid (Gd-DTPA), 57
Ganciclovir, in cytomegalovirus retinopathy, 402
  in retinal necrosis, 405
Gaze, cardinal positions of, 19, 134, *135*, 135t
Gd-DTPA (gadolinium-diethylene triamine pentacetic acid), 57
General anesthesia. *See* Anesthesia.
Gentamicin, cost of, 509t
  diffusion of, 507t
  endophthalmitis and, 501
    traumatic, 503, 508
  in corneal infections, 478
  in infectious conjunctivitis, 463
  in intraocular foreign body injury, 212
  in orbital cellulitis, 468
  in superficial punctate keratopathy, 246
Geometric field(s), in functional disorder testing, 445
Ghost cell glaucoma, 278
Giant cell arteritis, headaches and, 366t
  visual loss and, 418-419
Giemsa's stain, 79, 80-81, *81*, *82*
  in infectious conjunctivitis, 463, *464*
  procedure for, 82t
Gilles de la Tourette syndrome, 381
Glassblower cataract, 193, *194*
Glaucoma, 261-287
  angle-closure, findings in, 264-267, *265-267*
    phacomorphic glaucoma and, 272

534 Index

Glaucoma (*Continued*)
  angle-closure, postoperative, 272–273, *274*
    postoperative, 272–273, *274*
    primary acute, 263–269
    secondary acute, 269–274, *272*, *273*, *274*
    treatment of, 267–269, *268*
  blood-induced, 278–279
  diagnosis of, 262, 263t
  episcleral pressure and, 279
  ghost cell, 278–279
  history of, 269
  in lens emergencies, 256–259, *257*, *258*
  infantile or congenital, 279–283
    primary, 279–281, *280*, 281t, *282*
    secondary, 281–283, *283–285*, 285t
  lens particle, 277–278, *278*
  malignant, 273
  ophthalmologic referral in, 283
  phacolytic, 165, 277, *277*
  pigmentary dispersion syndrome in, 275, *276*
  pupillary block, 272, *272*, *273*
  secondary acute open-angle, 275–279
  trabecular meshwork in, *270*, 270–272, *271*
  traumatic lens-induced, 165
  uveitis with, 275, *276*
Glaucomaflecken, 265, *266*
Glaucomatocyclitic crisis. See Posner-Schlossman syndrome.
Glioma(s), optic nerve, 326
  child with, 71, 72, 310–311
    axial computed tomography in, *54*
Globe, ruptured, *66*
  smooth indentation of, 293
Glycerol, adverse effects of, 268
  in angle-closure glaucoma, 268
Goldmann applanation tonometry, 33, *35*
Goldmann lens, 31, *32*, 39
Gomori-methenamine-silver stain, of *Fusarium solani*, 83
Goniolens, Zeiss, 31, *31*
  angle-closure glaucoma and, 267, *268*
Gonioscopy, 31, *32*
  in angle-closure glaucoma, 265, *266*, *267*
Gonococcal ophthalmia neonatorum, 463–464
Gradenigo's syndrome, 349
Gradient echo, term of, 57
Gram's stain, 79–80, 81t
  in gonococcal infection, 464, *465*
Granulocytic sarcoma, 310
Granuloma, cat scratch fever and, *123*
  eosinophilic, 310
  Langerhans cells and, 310
  lethal midline, 320
  sarcoid, *421*
  Wegener's, 320
Guanethidine, 317

Guillain-Barré syndrome, Miller-Fisher bulbar variant of, 346
Gundersen flap, descemetocele and, 240, *240*

Haab's striae, 280
Haemophilus influenzae, endophthalmitis and, 508
  in animal and human bites, 499
  in child with infection, 298, 299
  in conjunctivitis, 463
  in endophthalmitis, 508
  in orbital fractures, 500
  in orbital infections, 466, 468
Hallucination(s), 449–450
  release, 374
  retinal disorders and, 373–375
Hamartoma(s), 295, 302–305, *303*, *305*
Hashish, 375
Hasner, valve of, 136, *218*, 219
Haverhill fever, 121–122
Headache, 363–372
  asthenopia and, 371–372
  cephalalgia, 368
  functional, 451
  tension, 371, 451
    differential diagnosis of, 290
  traction and inflammatory, 364–366, 365t–366t
  vascular, 367–371
    cluster, 370–371
    migraine, 367–370, 368t
Healon, 205
Hemangioma(s). *See also* Hemorrhage.
  capillary, *303*, 303–304
  cavernous, 323, 324
  choroidal, 69–70
  retinal, 69–70
Hemangiopericytoma(s), 323
Hematoma, subdural, headaches and, 365t
  shaken baby syndrome and, 99, *101*
Hemianopsia, monocular temporal, 444–445
Hemifacial spasm, 382, *382*
Hemorrhage. *See also* Hemangioma(s).
  child abuse and, 99
  choroidal, 69, *70*
    visual loss and, 427
  differential diagnosis in, 290
  headaches and, 365t
  intraparenchymal, 365t
  orbital, 138–140, 139t, *140*
  spontaneous, 320, *321*
  retinal. *See* Retina, hemorrhage in.
  retrobulbar, traumatic, 125–127, *126*
  subarachnoid, 365t
  subconjunctival, 153–155, *154*
    penetrating injury and, 197–198, *198*
  subretinal neovascular membrane, 422, *423*

Hemorrhage (*Continued*)
  thalamic, 77
  vitreous, blunt injury and, 166
    T_2-weighted image of, 69, *70*
  visual loss and, 411, 412t
Hereditary angioedema, 128
Herpes simplex, 478–481, *479–481*
  in infectious conjunctivitis, 464–466
  in ophthalmia neonatorum, 461
Herpes zoster ophthalmicus (HZO), 485, *486*
  cranial nerve palsy and, 346
  headaches and, 366t
Hertel exophthalmometer, *15*
Hirschberg light reflex test, 20
Hirtz view, of orbit, 49
Histamine, headaches and, 372
Histiocytoma(s), fibrous, 326–327
History, 5, 6
  in nontraumatic orbital disorders, 289–294
  of diplopia, 337–338
  of glaucoma, 263–264, *264*
  of lid injuries, 109
  of pupillary abnormalities, 354–355, *356*
  six Ps and, 290–293
HLA (human leukocyte antigen), 86
Hollenhorst plaque, 431, *431*
Homocystinuria, 253–254
Hordeola, 16
Horner's syndrome, anisocoria and, 357, *359*, 359–360
  differential diagnosis of, 361t
  pupillary abnormalities and, 355
Hounsfield unit(s), 52, 53t
Hruby lens, 39
Human bite(s), 120–122, *122*, *123*
  antibiotics in, 498–500, 499t
Human leukocyte antigen (HLA), 86
Human tetanus immune globulin, 112, 511
Hyaluronidase, 114
Hydrogen peroxide, 242
Hydrop(s), blunt injury and, 156
Hydroxyamphetamine (Paredrine), in neuron disorders, 360
Hydroxycobalamin, in Leber's optic neuropathy, 422
  in optic neuropathy, 429
Hyperosmotic agent(s), adverse effects of, 268
  in angle-closure glaucoma, 274
Hyperostosis, 48
Hyperplasia, lymphoid, 323–324
Hypertension, malignant, headaches and, 366t
  retinal hemorrhage and, 409–411, *410*
Hypertensive retinopathy, *38*
Hypertonic mannitol, 268
Hypertonic sodium chloride, in filamentary keratopathy, 247
  in recurrent corneal erosions, 245

Hyphema, blunt injury and, *159*, 159–162, 160t–162t
  diagnosis of, 158
Hypoparathyroidism, 381
Hypoplasia, optic nerve, 72
  plain film radiography of, 48
Hypotears, 233
Hysteria, term of, 441
HZO. *See* Herpes zoster ophthalmicus (HZO).

Illiterate E eye chart, 91, *92*
Illness, present, history of, 5
Illumination technique, slit lamp, *26*, 26–27
Image test, dissimilar, 21
Imaging technique(s), 62, 64t–66t. *See also* Diagnostic test(s).
Imipenem, cost of, 509t
  diffusion of, 507t
  endophthalmitis and, 484
  traumatic, 508
  penetration of, 508t
Imipenem-cilastatin (Primaxin) in endophthalmitis, 504, 505t, 508
Immunization, 510t, 510–511
Indirect ophthalmoscopy, 38, *40*
Indirect orbital floor fracture, term of, 142
Indirect traumatic optic neuropathy, posterior, 397
Indocin. *See* Indomethacin (Indocin).
Indomethacin (Indocin), in macular edema, 425
  in Posner-Schlossman syndrome, 275
  in scleritis, 490
Infant. *See also* Pediatric care.
  congenital nasolacrimal duct obstruction in, 219–220, *220*
  glaucoma in, 279–283, *280*, 281t, *282*
    secondary, 281–283, *283–285*, 285t
  papoose board restraint of, 91, *93*
Infarcted tissue, on palate, nasal mucosa, or skin, 293
Infection, 466–485
  Acanthamoeba keratitis and, 482–483, *483*
  conjunctival, 472–476, *473*. *See also* Conjunctivitis.
    viral, 472–475, *474*
  corneal, *477*, 477–478, *478*
  cranial nerve palsy and, 345–346
  differential diagnosis in, 290
  endophthalmitis and, 483–484, *484*, 485t
  fungal keratitis and, 481–482, *482*
  herpes simplex, 478–481, *479–481*
  herpes zoster ophthalmicus, 485, *486*
  in child, *294*, 297–300, 298t
  in neonate, 461–466, *462*

Infection (*Continued*)
  lacrimal, etiology of, *470*, 470–472, *471*
    evaluation and management of, 231–233, *232*
  ophthalmia neonatorum and, 461–466, *462*
    conjunctivitis in, 463–466, *464*, *465*
    evaluation of, 461–466, 462t
    silver nitrate in, 463
  orbital, 319–320
    child with, 295
    etiology of, 466–469, *467*
Infectious agent(s), stains and culture media for, 80t
Inferior oblique muscle, 133
Inferior orbital fissure, 133
Inflammation, 486–494
  anterior uveitis and, *490*, 490–491
  choroidal, 70, *70*
  corneal ulcer as, 237–239, *238*, 238t
  differential diagnosis of, 290
  episcleritis and, 486–487, *487*
  lid, *469*, 469–470
  ophthalmia neonatorum and, 461–466, *462*
    evaluation in, 461–466, 462t
    infectious conjunctivitis in, 463–466, *464*, *465*
    silver nitrate in, 463
  orbital, 73
  pars planitis and, 491, *492*
  pediatric, *300*, 300–301, *302*
    orbital, 295
  retinal, 70, *70*
  scleritis and, 487–490, *488*, *489*
  sympathetic ophthalmia and, 493–494
  toxoplasmosis and, 492–493, *493*, 493t
Infraorbital anesthesia technique, in lid lacerations, 114, *116*
Injury. *See* Trauma.
Innominate line, physical findings of, 293
  plain film radiography of, 48
INO. *See* Internuclear ophthalmoplegia (INO).
Internuclear ophthalmoplegia (INO), 339
  monocular nystagmus and, 375
  multiple sclerosis and, 346
Interstitial keratitis, 249–250, *251*
Intracerebral disorder, *76*, 76–78, *77*
Intracerebral tumor, 76
Intracranial aneurysm, 78
Intracranial pressure, cranial nerve palsy and, 346–347
Intracranial tumor, headaches and, 365t
  tests for, 76
Intraocular foreign body, *209*, *210*, 210–211
Intraocular hemorrhage, child abuse and, 99
Intraocular pressure, in chemical burn, 184
  in examination, 32–35, *33*, 34t, *35*, *36*, 36t

Intraocular pressure (*Continued*)
  measurement of, 95
  red eye and, 3
Intraorbital air, computed tomography of, 67
Intraorbital foreign body, 211–212, *212*
Intraparenchymal hemorrhage, 365t
Inversion recovery, term of, 57
Iodinated contrast agent(s), 78–79
  sensitivity to, 9–10, *10*
Iridocyclitis, glaucoma versus, 263t. *See also* Uveitis.
Iridodialysis, *158*, 158–159
Iris, blunt injury of, 157–159, *158*
  infarct or atrophy of, 361–362
  slit lamp examination of, 30
  transillumination of, 275, *276*
Iris bombé, glaucoma and, 272, *272*
Iritis, traumatic, 157–158
Irrigation, in chemical burns, 184, 185t
Irritative hallucination(s), 449
Irritative sympathetic lesion(s), 361–362
Irvine-Gass syndrome, 423
Ischemia, differential diagnosis of, 290
  in central retinal vein occlusion, 407–409, *408*
  in cerebrovascular disease, 365t
  in child, 295, 301–302
Ischemic optic neuropathy, 417t
  visual loss in, 419, *420*
Isosorbide, 268, 269
Itraconazole, 483

Jones dye test, *16*, 16–17
  in acquired lacrimal obstruction, 228, *229*

Keflex. *See* Cephalexin (Keflex).
Keratic precipitates, 275
Keratitis, *Acanthamoeba*, 482–483, *483*
  disciform, 480, *481*
  epithelial, 479
  fungal, 481–482, *482*
  herpes simplex, 479, *480*, *481*
  interstitial, corneal, 249–250, *251*
  metaherpetic, 480
  stromal, 480
  superficial punctate, 479
  Thygeson's, *247*
Keratoconjunctivitis, superior limbic, *247*
Keratoconjunctivitis sicca. *See* Dry eye syndrome.
Keratomalacia, 239
Keratopathy, exposure, 249
  superficial punctate keratopathy versus, *247*

Keratography (*Continued*)
 filamentary, 246–249, *248*
 neurotrophic, 249, *250*
 radiation, *247*
 superficial punctate, 246, 247t, *248*
 toxic, *247*
 traumatic posterior annular, 155–156
Ketoconazole, in *Acanthamoeba* keratitis, 483
 in endophthalmitis, 507t
 in fungal keratitis, 482
Kimura spatula, corneal infections and, *478*
Klebsiella pneumoniae, 463
Koeppe lens gonioscopy, 31
Krimsky test, 21
Krukenberg's spindle, 275

Laboratory study(ies), 79–83, 80t–82t, *80–83*
 in nontraumatic orbital disorders, 294, 317t
Laceration(s), conjunctival, 198–199
 blunt injuries and, 155
 corneal, 203–207, *204*, *206*
 lid, 111–120
  antibiotics in, 497–498
  evaluation and considerations for, 111–114, *112*
 optic nerve, 172
Lacrilube, in exposure keratopathy, 249
 in penetrating injuries, 201
 in superficial punctate keratopathy, 246
Lacrimal canaliculi, 218, *218*
 atresia of, 223
 inflammation of, 224–225
 obstruction of, 231
 stenosis of, 224
Lacrimal canaliculitis, 224–225
Lacrimal drainage system, 217–235. *See also* Lacrimal gland fossa.
 acquired disorder(s) in, 223–231
  causes of, 223–225, *224–226*
  epiphora as, 225–230, *228*, *230*
  treatment of, 230–231
 anatomy of, *218*, 218–219
 congenital disorders of, 219–223, *220*, *222*, *223*
 dry eye syndrome and, 233
 examination of, 16
 infection of, etiology of, *470*, 470–472, *471*
 evaluation and management of, 231–233, *232*
 nontraumatic orbital disorders and, 328–331, *330*
Lacrimal duct, 218, *218*, 219
Lacrimal gland fossa, 131
 calcification of, 293
 local compression of, 293

Lacrimal puncta, 134–135
 atresia of, 222–223
 stenosis of, 224
 treatment of, 231
Lacrimal sac, 131, 135–136, 218, *218*
Lacrimal sac fistula, 222, *223*
Lacrimal tumor(s), 328–329
Lacrisert, in chemical burns, 189
 in dry eye syndrome, 233
Lamina papyracea, fracture of, 146
Landolt C optotypes, 91
Langerhans cell granulomatosis, 310
Large pupil(s), 361–362
 bilateral, 363
Lasix (furosemide), in angle-closure glaucoma, 268
 in pseudotumor cerebri, 435
Lateral view, of orbit, 49, *51*, 63
Le Fort orbital fracture(s), *149*, 149–150
Lead, optic neuropathy and, 429
 pseudotumor cerebri and, 435
Leber's optic neuropathy, 421–422
Legal blindness, defined, 10–11
Lens, 39
 bandage. *See* Bandage lens.
 contact. *See* Contact lens.
 injury of, blunt, *163*, 163–165, *165*
  penetrating, 207–208
 nontraumatic emergencies of, 250–259
  cataracts in, 255–256, *256*
  ectopia lentis in, 251–255, *252–254*
  glaucoma in, 256–259, *257*, *258*
 slit lamp examination of, 30–31
 subluxation of, 251
Lens gonioscopy of Koeppe, 31
Lethal midline granuloma, 320
Leukemia, 310
Leukocoria, 383–387, *385–387*
Levator aponeurosis, repair of, *125*, *126*
Levobunolol, in hyphema, 161t
 in phacolytic glaucoma, 165
Levodopa, 362
Lid. *See* Eyelid.
Lidocaine (Xylocaine), in hemangioma, 304
 in lid laceration, 114, 114t
 in pediatric examination, 103t
Light reflex, pupillary, examination of, 17
 Hirschberg test in, 20
 pathway and parasympathetic fibers of, in pupillary abnormalities, 355–356
Limbic keratoconjunctivitis, superficial punctate keratopathy versus, *247*
Lipodermoid, 306, *307*
Lithium, cluster headache and, 371
 optic neuropathy and, 429
Local anesthesia, in lid lacerations, 114, 114t
 in pediatric examination, 103t

Log MAR, 9, *9*
Lorazepam (Ativan), 161t
Loss of vision, sudden and unexpected, 395–439
　amaurosis fugax in, 430–433, *431*, *432*
　sustained bilateral, 428–430
　sustained unilateral, 396–428, 398t, 399t, *400*
　　AIDS and, 401–405, *402–404*
　　choroidal disorder in, 427–428
　　cranial or other trauma and, 397–401, *401*
　　external ocular signs in, 396
　　macular disorder in, 422–427, *423–427*, 424t
　　optic neuropathy in, 415–422, 417t, *418*, *420*, *421*
　　posterior vitreous detachment in, 414–415
　　retinal disorder in, 405–414, *406–408*, *410*, *411*, 412t, 413t, *414*, *415*
　transient bilateral, 433t, 433–435
　transient unilateral, 430–433, *431*, *432*
Lowe's syndrome, 281
LSD (lysergic acid diethylamide), 363, 375
Lupus erythematosus, systemic, 419
Lyme disease, cranial nerve palsy with, 345
　optic neuropathy and, 422
Lymphadenopathy, hemifacial, *122*
Lymphangioma, 304, *321*
Lymphoid hyperplasia, 323–324
Lymphoma, 323–324, *325*
　Burkitt's, 310
　coronal computed tomography of, *54*
Lysergic acid diethylamide (LSD), 363, 375
Lysol, 429

Macropsia, defined, 25
Macula, age-related degeneration of, 422–423
　disk diameters of, 37
　edema of, 423–425, *425*
　sudden and unexpected loss of vision and, 422–427, *423–427*, 424t
Macular hole, traumatic, *169*, 169–170
　visual loss and, 426, *427*
Macular pucker, 426–427
Maculopathy, solar, 397
Maddox rod test, 21, 22
Magnetic resonance angiography, 59–60
Magnetic resonance imaging (MRI), 56–57, *58–60*
　advantages and disadvantages of, 62, 64t, 65t
　adverse effect of, 208
　in binocular diplopia, 340
Malignant glaucoma, 273

Malignant hypertension, headaches and, 366t
　retinal hemorrhage and, 409–411, *410*
Malignant neoplasm. *See also specific neoplasm.*
　melanoma as, *46*, 67
　of orbit, 295, 307–312, *308*, *309*, *311*
Malingering, 443
Malpractice suit(s), trauma-related, 63
Mannitol, adverse effects of, 268–269
　in hyphemia, 161t
　in phacolytic glaucoma, 165
Map-dot-fingerprint corneal dystrophy, 244, *245*
Marfan's syndrome, 253, *254*
Marijuana, hallucinations and, 375
　mydriasis and, 363
Mass(es). *See* Neoplasm(s); Tumor(s); *specific neoplasm.*
Mature cataract, 256, *257*
Maxillary sinus, 136, *137*
Medical history, 6
Medication(s), bottle top colors of, 5, 6t
　current, examination and, 6
Melanoma, malignant, *46*, 67
Membrane, Bruch's, fluorescein angiogram of fluid leakage from, *62*
　slit lamp examination of, 28
Meningioma(s), 326, *327*, *328*
　computed tomography of, 71, *71*
　in child, 311
Meningitis, carcinomatous, 341
　headaches and, 365t
　in bacterial conjunctivitis, 475
Meperidine (Demerol), 103t
Mepivacaine, 114t
Mercury, 429
Mescaline, hallucinations and, 375
　mydriasis and, 363
Mesenchymal sarcoma(s), 326–327
Mestinon (pyridostigmine), 353
Metabolic optic neuropathy, 429
Metaherpetic keratitis, 480
Metallic foreign bodies, plain film radiography of, 123, *124*
Metamorphopsia, 376–377, *377*
　defined, 25
Metastatic endophthalmitis, term of, 500
　visual loss in, 430
Metastatic orbital tumor(s), 327–328
Methanol, 429
Methasone acetate, 304
Methasone sodium phosphate, 304
Methohexital (Brevital), 103t
Methotrexate, in sarcoidosis, 421
　in scleritis, 490
　in Wegener's granulomatosis, 320
Methylcellulose, 47

Methylprednisolone, in macular edema, 425
  in pars planitis, 491
  periocular repository, 425
Methyltestosterone, 128
Methysergide, 369, 371
Metoclopramide, 369
Metronidazole (Flagyl), 468
Miconazole, in *Acanthamoeba* keratitis, 483
  in fungal keratitis, 482
Microbiologic culture media and stains, in diagnostic tests, 80t, 81–82
  in ophthalmia neonatorum, 462t
Microbiology Reference Laboratory (MRL), 345
Micropsia, defined, 25
Microvasculopathy, acquired immune deficiency syndrome and, 401, *402*
Migraine, 367–370, 368t
  classic, central retinal artery occlusion and, 407
  common, 368
  complicated, 368
  ophthalmoplegic, cranial nerve palsy and, 347
Migrainous optic neuropathy, 420
Millard-Gubler's syndrome, 347
Miller-Fisher variant, of Guillain-Barré syndrome, 346
Minocycline, 183
Miochol, 207
Miosis, traumatic, 157, 158
Miostat, 207
Miotics, in angle-closure glaucoma, 269, 274
  in anisocoria, 360
  in keratoconjunctivitis, 27
  in pigmentary dispersion syndrome, 275
Mixed tumor, benign, 328–329
Mnemonic, COWS, 22
  6Ps, 290–293
Monocular temporal hemianopsia, 444–445
Monocular visual loss, tests for, 443
Monosodium glutamate, 370, 372
Moore's lightning streak(s), 379
Morgagnian cataract, 256, *257*
Morphine, in pediatric examination, 103t
  miosis and, 362
Motility disorder(s), 74
MRL (Microbiology Reference Laboratory), 345
Mucocele, of lacrimal sac, 221–222, *222*
  orbital, 331, *332*
Mucomyst. *See* Acetylcysteine (Mucomyst).
Mucopyocele, 331
Mucor, 319, 468
Multiple sclerosis, cranial nerve palsy and, 346
  tests for, 77
Munchausen's syndrome, 455

Muscarinic antagonist(s), 272
Muscle cone, 133–134
Muscle contraction headache, 371
Muscular disorder(s), diplopia and, 352–353
Mutilation, self, 455–456
Myasthenia gravis, 340
  diplopia and, 352–353
Mydriacyl (tropicamide), 269, 273
Mydriasis, traumatic, 342
Mydriatic(s), in angle-closure glaucoma, 268, 269, 273
  in pupillary enlargement, 361
Myokymia, facial, 383
  superior oblique, 375–376

Nafcillin, in orbital cellulitis, 299, 468
  in preseptal cellulitis, 467
Nalidixic acid, 435
Nanophthalmos, 428
Narcissus Medical Foundation, 159
Narcotic(s), in pediatric examination, 103t
  in thermal burns, 191
Nasal mucosa, infarcted tissue of, 293
Nasolacrimal duct, 136
Nasolacrimal duct obstruction (NLDO), acquired, 223–224, 231
  congenital, 219–221, *220*
Nasopharyngeal carcinoma, 341
Natacyn (natamycin), 481–482
Natamycin (Natacyn), 481–482
National Registry of Drug-induced Ocular Side Effects, 6
Near reflex, spasm of, 363, 446–448, *447*, 448t
Near-vision chart, 7, *8*, 9t
Near-visual acuity conversions and percentage of central vision loss, 9t
Necrosis, retinal, acquired immune deficiency syndrome and, 403–405
Neisseria gonorrhoeae, in conjunctivitis, 464, 465, 475
  in corneal infection, 477
  in lacrimal infection, 470
  in ophthalmia neonatorum, 461
  silver nitrate and, 463
Neomycin, 128, 138
Neomycin-bacitracin-polysporin ointment, 138
Neoplasm(s). *See also specific neoplasm.*
  cranial nerve palsy with, 341–342
  malignant, melanoma as, *46*, 67
  pediatric orbital, 295, 307–312, *308*, *309*, *311*
  nasolacrimal duct or sac obstruction and, 224
Neosporin, in *Acanthamoeba* keratitis, 483
  in corneal infections, 478

540   Index

Neptazane, 161t
Neuralgia, trigeminal, 366t
Neurilemoma(s), 326
 in child, 305
Neuritis, optic, acquired immune deficiency syndrome and, 405
 postinfectious, 429
 visual loss and, 416–418, 417t, *418*
Neuro-ophthalmologic retinal emergency(ies), 335–393. *See also* Retina.
Neuroblastoma, 308–310, *309*
Neurofibroma, dysplasia of orbital bones in, 312, *313*
 in child, 304–305, *305*
 plexiform, 326
 infantile glaucoma and, 283, *284*
 simple, 324–326
Neurogenic disorder(s), cranial nerve, 346
Neuroimaging study(ies), in diplopia, 340, 341t
Neuropathy, optic. *See* Optic neuropathy.
Neurotrophic keratopathy, 249, *250*
Nevus, strawberry, 292, 303
Nitrate(s), 372
Nitroglycerin, 367
Nitrosurea(s), 429
NLDO (nasolacrimal duct obstruction), acquired, 223–224
 congenital, 219–221, *220*
Nodular granuloma, *123*
Noncontact lens, in retinal examination, 39
Nonhemorrhagic cerebral infarction(s), 76, *76*
Noninfectious corneal emergency(ies). *See* Cornea, nonpenetrating, noninfectious emergencies of.
Nonpenetrating corneal emergency(ies). *See* Cornea, nonpenetrating, noninfectious emergencies of.
Nonsteroidal anti-inflammatory agent(s), in recurrent corneal erosions, 245
 in scleritis, 487, 488–489
Nontraumatic emergency(ies), 215–457
 functional disorders in, 441–457. *See also* Functional and psychotic disorder(s).
 glaucoma in, 261–287. *See also* Glaucoma.
 of cornea, 237–250. *See also* Cornea.
 of lacrimal drainage system, 217–235. *See also* Lacrimal drainage system.
 of lens, 250–259. *See also* Lens.
 of orbit, 289–334. *See also* Orbit, nontraumatic disorders of.
 of retina, 335–393. *See also* Retina.
 psychotic disorders in, 441–457. *See also* Functional and psychotic disorder(s).
 sudden and unexpected loss of vision in, 395–439. *See also* Loss of vision, sudden and unexpected.
Norgesic (orphenadrine citrate), 383

Nutritional optic neuropathy, 429
Nystagmus, voluntary, 448

Oblique muscle, blurring of, as radiographic sign, 48, 293
 inferior, 133
 superior, 133
 myokymia of, 375
Oblique view, of orbit, 50, *53*
O'Brien anesthesia technique, 114–115, *116*
Observation of behavior, in disproving visual loss, 443–444
Obstetrical forceps injury(ies), *156*, 156–157
Obstruction, nasolacrimal duct, acquired, 223–225, 231
 congenital, 219–221, *220*
Occlusion, retinal artery, branch, 407, *407*
 retinal vein, branch, 409, *410*
 central, 407–409, *408*
Occucoat, 205
Ocular alignment, 19–23, 20t, 21t, *23*
Ocular and orbital trauma, blunt, 153–177. *See also* Blunt injury(ies).
 penetrating, 197–213. *See also* Penetrating injur(ies).
Ocular calcification, 293
Ocular cicatricial pemphigoid, 239
Ocular disorder(s), tests for, 63–78. *See also* Diagnostic test(s), disorders and.
Ocular emergency(ies), nontraumatic. *See* Nontraumatic emergency(ies).
Ocular examination, 3–43
 assessment of vision in, 4t, 6–12, *7–10*, 8t, 9t, 12t, *13*
 equipment for, *14*
 external, 4t, 12–17, *14–16*
 fundus in, 4t, 37–42, *38–41*, 40t, 41t
 intraocular pressure measurement in, 4t, 32–35, *33*, 34t, *35*, *36*, 36t
 ocular alignment and motility in, 4t, 19–23, 20t, 21t, *23*
 ophthalmic history in, 4t, 5–6, 6t
 pediatric, 91–105. *See also* Pediatric care.
 pupils in, 4t, 17t, 17–19, *18*
 referral indications and, 42
 slit lamp in, 4t, 25–31, *26*, *28*, *29*, *31*, *32*, 32t
 systemic history in, 4t, 6
 visual field, 4t, 23–25, *24*
Ocular flutter, 375
Ocular infection. *See* Infection.
Ocular inflammation. *See* Inflammation.
Ocular ischemic syndrome, 431
Ocular motility, 19–23, 20t, 21t, *23*, 137–138
 disorders of, 74
Ocular pursuit, diplopia and, 339, 340

Ocular trauma, blunt. *See* Blunt injury(ies).
  penetrating. *See* Penetrating injury(ies).
Oculocephalic test, 22
Oedipism, 455
Ophthalmia neonatorum, 461–466, *462*
  evaluation in, 461–466, 462t
  infectious conjunctivitis and, 463–466, *464, 465*
  silver nitrate and, 463
Ophthalmic history, 5
Ophthalmic vein, enlarged superior, 294
Ophthalmodynamometry, 39–42, *41*, 41t
Ophthalmologic disorder(s), functional and psychotic. *See* Functional and psychotic disorder(s).
Ophthalmologic referral, in glaucoma, 283
  of child, 42
Ophthalmoplegia, in orbital blunt injuries, 140–141, 141t
  in retinal disorders, 372–373
  internuclear, 339
    monocular nystagmus and, 375
    multiple sclerosis and, 346
Ophthalmoplegic migraine, 368–369
  cranial nerve palsy and, 347
Ophthalmoscopy, 38, *39, 40*
Opsoclonus, 375
Optic canal, 133
  enlargement of, 293
  plain film radiograph of, *53*
Optic chiasm, disorders of, 75
Optic disk, 37
Optic foramen, enlargement of, 311, *311*
Optic nerve, blunt injury of, 172–173, *173*
  disorders of, *71*, 71–72
  dysplasia of, 293
  enlargement of, 294
  glioma of, *54*, 310–311, 326
    axial computed tomography in, *54*
    magnetic resonance imaging of, *60*
  meningioma of, 326, *327*
Optic nerve sheath meningioma, 326, *327*
Optic neuritis, acquired immune deficiency syndrome and, 405
  postinfectious, 429
  visual loss and, 416–418, 417t, *418*, 429
Optic neuropathy, compressive, 422
  diabetic, 366t
  dominant, 429–430
  ischemic, 419, *420*
  Leber's, 421–422
  metabolic, 429
  migrainous, 420
  nutritional, 429
  radiation, 421
  sudden and unexpected loss of vision in, 415–422, 417t, *418, 420, 421*
  toxic, 429

Optic neuropathy (*Continued*)
  traumatic, 172
  posterior, indirect, 397
Optic sheath, disorders of, *71*, 71–72
Optociliary shunt vessel(s), at disc, 293
Oral contraceptive(s), optic neuropathy and, 429
  pseudotumor cerebri and, 435
Orbit, anatomy of, 131–137, *132*, 133t, *134–136*, 135t
  blunt injuries of. *See* Blunt injury(ies), orbital.
  calcifications of, 293
  cellulitis of. *See* Orbital cellulitis.
  emphysema of, 48
    fractures and, 141–142, *142*
  enlargement of, 48
  erosion of, 48
  evaluation of, *135*, 137–138
  fractures of. *See* Orbital fracture(s).
  hemorrhage of, 138–140, 139t, *140*
    spontaneous, 320–321, *321*
  infectious disorders of, 319–320, 466–469, *467*
    abscess in, 73–74, 299
    inflammation of, 73
  lymphoma of, *54*
  meningioma of, 326, *327, 328*
    pediatric, 311
  metastatic tumors of, 327–328
  nontraumatic disorders of, 289–334, *314*
    arteriovenous fistulas in, *321*, 321–322
    cavernous sinus thrombosis in, 322–323
    child with, 294–312, *296*. *See also* Pediatric care.
    diagnostic tests for, 63–78, 72t, *73, 74*
    fibrous dysplasia in, 331
    history and physical findings in, 289–294
    infectious. *See* Orbit, infectious disorders of.
    lacrimal gland in, 328–331, *330*
    mucoceles in, 331, *332*
    progression in, 290–291
    six Ps in evaluating, 290–293
    spontaneous hemorrhage in, 320–321, *321*
    thyroid ophthalmopathy in, 315–317, *316*, 317t, *318, 319*
    tumors in, 323–328, *324, 325, 327, 328*
    varices in, 321
    vasculitis in, 320
  pseudotumor of, headaches and, 366t
    papilledema and, 435
    pediatric, 300, *300*
  soft tissue injuries of, 138–141
  thyroid ophthalmopathy of, 315–317, *316*, 317t, *318, 319*
  varices of, 291, 321
  vascular malformations of, 74

542 Index

Orbital apex syndrome, 342
Orbital bruit(s), 14, 292
Orbital cellulitis, 467–468, *468*
 diagnostic tests for, *73*, 73–74, *74*
 pediatric, 297, *297*, 298t, 298–299
Orbital compartment syndrome, 142
Orbital fissure, inferior, 133
 superior, 132
  cranial nerve palsy and, *343*, 343–344
Orbital foramen, 131
Orbital fracture(s), 141–151
 antibiotics in, 500
 blowout, 142–146, *143–145*
 emphysema and, 141–142, *142*
 Le Fort, *149*, 149–150
 of medial wall, 146, *147*
 of superior wall, 146–147
 trimalar, 147–148, *148*
 tripod, 147–148, *148*
Orbital nerve(s), 132–133, *134*
Orbital scan, in computed tomography, 55–56, *56*
Orbital varix, 291, 321
Orbital venography, 60
Orbitopathy, thyroid, 315–317, *316*, 317t, *318*, *319*
Orphenadrine citrate (Norgesic), 383
Orthophoria, 20
Oscillopsia, 375–376
Osmotic(s), in angle-closure glaucoma, 268
 in dislocated lens, 255
Osteoblastic lesion, 293
Oxacillin, in animal bites, 499t
 in preseptal cellulitis, 467
Oxymethalone, 128

P's mnemonic, in nontraumatic orbital disease, 290–293
Pain, in nontraumatic orbital disorders, 290
 in retinal disorders, 372–373
Palate, infarcted tissue on, 293
Palianopia, 374
Palpation of orbit, in child, 14
 in nontraumatic disorders, 292
Papilla, 27–28
Papillary conjunctival reaction, 28, *29*
Papilledema, characteristics of, 417t
 visual loss and, 433t, 433–435, *434*
Papillopathy, diabetic, 420
Papoose board, 91, *93*
Paramomycin, 483
Paranasal sinus(es), *136*, 136–137
Paraneoplastic lesion, term of, 375
Parasellar abnormalities, 428
 tests for, 75
Parasympathetic antagonist(s), 272
Parasympathetic fiber(s), in pupillary abnormalities, 355–356

Paratrigeminal syndrome, Raeder's, benign, 370
Paredrine (hydroxyamphetamine), 360
Parinaud's syndrome, 339
 midbrain lesions and, 363
Pars planitis, 491, *492*
Pasteurella multocida, 498, 499, 500
Pedi cocktail, 103t
Pediatric care, 91–105. *See also* Infant.
 child abuse and, 99–102, 100t, *101*
 diagnostic tests in, 45–89. *See also* Diagnostic test(s).
 examination in, 3–43. *See also* Ocular examination.
 functional visual loss in, 445–446
 nontraumatic orbital disorders in, 294–312, *296*
  choristomas and, 305–307, *306*, *307*
  diagnostic tests for. *See* Diagnostic test(s).
  encephaloceles and, 312, *312*, *313*
  hamartomas and, 302–305, *303*, *305*
  infectious, *294*, 297–300, 298t
  inflammatory, *300*, 300–301, *302*
  ischemic, 295, 301–302
  malignant neoplasms and, 307–312, *308*, *309*, *311*
 ocular trauma and, 92–96
 sports-related, 96–98, *97*, *98*, 98t
 referral for, 42
 sedation and, 102–103, 103t, 104t
Pemphigoid, ocular cicatricial, 239
Penetrating injury(ies), 197–213
 corneal abrasions in, 201–203, *203*
 diagnostic tests in, 63–67, *66*, *67*
 foreign bodies in, corneal and conjunctival, 199–201, *200*, *202*
 intraocular, *209*, 210, 210–211
 intraorbital, 211–212, *212*
 lacerations in, conjunctival, 198–199
 corneal, 203–207, *204*, *206*
 of lens, 207–208
 of retina, 208–209, *209*
 subconjunctival hemorrhage in, 197–198, *198*
D-Penicillamine, 429
Penicillin, in lid injuries, 113, 122, 498
 in Lyme disease, 345, 422
 in orbital fractures, 500
 in pseudotumor cerebri, 435
 penicillinase-resistant, 121
Penicillin G, in animal bites, 499t, 500
 in lid injuries, 121
 in Lyme disease, 345
 in orbital cellulitis, 299
Penicillinase-resistant penicillin, 121
Peptococcus, 299
Periorbital changes, 292–293
Peripheral anterior synechia, *267*, 270
Perivasculitis, in pars planitis, 491, *492*

Perkins applanation tonometer, 91, *95*
  in infantile glaucoma, 280, *282*
Pertussis immunization, 510
  with tetanus prophylaxis, 511
Pesticide(s), 429
Peter's anomaly, 281, *283*
Phacoanaphylactic endophthalmitis, 278
Phacolytic glaucoma, 165
Phacomorphic glaucoma, 272
Phenergan (promethazine hydrochloride), in hyphema, 161t
  in pediatric examination, 103t
Phenylephrine, contraindications to, 186
  in angle-closure glaucoma, 268, 269
  in episcleritis, 486
  in malignant glaucoma, 273
  in pupillary block, 273
Phenylethylamine, 367, 370
Phosphate, in chemical burns, 186
Phosphene(s), 379
Phospholine iodide, 224
Photocoagulation, 407
Photophobia, functional, 450–451
  in retinal disorders, 377–379
  metamorphopsia and, 378–379
Photopsia, 379
Photostress recovery test, 11, 396
Phycomycosis, 319
Physical finding(s). *See also* Ocular examination.
  in nontraumatic orbital disorders, 289–294
  six Ps in orbital disease and, 290–293
Pigment epithelium detachment, ultraviolet light and, 194, *195*
  visual loss and, 414, *415*
Pigmentary dispersion syndrome, 275, *276*
Pilocarpine, anisocoria and, 360
  in Adie's pupil, 362
  in angle-closure glaucoma, 268, 269
  large pupil and, 450
Pinguecula, 28
Pithiatism, term of, 441
Pituitary abnormality(ies), apoplexy in, 341–342
  microadenoma in, 75
  visual loss and, 428
Plain film radiography, 48–50, *49–53*
  advantages and disadvantages of, 64t, 65t, 67
  ocular and orbital trauma and, 63
Plaque, Hollenhorst, 431, *431*
Plasma, in lid lacerations, 112
Plateau iris configuration, 265
Platelet(s), in lid lacerations, 112
Platelet-fibrin emboli, 431, *432*
Plexiform neurofibroma(s), 326
  in child, 304–305, *305*
  infantile glaucoma and, *284*
Poisoning, hallucinations and, 375

Polyarteritis nodosa, 320
Polymyxin B and trimethoprim (Polytrim), in bacterial conjunctivitis, 475
  in corneal abrasion, 203
  in corneal infections, 478
  in dacryocystitis, 472
  in endophthalmitis, 505t
  in nasolacrimal duct probe, 221
Polysporin ointment, 203
Polytrim. *See* Polymyxin B and trimethoprim (Polytrim).
Pontine angle lesion, 363
Portable slit lamp, 91, *94*
Positioning, in restraining toddler, 91, *93*
Posner-Schlossman syndrome, 275, 362
Posterior vitreous detachment (PVD), 379, 414–415
Postinfectious optic neuritis, 429
Postoperative complication(s), angle-closure glaucoma in, 272–273, *274*
Posttraumatic endophthalmitis, 502–509, 505t–508t
Posttraumatic fat embolism, 401, *401*
Potassium hydroxide, 179, 180t
Pred Forte. *See* Prednisolone acetate (Pred Forte).
Prednisolone, in hyphema, 161t
  in lupus erythematosus, 419
  in uveitis, 491
Prednisolone acetate (Pred Forte), in angle-closure glaucoma, 267, 269
  in chemical burns, 186
  in interstitial keratitis, 250
  in iritis, 158
  in macular edema, 425
  in phacolytic glaucoma, 165
  in sarcoidosis, 421
  in superficial punctate keratopathy, 246
Prednisolone sodium phosphate with sulfacetamide (Vasocidin), 246
Prednisone, in cluster headache, 370
  in lupus erythematosus, 419
  in macular edema, 425
  in sarcoidosis, 421
  in scleritis, 490
  in temporal arteritis, 419
  in thyroid ophthalmopathy, 317
  in toxoplasmosis, 492, 493t
  mydriasis and, 363
Present illness, history of, 5
Preseptal cellulitis, 466–467
  in child, 297, 298, 298t
Pressor agent(s), headaches and, 372
Pressure, intraocular. *See* Intraocular pressure.
Primary acute angle-closure glaucoma. *See* Glaucoma.
Primaxin (imipenem-cilastatin), 504, 505t, 508
Procainamide, myasthenia gravis and, 353

Procaine, in lid lacerations, 114t
Prochlorperazine (Compazine), in hyphema, 161t
  in migraine, 369
Promethazine hydrochloride (Phenergan), in hyphemia, 161t
  in pediatric examination, 103t
Propamidine isethionate (Brolene), 483
Proparacaine, in corneal ulceration, 184
  in lid laceration, 114
  in penetrating injuries, 201
Prophylaxis, antibiotic, 497–500
  antirabies, 113
  antitetanus, 112t, 112–113
  in exogenous endophthalmitis, 509
Propionobacterium acnes, 501, 504, 508
Propranolol, in migraine, 369, 407
  miosis and, 362
Proptosis, in examination, 12
  in pediatric nontraumatic orbital disorders, 291–292
  lacrimal sac mass and, *228*
Propulsion of eyeball, voluntary, 453
Prostigmine, 353
Protective eyewear, 97, *97*, *98*, 98t
Proteus, in conjunctivitis, 463
  in postoperative endophthalmitis, 501
Proton density, defined, 57
Pseudoepiphora, term of, 219
Pseudoisochromatic plate, 11, *13*
Pseudomembrane, slit lamp examination of, 28
Pseudomonas, 299
  in conjunctivitis, 463
  in postoperative endophthalmitis, 501
Pseudopapilledema, 417t
Pseudophakic pupillary block, 273, *274*
Pseudoproptosis, 291
  child with, 297
Pseudotumor. *See also* Tumor(s).
  orbital, headaches and, 366t
  papilledema and, 435
  pediatric, 300, *300*
Psilocin, 375
Psychotic disorder(s). *See* Functional and psychotic disorder(s).
Psychotic self-mutilation, 455–456
Pterygium, slit lamp examination of, 28
Ptosis, examination for, 14–15
  traumatic, 123–125, *125*, *126*
  lid ecchymosis and, *110*
Pulsation, in nontraumatic orbital disorders, 292
Punctate keratopathy, superficial, 246, 247t, *248*, 479
Pupillary abnormality(ies), Adie's tonic, 362
  amaurotic, 361

Pupillary abnormality(ies) (*Continued*)
  anatomy and, 355–356
  light reflex pathway and parasympathetic fibers in, 355–356
  sympathetic fibers in, 356, *357*
  anisocoria in, 356–362, *358*
  bilateral, 362–363
  large pupil, 361–362, 363
  physiologic, 357–359
  small pupil, *358*, *359*, 359–363, 361t
  Argyll-Robertson, 363
  functional, 450
  history of, 354–355, *356*
  in child, 17t, 17–19, *18*
  tadpole, 360
Pupillary block, aphakic, 273
  pseudophakic, 273, *274*
Pupillary block glaucoma, 272, *272*, *273*
Pupillary defect, relative afferent, 17–19, *18*
Pupillary dilation, in testing for functional disorder, 444
Pupillary light reflex, 17, 17t
Pupillary reaction, 17
  notations and abbreviations for recording, 17t
  paradoxical, 19
Purscher's retinopathy, 397–401
Pursuit, ocular, 339, 340
PVD (posterior vitreous detachment), 379
  sudden and unexpected loss of vision in, 414–415
Pyridostigmine (Mestinon), 353
Pyrimethamine, 403, 492, 493t

Quinidine, 353
Quinine, 363

Rabies prophylaxis, 113
Radiation injury, 192–194, *193–195*
  superficial punctate keratopathy versus, *247*
Radiography, in nontraumatic orbital disorders, 293–294
  plain film, 48–50, *49–53*
Raeder's paratrigeminal syndrome, 370
Rat bite fever, 121–122
Rectus muscle(s), 133
  injection over, 292
Recurrent corneal erosion(s), 243–246, *245*
Red eye, differential diagnosis of, *473*
  slit lamp examination in, 3
Red lens test, 21, 22
Referral, glaucoma and, 283
  of child, 42

Reflex, light. *See* Light reflex, pupillary.
  near, spasm of, 363, 446–448, *447*, 448t
  vestibulo-ocular, diplopia and, 339, 340
Refresh, in dry eye syndrome, 233
  in filamentary keratopathy, 247
  in inflammatory corneal ulcers, 239
  in soft contact lens reaction, 242
  in superficial punctate keratopathy, 246
Refresh PM, in dry eye syndrome, 233
  in exposure keratopathy, 249
  in filamentary keratopathy, 247
  in inflammatory corneal ulcers, 239
  in superficial punctate keratopathy, 246
Regional anesthesia, 114–115, *116*
Reid's line, 53–54, *56*
Relative afferent pupillary defect (RAPD), 17–19, *18*
Relaxation time(s), in magnetic resonance imaging, 57
Release hallucination(s), 374, 449
Reserpine, in migraine, 367
  mydriasis and, 363
Respiratory depressant(s), myasthenia gravis and, 353
Restraint(s), for pediatric examination, 91, *93*, *95*
Retina, 335–393
  blinking, blepharospasm, and lid twitching and, 381–383, *382*
  blunt injury of, 167–172, *168*, *169*, *171*
  detachments of, 69, *69*, 170
    ultraviolet light and, 194, *195*
    visual loss and, 414, *415*
    vitreous hemorrhage and, 411–413, 413t
  diplopia and, 336–353. *See also* Diplopia.
  edema of, 167–168
  examination of, 37
  floaters in, 380–381
  headaches and, 363–372. *See also* Headache.
  hemorrhage in, pediatric, 102
    shaken baby syndrome and, 99, *101*
    visual loss and, 397, 409–411
  in acquired immune deficiency syndrome, 401, *402*, 403–405
  leukocoria and, 383–387, *385*–
  metamorphopsia and, 376–377, *377*
  oscillopsia and, 375–376
  painful ophthalmoplegia and, 372–373
  penetrating injury of, 208–209, *209*
  photopsia and, 379
  presenting symptoms of, 336t
  pupillary abnormalities and, 353–363. *See also* Pupillary abnormality(ies).
  sudden and unexpected loss of vision and, 405–414, *406*–*408*, *410*–*415*
  visual field abnormality or, 387–388, 389t
  sudden onset of photophobia and, 377–379

Retina (*Continued*)
  tears of, 170–172
    vitreous hemorrhage and, 411–413
  tests of, 63–70, *69*, *70*
    detachments and, 69, *69*
    hemorrhage and, 69–70, *70*
    inflammatory diseases and, 70, *70*
    trauma and, 63–67, *66*, *67*
    tumors and, 67–69, *68*
    traumatic breaks in, 170. *See also* Retina, detachments of.
  vasculature of, examination of, 37–38
  visual hallucinations and, 373–375
Retinal artery occlusion, branch, 407, *407*
  central, 405–407, *406*
Retinal dialysis, 170, *170*
Retinal migraine, 368
Retinal vein occlusion, branch, 409, *410*
  central, 407–409, *408*
Retinitis, *Candida*, 403
Retinitis sclopetaria, 168–169
Retinoblastoma, 384, *386*
  diagnostic tests for, 68, *68*
Retinopathy, central serous, 413–414, *414*
  cytomegalovirus, 402, *403*
  diabetic, 411, *412*
  hypertensive, *38*
  Purscher's, 397–401
  stellate, 425–426, *426*
  venous stasis, 409
Retractor, Desmarre, 199, *200*
Retrobulbar anesthesia technique, 115, *116*
Retrobulbar hemorrhage, traumatic, 125–127, *126*
Retroillumination, 26, 27
Retropulsion, resistance to, 292
Rhabdomyosarcoma, 307, *308*
Rhese view, of orbit, 50, *53*
Rhizopus, 319
Riddoch phenomenon, 429
Rifampin, 320
Riley-Day syndrome, 362
Rocephin. *See* Ceftriaxone (Rocephin).
Rod test, Maddox, 21, 22
Rosacea, 246, *247*, *248*
  treatment of, 239
Rose bengal dye, 30
Rosenmueller, valve of, 218, *218*
Rubenstein-Taybi syndrome, 283, *285*
Rubeosis iridis, 270, *271*
Rupture, choroidal, 166
  corneal, 157
  globe, *66*
  scleral, 155

Saccades, in diplopia, 339, 340
Sagittal view, of orbit, 55, 56

546 Index

Salmon-colored mass, 292
Saran wrap moisture chamber, 127, *128*
Sarcoidosis, 420–421, *421*
Sarcoma, granulocytic, 310
   mesenchymal, 326–327
Saturation recovery, term of, 57
Schiotz tonometry, 32, 33, 34t
Schirmer test, 16, 228
Schwannoma(s). *See* Neurilemoma(s).
Sclera, blunt injury of, 153–155, *154*
   metallic foreign body embedded in, *209*
   rupture of, 155
   slit lamp examination of, 27
Scleral enhancement, in pseudotumor, 301, *302*
   physical findings of, 294
Scleritis, 487–490, *488*, *489*
Scleromalacia perforans, 488, *489*
Sclerosis, physical findings of, 293
Sclerotic scatter, *26*, 27
Scopolamine, hallucinations and, 375
   in anterior uveitis, 491
   in chemical burns, 185t, 186
   in iritis, 158
   in *Neisseria gonorrhea*, 464
   in recurrent corneal erosions, 245
   in sarcoidosis, 421
Scraping(s), in diagnostic test(s), 79
Scratch(es), of lid, 120–122, *122*, *123*
Secondary acute angle-closure glaucoma. *See* Glaucoma.
Sedation, in pediatric examination, 102–103, 103t, 104t
Seidel test, 204
Seizure(s), frontal, 381
Seldane, 476
Self-mutilation, psychotic, 455–456
Sella turcica, disorders of, 75
Sensory deprivation, 374
Serotonin, 367
Serratia marcescens, 463
Shaken baby syndrome, 99
Shigella, 477
Sickle cell disease, 301–302
   lid injuries and, 109
Silver nitrate, 463
Silver sulfadiazine, 127, 191
Simple neurofibroma(s), 324–325
Sinus(es), cavernous. *See* Cavernous sinus.
   opacification of, 294
   paranasal, *136*, 136–137
   physical findings of, 294
Sinus fistula, dural, 321
Sinus thrombosis, cavernous. *See* Cavernous sinus thrombosis.
Six Ps, in evaluating orbital disease, 290–293
Sixth nerve palsy, 347–349, *348*, 349t
Skin, black, crusted infarcted tissue on, 293
   of lid, avulsed, 138

Slit lamp, 25–31, *26*, *28*, *29*, *31*, *32*, 32t
   illumination techniques for, *26*, 26–27
   in foreign body removal, *202*
   in lid margin disorders, 227
   intraocular pressure and, 91, *95*
   notations and abbreviations to record findings with, 32t
   portable, 91, *94*
   red eye and, 3
Small pupil(s), *358*, *359*, 359–361, 361t
   bilateral, 362–363
Smear(s), in diagnostic test(s), 79
Smoking, cluster headache and, 371
Snellen acuity chart, 6–7, *7*, *8*
Snellen optotype(s), 8t
SOA (subperiosteal orbital abscess), 468
   in child, 299–300
Sodium chloride ointment, in filamentary keratopathy, 247
   in recurrent corneal erosions, 245
Sodium citrate, 185t, 188
Sodium hydroxide, 179, 180t
Sodium hypochlorite, 180t
Sodium tripolyphosphate, 180t
Sodoku fever, 122
Soft hydrogel contact lens, in recurrent corneal erosions, 245
Soft tissue injury(ies), of orbit, 138–141
Solar maculopathy, 397
Spasm of near reflex, 363, 446–448, *447*, 448t
Spatula, Kimura, *478*
Specular reflection, slit lamp technique of, *26*, 27
Sphenoid sinus, 136, *136*, 137
Sphenoid wing, absence of, 293
   elevation of, 48
   meningioma of, 326, *328*
Spin echo, term of, 57
Spiraling field(s), in functional disorder testing, 444
Spontaneous orbital hemorrhage, 320, *321*
Sports-related trauma, 96–98, *97*, *98*, 98t
SRNM (subretinal neovascular membrane), 422, *423*, 424t
s-shaped lid with bag of worms texture, 293
Stain(s), 79–83
   endophthalmitis and, 485t
   Giemsa's. *See* Giemsa's stain.
   Gram's. *See* Gram's stain.
   ophthalmia neonatorum and, 462t
Staphylococcus aureus, endophthalmitis and, 484
   exogenous, 508
   postoperative, 501
   posttraumatic, 502, 504
   in animal and human bites, 498, 499
   in conjunctivitis, 463
   in lid lacerations, 498

Index   547

Staphylococcus aureus (*Continued*)
   in orbital infections, 466, 468
   in pediatric infection, 298
Staphylococcus epidermidis, endophthalmitis
    and, 484, 501t
   exogenous, 508
   postoperative, 501
   posttraumatic, 502, 503, 504, 505t, 508
   in animal and human bites, 498, 499
   in lid lacerations, 498
   in orbital infections, 466
Stellate retinopathy, 425–426, *426*
Stenosis, lacrimal punctal, 224, 231
Steroid(s). *See also* Corticosteroid(s).
   endophthalmitis and. *See* Endophthalmitis.
   in acute setting, 510
   in allergic conjunctivitis, 476
   in anterior uveitis, 491
   in central retinal artery occlusion, 407
   in choroidal detachment, 427
   in collagen vascular disease, 239
   in corneal ulceration, 183
   in eosinophilic granuloma, 310
   in episcleritis, 487
   in hemangioma, 304
   in hypopituitarism, 323
   in interstitial keratitis, 250
   in migraine, 369
   in neovascular glaucoma, 274
   in pars planitis, 491
   in pupillary block, 273
   in sarcoidosis, 421
   in superficial punctate keratopathy, 246
   in systemic lupus erythematosis, 419
   in thyroid ophthalmopathy, 317
   in toxoplasmosis, 403
Strabismus, 20, 20t
Strawberry nevus, 292, 303
Streptococcus pneumoniae, in conjunctivitis, 463
   in orbital fractures, 500
   in orbital infections, 466, 468
   in pediatric infection, 298
   in posttraumatic endophthalmitis, 502
Streptococcus pyogenes, in orbital infection, 466
   in pediatric infection, 298
Streptococcus viridans, in endophthalmitis, 501, 501t, 502
Striated glass test of Bagolini, 22
Stromal keratitis, herpetic, 480
Sturge-Weber syndrome, 283, *284*
Stye, 16, *469*, 469–470
Subarachnoid hemorrhage, 365t
Subaxial view, of orbit, 49
Subcapsular cataract, posterior, 255–256, *256*
Subconjunctival hemorrhage, 153–155, *154*
   penetrating injury in, 197–198, *198*

Subdural hematoma, headaches and, 365t
   shaken baby syndrome and, 99, *101*
Submentovertex view, of orbit, 49, *52*
   in trauma, 63
Subperiosteal orbital abscess (SOA), 468
   in child, 299–300
Subretinal neovascular membrane (SRNM), 422, *423*, 424t
Succinylcholine, adverse effects of, 113
Sudden and unexpected loss of vision. *See* Loss of vision, sudden and unexpected.
Sudden onset of binocular diplopia, 336–353. *See also* Diplopia.
Sulfacetamide, in conjunctivitis, 463
   in corneal abrasion, 203
   in dacryocystitis, 471, 472
   in nasolacrimal duct probing, 221
   in prednisolone acetate with sulfacetamide (Blephamide), 246
   in prednisolone sodium phosphate with sulfacetamide (Vasocidin), 246
   in superficial punctate keratopathy, 246
Sulfadiazine, 403, 492, 493t
Sulfamethoxazole, 505t
Sulfinpyrazone, 370
Sulfuric acid, 180t
Superficial punctate keratopathy, 246, 247t, *248*, 479
Superior limbic keratoconjunctivitis, superficial punctate keratopathy versus, *247*
Supraorbital anesthesia technique, 114, *116*
Supraorbital notch, 131
Suprasellar mass, 75
Supratrochlear anesthesia, 114, *116*
Surgical history, 6
Swelling, of lid, 293
Swinging flashlight test, *18*
Sympathetic fiber(s), in pupillary abnormalities, 356, *357*
Sympathetic ophthalmia, 493–494
Sympathomimetic(s), action of, 6t
   in angle-closure glaucoma, 274
   pupillary block glaucoma and, 272
Synechia, peripheral anterior, *267*, 270
   posterior, angle-closure glaucoma and, 272
Syphilis, congenital, *251*
Systemic lupus erythematosus, 419

T_1- or T_2-weighted magnetic resonance imaging scan, 57, *58*, *59*
Tadpole pupil, 360
Tardive dyskinesia, 382
Tarsal anesthesia, 115
Td (diphtheria and tetanus immunization), 510, 511
Tear(s), artificial. *See* Artificial tear(s).
Tear film, slit lamp examination of, 30

548　Index

Teardrop sign, term of, 63
Tearing. *See* Epiphora.
Tears Plus, 233
Temporal arteritis, headaches and, 366t
　visual loss and, 418–419
Temporal hemianopsia, monocular, 444–445
Tensilon test, in diplopia, 340
　in myasthenia gravis, 353
Tension headache, 371, 451
　differential diagnosis of, 290
Teratoma, 307
Terson's syndrome, 397
Tetanus immune globulin (TIG), 112, 511
Tetanus immunization, 112t, 112–113, 510t, 510–511
Tetanus toxoid booster, 112
Tetracaine, in lid laceration, 114
　in penetrating injuries, 201
Tetracycline(s), in chalazion, 469
　in chemical burns, 186
　in chlamydial conjunctivitis, 476
　in conjunctivitis, 463
　in corneal ulceration, 183
　in Lyme disease, 345
　in pseudotumor cerebri, 435
　in rosacea, 239
　in toxoplasmosis, 403
Thalamic hemorrhage, *77*
Thermal burn, 127, *128*, 190–192
Thiamine, 429
Thioridazine, 363
Third nerve palsy, 351–352, *352*
Thorazine, 103t
Three-mirror gonioscopy, Goldmann, 31, *32*
Three-suture technique, in lid repair, 116–119, *118*
Thrombosis, cavernous sinus. *See* Cavernous sinus thrombosis.
Thygeson's keratitis, *247*
Thyroid function studies, 294
Thyroid ophthalmopathy, 315–317, *316*, 317t, *318*, *319*
　differential diagnosis of, 291
Tic douloureux, 381–382
TIG (tetanus immune globulin), 112, 511
Timolol (Timoptic), in chemical burns, 185t
　in hyphemia, 161t
　in infantile glaucoma, 280
　in myasthenia gravis, 353
　in phacolytic glaucoma, 165
Timoptic. *See* Timolol (Timoptic).
Titmus depth perception chart, 11, *13*
TNO random dot test, 11
Tobacco amblyopia, 429
Tobramycin, diffusion of, 507t
　in conjunctivitis, 463
　in corneal infection, 478
　in endophthalmitis, 505t

Tobramycin (*Continued*)
　in superficial punctate keratopathy, 246
　penetration of, 508t
Tolosa-Hunt syndrome, 300, 344
Tomography, 50
　computed. *See* Computed tomography (CT).
Tonometer, 32–35, *33*, 34t, *35*, *36*, 36t
　Perkins applanation, 91, *95*
　infantile glaucoma and, 280, *282*
　Schiotz, 32, 33, 34t
Toxic keratopathy, *247*
Toxic lid reaction, 128, *129*
Toxic optic neuropathy, 429
Toxocariasis, 384, *386*
Toxoplasma gondii, 492
Toxoplasmosis, 492–493, *493*, 493t
　in acquired immune deficiency syndrome, 403, *404*
Trabecular meshwork, glaucoma obstruction at, *270*, 270–272, *271*
Traction, inflammatory headaches and, 364–366, 365t–366t
Tram track sign, 71
Tranexamic acid, in hereditary angioedema, 128
　in hyphema, 160
Transient loss of vision, bilateral, 433t, 433–435
　unilateral, 430–433, *431*, *432*
Transillumination, of iris, 275, *276*
Trauma, 109–130
　annular keratopathy and, 155–156
　blunt. *See* Blunt injury(ies).
　burns in, 179–196. *See also* Burn(s).
　choroidal, 63–67, *66*, *67*
　contact lens and, 243
　corneal rupture and, 157
　cranial nerve palsy and, 342, *343*
　endophthalmitis after, 501t, 502–509, 505t–508t
　foreign bodies and. *See* Foreign body(ies); Penetrating injury(ies).
　iritis and, 157–158
　lid, 109–130. *See also* Eyelid, lacerations of.
　macular hole and, *169*, 169–170
　malpractice suits and, 63
　miosis and, 157, 158
　mydriasis and, 157, 158, 342
　obstetrical forceps in, *156*, 156–157
　optic neuropathy and, 172
　posterior indirect, 397
　pediatric, 92–96
　　sports-related, 96–98, *97*, *98*, 98t
　penetrating, 197–213. *See also* Penetrating injury(ies).
　ptosis and, 123–125, *125*, *126*
　lid ecchymosis and, *110*

Trauma (*Continued*)
  retinal, 63–67, *66*, *67*
    breaks and detachments in, 170
  retrobulbar hemorrhage and, 125–127, *126*
  sudden and unexpected loss of vision in, 397–401, *401*
  superficial punctate keratopathy versus, *247*
  whiplash, 77
Traumatic hyphema, *159*, 159–162, 160t–162t
Triamcinolone, in chalazion, 469
  in hemangioma, 304
  in pars planitis, 491
  in sarcoidosis, 421
Triaxone, 499
Trichiasis, 15, 225, *226*
Tricyclic(s), in migraine, 407
Trifluridine (Viroptic), in herpes simplex infections, 479, 480
  in neonate, 466
  in recurrent epithelial keratitis, 479
Trigeminal neuralgia, 366t
Trimalar fracture, 147–148, *148*
Trimethoprim. *See* Polymyxin B and trimethoprim (Polytrim).
Tripod orbital fracture(s), 147–148, *148*
Trisodium phosphonoformate hexahydrate (Foscarnet), 402
Trochlea, 131
Tropicamide (Mydriacyl), 269, 273
Tubercle of Whitnall, 131
Tubular field, 444
Tumor(s). *See also* Neoplasm(s); *specific neoplasm.*
  benign, mixed, 328–329
  ciliary body, 270–272
  differential diagnosis of, 291
  epiphora and, 227, *228*
  eyelid, 16
  in temple, 293
  intracranial, 76
    headaches and, 365t
  lacrimal, 328–329
  malignant. *See* Malignant neoplasm.
  orbital, 323–328, *324*, *325*, *327*, *328*
    metastatic, 327–328
  salmon-colored, 292
  superior nasal quadrant, 292
  superior temporal quadrant, 292
  suprasellar and parasellar, 75
  tests in, 64–69, *68*
  under conjunctiva, 292
Twitching, lid, 381–383, *382*
Two-person technique, of ophthalmodynamometry, *41*
Tyramine, 367, 370, 372

UGH (uveitis, glaucoma, and hyphema) syndrome, 275
Ulcer, corneal, in burns, *182*, 182–184
  inflammatory, noninfectious, 237–239, *238*, 238t
  soft contact lens and, 242–243, *244*
Ultrasonography, 45–48, *46*, *47*
  advantages and disadvantages of, 64t, 65t
  in nontraumatic orbital disorders, 294
  in ocular and orbital trauma, 63
  orbital masses differentiated by, 72t
Ultraviolet radiation injury, 192–194, *193–195*
Ultraviolet Wood's lamp, 91, *94*
Unexpected loss of vision. *See* Loss of vision, sudden and unexpected.
Urine vanillylmandelic acid, 294
Uveal effusion syndrome, 428
Uveitis, anterior, 293, *490*, 490–491
  glaucoma with, 275, *276*
  tests in, 83–86, 84t, 85t
Uveitis, glaucoma, and hyphema syndrome (UGH syndrome), 275

Valium, 103t
Valve, of Hasner, 136, *218*, 219
  of Rosenmueller, 218, *218*
van Lint anesthesia technique, 114, *116*
Vancomycin, cost of, 509t
  diffusion of, 507t
  in corneal infection, 478
  in endophthalmitis, 484, 505–507t
  in lid laceration, 498
  in orbital cellulitis, 299, 468
  in traumatic endophthalmitis, 504, 508
Vanillylmandelic acid, urine, 294
Varix, orbital, 291, 321
Vascular disorder(s), cranial nerve palsy in, 342–343
Vascular headache, 367–371
  cluster, 370–371
  migraine, 367–370, 368t
Vascular malformation(s), orbital, 74
Vasculitis, orbital, 320
Vasocidin (prednisolone sodium phosphate with sulfacetamide), 246
Vasocon-A (antazoline phosphate with naphazoline), 475, 476
Vasoconstrictor(s), in scleritis, 487
Vasodilator(s), in migraine, 367
Velosef. *See* Cephradine (Velosef).
Venography, orbital, 60
Venous stasis retinopathy, 409
Verapamil, in cluster headache, 371
  in migraine, 370
Vergence(s), 19–20

Vernal reaction, *247*
Version(s), 19
 diplopia in, 339, 339t
Vestibulo-ocular reflex, 339, 340
Vincristine, in optic neuropathy, 429
 in rhabdomyosarcoma, 308
Viral conjunctivitis, 472–475, *474*
 angle-closure glaucoma versus, 263t
 superficial punctate keratopathy versus, *247*
Viroptic. *See* Trifluridine (Viroptic).
Viscoat, 205
Viscoelastic agent(s), 205
Vision, assessment of, 6–12, *7–10*, 8t, 9t, 12t, *13*
 color, 11
 diagnostic tests for, 63–78. *See also* Diagnostic test(s).
 disproving loss of, 443–445
 double, 336–353. *See also* Diplopia.
 loss of. *See* Blindness.
  functional. *See also* Functional and psychotic disorder(s).
   adults with, 445
   child with, 445–446
  sudden and unexpected. *See* Loss of vision, sudden and unexpected.
Visual acuity, 6–12
 blunt injury and, 137
 functional loss of, 442–446
 recording of, 10, 12t
Visual field, 23–25, *24*
 functional loss of, 442–446
  abnormalities suggestive of, 444–445
 notations and abbreviations to record findings of, 36t
 retinal disorders and, 387–388, 389t
Visual hallucination(s), 449–450
 in retinal disorder, 373–375
Vitamin A, pseudotumor cerebri and, 435
Vitamin B_{12}, optic neuropathy and, 429
Vitamin C, in chemical burns, 185t, 186
 in corneal ulceration, 183
Vitamin K, in lid lacerations, 111
Vitreous, examination of, 37
Vitreous base, avulsion of, 170

Vitreous detachment, posterior (PVD), 379
 sudden and unexpected loss of vision in, 414–415
Vitreous hemorrhage, blunt injury in, 166
 T_2-weighted image of, 69, *70*
 visual loss and, 411, 412t
Volk 90 diopter lens, 39
Voluntary nystagmus, 448
Voluntary propulsion, of eyeball, 453
von Graefe sign, 316

Warfarin, 112
Waters view, of orbit, 49, *50*
 in blowout fracture, 144, *145*
Weber syndrome, 342, 351
Wegener's granulomatosis, 320
Weill-Marchesani syndrome, angle-closure glaucoma and, *273*
 dislocated lens and, *252*, 254
Westergren erythrocyte sedimentation rate (W-ESR), 340
Whiplash injury, 77
White pupil, 256
Whitnall, tubercle of, 131
Window level, term of, 52
Window width, term of, 52
Wood's lamp, 91, *94*
Worth's four dot test, 22

Xanthelasma, 16
Xylocaine. *See* Lidocaine (Xylocaine).

Yellow conjunctiva, 292

Zeiss goniolens, 31, *31*
 in angle-closure glaucoma, 267, *268*
Zinacef. *See* Cefuroxime (Ceftin, Zinacef).
Zinc deficiency, 429
Zinn, annulus of, 133–134
Zostrix, 485